Series Editors:
Alan G. Kamhi, Ph.D.
Rebecca J. McCauley, Ph.D.

Treatment of Autism Spectrum Disorder

Second Edition

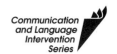
Communication
and Language
Intervention
Series

Treatment of
Autism Spectrum Disorder

Evidence-Based Intervention Strategies
for Communication & Social Interactions

Second Edition

edited by

Patricia A. Prelock, Ph.D.
Provost and Senior Vice President
Department of Communication Sciences and Disorders
University of Vermont
Burlington

and

Rebecca J. McCaulcy, Ph.D.
Professor
Department of Speech and Hearing Science
The Ohio State University
Columbus

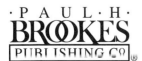
·P A U L·H·
BROOKES
PUBLISHING CO.

Baltimore • London • Sydney

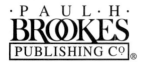

Paul H. Brookes Publishing Co.
Post Office Box 10624
Baltimore, Maryland 21285-0624
USA

www.brookespublishing.com

Typeset by Progressive Publishing Service, York, Pennsylvania.
Manufactured in the United States of America by Sheridan Books, Inc., Chelsea, Michigan.

The individuals described in this book are composites or real people whose situations are masked and are based on the authors' experiences. In all instances, names and identifying details have been changed to protect confidentiality.

The accompanying video clips that illustrate the interventions discussed in *Treatment of Autism Spectrum Disorder: Evidence-Based Intervention Strategies for Communication & Social Interactions, Second Edition*, were supplied by the chapter authors. Permission was obtained for all individuals shown in the footage.

Library of Congress Cataloging-in-Publication Data

Names: Prelock, Patricia A., editor. | McCauley, Rebecca Joan,
  1952– editor.
Title: Treatment of autism spectrum disorder : evidence-based intervention
  strategies for communication & social interactions / edited by Patricia
  A. Prelock, Provost and Senior Vice President, University of Vermont, Department of
  Communication Sciences and Disorders, Burlington and Rebecca J. McCauley, Ph.D.,
  Professor, Department of Speech and Hearing Science, The Ohio State University, Columbus.
Other titles: Treatment of autism spectrum disorders
Description: Second edition. | Baltimore, MD : Paul H. Brookes Publishing Co., [2021] |
  Series: Communication and language intervention series |
  Includes bibliographical references and index.
Identifiers: LCCN 2020056439 (print) | LCCN 2020056440 (ebook) |
  ISBN 9781681253985 (paperback) | ISBN 9781681254852 (epub) |
  ISBN 9781681254869 (pdf)
Subjects: LCSH: Autism spectrum disorders—Treatment. | Autism spectrum
  disorders in children—Treatment.
Classification: LCC RC553.A88 T735 2021 (print) | LCC RC553.A88 (ebook) |
  DDC 616.85/88200835—dc23
LC record available at https://lccn.loc.gov/2020056439
LC ebook record available at https://lccn.loc.gov/2020056440

British Library Cataloguing in Publication data are available from the British Library.

Contents

About the Videos and Downloads

For select interventions in *Treatment of Autism Spectrum Disorder: Evidence-Based Intervention Strategies for Communication & Social Interactions, Second Edition,* brief video clips that show the interventions in action are available for your review. Purchasers of this text may access and stream these videos for educational purposes only. Select tables from the book, specifically Table 15.7 Summary of Selected Research on Skillstreaming and Table 15.8 Summary of Selected Research on Social Competence Curricula (SCC) are also available to view and download for educational use.

To access the videos and downloads:

1. Go to the Brookes Publishing Download Hub:
   http://downloads.brookespublishing.com

2. Register to create an account or log in with an existing account.

3. Filter or search for the book title *Treatment of Autism Spectrum Disorder.*

Videos are available for the following chapters. See the end of each listed chapter for a brief summary of the video clip.

Chapter 4   Augmentative Alternative Communication Strategies: Manual Signs, Picture Communication, and Speech-Generating Devices

Chapter 5   The Early Start Denver Model (ESDM): Promoting Social Communication in Young Children With ASD

Chapter 6   Discrete Trial Instruction

Chapter 7   The Developmental, Individual-Difference, Relationship-Based (DIR) Model and Its Application to Children With ASD

Chapter 8   Functional Communication Training: Treating Challenging Behavior

Chapter 9   The JASPER Model for Children With Autism: Improving Play, Social Communication, and Engagement

Series Preface

The purpose of the *Communication and Language Intervention Series* is to provide meaningful foundations for the application of sound intervention designs to enhance the development of communication skills across the life span. We endeavor to achieve this purpose by providing readers with presentations of state-of-the-art theory, research, and practice.

In selecting topics, editors, and authors, we have not attempted to limit the contents of this series to viewpoints with which we agree or that we find most promising. We are assisted in our efforts to develop the series by an editorial advisory board consisting of prominent scholars representative of the range of issues and perspectives to be incorporated in the series.

Well-conceived theory and research on development and intervention are vitally important for researchers, educators, and clinicians committed to the development of optimal approaches to communication and language intervention. The content of each volume reflects our view of the symbiotic relationship between intervention and research: Demonstrations of what may work in intervention should lead to analysis of promising discoveries and insights from developmental work that may, in turn, fuel further refinement by intervention researchers. We trust that the careful reader will find much that is of great value in this volume.

An inherent goal of this series is to enhance the long-term development of the field by systematically furthering the dissemination of theoretically and empirically based scholarship and research. We promise the reader an opportunity to participate in the development of this field through debates and discussions that occur throughout the pages of the *Communication and Language Intervention Series*.

Editorial Advisory Board

About the Editors

Patricia A. Prelock, Ph.D., Provost and Senior Vice-President, University of Vermont, Burlington

Dr. Prelock is Provost and Senior Vice-President, University of Vermont. Formerly, she was the dean of the College of Nursing and Health Sciences at the University of Vermont for 10 years. She is also a professor of communication sciences and disorders and professor of pediatrics in the College of Medicine at the University of Vermont. Dr. Prelock has been awarded more than $11.9 million in university, state, and federal funding as a principal investigator (PI) or co-PI to develop innovations in interdisciplinary training supporting children and youth with neurodevelopmental disabilities and their families, to facilitate training in speech-language pathology, and to support her intervention work in ASD. She has more than 195 publications and 566 peer-reviewed and invited presentations/keynotes in the areas of autism and other neurodevelopmental disabilities, collaboration, interprofessional education, leadership, and language learning disabilities.

In 2019, she was named associate editor for the *Journal of Autism and Developmental Disorders.* Dr. Prelock received the University of Vermont's Kroepsch-Maurice Excellence in Teaching Award in 2000 and was named an ASHA Fellow in 2000 and a University of Vermont Scholar in 2003. In 2011, she was named the Cecil & Ida Green Honors Professor Visiting Scholar at Texas Christian University, and in 2015 Dr. Prelock was named a Distinguished Alumna of the University of Pittsburgh. In 2016, she received the ASHA Honors of the association, and in 2017, she was named a Distinguished Alumna of Cardinal Mooney High School. Dr. Prelock also received the 2018 Jackie M. Gribbons Leadership Award from Vermont Women in Higher Education. Dr. Prelock is a board-certified specialist in child language and was named a fellow in the National Academies of Practice (NAP) in speech-language pathology in 2018. She was the 2013 president for the American Speech-Language Hearing Association.

Rebecca J. McCauley, Ph.D., Professor, The Ohio State University, Columbus

Dr. McCauley is Professor in the Department of Speech and Hearing Sciences at the Ohio State University. Her research and writing have focused on assessment and treatment of pediatric communication disorders, with a special focus on speech sound disorders, including childhood apraxia of speech. She has authored or edited seven books on these topics and coauthored a test designed to aid in the differential diagnosis of childhood apraxia of speech. Dr. McCauley is a Fellow of the American Speech-Language-Hearing Association, has received honors of that association, and has served two terms as an associate editor of the *American Journal of Speech-Language Pathology.*

About the Contributors

Allison Bean, Ph.D., Associate Professor, The Ohio State University, Columbus

Allison Bean is an associate professor at The Ohio State University. Dr. Bean's research focuses on investigating the mechanisms underlying language development in minimally verbal children with autism. The ultimate goal for this work is to improve intervention for minimally verbal children with autism.

Ashley R. Brien, CCC-SLP, Speech-Language Pathologist and Doctoral Candidate, University of Vermont, Burlington

Ashley R. Brien is a speech-language pathologist in Vermont. She is pursuing her doctorate in interprofessional health sciences at the University of Vermont under the mentorship of Dr. Tiffany Hutchins and Dr. Patricia Prelock. Her research focuses on episodic memory and its relationship to theory of mind. She is currently designing interventions and treatment materials to support episodic memory and social cognition in children with ASD.

Tom Buggey, Ph.D., Retired, Siskin Chair of Excellence in Early Childhood Special Education, University of Tennessee at Chattanooga

Tom Buggey began research on self-modeling at Penn State in 1992, working with preschoolers with language delays. Following the urgings of two gifted graduate assistants, together they conducted their first research with children on the autism spectrum in 1995 with very positive results. Thereafter, children with autism became the focus of his research. Dr. Buggey was recruited to serve as the Siskin Chair of Excellence in the Special Education Department at UTC in 2007. The next 7 years were devoted to research on developing language and social skills with preschool-age children with autism. In his career as a researcher, he has conducted more than a dozen studies on the use of self-modeling, all which have appeared in major journals; published several book chapters of self-modeling and other aspects of early intervention; and published the only book on self-modeling, *Seeing is*

Believing (Woodbine House, 2007), which is currently being translated and published in Russia.

Erik W. Carter, Ph.D., Cornelius Vanderbilt Professor of Special Education, Vanderbilt University, Nashville, Tennessee

Erik W. Carter is Cornelius Vanderbilt Professor of Special Education at Vanderbilt University. Dr. Carter's research and writing focus on promoting inclusion and valued roles in school, work, community, and congregational settings for children and adults with intellectual disability, autism, and multiple disabilities.

Geraldine Dawson, Ph.D., Professor of Psychiatry and Behavioral Sciences, Duke University School of Medicine, Durham, North Carolina

Geraldine Dawson is the William Cleland Professor of Psychiatry and Behavioral Sciences at Duke University, director of the Duke Institute for Brain Sciences, and director of the Duke Center for Autism and Brain Development. Dawson is a licensed, practicing clinical psychologist and internationally renowned scientist whose work has focused on early detection and treatment of autism and brain development.

Abigail Delehanty, Ph.D., CCC-SLP, Assistant Professor, Duquesne University, Pittsburgh, Pennsylvania

Abigail (Abby) Delehanty is an assistant professor and program director for the Language Disorders and Autism Clinic in the Department of Speech-Language Pathology at Duquesne University. Dr. Delehanty has extensive clinical experience serving preschoolers, school-age children, and adolescents with communication disorders in a public-school setting. For the last 5 years of her career in the schools, she served as a speech-language pathologist on a multidisciplinary autism evaluation team, conducting weekly developmental screenings in the community and connecting more than 100 children with school-based services each year. Dr. Delehanty's research interests include studying and promoting social communication development in children with communication delays and autism and reducing the age of identification of communication delays and autism in young children from diverse cultural backgrounds and underserved areas.

V. Mark Durand, Ph.D., Professor of Psychology, University of South Florida St. Petersburg

V. Mark Durand is known worldwide as an authority in the area of ASD. He is professor of psychology at the University of South Florida–St. Petersburg, where he was the founding dean of Arts and Sciences and vice chancellor for Academic Affairs. He has authored more than 145 publications and more than a dozen books, including *Optimistic Parenting: Hope and Help for You and Your Challenging Child* and, most recently, *Autism Spectrum Disorder: A Clinical Guide for General Practitioners.*

Elizabeth A. Fuller, Ph.D., Vanderbilt University, Nashville, Tennessee

Dr. Fuller specializes in early intervention and behavioral therapy for children with autism and developmental disabilities. She received her doctorate from Vanderbilt University in early childhood special education and is a board-certified behavior analyst (BCBA). She has over ten years of experience in play and behavior therapies and in coaching parents to implement effective strategies with their children.

Sima Gerber, Ph.D., CCC-SLP, Professor, Queens College, City University of New York

Sima Gerber is a professor of speech-language pathology in the Department of Linguistics and Communication Disorders of Queens College, City University of New York. She has been a speech-language pathologist for more than 40 years, specializing in the treatment of children with ASD and other developmental challenges. Dr. Gerber has presented nationally and abroad (China, Italy, The Netherlands, South Africa, Israel, Georgia) on language acquisition and developmental approaches to assessment and intervention for children with language and communication disorders. Dr. Gerber is a Fellow of the American Speech-Language-Hearing Association.

Jodi K. Heidlage, Ph.D., BCBA, Project Director, Vanderbilt University, Nashville, Tennessee

Jodi K. Heidlage is a special educator with expertise in behavioral and naturalistic interventions for children with autism and significant learning challenges. She has more than 10 years of experience providing direct services for young children with ASD and has served as a therapist and parent interventionist on several clinical trials. She currently is the project director for an early reading intervention for children with intellectual and developmental disabilities at Vanderbilt University.

Renee Daly Holland, M.S., CCC-SLP, Assistant Director of Early Intervention Services Research, Florida State University, Tallahassee

Renee Daly Holland is the assistant director of Early Intervention Services Research for the Autism Institute in the College of Medicine at Florida State University. Mrs. Holland's clinical experience over the past 27 years has focused on home- and community-based early intervention for children with autism spectrum and speech and language disorders. As the lead interventionist for the Early Social Interaction Project (ESI), she currently oversees the fidelity implementation and supervision of the ESI model used in randomized controlled trials across multiple sites. An author of the Autism Navigator collection of Web-based courses and tools, Mrs. Holland also serves as an Autism Navigator Global Trainer and supports professionals within early intervention systems to deliver effective, evidence-based intervention in natural environments.

Jill Howard, Ph.D., Assistant Professor, Licensed Psychologist, Duke University School of Medicine, Durham, North Carolina

Jill Howard is a licensed psychologist and assistant professor at the Duke Center for Autism and Brain Development in the Department of Psychiatry and Behavioral Sciences. She specializes in conducting comprehensive diagnostic assessments and delivering intervention services to individuals and families affected by ASD. Dr. Howard's primary research interests involve the early identification of and evidence-based treatments for ASD, as well as the development of social attention and behavior. Dr. Howard is certified as an Early Start Denver Model therapist and trainer.

Tiffany L. Hutchins, Ph.D., Associate Professor, University of Vermont, Burlington

Dr. Hutchins conducts research in social cognition and language development in autism, attention-deficit/hyperactivity disorder, hearing loss, and childhood trauma. She also teaches courses in measurement, language disorders, and psycholinguistics. Dr. Hutchins is primary author of the Theory of Mind Inventory and the Theory of Mind Atlas.

Ann P. Kaiser, Ph.D., Susan W. Gray Professor of Education and Human Development, Department of Special Education, Peabody College, Vanderbilt University, Nashville, Tennessee

Ann P. Kaiser is the Susan W. Gray Professor of Education and Human Development at Vanderbilt University. She is the author of more than 175 articles on early intervention for children with autism and other development communication disabilities. Her research focuses on therapist- and parent-implemented naturalistic interventions.

Connie Kasari, Ph.D., Professor of Human Development and Psychiatry, University of California Los Angeles

Dr. Kasari received her doctorate from the University of North Carolina at Chapel Hill and was a National Institute of Mental Health postdoctoral fellow at the Neuropsychiatric Institute at UCLA. Since 1990, she has been on the faculty at UCLA, where she teaches both graduate and undergraduate courses and has been the primary advisor to more than 60 doctoral students. She is a founding member of the Center for Autism Research and Treatment at UCLA. Her research aims to development novel, evidence-tested interventions implemented in community settings. Recent projects include targeted treatments for early social-communication development in at-risk infants, toddlers, and preschoolers with autism and peer relationships for school-age children with autism. She leads several large multisite studies, including a network on interventions for minimally verbal school-age children with ASD, and a network that aims to decrease disparities in interventions for children with ASD who are underrepresented in research trials. She is on the science advisory board of the Autism Speaks Foundation and regularly presents to both academic and practitioner audiences locally, nationally, and internationally.

Shubha Kashinath, Ph.D., CCC-SLP, Associate Professor, California State University, East Bay, Hayward

Shubha Kashinath is currently chair of the Department of Speech Language and Hearing Sciences at Cal State East Bay. Her academic and professional interests focus on autism across the life span, treatment efficacy, caregiver-focused interventions, and personnel preparation. She has more than 20 years of experience as a speech language pathologist serving individuals with disabilities and their families.

Amanda Kazee, M.A., School Psychology Extern, Registered Behavior Technician, Ball State University, Muncie, Indiana

Amanda Kazee is a doctoral candidate in the School Psychology program with a specialization in applied behavior analysis at Ball State University. Amanda has presented and published scholarly work alongside Dr. Susan Wilczynski on evidence-based practice. She currently serves as a registered behavior technician and school psychology extern at a local school district.

Lynn Kern Koegel, Ph.D., CCC-SLP, Clinical Professor, Stanford University School of Medicine, California

Dr. Lynn Kern Koegel and her husband developed Pivotal Response Treatment®, an intervention used worldwide for the treatment of ASD. She has published well over 100 articles and chapters, field manuals, and eight books, including *Overcoming Autism* and *Growing Up on the Spectrum* with parent Claire LaZebnik, published by Viking/Penguin and available in most bookstores. The Koegels have received many awards, including the first annual Children's Television Workshop Sesame Street Award for Brightening the Lives of Children, the first annual Autism Speaks award for Science and Research, and the International ABA award for enduring programmatic contributions in behavior analysis. Dr. Lynn Koegel has appeared on numerous television and radio shows discussing autism, including the Discovery Channel, and ABC's hit show *Supernanny*, working with a child with autism. The Koegels' work has also been showcased on ABC, CBS, NBC, and PBS, and they are the recipients of many state, federal, and private foundation gifts and grants for developing interventions and helping families with ASD.

Amy C. Laurent, Ph.D., OTR/L, Developmental Psychologist, Educational Consultant, Pediatric Occupational Therapist, Autism Level UP!, North Kingston, Rhode Island

Amy Laurent specializes in the education of autistic children. Her work involves creating learning environments designed to facilitate children's active engagement at home, in schools, and throughout their communities. She is a coauthor of The SCERTS Model and frequently lectures around the globe. She is passionate about neurodiversity and helping others to honor and understand the implications of "different ways of being" in relation to navigating the physical and social world.

Maria Martino, M.A., Clinical Project Coordinator, University of Alabama, Tuscaloosa

Maria Martino received her master's in clinical psychology from Ball State University. Maria has focused on evidence-based practice and identifying abuse for populations with ASD under the supervision of Dr. Susan Wilczynski. Maria is currently coordinating an NIH-funded study examining reading comprehension and neural connectivity in children with ASD under Dr. Rajesh Kana at the University of Alabama.

Lauren J. Moskowitz, Ph.D., Assistant Professor, St. John's University, Queens, New York

Lauren Moskowitz is an associate professor in the Department of Psychology at St. John's University. She earned her bachelor of science degree from Cornell University, her master's and doctorate in clinical psychology from Stony Brook University, and completed her clinical internship and postdoctoral fellowship at NYU Child Study Center. Her research focuses on behavioral assessment and intervention for problem behavior and anxiety in children with ASD and developmental disabilities. Dr. Moskowitz has coauthored several papers and book chapters; has presented at numerous international, national, and regional conferences; has taught several undergraduate and graduate courses covering ASD and developmental disabilities, applied behavior analysis, and positive behavior support, and has been on the editorial board for the *Journal of Positive Behavior Interventions* since 2013.

Nicholas L. Mundell, B.S., Graduate Research Assistant, Ball State University, Muncie, Indiana

Nicholas (Nick) Mundell is a dual-degree master's student in the Clinical and Quantitative Psychology programs at Ball State University. Nick serves as a graduate research assistant in the Department of Special Education. In his spare time, Nick enjoys playing videogames, watching movies, and playing disc golf.

Elizabeth Ponder, M.A., BCBA, Clinical Supervisor, PRT Trainer, Stanford Autism Center, California

Elizabeth began her training in Pivotal Response Treatment (PRT) as a research assistant at the Koegel Autism Center while completing her bachelor of arts in psychology at the University of California, Santa Barbara. After graduating, Elizabeth expanded her knowledge and skills pertaining to ASD and PRT by working as an interventionist. In 2009, she entered the Special Education, Disabilities and Developmental Risk Studies (SPEDDR) graduate program at the University of California, Santa Barbara, with Dr. Robert Koegel as her advisor. After receiving her master's degree in 2011, she went on to become a BCBA and has continued her work with individuals on the spectrum, with a focus on parent and professional education and training.

Barry M. Prizant, Ph.D., CCC-SLP, Adjunct Professor, Brown University, Director, Childhood Communication Services, Providence, Rhode Island

Dr. Barry Prizant has 45 years' experience as a speech-language pathologist, author, researcher, and international consultant. He is an adjunct professor at Brown University and director at Childhood Communication Services, a private practice. Barry is a codeveloper of The SCERTS Model, an educational framework now being implemented in more than a dozen countries. His recent book is *Uniquely Human: A Different Way of Seeing Autism* (Simon & Schuster, 2015), which has received the Autism Society of America's Dr. Temple Grandin Award for the Outstanding Literary work in autism and is published in 16 languages.

Molly Quinn, M.A., Behavior Analyst, Ball State, University, Muncie, Indiana

As a professional, Molly Quinn has been defined as a teacher, a behavior analyst, a parent-training consultant, and a researcher. She has worked with people between the ages of 2 years and 30 years who were diagnosed with a developmental disability, within their homes, schools, and communities, for the last 15 years. In her personal life, Molly is a mother of three and a foster mom to two children, living in Plainfield, Indiana. If given the opportunity for leisure, Molly enjoys reading and is passionate about traveling and interior decorating.

Emily Rubin, M.S., CCC-SLP, Director, Educational Outreach Program, Marcus Autism Center, Atlanta, Georgia

Emily Rubin is the director of the Educational Outreach Program at the Marcus Autism Center in Atlanta, Georgia. She is a speech-language pathologist specializing in autism, Asperger syndrome, and social-emotional learning. She is a coauthor of The SCERTS Model, a criterion-referenced assessment tool and educational framework for social communication and emotional regulation. Her current work is focused on building the capacity of public-school systems to embed interpersonal and learning supports that benefit all students and young children.

Kyle Sterrett, M.A., Doctoral Candidate, University of California Los Angeles

Kyle Sterrett's research interest lies in the optimization of evidence-based interventions through the understanding of their active ingredients using quantitative methods—for example, understanding of the role of speech-generating devices within efficacious interventions for language learners with autism. He has been involved as a clinician in a number of recent intervention trials, implementing interventions for children with autism and developmental delays within schools and in home settings through parent training in the JASPER intervention model.

Kristen Strong, Ph.D., Psychologist, Acacia Counseling and Wellness, Isla Vista, California

Dr. Strong is a clinical psychologist and received her doctoral degree from the University of California at Santa Barbara. She worked with Drs. Robert and Lynn Koegel and has significant experience working with individuals with ASD across the life span.

Shawnna Sundberg, M.A., Ball State University, Muncie, Indiana

Shawnna received a bachelor of arts degree in psychology from Purdue University in 2008, and a master's degree in special education with certifications in applied behavior analysis (ABA) and autism from Ball State University in 2015. Shawnna is a board-certified behavior analyst with more than 10 years of experience working in the mental health and ABA/verbal behavior (VB) field. Shawnna has worked as a child and adolescent home-based case manager, ABA/VB therapist, training specialist, parent-training coordinator, and behavior consultant.

Jane R. Wegner, Ph.D., Clinical Professor, Clinic Director, Schiefelbusch Speech-Language-Hearing Clinic, University of Kansas, Lawrence

Dr. Wegner is a clinical professor and director of the Schiefelbusch Speech-Language-Hearing Clinic at the University of Kansas (KU). She directs the Pardee Augmentative and Alternative Communication Resource and Research Laboratory on the Lawrence campus of KU. Dr. Wegner directed numerous personnel preparation projects funded by the U.S. Department of Education, Office of Special Education Programs, including the Communication, Autism, and Technology Project and the Augmentative Communication in the Schools Project. She has authored numerous articles and book chapters on Augmentative and Alternative Communication. Dr. Wegner is a Fellow of the American Speech-Language-Hearing Association and served on the ASHA Ad Hoc Committee on Autism Spectrum Disorders that developed the ASHA policy documents for practice with people with ASD.

Amy Wetherby, Ph.D., CCC-SLP, Distinguished Research Professor, Department of Clinical Sciences, College of Medicine, Florida State University

Amy M. Wetherby is a Distinguished Research Professor in the Department of Clinical Sciences, director of the Autism Institute in the Florida State University College of Medicine, and the Laurel Schendel Professor of Communication Disorders in the Florida State University College of Communication and Information. She has 30 years of clinical experience and is a Fellow of the American Speech-Language-Hearing Association. Dr. Wetherby has published extensively and gives presentations regularly at national conventions on early detection of children with ASD and intervention for children with ASD using The SCERTS Model. She is the project director of a doctoral leadership training grant specializing in autism and funded by the U.S. Department of Education. She served on the National Academy of Sciences Committee for Educational Interventions for Children with Autism and is executive director of the Florida State University Center for Autism and Related Disabilities. Dr. Wetherby is project director of the FIRST WORDS Project, a longitudinal research investigation on early detection of ASD and other communication disorders, funded by the U.S. Department of Education, National Institutes of Health, and Centers for Disease Control and Prevention. She is also the principal investigator of an early treatment study, funded by Autism Speaks and the National Institutes of Health, teaching parents of toddlers with ASD how to support social communication and play in everyday activities.

Susan M. Wilczynski, Ph.D., BCBA-D, Professor, Ball State University, Muncie, Indiana

Dr. Wilczynski is the Plassman Family Distinguished Professor of Special Education and Applied Behavior Analysis and the former executive director of the National Autism Center. Dr. Wilczynski has edited or written multiple books and published scholarly works in *Behavior Analysis in Practice, Journal of Applied Behavior Analysis, Behavior Modification, Focus on Autism and Other Developmental Disabilities*, and *Psychology in the Schools.* Dr. Wilczynski is a licensed psychologist and a board-certified behavior analyst.

Juliann J. Woods, Ph.D., CCC-SLP, Professor Emeritus, Florida State University, Tallahassee

Juliann J. Woods is professor emeritus and consultant, Communication and Early Childhood Research and Practice Center in the School of Communication Science and Disorders, and associate director of research to practice in the Autism Institute at Florida State University. Throughout her career, she has emphasized the translation of research to practice, has published extensively, and presents regularly at national conferences on early communication and intervention for young children and their families, early identification and intervention in autism, coaching and professional development, and the use of technology.

Foreword

This comprehensively revised and updated second edition of *Treatment of Autism Spectrum Disorder* (and accompanying videos and case studies) overviews what we know, and what remains to be done, about the practice and evidence base for social communication interventions for children and young people with autism spectrum disorder (ASD). Its overriding aim is to make the research and clinical literature accessible to a wide range of audiences—frontline professionals working with children and families, students and professors who are learning about or study ASD, and parents and families of children with ASD. It is firmly based in two sometimes unaligned arenas; first, the evidence base for what works the children with ASD and, second, the everyday world of professional practice. Since the first edition published, the term Naturalistic Developmental Behavioral Interventions (NDBIs) has been coined, which describes the key theoretical and practical underpinning of many of the approaches included here. This edition is a tour de force summary of the state of the art and has a stellar line up—a veritable *who's who* of applied practitioners and researchers in the field.

The introduction by Prelock and McCauley (**Chapter 1**) summarizes the revolution that has occurred over the past two decades and recognizes that social-pragmatic developmental interventions are appropriate—indeed even essential—for children and young people with ASD, alongside the more traditional behavioral approaches. It starts out by recapitulating the important changes in conceptualization and practice that were realized and indeed proceeded the publication of DSM-5 in 2013, most notably the formalization of ASD as the overarching diagnostic term for all individuals on the autism spectrum and the important addition of the clinical specifiers that are often more informative about the intervention support needs of an individual than the diagnosis itself. Given that difficulties with social communication are the core features that characterize children with ASD, and in particular young children, including those who are nonverbal or who have minimal language skills, this might seem obvious, but it is only over the last 20 years that a secure evidence base has emerged for such approaches. This edition aims to translate the updated National Autism Center (NAC) 2015 report on the National Standards Project— a seminal but also very technical and very long review of interventions for children and young people with ASD—into an accessible and practical manual. Each chapter not only explains the theoretical basis of a particular intervention approach and the evidence for its effectiveness, but also highlights the practical requirements needed to implement it (i.e., time, training, expertise) and describes how practitioners and parents can evaluate whether the intervention is working for any particular child or young person. The use of case studies and the accompanying videos of several of the key social communication intervention approaches, including Early Start Denver Model (ESDM), SCERTS®, and video modeling, to illustrate the different interventions makes this text a manual for practice and one with an unusually close eye on evidence, which is as it should be to best serve children and young people with autism and their families.

The new **Chapter 2** by McCauley, Bean, and Prelock on *Assessment for Treatment Planning and Progress Monitoring* amplifies the important tenant that good evidence-based practice starts with a comprehensive assessment and profiling of an individual's strengths and needs. The authors cover key areas to consider in a social communication assessment that both relate to the heterogeneous presentation seen in individuals with ASD, but also other factors including common co-occurring conditions that can impact on social communication itself and also need to be taken into account in modifying intervention programs to best suit the individual. They also emphasize the critical need to consider individual factors ranging from developmental level to cultural, family and social-environmental factors that need to be considered in the personalization of both the assessment and the subsequent intervention itself. Chapter 2 also highlights how all of these factors need to be part of ongoing monitoring process once intervention is initiated, in order to assess its effectiveness for the individual in relation to the targeted outcomes, and then to revise and refine the approach based on this evidence. They outline some of the tools that are available for different social communication intervention approaches to do just this.

Another new chapter by Brien and Prelock (**Chapter 3**) breaks down different components of social communication abilities that can all be appropriately targeted by social communication interventions for individuals with ASD. These components range from understanding what intentional communication is and what it is for; to different preverbal social communication skills such as imitation, play, and joint attention; to the more structural aspects of language and communication use including semantic, syntactic, and phonological development. In each of these sections, the authors provide a helpful contrast between what we know from developmental studies of typical development and how such communication can be different for individuals with ASD. This links back to one of the overarching themes of the whole book in that evidence-based and effective interventions for individuals with ASD should be based on a good understanding in training about both theory and practice of what social communication is. The chapter also emphasizes the need for collaborative and partnership work with parents and caregivers and the way in which this is a key component of many well evidenced programs.

Wegner summarizes the evidence for augmentative and alternative communication (AAC) strategies (**Chapter 4**). These are approaches used with children and young people who are nonverbal or minimally verbal—a significant minority of individuals with ASD. Some of the most widely used systems are the Picture Exchange Communication System (PECS), graphic communication systems, sign language, and speech-generating devices (SGDs). As with any successful intervention, but perhaps particularly so for AAC approaches, the fit between the communication needs of an individual child or young person and the particular intervention implemented is the key. Many of the interventions reviewed in the chapter use overarching frameworks such as the Participation Model, the Social Networks tool, or The Social Communication, Emotional Regulation, and Transactional Supports (SCERTS®) Model, all of which emphasize the need for AAC approaches to be person and family centered and place an emphasis on natural environments and meaningful contexts. By their nature, these approaches are time and labor intensive and require both considerable expertise (usually from a speech-language pathologist [SLP]) and a team approach to ensure the consistency of approach that is critical for them to be successful. Clinical examples with a child and adult ground these principles in the real-world application of PECS and SGDs, respectively. The chapter also highlights how considerations about inclusive practice and cultural and linguistic diversity are components of successful augmentation.

Chapter 5 by Howard and Dawson gives an overview of the Early Start Denver Model (ESDM) one of the better-established and better evidence-based NDBIs for young children with ASD. ESDM combines both behavioral theory and behavioral techniques with a developmental and dyadic (relationship and interaction) stage-based approach to promoting social interaction and functional communication abilities as key targeted outcomes. The authors summarize the evidence for different versions of delivery of ESDM, ranging from intensive direct therapist- and parent-delivered intervention, to a 12-week parent coaching model to group implementation in the community and in school settings. Variants of ESDM have also need used via telehealth—important in the context of the current COVID-19 pandemic—and increasingly in global settings, including low- and middle-income countries. Measuring implementation fidelity and monitoring progress are key structural components built into the ESDM program, and materials are provided with the manuals for practitioners to use in their everyday practice.

Kazee, Wilczynski, Martino, Sundberg, Quinn, and Mundell describe the long-established discrete trial instruction (DTI) approach (**Chapter 6**). This method is based on behavioral approaches that date back to the original work of B. F. Skinner on operant conditioning. The fundamental principles of DTI are clearly laid out—a discriminative stimulus, a response, a consequence (reinforcement), and an inter-trial interval. This approach has been applied to many aspects of development and behavior in children and young people with ASD, including in broader, comprehensive programs, pioneered by Ivar Lovaas, which are sometimes called the applied behavioral analysis (ABA) approach or, more recently, early intensive behavioral intervention (EIBI). Many of the programs covered in other chapters in the volume, including those on ESDM and Pivotal Response Treatment (PRT), incorporate some of the DTI principles into their approaches, with justification since it is a tenant of behavioral psychology and learning theory. The authors illustrate how DTI approaches can be used to promote prelinguistic skills, such as joint attention, as well as language in more formal verbal behavior programs. One important contribution from the DTI and wider ABA field has been the strong emphasis placed on routinely measuring responses and outcomes and the accompanying development of a suite of tools for practitioners to use to assess intervention response, such as the widely used Verbal Behaviour Milestones and Placement Program (VB-MAPP; Sundberg, 2008). Practice examples and checklists of many of these components of DTI are threaded throughout this comprehensive summary.

Gerber outlines the ASD-specific intervention developed by Stanley Greenspan, the Developmental, Individual-Difference, Relationship-Based (DIR) Model (**Chapter 7**). This approach emphasizes interpersonal development and draws on a wide range of theoretical foundations, most notably contemporary theories of developmental psychology. The functional emotional developmental levels characterize social communication and cognitive problem solving seen in typically developing children in the early years. Using the intervention strategy known as Floortime, the DIR approach emphasizes spontaneous interactions alongside semi-structured and structured learning activities and includes sensory and perceptual-motor targets and activities that commonly present difficulties for children and young people with ASD. Helpfully, the chapter also emphasizes the overlap between the DIR approach and other developmental social communication interventions such as The SCERTS Model and the Hanen More Than Words program. DIR practitioners, mostly SLPs, use the Functional Emotional Assessment Scales (FEAS) to determine the child's functional emotional developmental levels, as well as the nature of the interactions between the child and his or her caregivers, to create a treatment plan based on the child's individual profile and provides a baseline for measuring his or her progress. The chapter also places the DIR model within a broader framework of an interdisciplinary team of professionals working with a child and their parents or carers.

In **Chapter 8**, Durand and Moskowitz outline the well-established behavioral approach known as functional communication training (FCT). This application of behavioral techniques is specifically designed to reduce challenging behaviors such as tantrums, aggression, or self-injury. The authors highlight that such difficulties are common and enduring in individuals with ASD and have a significant impact upon them and their families. In common with other behavioral approaches, a functional behavioral assessment is the starting point for developing an individually tailored behavioral intervention. The principle of functional equivalence is central to the FCT approach in that an alternative, more adaptive behavior can serve the same function for an individual as the maladaptive, challenging behavior. The authors summarize the many studies that have provided positive evidence for the benefits of FCT, most of which are single-case designs or small case series. A summary of the seven components of FCT is given, from assessing the function of a behavior to modifying the environment. In closing, the authors raise an important caveat that also applies to all interventions covered by the volume: Some teachers and parents do not find FCT easy to carry out effectively; and working on parental (and teacher) understanding and acceptance of the role that their own attitudes and feelings towards their child's challenging behavior may play is an important component of support and successful implementation of FCT. Not all interventions will suit all practitioners and families, and alongside consideration of the evidence base for any approach it is important to consider the fit between the approach and the individual implementing the intervention.

Kasari and Sterrett summarize the evidence for the Joint Attention, Symbolic Play, Engagement, and Regulation (JASPER) intervention (**Chapter 9**) that specifically targets critical prelinguistic social communication skills that is a particular area of impairment for many young children with ASD. Similar to the DIR approach, joint attention interventions have a theoretical foundation in developmental psychology. Joint attention, joint action routines (e.g., nursery rhymes), and symbolic play are interactive activities through which typically developing young children learn preverbal social communication and social interaction skills, typically in interactions with their parents and other caregivers. Because JASPER is based heavily in play and activity, it is appropriate for children up to age 9 who are minimally verbal or preschool children. The authors summarize the findings from the now more than 10 randomized controlled trials (RCTs) of the JASPER program that have been published—more trials than of any other program included in the volume. Studies have found that joint attention and joint engagement skills improved in interactions both with therapists and with parents and, in one study at a 12-month follow-up, language skills had improved. In common with ESDM, therapist-, parent-, and teacher-mediated variants of JASPER have now been tested with some evidence of benefit, at least in proximal outcomes and skills. In common with all chapters in the volume, the authors include a section on considerations for children from culturally and linguistically diverse backgrounds, but uniquely Kasari and Sterrett have actually run trials in socially deprived and underserved communities, and studies are now also underway of the program in low-and-middle income countries. However, the authors note that there are cultures differences in some aspects of parent–child interaction and expectations and these need to be taken into account when working with these populations.

Kaiser, Fuller, and Heidlage introduce the Enhanced Milieu Teaching (EMT) approach (**Chapter 10**). This approach is specifically tailored for young children with ASD who have foundational verbal or pre-verbal language skills. By using a combination of contemporary ABA and developmental pragmatic techniques, the therapist (who can be a parent) works on expanding and modeling the child's emerging language abilities. EMT has been used with young language learners with intellectual disability, specific language impairment and Down syndrome, as well as ASD. The six core components of EMT are 1) environmental arrangement, 2) responsive interaction, 3) language modeling, 4) language expansions, 5) time delays, and 6) milieu teaching prompts. The milieu around the child varies in the level of prompting, following a most-to-least support strategy, so that the child progresses from imitating language to independently initiating language interactions. An increasing number of trials by the chapter authors and others have demonstrated its effectiveness. In the *Future Directions* section of the chapter, the authors mention recent trials undertaken combining EMT with the use of SGDs with 5 to 8-year-olds who are minimally verbal, despite 2 years of conventional intervention with promising results emerging.

Woods, Wetherby, Delehanty, Kashinath, and Holland describe the development and evidence for the Early Social Interaction (ESI) model (**Chapter 11**) which is a social communication intervention for toddlers as young as 18 months of age diagnosed with, or at familial risk of, ASD. The authors summarize the developmental foundations and evidence base for the ESI approach. In common with many of the modern NDBIs approaches to intervention for children with ASD covered in the volume (e.g., DIR, EMT), ESI combines elements from developmental-pragmatic and behavioral intervention approaches. The model adopts a collaborative coaching approach to support parent learning and generalization and in tandem it also emphasizes the importance of the family system around the child and the need for family-centered services and supports. In common with other parent-implemented social communication approaches, the intervention strategies are embedded in everyday caregiving interactions and family daily routines (e.g., mealtimes, bath time, bedtime). In using such approaches, the goal is to be able to deliver several hours per day of intervention with the child for only a few hours of direct, professional input per week. One emphasis throughout the volume is the need for programs to be both accessible and universally available across communities, and the ESI approach sets out to make this goal realizable. Resources and support linked to the ESI program—including training and demonstration videos and example activity schedules—are available via a website (https://autismnavigator.com) providing an infrastructure for a scalable and widely accessible intervention.

Carter summarizes the evidence base for peer-mediated interventions (**Chapter 12**). These are usually school-based programs that use behavioral and social learning theory approaches in which the assistance of typically developing peers in inclusive education settings is engaged to promote social interaction and learning. The peers are trained and supported to prompt, model, and reinforce the social and academic learning targets for the child or children with ASD. The author systematically summarizes the nearly 30 published empirical studies that have used the peer-mediated model. Different programs use different approaches, ranging from peer interaction training and peer networks (for promoting social behaviors) to cooperative learning groups and peer tutoring (for promoting academic learning). General and special educators require training in how to implement such approaches, as the specific psychological theory that underpins peer-mediated approaches may not have been part of their original education training. In common with the previous chapter, although some input from expert professionals is required, the economic model behind peer-mediated approaches may allow the possibility of wide implementation. Importantly in a setting—both school and with age peers—in which many young children with ASD will spend a lot of time. In some communities around the globe, including here in the UK, there is a move for services and support for ASD children to be located in the community, including in schools, as opposed to clinical settings; and peer-mediated interventions should play a role in these developments.

Koegel, Koegel, and Ponder outline another social communication intervention that draws both on behavioral and developmental principles—perhaps the longest established model in the field and in some ways the forerunner of many of the other programs and approaches included in the volume—the Koegel's Pivotal Response Treatment (PRT; **Chapter 13**). In common with other similar interventions, PRT emphasizes working within the child's natural environment and centrally involving parents as interventionists, often alongside therapists. The emphasis on *pivotal areas* in the child's behavioral repertoire is intended to take advantage of the cascading collateral effects on responding and functioning that can follow. These pivotal areas include identifying motivational strategies that engage the child, using multiple cues to overcome the overselectivity that characterizes some children with ASD, promoting self-initiations and not prompted behaviors, and self-management—helping the child to monitor his or her own behavior. Although there has long been an evidence base from single cases and case series studies and some uncontrolled trials, the past decade has also seen a number of independent RCTs demonstrating effectiveness for social communication outcomes, which the authors summarize. The authors highlight one collateral benefit from a parent training intervention such as PRT, which is that studies have shown reduced parental stress after having been through the training program—their central involvement in the program is support for themselves as parents as well as for their child.

Another new addition (**Chapter 14**) by Laurent, Rubin, and Prizant summarizes the well-known Social Communication, Emotional Regulation, and Transactional Supports (SCERTS®) Model. SCERTS is described by the authors as a comprehensive educational approach and has in some ways a broader overarching framework and philosophy than some of the other models in this book, which focus on particular techniques of social communication practice or development. The assumptions, practices, and outcomes that underpin the transdisciplinary model are outlined in the chapter and the empirical evidence helpfully reviewed. In common with other programs, there is a dedicated SCERTS® Assessment Process (SAP) observation tool that can be used by practitioners during the assessment (of need) and monitoring (of outcome). SCERTS is widely used in many educational settings for children and young people with ASD, and the evidence base has grown significantly over the past decade.

In **Chapter 15,** Prelock and Brien review broader social skills intervention programs, of which there are many, which support a child's appropriate use of gestures, eye gaze, reciprocity, and initiating, sustaining, and finishing an interaction with others. They review the content and research on 10 programs, perhaps the best known and researched of which are Children's Friendship Training (CFT) and Program for the Education and Enrichment of Relational Skills (PEERS®). In contrast to many approaches in the this edition, social skills interventions are primarily for school age children and young people through adolescence and even into adulthood. The authors review the key components and tools for assessment and planning and monitoring progress—that overlap but also differ from program-to-program—of each program, including more recently developed innovations such as the Virtual Reality-Social Cognition Training (VR-SCT). Picking up an important caution that applies to other approaches in the volume, the authors highlight that sustained performance of social skills learned via such approaches do not always sustain once the intervention is no longer being implemented. The issue of both generalization and maintenance of intervention outcomes is one key critical challenge for both the practice and the research fields.

Hutchins provides a comprehensive and up-to-date review of the evidence base for Carol Gray's Social Stories™ (**Chapter 16**). These are written-out, individualized stories that are aimed to facilitate social understanding by providing direct access to social information. This intervention addresses the difficulties in social cognition and social understanding that characterize individuals with ASD. Gray's Social Stories approach draws on a wide range of contemporary psychological theories of ASD, including impairments in theory of mind or mentalizing abilities and the cognitive style of weak "central coherence" or gestalt. The contextual approach that the Social Stories intervention takes emphasizes that social impairments in ASD are located in the social space between people and not inherently located in the individual him- or herself. For practitioners and families there are online resources: (https://carolgraysocialstories.com) that offer information and training to support effective strategies for developing Social Stories that adhere to Gray's guidelines. Alongside a thorough review of the evidence for the Social Stories approach, the author highlights two issues that apply to many of the interventions included in the volume. The authors ends with a note of caution: as with many other programs, although there is promising (emergent) evidence for their effectiveness, we know much less about the generalizability and maintenance of treatment effects.

Buggey reviews the literature on the fairly recently emerged technique of video modeling (**Chapter 17**). Its theoretical basis is learning theory and Bandura's social learning theory, and it builds on the notion that people with autism tend to be visual thinkers as opposed to language-based thinkers. The video modeling approach can be applied to a wide range of target behaviors, including social skills and behaviors, learning about emotions, perspective-taking skills, and language.

Most programs have used adult or peer models, but more recently people have begun to use self-modeling (where the individual him- or herself acts as the model) and animations. The author usefully summarizes the practical advantages and disadvantages of these different formats in a table. In line with its relatively recent emergence, there is a limited but increasing literature on the effectiveness of video modeling approaches. In the chapter's *Future Directions* section, the author highlights the coming potential for new technologies like virtual reality (VR) to provide a three-dimensional world where interactive video modeling can take place to train social and functional skills but the technology and cost is only making such potential now realizable.

In their closing overview, the editors McCauley and Prelock set out future directions for the field of social communication intervention for individuals with ASD (**Chapter 18**). Without repeating in full, the thoughtful but also challenging directions that they outline for researchers, practitioners, and families, I will highlight some of the ideas that most strongly caught my attention. There is wide agreement, though disappointingly slower progress, that we need to develop better measures of meaningful outcomes against which to test different interventions. However rigorous the design and conduct of future research studies, if we are not measuring the right outcomes, we will not be doing the best for individuals with ASD and their families. Another challenge is to find out more about *who* benefits from *which* treatments so that packages of interventions can be individually tailored (personalized) to an individual's and family's needs. Finally, the authors emphasize the research-to-practice gap: Even if research provides strong evidence for particular programs, how do we ensure that these programs are implemented correctly in the community and made accessible and acceptable to all members of the community? Important considerations are how to ensure cultural, linguistic, and social appropriateness and accessibility, as well as the potential for scalable models of intervention programs that can be adapted for use in low-and middle-income countries and in underserved communities. The modern practice of implementation science is only just emerging in the field of ASD intervention research. The authors end with another useful practical service by pointing out the increasing number of useful, balanced, and fair web sites where practitioners and family members can go to learn about the evidence base for interventions for individuals with ASD.

I am sure that readers of this excellent text, once they have learned much from its contents, will use these resources as they continue their journey to improve the life outcomes for people with ASD.

Tony Charman, Ph.D.
Institute of Psychiatry,
Psychology & Neuroscience,
King's College, London

REFERENCE

Sundberg, M. L. (2008). *VB-MAPP Verbal Behavior Milestones Assessment and Placement Program: A language and social skills assessment program for children with autism or other developmental disabilities: Guide.* AVB Press.

Acknowledgments

This second edition of our intervention book has taken its final shape as a result of the diligent and creative efforts of a large number of individuals. In particular, we would like to acknowledge the authors of the intervention chapters for their contributions. Through their writing, and the research and practice that led to it, they have demonstrated a remarkable dedication to recommended practices for individuals with ASD and their families, a dedication that is certain to guide others who share a similar desire to make a difference. The writing task they took on for this project asked them not only to offer their best insights into the interventions but to include additional evidence for the interventions while following a framework that offered practical information and case examples for our readers. Without our authors, there would be no book.

We are especially grateful to all those at Paul H. Brookes Publishing Company who have supported every step of the process involved in the making of this book—from the thoughtful planning of this second edition to guiding needed updates to preparing the book for its final editing and production. The resulting pages have benefited from their efforts, and the contributing authors and we as editors have benefited personally from their skillful advice, encouragement, and patience. First, Astrid Zuckerman, with her extensive knowledge of this book from the first edition, then Liz Gildea, with her encouraging steadiness when the work progressed more slowly than one might have hoped—we could not have been more fortunate in these colleagues at Brookes! The bittersweet loss of Astrid to doctoral studies was tempered by the pleasure of our work with Liz. We also deeply appreciate the first-rate work of our project manager, MaryBeth Winkler, and the help provided by everyone to create books that show the meticulous attention all have brought to this project.

In Vermont, Patty acknowledges the constant support of her husband and family, who gave up their time with her so she could write. She also wishes to thank the authors for their diligence and expert contributions that enriched the quality of the final product. Patty especially appreciated the opportunity to work with Ashley Brien, a doctoral student at the University of Vermont, who offered significant contributions to this book.

In Ohio, Rebecca wants to offer special thanks to all of her colleagues and students at Ohio State University and to her friends and sisters in various locations for their continuing support, but especially to her sister Ruth, who has heard more about the excitement of developments in autism research than she might ever have imagined. In addition, Rebecca would like to express special appreciation for the support and expertise of her colleague Allison Bean in navigating the complex and fast-moving literature on autism.

Finally, we offer our most heartfelt thanks to those individuals with ASD and their families, who continually inspire us to understand more about how knowledgeable and caring clinicians and others can assist them in their efforts to engage in more satisfying social interactions and communicate more effectively.

To the children, adolescents, and adults with autism and their families from whom we have had the privilege to learn over the years

1

Introduction to Treatment of Autism Spectrum Disorder (ASD)

Patricia A. Prelock and Rebecca J. McCauley

INTRODUCTION

This book is intended to introduce readers who have some familiarity with autism spectrum disorder (ASD) and its core impairments to a group of interventions focused on social communication and social interaction. Because the diagnostic category for autism has undergone modification since the first edition of this text, this chapter describes these changes and briefly highlights some implications for these changes. The chapter then provides updates on national reviews of interventions considered to be established in support of the social communication and social interaction of children with ASD.

CHANGES TO THE DSM-5

When the *Diagnostic and Statistical Manual of Mental Disorders, Fourth Edition-Text Revision* (DSM-IV-TR; American Psychiatric Association [APA], 2000) was updated to DSM-5 (APA, 2013), pervasive developmental disorder/autism, with its subthreshold diagnoses, changed to autism spectrum disorder. The diagnostic criteria also moved from three primary diagnostic categories to two: 1) social communication and social interaction and 2) restricted, repetitive, and stereotyped patterns of behavior. Expansion within each category also occurred. Table 1.1a summarizes differences between the earlier (DSM-IV-TR, APA, 2000) and the current characterization of ASD (DSM-5; APA, 2013). A particularly significant change is that language and cognition are now considered to be potential comorbid conditions and require a separate assessment to ensure deficits in these areas cannot be better explained by an intellectual disability (ID) or a global developmental delay.

Table 1.1a. A summary of changes associated with autism spectrum disorder (ASD) diagnoses based on the *Diagnostic and Statistical Manual of Mental Disorders, Fourth Edition-Text Revision* (DSM-IV-TR; American Psychiatric Association [APA], 2000) and *Fifth Edition* (DSM-5; APA, 2013)

	DSM-IV-TR	DSM-5
Possible diagnoses	Autism spectrum disorders with pervasive developmental disorder-not otherwise specified (PDD-NOS), autistic disorder, Asperger disorder, childhood disintegrative disorder	Autism spectrum disorder is the sole diagnosis and should be used for individuals with well-established diagnoses of autistic disorder, Asperger disorder, or PDD-NOS by using the DSM-IV-TR criteria.
Diagnostic criteria for ASD	Clinically significant, persistent deficits in social communication and interactions (must meet two of the social and one of the communication criteria) Restricted repetitive patterns of behavior, interests, and activities (must meet one of the behavior criteria) Symptoms must be present in early childhood (but may not become fully manifest until social demands exceed limited capacities).	Deficits in social communication/interaction (must meet all three of the social criteria) Restricted and repetitive interests (must meet two of the four behavior criteria)
Onset	Must have been seen before age 8	Symptoms must have been present since early development, even if only recognized later.
Possible co-occurring diagnoses	—	Attention-deficit/hyperactivity disorder; speech sound disorder, language disorder, childhood-onset fluency disorder; NOT social (pragmatic) communication disorder
Possible specifications	—	With or without accompanying intellectual impairment With or without accompanying language impairment Associated with a known medical or genetic condition or environmental factor
Severity level description	Severity level description was not specified.	Severity level described in three levels. See Table 1.1b for a description of each level.

Source: American Psychiatric Association [APA], 2000 and 2013.

Table 1.1b describes the severity levels now associated with each of the two primary diagnostic categories (DSM-5; APA, 2013).

Several implications are discussed in the literature regarding the application of the new DSM-5 criteria. For example, Young and Rodi (2014) found only 57.1% of those with pervasive developmental disorders (PDDs) on the DSM-IV met the criteria for DSM-5, whereas 50%–75% maintained diagnoses in a review completed by Smith and colleagues (2015). In both studies, children with a diagnosis of PDD-not otherwise specified (PDD-NOS) and Asperger's disorder were less likely to meet the DSM-5 criteria, specifically all three social communication and social interaction criteria. However, a case was made to ensure students who may not qualify under

Table 1.1b. Severity levels associated with the two diagnostic criteria for autism spectrum disorder in the DSM-5

Severity level	Social communication	Restricted, repetitive behaviors
Level 3: Requiring very substantial support	Severe deficits in verbal and nonverbal social communication skills cause severe impairments in functioning, very limited initiation of social interactions, and minimal response to social overtures from others (e.g., a person with few words of intelligible speech who rarely initiates interaction and, when he or she does, makes unusual approaches to meet needs only and responds to only very direct social approaches)	Inflexibility of behavior, extreme difficulty coping with change, or other restricted/repetitive behaviors markedly interfere with functioning in all spheres Great distress/difficulty changing focus or action
Level 2: Requiring substantial support	Marked deficits in verbal and nonverbal social communication skills Social impairments apparent even with supports in place Limited initiation of social interactions; and reduced or abnormal responses to social overtures from others (e.g., a person who speaks simple sentences, whose interaction is limited to narrow special interests, and has markedly odd nonverbal communication)	Inflexibility of behavior, difficulty coping with change, or other restricted/repetitive behaviors appear frequently enough to be obvious to the casual observer and interfere with functioning in a variety of contexts Distress and/or difficulty changing focus or action
Level 1: Requiring support	Without supports in place, deficits in social communication cause noticeable impairments Difficulty initiating social interactions, and clear examples of atypical or unsuccessful response to social overtures of others May appear to have decreased interest in social interactions (e.g., a person who is able to speak in full sentences and engages in communication but whose to-and-fro conversation with others fails and whose attempts to make friends are odd and typically unsuccessful)	Inflexibility of behavior causes significant interference with functioning in one or more contexts Difficulty switching between activities Problems of organization and planning hamper independence

the new criteria continue to receive the intervention services they require (Smith et al., 2015; Young & Rodi, 2014).

A study with 185 children under 5 years old indicated that children with autism on the *Diagnostic and Statistical Manual of Mental Disorders, Fourth Edition, Text Revision* (DSM-IV-TR; APA, 2000) were also diagnosed with ASD on the DSM-5, but children with previous PDD-NOS diagnoses had fewer comorbid and emotional behaviors and insufficient symptoms in the restricted repetitive patterns of behavior category to qualify for an ASD diagnosis (Christiansz et al., 2016). Another study (Zander & Bolte, 2015) of younger children between 20 and 47 months found that 12%–07% of the children who met the DSM-IV-TR criteria did not meet the DSM-5 criteria, although diagnosis was influenced by severity level, leading to less consistent diagnosis. Reports by the Centers for Disease Control and Prevention (Baio et al., 2018), however, indicate the number of children meeting the DSM-5 criteria for ASD as compared to the DSM-IV-TR criteria are fairly similar, with DSM-IV-TR cases exceeding DSM-5 cases by less than 5% and with an 86% overlap between the two definitions. It remains unclear what the impact has been or will be to the prevalence of ASD diagnoses with the addition of social communication disorder (APA, 2013). Although this disorder is characterized by challenges in the social use of both verbal and nonverbal communication similar to ASD, there is no evidence of restricted and repetitive patterns of behaviors, interests, or activities. Whatever the ultimate impact is of the application of the DSM-5 on the diagnosis of ASD, children still require evidence-based interventions that address their social communication and social interaction impairments, as prevalence numbers continue to rise with 1 in 59 children receiving a diagnosis (Baio et al., 2018).

BACKGROUND ON INTERVENTION STRATEGIES FOR COMMUNICATION AND SOCIAL INTERACTION

Since 2000, thinking has evolved about which intervention approaches are most appropriate for supporting the social interaction and communication needs of children with ASD as well as children with social pragmatic disorders who may not meet the ASD diagnosis. Although **traditional behavioral interventions** are plentiful in the literature (e.g., Cooper et al., 2007) and tremendously influential in a variety of settings (Downs et al., 2007; Lafasakis & Sturmey, 2007; Taubman et al., 2001), **social-pragmatic developmental interventions** continue to gain traction, including those that involve parent training, in part because they emphasize opportunities for people with ASD to establish positive social connections and generalize their skills in the natural environment. Interest in these approaches has also arisen in response to limitations identified in traditional behavioral approaches to ASD in terms of generalization of targeted behaviors, particularly those related to the social use of communication and language (Wetherby & Woods, 2006, 2008). This book focuses primarily on such approaches because of their special promise in addressing the social communication and social interaction challenges at the core of ASD and their potential to minimize barriers to the functional application of learning.

In the traditional behavioral approach, practitioners teach skills one-to-one with a predetermined correct response (Karsten & Carr, 2009; Newman et al., 2009; Prelock & Nelson, 2012) and a highly prescribed teaching structure (e.g., discrete trial training [Cooper et al., 2007]). In contrast, in a social-pragmatic developmental approach, the interventionist follows the child's lead, fosters initiation and spontaneity, and reinforces contingent responses. Several strategies consistent with these approaches have long been implemented as part of naturalistic communication and language interventions for children with a variety of communication and language challenges (Girolametto et al., 1996; Kaiser et al., 2000; Kaiser & Hester, 1994) and have more recently been elaborated upon and modified to address the special challenges presented by ASD.

Several of the interventions described in this text capitalize on the value of integrating the best of behavioral and developmental approaches to achieve functional and relevant social and communicative outcomes for children, adolescents, and adults with ASD. For example, Prizant and Wetherby (1998), recognizing the contributions of both a traditional behavioral and older developmental approaches to intervention, proposed **contemporary behavioral interventions** (i.e., middle ground interventions) to support the communication and social interaction needs of children with ASD. In particular, they described the value of giving children choices, sharing communication opportunities between the interventionist and the child, and using preferred activities and materials—strategies that characterize pivotal response training (Koegel, Koegel, Harrower, & Carter, 1999; Koegel, Koegel, Shoshan, & McNerney, 1999).

As intervention approaches have evolved, so too have comprehensive guidelines for best practices. In 2001, the National Research Council (NRC) offered a description of best practices for children with ASD through the early childhood years. A number of intervention guidelines emerged from a comprehensive review of the literature, including initiating treatment as soon as possible; ensuring active engagement during intensive instruction; using developmentally appropriate, goal-based, and systematically planned activities; implementing planned teaching opportunities throughout the day; and involving families and peers in the intervention to facilitate generalized skill learning. Many early intervention programs have used these best practices to design comprehensive educational programs for young children with ASD.

As a follow-up to the NRC (2001) description, Iovannone and colleagues (2003) proposed six educational practices as appropriate and effective for school-age children with ASD: 1) providing individualized supports and services that matched a student's profile as defined through the individualized education program (IEP) process; 2) offering systematic, carefully planned, and defined instructional procedures to achieve valid goals with a process for measuring outcomes; 3) creating a structured learning environment; 4) adding specialized curriculum content in the area of social engagement and recreation and leisure skills; 5) defining a functional approach to problem behaviors; and 6) engaging families in their student's educational success. Challenges remained, however, in determining the most effective instructional procedures for children of varying ages, language abilities, and cognitive levels with diagnoses of autism and subthreshold diagnoses, such as Asperger syndrome and PDD-NOS.

To address the gaps in the intervention effectiveness literature for the large heterogeneous group of children with ASD, in 2009 the National Autism Center (NAC) (https://www.nationalautismcenter.org) released a report of a comprehensive review of 775 intervention studies since 1957. In that report, the authors categorized the current level of evidence for several interventions typically used in the treatment of individuals with ASD (0–21 years). The interventions fell into one of four groups: established, emerging, unestablished, or ineffective/harmful, although no interventions were identified in the ineffective/harmful group. Behavioral treatments were identified as having the strongest support, and nonbehavioral approaches were identified as making a significant contribution but requiring more research (NAC, 2009).

In 2015, the NAC published a second report, examining research from 2007 to 2012, including any intervention research for those with ASD over 22 years of age (from 1987 to 2012), collapsing a couple of the behavioral packages under behavioral interventions and adding a couple of intervention categories. Their findings continued to support behaviorally based interventions, although limited research was found for adults over 22, with only 28 studies meeting the inclusion criteria, finding one established, one emerging, and four unestablished interventions for adults with ASD. Notably, however, the 2015 NAC report added three interventions to the established category for individuals from birth to age 21: 1) language training (specifically language production using behavioral principles); 2) parent training; and 3) a social skills package. The report's chapter on behavioral interventions speaks to some of the more recent work in language production training. This second edition of *Treatment of Autism Spectrum Disorder* includes two new chapters that involve parent training, which adds to the three chapters from the first edition that already focus on the value of parent training, and this edition also features a new chapter on social skills training.

Table 1.2 lists the 14 interventions included in this book according to their level of evidence at the time of the most recent publication of the National Standards Project (NAC, 2015). Established treatments are those identified with sufficient evidence leading to positive outcomes. Emerging treatments are those with one or more studies yielding positive outcomes but requiring additional high-quality studies to show consistent results. Unestablished treatments are those with little evidence and that consequently require additional research. No treatments are those judged to be ineffective or harmful. Interventions described in this book fall primarily within the top two categories of evidence—established and emerging; only one intervention (DIRFloortime, Chapter 7) is considered unestablished, although it involves parent

Table 1.2. Levels of evidence for interventions included in this book based on the National Standards Project

Level of evidence	Level description	Chapter	Intervention
Established (14 interventions identified)	Sufficient evidence that the intervention leads to positive outcomes	6	Behavioral intervention strategies
		9	Joint attention intervention
		10	Enhanced Milieu Teaching (EMT)
		12	Peer-mediated support strategies
		13	Pivotal Response Treatment (PRT)
		15	Social skills training
		16	Social Stories
		17	Video modeling
Emerging (18 interventions identified)	One or more studies yielding positive outcomes, but study quality and results are inconsistent	4	Augmentative and alternative communication (AAC), including Picture Exchange Communication System (PECS)
		8	Functional communication training
Unestablished (13 interventions identified)	Little evidence and requiring additional research	7	Floortime and the Developmental, Individual-difference, Relationship-based (DIR) model
Not specifically named in the NAC report but all involve parent training, which is an established intervention	—	5	Early Start Denver Model
		11	Early Social Interaction Project
		14	The SCERTS® Model

From National Autism Center (2009). *National Standards Project—findings and conclusions: Addressing the needs for evidence-based practice guidelines for autism spectrum disorders.* Randolph, MA: Author; adapted by permission.

training, which is an established intervention. Also, three interventions are included that relate specifically to parent training (i.e., Early Denver Start Model [Chapter 5], Early Social Interaction Project [Chapter 11], and The SCERTS® Model [Chapter 14]) that were not specifically named in the 2015 NAC National Standards Project report. With the National Standards Project as a guide for evidence-based practice with children and youth affected by ASD, this text is timely because it emphasizes key established and emerging interventions used to facilitate the communication and social interaction of individuals with ASD and highlights those interventions with parents playing a key role.

PURPOSE OF THE BOOK

This book describes and critically analyzes specific treatment approaches used to address the communication and social interaction challenges of children, adolescents, and adults with ASD. Although these challenges are of specific interest to speech-language pathologists, providers across disciplines have a stake in using evidence-based intervention to respond to these core areas of impairment for individuals with ASD. Approaches selected for inclusion have empirical evidence of efficacy or effectiveness established through systematic reviews or at least two peer-reviewed articles that indicate the approaches are well-established, probably efficacious or promising emerging interventions (e.g., Chambless et al., 1998; Chorpita et al., 2002; NAC, 2015).

Traditionally, randomized control trials (RCTs) are considered the gold standard for evaluating treatment efficacy. RCTs, however, are rare in many clinical fields. In contrast, single-subject experimental designs are underacknowledged in evaluating treatment efficacy (Barlow et al., 2009; Perdices & Tate, 2009), yet they constitute the majority of credible evidence in the intervention research in autism (Debodinance et al., 2017; Odom et al., 2003). Single-subject designs make important contributions to the research base on treatment when they 1) are replicated across behaviors, participants, and contexts; 2) measure change reliably and systematically; 3) have established implementation fidelity; and 4) are socially valid. In fact, results from many single-subject designs indicate that specific interventions are associated with positive learning outcomes for individuals with ASD (Lord et al., 2005). Therefore, the effectiveness of selected treatments included in this book has been established primarily through single-subject experimental designs, although instances of randomized control trials do exist (e.g., joint attention training using the JASPER model).

Table 1.3 provides a summary to facilitate the reader's understanding of the similarities and differences among the interventions in terms of basic principles, techniques, teaching methods, treatment targets, and ages for which evidence has been established. This table also identifies the evidence rating provided by the National Autism Center (2015). In addition, to make the treatments accessible to the reader and to facilitate their comparison, the table's descriptions were standardized using a template adapted from that used in McCauley and Fey (2006) in which critical features of each treatment are highlighted. Treatments are also illustrated by a short video example, which can be accessed on the Brookes Download Hub (see the About the Videos and Downloads page in the front matter for guidance on how to access the video clips).

Readers will learn that the interventions emphasize somewhat different principles, techniques, and teaching methods to foster communication and social

Table 1.3. National Autism Center (2015) categorization of featured interventions

Interventions	NSP rating[a]	Basic principles	Methods	Targets	Ages
AAC including PECS (Chapter 4)	Emerging	Social-pragmatic and behavioral	Assessment of partner and environmental influence AAC system and target vocabulary selection Meaningful contexts Responsive partners Natural environment Family and person centered Systematic teaching Time delay Direct, natural reinforcement Shaping Modeling Prompting Visually based	Enhance existing communication skills Expand language Replace speech Provide structure to support language development Initiate requests spontaneously Request reinforcing items or activities, help, or a break Reject offers for undesired items or activities Affirm offers for desired items or activities Follow a direction to wait Respond to directions Follow transitional cues and visual schedules	Toddler through adult
Early Start Denver Model (Chapter 5)	Not specifically reported but is parent training focused, which is established	Developmental and behavioral	Play Relationship building Applied behavior analysis techniques Naturalistic developmental behavioral techniques including natural interactions, shared control, natural contingencies Group-delivered ESDM Parent-delivered ESDM Implementation fidelity	Receptive and expressive language Social skills with adults and peers Joint attention Imitation Play	1–5 years

8

Intervention	Status	Approach	Characteristics	Targets	Age range
Behavioral intervention strategies: discrete trial learning, differential reinforcement, and shaping (Chapter 6)	Established	Behavioral	Adult-directed, individualized one-to-one instruction Predetermined correct responses Contingent or differential reinforcement Shaping behaviors Operant conditioning Massed trials Maintenance trials Mand-modeling	Communication, social, and adaptive skills Use of verbal operants (e.g., mands, tacts, echoics, intraverbals)	3–21 years
DIR Floortime (Chapter 7)	Unestablished	Developmental	Family based Child directed Interpersonal development Individual differences Caregiver–child relationships Parent and clinician implemented	Shared attention and regulation Engagement and relating Two-way intentional communication Complex problem solving Creative representations and elaboration Representational and emotional thinking	18 months–9 years
Functional communication training (Chapter 8)	Emerging	Behavioral	Functional behavior assessment Selection of an alternative behavior Fading prompts Response match, success, efficiency, acceptability, recognizability, and milieu Natural communities of reinforcement	Replacement of aggression, self-injury, elopement, and inappropriate sexual behavior with functional communication forms	3–21 years
Joint attention: JASPER Model (Chapter 9)	Established	Behavioral and developmental	Directed instruction Individualized Intensive Milieu teaching Parent and clinician implemented	Response to and spontaneous initiation of joint attention	3–5 years
Enhanced Milieu Teaching (Chapter 10)	Established	Behavioral and developmental	Environmental arrangement Responsive interaction Language modeling Milieu teaching Parent and clinician implemented	Productive, spontaneous, and meaningful use of new language forms Initiations and responses	3–9 years

(continued)

Table 1.3. *(continued)*

Interventions	NSP rating[a]	Basic principles	Methods	Targets	Ages
Early Social Interaction (Chapter 11)	Not specifically reported but is parent training focused which is established	Developmental	Family based Child directed Environmental arrangement Responsive interactions Preferred activities and materials Routine based Natural environment	Social communication from preverbal to multiword stage Gesture use Initiation of and response to joint attention Word knowledge Reciprocity	18 months–3 years
Peer mediation (Chapter 12)	Established	Behavioral	Peer interaction training Peer network strategies Regular opportunities to interact within and outside instructional settings Adult coaching, guidance, and support Inclusive environment Communities of reinforcement Instructional arrangements (e.g., cooperative groups, peer support arrangements)	Initiating and maintaining conversation Exchanging compliments Turn-taking Helping behaviors Sharing materials Collaborating on assignments Making introductions Conversing about shared interests	3–14 years
Pivotal Response Treatment (Chapter 13)	Established	Behavioral and developmental	Play based Family based Natural environment Routine based Child choice Turn taking Shared control of teaching opportunities Direct and natural reinforcement Reinforcing communication attempts Preferred activities and materials Interspersing maintenance tasks within teaching sessions	First words Basic social skills Sophisticated language and social skills Pivotal behaviors (e.g., motivation, responsivity to multiple cues, self-management, self-initiations)	3–9 years

Intervention (Chapter)	Evidence	Approach	Key components	Goals	Age range
Social Stories (Chapter 16)	Established	Social-pragmatic	Visually based Situation specific Individualized instructional strategy (determine topic, gather information, develop the story, consider additional supports, critical review, introduce story, generalization training, maintenance and fading)	Reduction of disruptive behaviors (e.g., tantrums, aggression, self-injurious acts) Establish routines Introduce changes in routines Understanding of a new or unfamiliar event Social skills (e.g., getting a peer's attention, making choices, playing independently, peer engagement and participation) Communication (e.g., reduction of echolalia, interrupting, and loud talking)	6–14 years
Video modeling (Chapter 17)	Established	Behavioral and developmental	Visually based Viewing positive video models Adult anc peer modeling Point-of-view modeling Self-modeling including feed forward and positive self-review	Teach new skills or improve existing skills across developmental domains (e.g., self-help skills—dressing, feeding, washing; cognitive skills—play, perspective taking, attention; social skills—conversation, prosody, turn-taking; language skills—question asking and answering, greeting, comprehending stories) Replace or extinguish maladaptive behavior	3–18 years
The SCERTS® Model (Chapter 14)	Not specifically reported but is parent training focused which is established	Developmental	Collaboration Curriculum-based assessment Natural routines	Social communication Emotion regulation Transactional supports	Preschool through school age
Social skills interventions (Chapter 15)	Established	Social-pragmatic and behavioral			

aSource: National Autism Center. (2015).
Key: AAC, augmentative and alternative communication; ESDM, Early Start Denver Model; JASPER, Joint Attention, Symbolic Play, Engagement, and Regulation; PECS, Picture Exchange Communication System; SCERTS, Social Communication, Emotional Regulation, and Transactional Supports.

development in children, adolescents, and adults with ASD; therefore, there is not one best approach for all individuals. Instead, there are profiles of individuals affected by ASD who are likely to benefit most from each intervention guided by the evidence. Early, intensive, and structured intervention as well as a collaborative approach to working in home, educational, and community settings appear to be critical features of effective intervention. Further, this book emphasizes the importance of addressing the core deficits of social interaction and social communication.

HOW TREATMENTS ARE DESCRIBED

Authors prepared their intervention chapters, Chapters 4–17, using a template, with sections indicated by the headings provided in Table 1.4. Each chapter begins with a brief introduction summarizing the treatment approach and defining the subgroups of individuals with ASD for whom the treatment is designed. The chapter also includes the age, developmental level, language level, and service delivery model the treatment entails, including its basic focus and methods. In the description of the subgroups for whom the intervention is appropriate, the authors consider not only the specific diagnoses (e.g., autism spectrum disorder, social communication disorder) but also the individual's level of verbal skills and cognitive abilities.

The next section in each chapter includes the theoretical basis for the treatment approach. Here the authors discuss four main components. The first component is a theoretical explanation or rationale for the treatment. The second component includes underlying assumptions regarding the nature of the communication and social interaction impairment being addressed by the treatment. The third component describes the functional outcomes or desired consequences (e.g., increase joint attention, facilitate social interaction, foster communication and symbol use) being addressed. The final component highlights the treatment target (e.g., language or social functioning).

The theoretical basis is followed by a summary of research providing an empirical basis for the treatment. In this section, the authors summarize and interpret studies providing evidence that supports the use of the treatment. Authors have prepared a level of evidence table in which they present the major research designs used to examine the intervention and the outcomes reported for both group and single-subject research. Where possible, effect sizes are reported as originally published or computed for the chapter when means and standard deviations were given.

To support practitioners' use of the described interventions in their specific settings, in the next section of each chapter, authors outline some practical requirements for implementing the treatment. This section of each chapter includes a discussion of time demands, training, or expertise required by clinicians wishing to use the intervention and any materials or equipment needed for treatment implementation.

Practical requirements are followed by a description of the key components of the intervention approach. The goal for this section is to ensure the reader has a strong, preliminary understanding of the procedures. Authors provide information about the nature of the goals addressed by the intervention, how multiple goals are addressed over time (e.g., sequentially, simultaneously, cyclically), a procedural or operational description of activities within which the goals are addressed, and the nature of involvement of participants beyond the clinician and child (e.g., peers, siblings, teachers, primary caregivers). (Several of the authors also reference training

Table 1.4. Description of the topics addressed in each section of the treatment chapters

Section	Content
Introduction	Overview of the intervention is provided, including the specific individuals for whom it is designed and their age (i.e., infants/toddlers, children, adolescents, adults), developmental level, and language level. The service delivery model involved, the intervention's basic focus, and its primary methods are highlighted.
Target populations	Description of those subgroups on the autism spectrum (i.e., autistic disorder, Asperger disorder, pervasive developmental disorder-not otherwise specified, Rett disorder, and childhood disintegrative disorder) for whom the intervention is primarily designed and for whom there is empirical support for its use. Level of verbal skills and cognitive abilities are also discussed. Assessment methods used to establish the appropriateness of the treatment for an individual child, adolescent, or adult with autism spectrum disorder (ASD) are presented.
Theoretical basis	Description of the dominant theoretical explanation or rationale for the treatment approach, underlying assumptions regarding the nature of communication and social interaction impairment being addressed by the treatment, the functional outcomes being addressed, and the area of treatment being targeted.
Empirical basis	Comprehensive summary and interpretation of studies providing evidence that supports the use of the intervention, including descriptions of the experimental design and treatment effects for both group and single-subject research, the nature of outcome data reported (e.g., standardized testing vs. naturalistic probes), intervention fidelity, maintenance and generalization of treatment effects, and social validity
Practical requirements	Description of the time and personnel demands for the primary clinician and related other participants, whether or not a team approach is used, required training of personnel involved, or materials required
Key components	Description of the goals addressed by the intervention, how multiple goals are addressed over time (e.g., sequentially, simultaneously, cyclically), activities within which the goals are addressed, and involvement of participants beyond the clinician and child (e.g., peers, siblings, teachers, primary caregivers)
Assessment for treatment planning and progress monitoring	Description of the major assessments and assessment points used to reach decisions about 1) the appropriateness of the intervention; 2) initial and subsequent treatment targets, etc.; 3) advancement through treatment; and 3) treatment termination
Considerations for children from culturally and linguistically diverse backgrounds	Discussion of the applicability of the intervention to children from linguistically and culturally diverse backgrounds and ways in which the intervention might be modified to be most appropriate
Application to a child	Description of a real or hypothetical case of a child illustrating the implementation and effectiveness of the treatment approach
Application to an adolescent or adult	Description of a real or hypothetical case of an adolescent or an adult, illustrating the implementation and effectiveness of the treatment approach
Future directions	Discussion of additional research needed to advance the refinement or ongoing validation of the intervention across populations of individuals with ASD and related neurodevelopmental disabilities
Suggested readings	Summary of a few readings of greatest use to readers who might want to know more about the specific intervention
Learning activities	Topics for further discussion, ideas for projects, questions to test integration of the reading material, and possible writing assignments to facilitate the readers' learning

manuals, which can support a more thorough understanding of the procedures involved in the intervention they describe.)

Assessment methods used to establish the appropriateness of the treatment plan and progress monitoring for an individual child, adolescent, or adult with ASD are presented in the next section. Recognizing the critical role of data to guide practice, this section of each chapter also describes data collection methods to support decision making. The authors provide descriptions of how data are collected, ways to evaluate progress, strategies for determining when and how adjustments should be made, and when the intervention approach should be terminated. They explain how data collection is used to guide ongoing treatment decision making and to assess immediate and long-term outcomes.

This section is followed by implications for inclusive practice, offering examples where the intervention can be applied in the home, school, work, and/or community setting. Considerations for implementing the intervention for children from culturally and linguistically diverse backgrounds are described in the final section before specific applications are made to children, adolescents, or adults. The authors offer guidance in planning modifications related to the particular cultural and personal factors affecting an individual child, adolescent, or adult while ensuring consistency in the treatment approach.

In the next two sections, the authors provide a description of potential applications of the intervention to a child and to an adolescent or adult. They offer two brief case studies: one of a younger individual with ASD for whom the treatment is considered appropriate and effective and one of an adolescent or adult for whom the treatment is considered appropriate and effective if, in fact, the intervention is appropriate for older individuals.

The final content section of each chapter is a description of directions for future research needed to advance the development or ongoing validation of the intervention approach across populations of individuals with ASD and related neurodevelopmental disabilities. This is followed by three to five suggested readings the authors believe represent important further details or background about the intervention as well as learning activities the authors pose to facilitate further discussion, ideas for projects, questions to test integration of the reading material, and possible writing assignments. In addition to a comprehensive set of references at the end of each chapter, a glossary of key words is provided at the end of the book, with these key words bolded in the text to inform readers that more information about them is available in the glossary. Finally, a summary of the video clip to illustrate the intervention is provided.

NEW COMPONENTS

This book includes two new chapters beyond the intervention chapters to facilitate the reader's use of the book. Chapter 2 highlights the importance of assessment to treatment planning and progress monitoring. The context for assessment is discussed recognizing the importance of a family-centered, culturally informed approach that is both interdisciplinary and comprehensive. The role of screening and diagnostic testing to identify the presence of ASD and comorbid conditions is also described, but more briefly. This chapter includes approaches to identifying severity and creating profiles of social communication and social interaction challenges. Most important, this chapter provides strategies for monitoring change over time.

Chapter 3 highlights the language and communication strengths and challenges most often seen in children with ASD, as these have implications for intervention. Early communication challenges are discussed, including intentional communication, gesture use, word learning, and the use of unconventional verbal behavior. The chapter emphasizes those challenges that specifically impact language development, social communication, and social interaction, such as impairments in joint attention, play, and theory of mind. This chapter is designed to help the reader understand what researchers know about the syntactic, semantic, phonological, and pragmatic development of children with ASD and what the implications are for intervention.

In addition to these changes in the content included in this second edition, a companion resource, *Case Studies for the Treatment of Autism Spectrum Disorder* (Prelock & McCauley, 2021), is offered as an optional supplementary resource. Through 14 individual cases, readers are introduced to hypothetical but instructive scenarios posing the kinds of clinical problems that face clinicians who wish to devise comprehensive services for clients with ASD. Although there is particular focus on social communication and social interaction difficulties, the multitude of co-occurring problems that so often complicate the decision making required for effective management in ASD are incorporated to provide a real-world flavor. Alongside decisions recommended by experts, the casebook includes decision-making exercises that can enrich readers' understanding of social communication and social interaction challenges as well as the possible strategies that can help address them.

REFERENCES

American Psychiatric Association. (2000). *Diagnostic and statistical manual of mental disorders, fourth edition, text revision* (DSM-IV-TR). Author.

American Psychiatric Association. (2013). *Diagnostic and statistical manual of mental disorders, fifth edition* (DSM-5). Author.

Baio, J., Wiggins, L., Christensen, D. L., Maenner, M. J., Daniels, J., Warren, Z., Kurzius-Spencer, M., Zahorodny, W., Rosenberg, C. R., White, T., Durkin, M. S., Imm, P., Nikolaou, L., Yeargin-Allsopp, M., Lee, L.-C., Harrington, R., Lopez, M., Fitzgerald, R. T., Hewitt, . . . K., Dowling, N. F. (2018). Prevalence of autism spectrum disorders among children aged 8 years—Autism and Developmental Disabilities Monitoring Network, 11 sites, United States, 2014. *Morbidity and Mortality Weekly Report, 67*(SS-6), 1–23.

Barlow, D. H., Nock, M. K., & Hersen, M. (2009). *Single case experimental designs: Strategies for studying behavior change* (3rd ed.). Pearson/Allyn & Bacon.

Chambless, D. L., Baker-Ericzen, M. J., Baucom, D., Beutler, L. E., Calhoun, K. S., Crits-Christoph, P., Daiuto, A., DeRubeis, R. L., Detweiler, J., Haaga, D., Bennett Johnson, S., Mccurry, S. M., Mueser, K., Pope, K. S., Sanderson, W. C., Shoham, V., Stickle, T., Williams, D. A., & Woody, S. R. (1998). Update on empirically validated therapies: II. The Clinical Psychologist, 51(1), 3–16.

Chorpita, B. F., Yim, L. M., Donkervoet, J. C., Arensdorf, A., Amundsen, M. J., McGee, C., Serrano, A., Yates, A., Burns, J. A., & Morelli, P. (2002). Toward large-scale implementation of empirically supported treatments for children: A review and observations by the Hawaii empirical basis to services task force. *Clinical Psychology: Science and Practice, 9*(2), 165–190.

Christiansz, J. S., Gray, K. M., Taffe, J., & Tonge, B. J. (2016). Autism spectrum disorder in the DSM-5: Diagnostic sensitivity and specificity in early childhood. *Journal of Autism and Developmental Disorders, 46*(6), 2054–2063.

Cooper, J. O., Heron, T. E., & Heward, W. L. (2007). *Applied behavior analysis* (2nd ed.). Pearson/Merrill-Prentice Hall.

Debodinance, E., Malijaars, J., Noens, I., & Van den Noortgate, W. (2017). Interventions for toddlers with autism spectrum disorder: A meta-analysis of single-subject experimental studies. *Research in Autism Spectrum Disorders, 36*, 79–92.

Downs, A., Downs R. C., Johansen, M., & Fossum, M. (2007). Using discrete trial teaching within a public preschool program to facilitate skill development in students with developmental disabilities. *Education and Treatment of Children, 30*(3), 1–27.

Girolametto, L., Pearce, P., & Weitzman, E. (1996). Interactive focused stimulation for toddlers with expressive vocabulary delays. *Journal of Speech and Hearing Research, 39*, 1274–1283.

Iovannone, R., Dunlap, G., Huber, H., & Kincaid, D. (2003). Effective educational practices for students with autism spectrum disorders. *Focus on Autism and Other Developmental Disabilities, 18*(3), 150–165.

Kaiser, A., Hancock, T., & Nietfeld, J. (2000). The effects of parent-implemented enhanced milieu teaching on the social communication of children who have autism. *Early Education and Development, 11*, 423–446.

Kaiser, A. P., & Hester, P. P. (1994). Generalized effects of enhanced milieu teaching. *Journal of Speech and Hearing Research, 37*, 1320–1340.

Karsten, A. M., & Carr, J. E. (2009). The effects of differential reinforcement of unprompted responding on the skill acquisition of children with autism. *Journal of Applied Behavior Analysis, 42*, 327–334.

Koegel, L. K., Koegel, R., Harrower, J. K., & Carter, C. M. (1999). Pivotal response intervention I: Overview of approach. *Journal of the Association for Persons with Severe Handicaps, 24*, 174–185.

Koegel, L. K., Koegel, R. L., Shoshan, Y., & McNerney, E. (1999). Pivotal response intervention II: Preliminary long-term outcomes data. *Journal of The Association for Persons with Severe Handicaps, 24*, 186–198.

Lafasakis, M., & Sturmey, P. (2007). Training parent implementation of discrete-trial teaching: Effects on generalization of parent teaching and child correct responding. *Journal of Applied Behavior Analysis, 40*, 685–689.

Lord, C., Wagner, A., Rogers, S., Szatmari, P., Aman, M., Charman, T., Dawson, G., Durand, M., Grossman, L., & Guthrie, D. (2005). Challenges in evaluating psychosocial interventions for autistic spectrum disorders. *Journal of Autism and Developmental Disorders, 35*, 695–708.

McCauley, R. J., & Fey, M. E. (2006). *Treatment of language disorders in children*. Paul H. Brookes Publishing Co.

National Autism Center. (2009). *National Standards Project, Phase 1: Addressing the need for evidence-based practice guidelines for ASD*. Author.

National Autism Center. (2015). *National Standards Project, Phase 2: Addressing the need for evidence-based practice guidelines for ASD*. https://www.nationalautismcenter.org

National Research Council. (2001). *Educating children with autism*. National Academy Press.

Newman, B., Reinecke, D., & Ramos, M. (2009). Is a reasonable attempt reasonable? Shaping versus reinforcing verbal attempts of preschoolers with autism. *Analysis of Verbal Behavior 25*, 67–72.

Odom, S. L., Brown, W. H., Frey, T., Karasu, N., Smith-Canter, L. L., & Strain, P. (2003). Evidence-based practices for young children with autism: Contributions for single-subject design research. *Focus on Autism & Other Developmental Disabilities, 18*(3), 166–175.

Perdices, M., & Tate, R. L. (2009). Single-subject designs as a tool for evidence-based clinical practice: Are they unrecognised and undervalued? *Neuropsychological Rehabilitation, 19*(6), 904–927.

Prelock, P. A., & McCauley, R. J. (2021). *Case studies for the treatment of autism spectrum disorder*. Paul H. Brookes Publishing Co.

Prelock, P. A., & Nelson, N. (2012). Language and communication in autism: An integrated view. *The Pediatric Clinics of North America, 59*(1), 129–145.

Prizant, B. M., & Wetherby, A. M. (1998). Understanding the continuum of discrete-trial traditional behavioral to social-pragmatic developmental approaches in communication enhancement for young children with autism/PDD. *Seminar in Speech and Language, 19*, 329–352.

Smith, I. C., Reichow, B., & Volkmar, F. (2015). The effects of DSM-5 criteria on number of individuals diagnosed with ASD: A systematic review. *Journal of Autism and Developmental Disorders, 45*, 2541–2552.

Taubman, M., Brierley, S., Wishner, J., Baker, D., McEachin, J., & Leaf, R. B. (2001). The effectiveness of a group discrete trial instructional approach for preschoolers with developmental disabilities. *Research in Developmental Disabilities, 22*, 205–219.

Wetherby, A., & Woods, J. (2006). Effectiveness of early intervention for children with autism spectrum disorders beginning in the second year of life. *Topics in Early Childhood Special Education, 26*, 67–82.

Wetherby, A., & Woods, J. (2008). Developmental approaches to treatment of infants and toddlers with autism spectrum disorders. In F. Volkmar, A. Klin, & K. Chawarska (Eds.), *Autism spectrum disorders in infancy and early childhood* (pp. 170–206). Guilford Press.

Young, R. L., & Rodi, M.L. (2014). Redefining ASD using DSM-5: The implications of the proposed DSM-5 criteria for ASD. *Journal of Autism and Developmental Disorders, 44*, 758–765.

Zander, E., & Bolte, S. (2015). The new DSM-5 impairment criterion: A challenge to early autism spectrum disorder diagnosis. *Journal of Autism and Developmental Disorders, 45* (11), 3634–3643.

2

Assessment for Treatment Planning and Progress Monitoring

Rebecca J. McCauley, Allison Bean, and Patricia A. Prelock

INTRODUCTION

Assessments that aid in treatment planning and progress monitoring are crucial to the effective management of challenges associated with autism spectrum disorder (ASD). Carefully designed assessments help clinicians describe specific communication and interaction difficulties and identify individual strengths as well as personal interests and relevant environmental factors. This information can then be used to guide intervention decisions about skills and environmental factors that should be considered to achieve desired outcomes. Ongoing assessments to monitor progress help the clinician track progress toward specific goals as well as overall progress to determine whether the current treatment plan is effective, needs to be modified, or even needs to be replaced.

The appropriateness of particular assessment methods depends on the purpose for which the testing will be used (e.g., diagnosis, treatment planning, progress monitoring) and on the characteristics of the person being tested (e.g., development level, areas of impairment). For treatment planning, relevant questions include the following:

- What areas of communication and social interaction are difficult for this person?

- What kinds of assistance might be helpful in a given area?

- What personal strengths and interests should be considered when planning treatment?

For progress monitoring, relevant questions include the following:

- Is progress being made on a specific goal?

- Have improvements been seen in broader areas of difficulty?

- Is an observed change likely to be due to treatment?

In this chapter, we outline those factors affecting the assessment needs of individuals with ASD, describe the use of assessments for basic treatment planning and monitoring, identify the characteristics of desirable assessments, and introduce a selection of measures that authors of the intervention chapters in this book recognize as important for their interventions. Finally, we consider each testing purpose and introduce a selection of measures to consider for these purposes—some already introduced in relation to specific chapters and others based on other sources in the research and clinical literature.

FACTORS AFFECTING ASSESSMENT NEEDS

Personal characteristics that need to be considered when choosing assessments are 1) overall problem severity, 2) communication domains affected, and 3) the affected individual's age and developmental stage.

Differences in Overall Problem Severity

Communication and social interaction problems can range from mild to profound in their impact on people with autism. Some individuals with ASD experience very severe communication problems; current estimates suggest that about 30% of individuals with ASD will be minimally verbal or nonverbal at school age (Tager-Flusberg & Kasari, 2013). Consequently, the assessment needs of more severely affected individuals will typically center on the identification of social interaction patterns, gestural use, and other precursors or early correlates of linguistic communication with interventions designed to increase requests and responses to and initiations of joint attention (Crais et al., 2009). In contrast, some people with autism experience milder communication challenges that may be interpreted by others as social aloofness or awkwardness. These challenges may be barely noticed by unfamiliar conversational partners despite being keenly felt by the individuals themselves (Maddox & White, 2015). The assessment needs for more verbal children will likely involve their understanding of the social code for interaction and more advanced aspects of theory of mind with interventions designed to support their social engagement and interactions with peers. Ultimately, assessments should be uniquely designed to tap the variability of communication strengths and challenges associated with autism. The severity of communication needs is likely to be influenced by the presence and degree of cognitive impairment (Matson & Shoemaker, 2009). Clinicians must prioritize the social communication and social interaction domains requiring attention as well as pinpoint assessment strategies that might prove productive in obtaining the needed information.

Differences in Affected Communication Domains

Four language domains—phonology, semantics (especially lexical), grammar, and pragmatics—are viewed as particularly important targets for assessment in younger children from about 1 to 4 years of age (Tager-Flusberg et al., 2009). At older ages, these same domains may require initial or ongoing assessment, depending on the individual's persisting or emerging problems and developing skills. In particular, for adolescents and adults with ASD but without cognitive impairment, phonology (especially **suprasegmental aspects of speech production**) as well as some semantic and pragmatic skills are likely to be more problematic than vocabulary and grammar (Magiati, 2016). In fact, the latter domains are likely to be on par with those of nonaffected peers. Nonetheless, some older individuals with both ASD and cognitive impairment may require broader language and communication assessments because of more persistent widespread difficulties.

As part of the assessment of communication for individuals with autism, **challenging behaviors** are often a focus, as they provide one mechanism for a person with ASD to communicate an immediate need, desire, frustration, and so on. They often serve communicative purposes (e.g., protesting, seeking attention), although they do so in unconventional, ineffective, and frequently antisocial ways (e.g., aggression toward self or others; Kanne & Mazurek, 2011). Challenging behaviors can include difficult or socially unacceptable behaviors on the less severe end and self-injury, destructive behavior, and aggression on the more severe end of the continuum. Challenging behaviors may require assessment among about 10% of people with autism, with higher frequency in those with intellectual disability and more severe autism (Murphy et al., 2009). In fact, evidence suggests that in individuals with intellectual disability who also have autism, challenging behaviors may affect as many as 36% of individuals (Holden & Gitlesen, 2006).

When challenging behaviors include aggression, caregivers and teachers experience high levels of stress (Lecavalier et al., 2006), which increases the risk of physical abuse (Kanne & Mazurek, 2011). Although many speech-language pathologists (SLPs) may not be well trained to deal with such behaviors, those who wish to work effectively with individuals with ASD need to develop both assessment and intervention skills in this area (Matson & Nebel-Schwalm, 2007). However, owing to the complicated nature of these behaviors and the complexity of some of the available assessment methods (Lloyd & Kennedy, 2014), the management and assessment of these behaviors should be conducted by an interdisciplinary team that includes SLPs and other professionals, such as psychologists and behavior analysts.

Differences in Age and Developmental Stage

Given the lifelong nature of ASD, varied assessments are needed for individuals across age and developmental stage. As individuals with autism develop and change across the lifespan, the demands and opportunities presented by their social environments also change. Therefore, both individual and contextual factors influence the selection of assessment strategies across the lifespan.

At younger ages, clinicians should focus on assessing prelinguistic nonverbal communication and social interaction skills as well as emerging verbal productions. In particular, observations have been made that "useful speech by age 5 consistently predicts better social and adaptive functioning later in life" (Tager-Flusberg & Kasari, 2013, p. 2). Failing to meet that benchmark decreases the likelihood the child will acquire significant linguistic skills thereafter (Tager-Flusberg et al., 2005). Therefore, intervention efforts designed to promote spoken language have focused not only on children with emerging verbal communication but also on the 25%–30% of children who might be described as nonverbal or minimally verbal when entering kindergarten. Children with ASD and minimal verbal communication have been found to vary significantly in both their cognitive and receptive language skills, suggesting the need for a variety of assessment and intervention strategies, including those focused on both spoken and alternative means of communication (e.g., voice output communication aids, sign language).

For school-age children with ASD who are developing communication and language skills more successfully, written as well as oral communication become potentially important assessment domains. Further, the increasing likelihood that the child is spending much of each day in a school setting introduces a significant change in social contexts, which may reveal new or intensified challenges. Assessments for individuals in this context are steadily being researched, although many of the tools that are currently used still have relatively modest evidence about their validity when used for children with ASD (Tager-Flusberg et al., 2009) despite the evidence for their use with other children at risk for language impairment.

Later in development, assessments for adolescents with autism transitioning from educational to adult services and/or from family to independent living have been described as "sorely lacking" (Williams & Matson, 2016, p. 455). Even access to appropriate diagnostic services for older adults with autism or suspected autism is limited by systems failures, inadequate numbers of trained professionals, and a dearth of appropriate measures (Murphy et al., 2016; Trammel et al., 2013). Further, the lack of appropriate assessments for adolescents and adults has recently been identified as an urgent target for research (National Autism Center, 2015; Saulnier & Ventola, 2012; Wehman et al., 2009; Williams & Matson, 2016). Despite increased interest in research with a focus on adults with autism (Cottle et al., 2016), assessments for adolescents and adults represent an area of great need in treatment planning and progress monitoring. This remains especially true for individuals who do not receive a diagnosis of ASD until adulthood either because they present with more subtle problems (Heijnen-Kohl et al., 2016) or because they have been wrongly or inadequately diagnosed (Magiati, 2016). For example, an adult may have been diagnosed with anxiety disorder when an additional diagnosis of ASD was also warranted, or a diagnosis of language impairment may have been given when a diagnosis of ASD would have been more accurate. These missed or inaccurate diagnoses have consequences, particularly in the range of services available to the affected individuals.

In sum, because of the diversity of problem severity, affected communication domains, age, and developmental stages of individuals with autism, finding useful assessment tools for SLPs and other professionals is a challenging endeavor. The complexity of assessment in ASD also presents challenges in assessment tool selection and administration, warranting several recent books on the subject (e.g., Kroncke et al., 2016; Matson, 2016). Given space limitations and this book's emphasis on intervention, in this chapter, we focus our discussion on assessments for treatment planning and progress monitoring for children and youth up to age 21.

CONSIDERATIONS FOR TREATMENT PLANNING AND PROGRESS MONITORING

Although standardized measures, observational methods, and clinical expertise are linchpins to the *diagnosis* of communication and other problems, different but equally varied measures often come into play during treatment planning and progress monitoring. This is the case for at least two reasons. First, although some

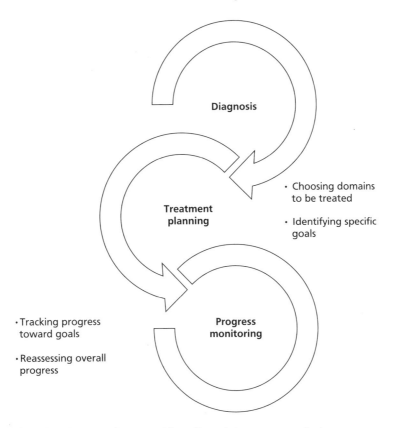

Figure 2.1. Purposes of assessment from diagnosis to progress monitoring.

diagnostic tests have been developed to include components that may help in treatment planning and progress monitoring, measures for treatment planning and monitoring usually focus on a broader range of specific behaviors rather than on the smaller group of discriminative behaviors that can prove useful in screening or diagnosis. Second, when progress monitoring is the purpose, appropriate measures need to be sensitive to change (McCauley, 2001; Tager-Flusberg et al., 2009). Although test developers are able to develop tools that can be used both for initial diagnoses and treatment planning and progress monitoring, the additional complexity and subsequent cost of doing so are usually prohibitive. Figure 2.1 illustrates the changing sequence of assessment purposes from diagnosis to progress monitoring, which may be repeated frequently across the lifespan of a person with ASD.

RECOMMENDED CHARACTERISTICS OF ASSESSMENT FOR TREATMENT PLANNING AND PROGRESS MONITORING

Many readers will recall (and others benefit from being reminded) that two critical characteristics of any measure are reliability and validity for a given purpose and person (McCauley, 2001, Messick, 1989). Reliability is the relative constancy of a measurement result for tested individuals across conditions that should *not* have any significant effect on the outcome being measured (conditions such as who is administering the measure, when it is being measured, etc.). Validity is the ability of the measure to actually measure what it purports to measure. Although validity is specific to a given testing purpose, it also depends on reliability; however, reliability, does not assure validity. For example, a measure of expressive vocabulary may be highly reliable upon retest or when made by various examiners but have very low validity as a predictor of broader communication skills in any population.

Because reliability and validity are specific to the purpose of testing and the person being tested, a measure cannot be declared unequivocally valid or reliable. For example, a test that is valid for diagnosing ASD may not be as valid for planning treatment or monitoring symptom severity. In fact, the two purposes of greatest importance in the context of this book—helping identify reasonable targets for intervention and assessing progress towards a treatment goal or overall changes in problem severity—often require important differences in item selection and test development from those required by diagnostic or screening measures (McCauley, 1996, 2001).

Along with using individual instruments with high reliability and validity for their intended purpose and target test taker, clinicians should strive to include four additional characteristics in the overall assessment *process* used in treatment planning and progress monitoring for individuals with ASD. Specifically, the entire process of assessment should be interdisciplinary, comprehensive, culturally informed, and family centered. Although all of these characteristics are vital to gaining more accurate and reliable information on which to base decision making, each characteristic places additional learning and implementation demands on the professionals involved. In this section, we describe why each of these four characteristics is desirable and what each entails.

Interdisciplinary Assessment

Whereas an interdisciplinary assessment is needed initially to help differentially diagnose ASD (Gerdts et al., 2018), it is equally valuable as a basis for planning and monitoring individualized treatment for several reasons. First, interdisciplinary assessments tend to lead to well-coordinated and efficient service delivery through interdisciplinary planning and practice (Odom et al., 2010; Odom et al., 2014). Second, interdisciplinary assessments have the potential to identify coexisting difficulties or disorders, relative strengths, interests, and contextual effects that can provide important background information for treatment planning. Table 2.1 lists several important areas in which co-occurring disorders have been identified through an interdisciplinary approach to assessment. Although most of the references and risk levels recorded in Table 2.1 come from studies of children with autism, research also suggests that many of these risks are at least as high or perhaps higher in adults with autism (Gardner et al., 2016).

A third reason to incorporate interdisciplinary team management as part of treatment planning stems from the particular demands and available supports associated with different intervention contexts. For example, public school settings require that in addition to working closely with parents, SLPs should work in alliance with school psychologists, special and regular educators, occupational therapists (OTs), and other school professionals. Not only will an interdisciplinary team be useful in establishing the diagnosis and the evidence of negative educational impact required for the child or youth to receive services, the effectiveness of educational as well as communication interventions will benefit from interdisciplinary input (Individuals with Disabilities Education Act, 2004; McClain et al., 2018; Odom

Table 2.1.   Risk for co-occurring disorders in autism spectrum disorder

Problem area	Risk[a]	Selected references
Medical		
Epilepsy	20%	Amiet et al. (2008); Besag (2018)
Gastrointestinal problems	Threefold risk of children with typical development	McElhanon et al. (2014)
Sleep problems	44%–83%	Gail-Williams et al. (2004); Liu et al. (2006); Williams et al. (2004)
Ear infections	General finding of increased risk	Adams et al. (2016); Niehus & Lord (2006)
Cognitive		
Cognitive impairment	49%–70%	Carlsson et al. (2013)
Attention-deficit/ hyperactivity disorder	30%–50%	Leitner (2014); Zachor & Ben-Itzchak (2019)
Sensory integration	90%	Suarez (2012)
Psychological or psychiatric		
Psychiatric diagnoses	70%	Trammel et al. (2013)

[a] Percentage of occurrence or level of increased risk compared to individuals without autism spectrum disorder.

et al., 2014; Prelock et al., 2003). Despite significant increases in the number of children with ASD who are being served in schools (Wilkinson, 2016), school psychologists and teachers in whose class children with autism may be included have relatively little training or expertise in working with this population (McClain et al., 2018). Therefore, they will benefit greatly from the participation of a knowledgeable SLP. In addition, ready access to consultations and even co-treatment with an OT may provide important strategies for addressing sensory needs that can otherwise interfere with productive treatment in other areas of need (Ashburner et al., 2008).

In summary, children and adults with ASD may demonstrate differing talents and needs as well as differing demands associated with particular social, educational, or work contexts. Input from relevant experts as part of an interdisciplinary team can tailor treatment to each individual's pattern of strengths and weaknesses. When SLPs become aware of some of the noncommunication challenges and assets a person with ASD may have, they can plan interventions that will address communication and social interactions within the context of the person's health, abilities, and needs. Finally, coordination of the various kinds of interventions that a person with ASD may be receiving can be more effective and efficient given successful interdisciplinary collaboration (Odom et al., 2010). Although such collaborations may differ greatly across settings, there is increasing knowledge about underlying principles of team structure and team process that lead to good outcomes (Nancarrow et al., 2013).

Comprehensive Assessment

A comprehensive assessment is one that uses a variety of methods to obtain information, takes into consideration the full range of affected language and communication domains, and includes attention to the various functional impacts associated with ASD. The characteristics of a comprehensive assessment are addressed briefly in the next three sections.

Use a Variety of Methods to Describe Strengths and Challenges   For diagnostic assessments involving children, best practices indicate that a comprehensive evaluation should include the following components: "1) parent or caregiver interview, 2) review of relevant medical, psychological and/or school records, 3) cognitive/developmental assessment, 4) direct play observation, 5) measurement of adaptive functioning, and 6) comprehensive medical examination" (National Autism Center, 2015, p. 12). Whereas adolescents and young adults with autism may require attention to different content, their assessment is nonetheless likely to benefit from naturalistic observations of the communication difficulties the person experiences and from input provided by familiar communication partners (Paul et al., 2014; Wetherby & Prizant, 2006). Using multiple assessments can help prevent poor decision making caused by insufficient data from too few social contexts and can contribute to an understanding of how reactive or responsive the individual is to differences across settings (e.g., Floyd et al., 2015).

Consider the Range of Communication and Language Domains Likely to Be Affected   Approximately 76% of children with ASD also are diagnosed with a language disorder, with a much smaller number identified with speech problems (Kjelgaard & Tager-Flusberg, 2001). Speech and language problems are more common among individuals with autism and cognitive impairment, which occurs in 40%–70% of children with ASD (Autism and Developmental Disabilities Monitoring Network, 2012; Frombonne, 2003) and may require special considerations in assessment (e.g., Matson & Shoemaker, 2009; Matson et al., 2008). Most important, by definition, children, youth, and adults with ASD experience difficulties with pragmatics and social interaction. Thus, although all areas of language remain of interest across the lifespan, pragmatics and social interaction probably warrant the greatest attention. Frequently, assessment in this area includes assessment of theory of mind (Beaudoin et al., 2020; Sprung, 2010), a construct that can include understanding of mental states and social situations, including "emotions, desires, intentions, percepts, knowledge, beliefs and mentalistic understanding of non-literal communication" (Beaudoin et al., 2020, p. 1).

Speech sound disorders identified in children with ASD and without significant cognitive impairments often have only small effects on intelligibility and can be described as involving articulation, that is, errors on a relatively small number of sounds that tend to occur later in typical development, as well as differences in prosody, including speech that is overly loud, higher pitched than expected, or marked by misplaced stress (e.g., Broome et al., 2017; Shriberg et al., 2011). Although phonological disorders and motor speech disorders have also been described as prevalent in children with autism, research support for these ideas is limited (e.g., Shriberg et al., 2011). Recommendations for phonological assessment methods have recently been proposed subsequent to a systematic review of research practices (Broome et al., 2017). Broome and colleagues' recommendations include standard collection of an oral-motor assessment and a connected speech sample of 50 or more speech-like utterances; a single word naming task of greater than 100 words; a probe for stimulability; and, depending on the child's level of skill, a task requiring multisyllabic words.

Broome and colleagues (2017) provide additional recommendations regarding minimal as well as possible additional analyses that are considered desirable for use by both researchers and practicing clinicians. For children who are considered prelinguistic, the minimum data analysis the authors recommend is the description of the child's phonetic repertoire, syllable shapes, and stress patterns. In contrast, for children who are verbal, intelligibility is also considered part of a core set of analyses, which also includes sentence imitation and, if possible, the comparison of imitated versus spontaneous productions.

Obtain Information About the Functional Impacts of ASD   The *International Classification of Functioning, Disability and Health* (ICF; World Health Organization [WHO], 2001) provides another perspective on what it means to describe an assessment plan as comprehensive. Representing a biopsychosocial model of functioning (Bölte et al., 2014), the classification system embodied in these two versions has been designed to examine functional impacts on both activities (e.g., talking, learning) and on participation in social roles (e.g., friendships, family life). Although use of the ICF approach is somewhat more common in research with children than with adults, no well-developed method for implementing it clinically exists for either group despite ongoing efforts (e.g., Gan et al., 2013). Nonetheless, the ICF is in accord with the universally acknowledged need to include a focus on functional outcomes for individuals with autism (Schiariti et al., 2018). Measures that examine quality of life in individuals with ASD and their families or that examine their ability to participate in particular settings can be used to identify valued outcomes and to track performance.

Undertake Culturally Informed Assessment

As it is in all areas of clinical practice, sensitivity to the cultural background of individuals with ASD is necessary for ethical, effective practice. This need is underscored for people with ASD because research has suggested that ASD, especially when accompanied by cognitive impairment, is often misdiagnosed or undiagnosed in some racial/ethnic groups (e.g., Mandell et al., 2009; Sullivan, 2013). Using a dataset that included 65.9 million children based on the 2008 child count data required by the Individuals with Disabilities Education Act (IDEA; §618, Part B) and 2008 school census data by state, Sullivan (2013) found that Hispanic and American Indian/Alaskan Native students were identified less often than majority white students, whereas Asian/Pacific Islander students were more likely to be identified than white students. Further, whereas earlier age of diagnosis is facilitated by higher socioeconomic status in the United States, that relationship is not seen in Sweden, possibly owing to universal access to health care in the latter country (Klaiman et al., 2015).

Despite such indications that an individual's social background may affect outcomes, this topic has been the focus of remarkably little research. For example, in a systematic review identifying 30 articles addressing ASD assessment and evaluation research in 10 school psychology journals from 2007 to 2017, McClain and colleagues (2018) identified a single article by Sullivan (2013) that focused on issues of cultural and linguistic diversity. At present, this lack of evidence makes it impossible to determine the degree to which observed differences in identification rates for different groups stem from test bias, practitioner bias, differential access to or usage of assessment services, or socioeconomic stressors often associated with minority status (Begeer et al., 2009).

In 2014, Harris and colleagues evaluated five ASD diagnostic and six screening tools for cultural and linguistic responsiveness using a 16-item checklist (with higher scores indicating greater cultural responsiveness). The researchers found the scores on the checklist ranged from only 2 to 9, respectively, for the Autism Diagnostic Observation Schedule–Second Edition (ADOS-2; Lord et al., 2012) and the Ages and Stages Questionnaire: Social-Emotional™ (ASQ:SE™; Squires et al., 2003), with both diagnostic and screening measures averaging scores of 5 out of the possible total of 16. Harris and colleagues (2014) pointed to the pressing need for improved tools and assessment practices for children from culturally and linguistic diverse populations. The extent to which concerns regarding bias extend beyond screening and diagnostic methods to methods used for treatment planning and progress monitoring is uncertain, but these findings nonetheless suggest the need for clinical vigilance.

The possibilities of bias and reduced access to effective assessments for individuals with ASD who are also from underrepresented groups means that increased cultural competence needs to be a paramount concern of all SLPs working with ASD. **Cultural competence** can be viewed as including "an awareness of one's own cultural biases and beliefs and how they may come into conflict with those from other backgrounds" (ASHA, n.d.). In addition, cultural competence involves seeking greater knowledge and deeper understandings of the traditions, values, beliefs, and social contexts that inform client experiences and therefore should inform clinical practices. Although a clinician's cultural competence cannot completely undo the possible effects of tools poorly developed for this population, it can cause the clinician to make use of rich and diverse sources of information to aid in their decision making about interventions and meaningful ways to evaluate progress.

Family-Centered Assessment

The terms *person-centered* and *family-centered* require yet another level of appreciation for the uniqueness of each person and family within any culture. In the case of children, family is defined as biologic, foster or adoptive, nuclear, and extended family members; for adults, it may be defined as sexual partners, friends, or neighbors. As clinicians face family compositions, values, and practices that differ from their own, they need to attend to not only the person with ASD but also the family of the individual, who are experts on that person. Both person- and **family-centered** assessment incorporates a strength-based approach that places individuals with disorders and their families as key partners and decision makers with professionals in service delivery rather than as passive recipients (Beatson, 2006; Prelock et al., 2003).

The importance of family involvement extends beyond their role in decision making for the child with autism. Difficulties that parents and family members of children with autism experience include reduced parental self-efficacy, increased parenting stress, decreased mental and physical health, higher divorce rates, and suspected strains on sibling relationships (Karst & Van Hecke, 2012). Resources may also be stressed both financially and in the family time available for rest and relaxation given the demands of the child's care (Karst & Van Hecke, 2012). Not surprisingly, evidence suggests that the impact of this stress on the family may create a vicious cycle of negative outcomes for the child with autism.

In recent formulations of person- and family-centered care (e.g., Baas, 2012; Committee on Hospital Care and Institute for Patient- and Family-Centered Care, 2012), the concept of family has been revised from conventional notions of family to focus on family as the people whom the individual with ASD perceives as his or her source of greatest support.

Family participation in assessment typically has been described as the involvement of parents of children with autism who complete checklists and observational tools and frequently observe structured testing (Prelock et al., 2003). However, families can also play a considerable role in diagnosis and treatment planning for adults with autism (Heijnen-Kohl et al., 2016). For all ages, families may help define the scope of assessment, contribute data, aid in the interpretation of data, and actively participate in decisions regarding future programming and intervention planning (Prelock, 2019). Such participation paves the way for the development of strong relationships that lead to effective intervention and ongoing progress monitoring.

To help set the stage for effective alliances with families, clinicians may want to systematically assess 1) the family's composition and 2) its connections to the community. The goal of these assessments is to help the clinician (and sometimes the client or the client's family) develop a richer understanding of the client's most important relationships and the family's access to broader community resources (Friedman & Neuman Allen, 2011; Goldrick & Gerson, 1985; Rempel et al., 2007). Two descriptive tools that have been drawn from social work and used for these purposes in interdisciplinary interventions involving ASD are genograms and ecomaps (e.g., Goodluck, 1990; Prelock & Beatson, 2019; Prelock et al., 2003; Prelock et al., 1999; Tobias, 2018). Similar to a family tree, the **genogram** visualizes family history (e.g., identifying people living in the home, the presence of specific illnesses) currently and over time, usually up to three generations. The **ecomap** describes the family's larger social context, including organizations that may affect the client directly or indirectly and thus may support or complicate the family's and client's best functioning. Applications of these methods can be found in the casebook associated with this volume (Prelock & McCauley, 2021).

ASSESSMENT TOOLS FOR TREATMENT PLANNING AND PROGRESS MONITORING—OUR AUTHORS' CONTRIBUTIONS

The intervention chapters in this book not only include detailed descriptions of individual interventions or sets of related interventions but also allude to specific assessment tools that have often been integral to clinical decision making regarding treatment planning and progress monitoring described for that intervention. In this section of the chapter, we briefly highlight assessment tools and strategies identified by these skilled clinicians and clinical researchers. Table 2.2 assembles strategies highlighted in each chapter. Usually, these strategies are found under the heading "Assessment for Treatment Planning and Progress Monitoring," but occasionally, under the heading "Target Populations," "Application to a Child," or "Application to an Adolescent or Adult," they are discussed in more detail and individual examples are given.

Assessments in Table 2.2 include the many variations of probe data that may be used to baseline specific target behaviors, then track a client's progress, using more informal methods or methods from single case experimental designs that could in some cases better establish the role of the intervention in contributing to observed

Table 2.2.   Assessments identified in intervention chapters

Chapter number	Chapter title	Purpose	Assessment measures
4	Augmentative and Alternative Communication Strategies	Both treatment planning and progress monitoring	• **The SCERTS® Model** (Prizant et al., 2006a, 2006b): Questionnaires, interviews, and observational data that are designed for use across the lifespan • **Social Networks Inventory** (Blackstone & Hunt Berg, 2003): Interviews that are designed for use across the lifespan • **Augmentative & Alternative Communication Profile: A Continuum of Learning Tool** (Kovach, 2009): Observational data and rating scales that are designed for use across the lifespan • **Interviews, surveys, and observations** of the individual and their communicative partners in daily activities
		Treatment planning only	• **Participation model** (Beukelman & Mirenda, 2013): Observational data, interviews, inventories, and specific capabilities assessments
		Progress monitoring only	—
5	The Early Start Denver Model (ESDM)	Both treatment planning and progress monitoring	—
		Treatment planning only	• **ESDM Curriculum Model Checklist for Young Children with Autism** (Rogers & Dawson, 2009): Curriculum-based assessment related to developmental sequences of skills within targeted domains
		Progress monitoring only	• **Observations** at set time intervals (e.g., every 15 min) that are recorded on a daily data sheet
6	Discrete Trial Instruction	Both treatment planning and progress monitoring	—
		Treatment planning only	• **Verbal Behavior Milestones and Placement Program** (VB-MAPP; Sundberg, 2008): Assessment and curriculum guide for language skills that is designed for developmental levels up to 48 months • **Promoting the Emergence of Advanced Knowledge Relational Training System** (PEAK; Dixon et al., 2015): Two versions, one for children with skills demonstrated by children up to 8 years; the other for children with skills demonstrated by children 11 years or younger

Table 2.2.   *(continued)*

Chapter number	Chapter title	Purpose	Assessment measures
		Progress monitoring only	• **Trial-by-trial recording of correct, incorrect or prompted responses** (Nopprapun & Holloway, 2014) • **Percentage of correct responses** (Carroll et al., 2016): Responses compared against mastery criteria, which usually are set at 80% or higher for correct responses across two consecutive sessions • **Visual analysis of treatment data** • **Ongoing collection of generalization data**
7	The Developmental, Individual-Difference, Relationship-Based (DIR) Model	Both treatment planning and progress monitoring	• **Functional Emotional Assessment Scales** (Greenspan et al., 2001): Described as the primary assessment tool for this intervention • **Social-Emotional Growth Charts** (Greenspan, 2004) • **Individual Processing Profile:** A component of the *Diagnostic Manual for Infants and Children* (Interdisciplinary Council on Developmental Learning Disorders, 2005)
		Treatment planning only	• **The SCERTS Model curriculum assessment plan** (Prizant et al., 2006a and b)
		Progress monitoring only	• **Ongoing data collection methods,** described in some detail in Table 7.5
8	Functional Communication Training	Both treatment planning and progress monitoring	• **Functional behavioral assessment,** including informal observations, antecedent-behavior-consequence (ABC) charts, a variety of rating scales such as **Motivation Assessment Scale** (Durand & Crimmins, 1992) and others (see Chapter 8 for more details) • **Functional analyses** (Hanley et al., 2003)
		Treatment planning only	• **Scales of Independent Behavior–Revised** (Bruininks et al., 1996)
		Progress monitoring only	• **Data on challenging behavior, communication, and educational progress,** including sample data forms (Durand & Hieneman, 2008)
9	The JASPER Model for Children With Autism	Both treatment planning and progress monitoring	• **Early Social Communication Skills** (Mundy et al., 2003) • **Structured Play Assessment** (SPA; Lifter et al., 1993; Ungerer & Sigman, 1981)
		Treatment planning only	—
		Progress monitoring only	• **Short Play and Communication Evaluation** (SPACE; Shire et al., 2018)

(continued)

Table 2.2.   *(continued)*

Chapter number	Chapter title	Purpose	Assessment measures
10	Enhanced Milieu Teaching	Both treatment planning and progress monitoring	• **Direct observation** and analysis of communication and language (language sampling) in natural environments and observations of specific targets within a specific time interval (e.g., variety of communication functions used, level of prompting needed) • Use of a **global language measure** (e.g., Preschool Language Scale–Fifth Edition, Zimmerman et al., 2011) as well as more targeted standardized measures of communication and observational assessments (e.g., Peabody Picture Vocabulary Test–Fourth Edition, Dunn & Dunn, 1959–2019) • Caregiver questionnaires (e.g., McArthur-Bates Communication Development Inventory–Second Edition; Fenson et al., 2007) and interviews (e.g., a Routines-Based Interview; McWilliam et al., 2009)
		Treatment planning only	—
		Progress monitoring only	—
11	Early Social Interaction	Both treatment planning and progress monitoring	• **The SCERTS Model** (Prizant et al., 2006a): Questionnaires, interviews, and observational data that are designed for use across the lifespan
		Treatment planning only	• **Developmental model for goal setting** and intervention planning
		Progress monitoring only	—
12	Peer-Mediated Support Interventions	Both treatment planning and progress monitoring	• **Direct observations in educational settings** (e.g., specific classrooms, extracurricular activities, cafeteria, hallways, playground) and **instructional contexts** (e.g., large-group lecture or discussion, small-group activities, independent seat work); often, for research purposes, used in conjunction with single case experimental designs
		Treatment planning only	—
		Progress monitoring only	—
13	Pivotal Response Treatment	Both treatment planning and progress monitoring	• **Direct observation of language (language sampling) and other behaviors across multiple environments** • **Vineland Adaptive Behavior Scales** (Sparrow et al., 2005) • **Probe data for ongoing monitoring of progress and intervention effectiveness**

Table 2.2.   *(continued)*

Chapter number	Chapter title	Purpose	Assessment measures
		Treatment planning only	—
		Progress monitoring only	—
14	The SCERTS Model	Both treatment planning and progress monitoring	• **The SCERTS Model curriculum assessment plan** (Prizant et al., 2006a and b)
		Treatment planning only	—
		Progress monitoring only	• **Individual forms for data collection** regarding social communication targets, emotional regulation targets, and transactional supports included
15	Social Skills Interventions	Both treatment planning and progress monitoring	• **Social Skills Improvement System Rating Scales** (Gresham & Elliott, 2008) • **Theory of Mind Inventory-A-SR:** An adult self-report measure (Hutchins et al., 2020) • **Theory of Mind Inventory–2:** Parent informant measure (Hutchins & Prelock, 2016)
		Treatment planning only	—
		Progress monitoring only	• **Theory of Mind Task Battery:** Child performance measure (Hutchins & Prelock, 2016)
16	Social Stories	Both treatment planning and progress monitoring	• A wide range of **probe types** have been used in research on Social Stories, including behavior frequency per activity or per time period, percentage time engaged in an activity, interviews, etc. (see Chapter 16, especially Table 16.1). Often used within an AB or more extensive single case experimental design
		Treatment planning only	—
		Progress monitoring only	—
17	Video Modeling for Persons With ASD	Both treatment planning and progress monitoring	• **Observational data** collected within a single case experimental design or curriculum assessment context
		Treatment planning only	• **Observations** designed to assess individual's interest in and attention toward video content
		Progress monitoring only	—

change (Byiers et al., 2012). Also included are a variety of curriculum-based assessments, especially for interventions that target a greater number of domains as well as structured interviews, surveys, and checklists. When indicated by chapter authors, the age range of the specific tools is also shared in the table.

Because authors have been asked in their respective chapters to communicate both the research base for the intervention they describe and its clinical applications, some of the assessments that are specified may require expertise, training, or time away from intervention that would be burdensome or problematic in some practice contexts, although integral to research. Nonetheless, this list of assessment tools may provide a starting point for clinicians who wish to enlarge their tool kit for describing the needs of their clients and for gauging treatment progress. In addition, this table can provide a starting point for thinking about how well-developed interventions depend on establishing strategies for decision making such as those conveyed in particular assessments.

ASSESSMENT TOOLS FOR TREATMENT PLANNING—OTHER SOURCES

As another source of information regarding specific tools, we searched the literature for thoughtful and, ideally, evidence-based recommendations about useful measures. Although this literature is not large, it was substantial enough to provide a starting point. When planning treatment, two major questions arise: What content should be targeted in treatment? and How should it be targeted? The first question is typically addressed using standardized measures and analyses of samples of speech, language, and/or social interaction to identify intervention targets. The second question involves identifying *what kinds of supports* may facilitate learning and improved functioning, either directly through interventions with the individual or indirectly through alterations to the individual's environment. To answer the second question, dynamic assessments increasingly are being seen as an effective strategy. Therefore, to introduce measures that may be most helpful in planning treatment, we first describe tools available to help identify targets—primarily standardized tests and language analyses; then we describe dynamic assessment as a method available to help examine initial responsiveness to an intervention.

Deciding What to Target

Major guidance for our discussion of decisions regarding targets comes from the communication *phases* and main communication *domains* described in a seminal paper by Tager-Flusberg and colleagues (2009) that was an outgrowth of a working group convened by the National Institute on Deafness and Communication. These authors identified specific *expressive* language achievements, or benchmarks for infants through preschoolers, along with the methods by which they could be assessed for widespread research and clinical use. Expressive language, rather than receptive language, was the focus of these recommendations because the authors viewed it as the more frequent focus of intervention as well as the more reliably measured domain (Tager-Flusberg et al., 2009). They described five developmental phases: *prelinguistic/minimally verbal, first words, word combinations, early grammar use*, and *more advanced language* (Tager-Flusberg et al., 2009). A brief description of each of these stages is included in Table 2.3.

Recommendations by Tager-Flusberg and colleagues (2009) for expressive measures covered only the three phases of communication expected to occur

Table 2.3. Developmental communication phases

Phase	Age	Defining characteristics
1: Preverbal communication	6–12 months	Gestures and babbling to communicate intent
2: First words	12–18 months	Spontaneous single words to communicate about objects and events
3: Word combinations	18–30 months	Increased vocabulary using nouns, verbs, and describing words to refer to objects and events; combining two and three words to communicate multiple functions
4: Sentences	30–48 months	Combine words into clauses or simple sentences; some use of morphological endings (e.g., plurals, prepositions, verb tense); vocabulary adequate to communicate in daily situations
5: Complex language	After 48 months	Large vocabulary communicating on a range of topics with complex grammatical constructions in conversation

Source: Adapted from Tager-Flusberg et al. (2009).

Note: Phases indicated with shading are those for which the authors described benchmarks for describing a child's language level. Age ranges are those usually seen in children with typical development.

during the preschool years in children with the typical development: first words, word combinations, and early grammar use. Because interventions discussed in this book include interventions that might be used for individuals with ASD who have more advanced language, we relied not only on the expressive language recommendations of Tager-Flusberg and colleagues but also on those offered by other sources (e.g., Broome et al., 2017; Kasari et al., 2013; Luyster et al., 2008). In addition, we included measures for receptive language across all five phases while reminding readers that Tager-Flusberg and colleagues (2009) chose not to include receptive language assessments because of reliability concerns.

Three tables identify measures that can be used for descriptive purposes across a wide range of language, communication, and social interaction domains as well as across developmental communication phases. Table 2.4 lists measures that cover several developmental domains, including language. Table 2.5 lists measures that are omnibus communication measures and Table 2.6 lists measures that are relatively domain specific (e.g., measures of pragmatics or phonology).

Table 2.7 lists tools for measuring domains that are often not included in typical speech and language evaluations but may be particularly helpful in identifying behaviors or skills that may nonetheless be a treatment target for the SLP or other members of an interdisciplinary team working with a person with autism. These tools assess challenging behaviors and quality of life. Table 2.7 describes widely used or recommended measures appropriate for specific ages or developmental levels. Citations are also included for sources that discuss the strengths and weaknesses of the particular measures.

The sheer number of tools cataloged in Tables 2.4 to 2.7, as well as those listed in Table 2.2, hint at how difficult it can be to decide which tools to include in a battery used to describe a child's current status. The child's areas of greatest need, areas in which treatment or other kinds of management may be provided, as well as practical considerations (e.g., available time and expertise) bear heavily on such decisions. At the end of the chapter, we include a small set of learning activities

Table 2.4. Measures targeting multiple domains, including communication

Measure	Type	Intended ages	Communication and other domains						Functional communication phase[a]				
			Communication					Other	Preverbal	1st wd	Wd comb	Sentences	Complex lang
			Ges	Phon	Vocab	Gram	Prag						
Natural language or communication sample	Naturalistic observation	Any age	E	E	E	E	E	—	x	x	x	x	x
Communication and Symbolic Behavior Scale (Wetherby & Prizant, 2006)	Parent report/direct observation	6–24 months functional communication age	E	—	—	—	E	Eye gaze, facial expressions, play	x	x	—	—	—
MacArthur-Bates Communication Development Inventories (Fenson et al., 2007) • CDI Words and Gestures	Standardized parent report	8–18 months[b]	E/R	—	E/R	—	—		x	x	—	—	—
• Words and Sentences	Standardized parent report	16–30 months		E	E	E				x	x	x	
Preschool Language Scales–Fifth Edition (Zimmerman et al., 2011)	Standardized	Birth–7;11	E	E/R	E/R	E/R	—	Play, emergent literacy	x	x	x	x	x
Vineland Adaptive Behavior Scales–Third Edition (Sparrow et al., 2016)	Interview; parent/caregiver form; teacher rating form	Birth–90 years	—	—	—	—		Daily living skills, socialization skills, motor skills, maladaptive behavior	x	x	x	x	x

[a]Source: Tager-Flusberg, et al. (2009). [b]Not validated for school-age children but has been used in research for older CWA (Kasari et al., 2013).

Key: 1st wd, first words; Complex lang, complex language; E, expressive language; Ges, gesture; Gram, grammar; Phon, phonology; Prag, pragmatics; Preverbal, preverbal communication; R = receptive language; Vocab, vocabulary; Word comb, word combinations.

Table 2.5. Measures that primarily target communication, often providing more specific information on specific domains

Measure	Type	Ages	Communication domain				Functional communication phase[a]				
			Phon	Vocab./Seman	Gram/Syn	Prag	Preverbal	First wds	Word comb	Sentences	Complex lang
Children's Communication Checklist–Second Edition (CCC-2; Bishop, 2006	Parent or caregiver rating scale	4;0–16;11	E/R	E/R	E/R	E/R	—	—	—	X	X
Clinical Evaluation of Language Fundamentals–Fifth Edition (CELF-5; Wiig et al., 2013)	Standardized test	5;0–21;11	E/R	E/R	E/R	E/R	—	—	X	X	X
Systematic Analysis of Language Transcripts (SALT; Miller & Iglesias, 2012)	Standardized analysis method based on transcriptions of language samples	3;0–16:0	E	E	E	E	—	X	X	X	X
Test of Language Competence–Expanded (TLC-Expanded; Wiig & Secord, 1989)	Standardized test	5;0–18;0	—	E	E	Metalinguistics (inferencing, figurative language)	—	—	—	—	X

Source: Tager-Flusberg et al. (2009).

[a]

Key: 1st wd, first words; Complex lang, complex language; E, expressive language; Ges, gesture; Gram, grammar; Phon, phonology; Prag, pragmatics; Preverbal, preverbal communication; R, receptive language; Seman, semantics; Syn, syntax; Vocab, vocabulary; Word comb, word combinations.

Table 2.6. Measures that target specific communication domains of gesture, phonology, vocabulary, syntax, discourse, pragmatics, including theory of mind

Measure	Type	Intended ages	Domain	Functional communication phase[a]				
				Preverbal	1st wd	Word comb	Sentences	Complex lang
Goldman-Fristoe Test of Articulation (Goldman & Fristoe, 1969–2015)	Standardized test	2;0–21;11	Phonology–expressive	—	×	×	×	×
Profiling Elements of Prosodic Speech in Children (PEPS-C; Peppé & McCann, 2003)	Descriptive, nonstandardized test	4;0+	Phonology–prosody–expressive and receptive	—	—	×	×	×
Expressive Vocabulary Test (Williams 1997–2007)[b]	Standardized test	2;6–90;0	Vocabulary–expressive	—	×	×	×	×
Peabody Picture Vocabulary Test–Third Edition (PPVT-3; Dunn & Dunn, 2007)[b]	Standardized test	2;6–90;0+	Vocabulary–receptive	—	×	×	×	×
Test of Grammatical Impairment (Rice & Wexler, 2001)	Standardized test	3;0–9;0	Syntax, grammatical morphology	—	—	×	×	×
Joint Attention Protocol (Nowell et al., 2018; Watson et al., 2003)	Live-coded behavioral measure	2;0–12;0	Joint attention (nonverbal gestures and eye gaze)	×	—	—	—	—
Language Use Inventory for Young Children (O'Neill, 2007, 2009)	Standardized parent-report questionnaire	18–47 months	Pragmatics	×	×	×	×	×
Test of Language Competence–Expanded (TLC-Expanded; Wiig & Secord, 1989)	Standardized test	5;0–9;0 (level 1) and 10;0–18;0 (level 2)	Metalinguistics (ambiguous sentences, making inferences, re-creating speech acts, figurative language, and a supplemental memory subtest)	—	—	—	—	×
Test of Narrative Language–Second Edition (Gillam & Pearson, 2004–2017)	Standardized test	4;0–15;11	Narrative skills–expressive and receptive	—	—	—	—	×
Theory of Mind Inventory-2 (Hutchins et al., 2016)	Parent questionnaire	2;0–18;0	Theory of mind	—	—	×	×	×
Theory of Mind Task Battery (Hutchins & Prelock, 2016)	Child performance measure	2;0–12;0	Theory of mind	—	—	×	×	×

Source: [a]Tager-Flusberg et al. (2009). [b]Recommended in Magiati (2016).

Key: 1st wd = first words; Complex lang = complex language; Preverbal = preverbal communication; Word comb = word combinations.

Table 2.7. Measures of domains of possible interest for individuals with autism spectrum disorder, including problem behaviors and quality of life

Domain	Tool	Type	Intended ages/ developmental level	Sources mentioning the measure
Problem behaviors	Child Behavior Checklist (CBCL; Achenbach & Rescorla, 2000)	Caregiver-report questionnaire	1;6–5;0	Handratty et al.,2015
	Child Behavior Checklist (CBCL; Achenbach & Rescorla, 2001)	Caregiver-report questionnaire	6;0–18;0	Handratty et al., 2015
	Home Situations Questionnaire–Autism Spectrum Disorders (HSQ-ASD)	Caregiver rating scale	4;0–14;0	Chowdhury et al., 2015; Handratty et al., 2015
Quality of life	Pediatric Quality of Life Inventory (PedsQL), Version 4.0 (Varni et al., 2001).	Child self-report and parent-proxy report	Parent report (2;0–18;0) child report (5;0–7;0; 8;0–12;0; 13;0–18;0)	Eapen et al., 2016; Ikeda et al., 2014
	WHOQoL-BREF (World Health Organization Quality of Life Group, 1998); contains four subscales: physical, psychological, social, and environment	Self-report questionnaire	Adults, as culturally defined	Eapen et al., 2016; Mason et al., 2018

designed to allow readers to reflect on differences in the choice of specific measures based on client characteristics and circumstances.

Deciding How to Intervene

To a great extent, the selection of a treatment approach entails adoption of the intervention's procedures that, by definition, are intended to support the client's learning. Nonetheless, sometimes the identification of linguistic or environmental variables (physical environment, type of activity in which it is embedded), especially those that might be used in a cuing hierarchy, may ease the learning task. Dynamic assessment (Hasson & Joffe, 2007) has been used to help identify such variables for phonological skills (Glaspey, 2012; Glaspey & Stoel-Gammon, 2007), narrative skills (Gillam et al., 1999), and other language skills for children with a variety of diagnoses (e.g., Bain & Olswang, 1995). Most prominently, however, dynamic assessments are being used for children from culturally and linguistically diverse backgrounds, where the child's lack of experience may undermine his or her ability to demonstrate skills when static assessment is used (Peña et al., 2014). Despite that dynamic assessment was initially developed to provide more valid assessment methods for children who were difficult to test, it is only infrequently used for children with ASD (e.g., Donaldson & Olswang, 2007) and more often is used to tackle the question of language difference versus language disorder associated with children from diverse linguistic or cultural backgrounds. Still, given the benefits of dynamic assessment, it seems worth mentioning in the context of this chapter as a potential area for further exploration.

ASSESSMENT TOOLS FOR MONITORING PROGRESS

Usually, tools used for monitoring progress can be thought of as examining change across two timescales. The first timescale relates to longer intervals between measurements for which the purpose is often the examination of changes in severity of ASD symptoms or impairments as well as changes in participation and quality of life. The second timescale involves repeated measurements to provide continuous monitoring useful to ongoing decision making within an intervention, often to determine whether specific shorter-term objectives are met so that others can be targeted in turn. Because different measures tend to be used for each of these timescales, we talk about each in turn.

Measuring Longer-Term Progress

Many of the same measures used during diagnosis and the initial description of the impairments and functioning of the person with autism (i.e., those listed in Tables 2.2, 2.4–2.7) are routinely used to examine change related to long-term goals (e.g., improved social interaction, decreased challenging behavior) at fairly lengthy time intervals. Such timescales are intended to be long enough that significant changes in symptoms, abilities, and skills may be observed, thereby justifying the time required to administer them. Guidelines concerning the frequency of such testing are often dictated by the educational or clinical placement of the person with ASD. One relatively recent recommendation concerning the frequency of such testing of individuals with ASD is at least once every 6 months (Eapen et al., 2016).

As an example, imagine Gabe, a 5-year-old child with ASD who is included in a public school kindergarten class. Applying the Tager-Flusberg and colleagues framework (2009) introduced in Table 2.3, Gabe is functioning at the word combination phase of communication development, but he demonstrates reduced social interaction and challenging behaviors that include regularly grabbing toys from other children and meltdowns that occur when there are changes to classroom routines. Measures that might have been used as part of his initial diagnosis and would be repeated at a 1-year evaluation could be the following: the McArthur-Bates Communicative Development Inventories (MB-CDI) Words and Sentences (Fenson et al., 2007), the Vineland Adaptive Behavior Scales–Second Edition (Sparrow et al., 2016), and the Clinical Evaluation of Language Fundamentals–Fifth Edition (CELF-5; Wiig et al., 1980–2013). In addition, a language sample analysis might be used to examine the complexity of his emerging language in a more naturalistic context. Finally, an appropriate battery might also include slightly more focused measures to determine progress on specific social interaction or linguistic goals as well as measures to assess management of Gabe's challenging behaviors. A battery of this kind brings to light developments that would result in shifting priorities (e.g., from lexical to syntactic language goals) or enabling different intervention strategies to be pursued (e.g., group sessions that had not been possible previously because a particular challenging behavior had been insufficiently controlled).

Despite their familiarity, the reuse of standardized and other assessments presents several challenges (Eapen et al., 2016). First, many standardized speech and language measures were not developed with a person with autism in mind, and therefore, they may not reflect patterns of change in autism. Second, measures that are currently used for examining major symptoms of autism and language abilities are not necessarily backed by evidence that they are sensitive to change. In a systematic review of outcome measures used in the research literature for children with ASD up to age 6, McConachie and colleagues (2015) set out to examine the quality, including sensitivity to change, of 132 measures, using the Consensus-Based Standards for the Selection of Health Status Measurement Instruments (COSMIN) rating system (Mokkink et al., 2010). The measures covered outcomes across "core ASD impairments, such as communication, social awareness, sensory sensitivities and repetitiveness; social skills such as social functioning and play; participation outcomes such as social inclusion; and parent and family impact" (p. vii). Only 75 of these 132 measures were associated with studies meeting inclusion criteria, so only that subset of measures was evaluated.

At the end of their review, McConachie and colleagues (2015) found only 12 measures with relatively strong supporting evidence for their use, the majority of which focused on autism characteristics and problem behaviors. Even among these 12 measures, the authors indicated "little evidence that the identified tools would be good at detecting change in intervention studies." However, two widely used measures were among those 12. First, the Vineland Adaptive Behavior Scales screener (Sparrow et al., 2005) demonstrated moderately strong evidence that it could identify change on targeted domains. Second, the MB-CDI (Fenson et al., 2007) showed strong evidence of content validity and moderate evidence of construct validity.

In addition, McConachie and colleagues (2015) identified a measure that was part of the development of the ADOS-2 (Lord et al., 2012), the Brief Observation of Social Communication Change (BOSCC; Grzadzinski et al., 2016), as a potentially robust tool for capturing social behavior change in children up to age 6. The BOSCC has been shown to exhibit not only sensitivity to change but also high interrater agreement (e.g., Kitzerow et al., 2016; Pijl et al., 2018).

Given McConachie and colleagues' (2015) findings, it is clear that more work needs to be done in studying widely used language tests for their sensitivity to change as well as their applicability to individuals with autism. In the meantime, however, we recommend that clinicians look in test manuals for information about sensitivity to change, search the research literature, and recognize that at times they may be in the position of stressing a client's current status upon retesting rather than the degree to which any apparent change is both real and meaningful. Input from families and individuals with autism as well as other caregivers and professionals may provide additional sources of evidence that can contribute to valuable observations about progress on this longer timescale.

Measuring Shorter-Term Progress

Progress monitoring on a shorter timescale is used to guide day-to-day decisions in treatment. Measures for such purposes are often informal, criterion referenced, and constructed by the clinician to track a client's performance toward immediate treatment objectives (McCauley, 1996). A criterion, such as a specified percentage accuracy or response latency, is used rather than norms to aid interpretation. Table 2.2 documents the large number of interventions described in this book that rely on these sorts of measures for progress monitoring.

For example, a clinician using an intervention to increase the rate of initiations made by a child with ASD might use a criterion of 10 initiations in 5 minutes to trigger the decision to increase treatment task difficulty or to shift to another objective altogether. Among the data that might be used for this kind of monitoring are

1) treatment data on initiations observed during the session (e.g., evaluation of the rate of initiations occurring during a treatment session in which a group of preferred objects are used as communication temptations), 2) a probe obtained outside of treatment (e.g., evaluation of the rate of initiations during a 5-minute period occurring in a nontreatment setting in which most treatment supports are absent but with the same objects available), or 3) both. Whereas treatment data would suggest that the treatment conditions actually facilitate better performance in the moment, the probe data would suggest that generalization associated with more robust learning is occurring (Olswang & Bain, 1994).

Because such measures are tailored to the assessment purpose, they have some claim to content validity; however, reliability and other aspects of validity are not necessarily assured (McCauley, 1996; Yoder et al., 2018). When such measures are used widely, for example, by an intervention team or clinical group, steps can and should be undertaken to examine their reliability at the very least (Gillam et al., 2017; Vetter, 1988; Yoder et al., 2018). Much of the thinking about how such measures should be developed, such as the importance of baseline data, stems from their use as part of single case experimental designs. Single case experimental designs represent an important strategy for facilitating clearer interpretations of progress on the smaller timescale (Kazdin, 2010) and are encouraged by a number of interventions described in this volume.

CONCLUSION

The process of assessment for individuals with ASD remains crucial well after their initial diagnosis. Guidance for SLPs and their interdisciplinary teams, as well as for individuals with autism and their families, will continue to depend on reliable and valid descriptions of their current strengths and weaknesses as well as changes that may be occurring as the result of development, active management, or alterations in their daily lives. Clearly, continuing efforts are needed to improve the quality of tools available to help provide such guidance, but in the meantime, the integration of information across a variety of sources can provide a valuable starting point for decision making.

Learning Activities

Following are three case examples that could help readers working in small groups or individually learn to apply the concepts discussed in this chapter.

1. **Toddler at Risk for ASD:** Chad is an 18-month-old boy whose older brother has a diagnosis of autism. Chad currently has a limited consonant repertoire and uses only gestures for requesting items. He does not use gestures to initiate joint attention and responds to his parents' initiations of joint attention inconsistently. Chad has been approved for speech and language services through early intervention and is currently on the waiting list for an interdisciplinary evaluation to determine whether or not he will receive an autism diagnosis. Given these concerns, what evaluations would be appropriate for long-term treatment planning?

2. **Preschooler With ASD Who Is Entering an Inclusive Educational Setting:** Ben is 5 years of age and received a diagnosis of autism at age 3. He has made remarkable gains in his speech and language development after 2 years of intensive speech and language services. He was in a self-contained preschool

classroom for children with autism. Testing at the end of the year revealed that his receptive and expressive language skills were within age expectations; however, he still demonstrated significant impairments in his social communication (e.g., telling narratives, deviating from scripted play schemas). Because of the gains in his skills, his team determined that he should go into an inclusion classroom as he starts kindergarten. What evaluations would be appropriate for treatment planning and progress monitoring during his kindergarten year of school?

3. **Adolescent Who Uses Augmentative and Alternative Communication as His Primary Mode of Communication:** Mark is a 14-year-old boy diagnosed with ASD and cognitive impairment who uses a speech-generating device (SGD) as his primary mode of expressive communication. He currently produces two- to three-word phrases on his device and uses his device primarily to request his wants and needs. His current individualized education program (IEP) focuses on expanding his use of his SGD for a variety of communicative functions, such as commenting and protesting as well as increasing his mean length of utterance. What evaluations would be appropriate for progress monitoring?

REFERENCES

Achenbach, T. M., & Rescorla, L. A. (2000). *Manual for Achenbach System of Empirically Based Assessment (ASEBA) Preschool Forms and Profiles.* University of Vermont, Research Center for Children, Youth and Families.

Achenbach, T. M., & Rescorla, L. A. (2001). *Manual for ASEBA School-Age Forms and Profiles.* University of Vermont, Research Center for Children, Youth and Families.

Adams, D. J., Susi, A., Erdie-Lalena, C. R., Gorman, G., Hisle-Gorman, E., Rajnik, M., Elrod, M., & Nylund, C. M. (2016). Otitis media and related complications among children with autism spectrum disorders. *Journal of Autism and Developmental Disorders, 46,* 1636–1642.

American Speech-Language-Hearing Association. (n.d.). *Cultural competence.* Accessed December 14, 2018, https://www.asha.org/practice-portal/professional-issues/cultural-competence

Amiet, C., Gourfinkel-An, I., Bouzamondo, A., Tordjman, S., Baulac, M., Lechat, P., Mottron, L., & Cohen, D. (2008). Epilepsy in autism is associated with intellectual disability and gender: Evidence from a meta-analysis. *Biological Psychiatry, 64*(7), 577–582.

Ashburner, J., Ziviani, J., & Rodger, S. (2008). Sensory processing and classroom emotional, behavioral, and educational outcomes in children with autism spectrum disorder. *American Journal of Occupational Therapy, 62,* 564–573.

Autism and Developmental Disabilities Monitoring Network Surveillance Year 2008 Principal Investigators. (2012). Prevalence of autism spectrum disorders—Autism and Developmental Disabilities Monitoring Network, 14 Sites, United States, 2008. *Morbidity and Mortality Weekly Report, 61*(SS-03), 1–19.

Baas, L. S. (2012). Patient- and family-centered care. *Heart and Lung, 41*(6), 534–535.

Bain, B. A., & Olswang, L. B. (1995). Examining readiness for learning two-word utterances by children with specific expressive language impairment: Dynamic assessment validation. *American Journal of Speech-Language Pathology, 4,* 81–91.

Beatson, J. (2006). Preparing speech-language pathologists as family-centered practitioners in assessment and program planning for children with autism spectrum disorder. *Seminars in Speech and Language, 27*(1), 1–9.

Beaudoin, C., Leblanc, E., Gagner, C., & Bauchamp, M. H. (2020). Systematic review and inventory of theory of mind measures for young children. *Frontiers in Psychology.* https://doi.org/10.3389/fpsyg.2019.02905

Begeer, S., El Bouk, S., Boussaid, W., Terwogt, M. M., & Koot, H. M. (2009). Underdiagnosis and referral bias of autism in ethnic minorities. *Journal of Autism and Developmental Disabilities, 39,* 142–148.

Besag, F. M. C. (2018). Epilepsy in patients with autism: Links, risks, and treatment challenges, *Neuropsychiatric Disease and Treatment, 14*, 1–10.

Beukelman, D. R., & Mirenda, P. (2013). *Augmentative and alternative communication: Supporting children and adults with complex communication needs* (4th ed.). Paul H. Brookes Publishing Co.

Bishop, D. V. M. (2006). *Children's Communication Checklist-2: United States Edition.* Pearson.

Blackstone, S., & Hunt Berg, M. (2003). *Social networks: A communication inventory for individuals with complex communication needs and their communication partners.* Augmentative Communication.

Bölte, S., de Schipper, E., Robinson, J. E., Wong, V. C. N., Selb, M., Singhal, N., de Vries, P. J., & Zwaigenbaum, L. (2014). Classification of functioning and impairment: The development of ICF core sets for autism spectrum disorder. *Autism Research, 7*, 167–172.

Broome, K., McCabe, P., Docking, K., & Doble, M. (2017). A systematic review of speech assessment for children with autism spectrum disorder: Recommendations for best practice. *American Journal of Speech-Language Pathology, 26*, 1011–1029.

Bruininks, R. H., Woodcock, R. W., Weatherman, R. F., & Hill, B. K. (1996). *Scales of Independent Behavior—Revised.* Riverside.

Byiers, B. J., Reichle, J., & Symons, F. J. (2012). Single-subject experimental design for evidence-based practice. *American Journal of Speech-Language Pathology, 21*(4), 397–414.

Carlsson, L. H., Norrelgen, F., Kjellmer, L., Westerlund, J., Gillberg, C., & Fernell, E. (2013). Coexisting disorders and problems in preschool children with autism spectrum disorders. *The Scientific World Journal*, 2013, Article ID 213979. https://doi.org/10.1155/2013/213979

Carroll, R. A., Kodak, T., & Adolf, K. J. (2016). Effect of delayed reinforcement on skill acquisition during discrete-trial instruction: Implications for treatment-integrity errors in academic settings. *Journal of Applied Behavior Analysis, 49*(1), 176–181.

Chowdhury, M., Aman, M. G., Lecavalier, L., Smith, T., Johnson, C., Swiezy, N., McCracken, J. T., King, B., McDougle, C. J., Bearss, K., Deng, Y., & Scahil, L. (2015). Factor structure and psychometric properties of the revised Home Situations Questionnaire for autism spectrum disorder: The Home Situations Questionnaire-Autism Spectrum Disorder. *Autism*, 1–10. https://doi//10.1177/1362361315593941

Committee on Hospital Care and Institute for Patient- and Family-Centered Care. (2012). Policy statement: Patient- and family-centered care and the pediatrician's role. *Pediatrics, 129*(2), 394–404.

Cottle, K. J., McMahon, W. M., & Farley, M. (2016). Adults with autism spectrum disorders: Past, present, and future. In S. D. Wright (Ed.), *Autism spectrum disorder in mid and later life* (pp. 30–50). Jessica Kingsley Publishers.

Crais, E. R., Watson, L. R., & Baranek, G. T. (2009). Use of gesture development in profiling children's prelinguistic communication skills. *American Journal of Speech-Language Pathology, 18*, 95–108.

Dixon, M. R., Belisle, J., Stanley, C., Rowsey, K., Daar, J. H., & Szekely, S. (2015). Toward a behavior analysis of complex language for children with autism: Evaluating the relationship between PEAK and VB-MAPP. *Journal of Developmental and Physical Disabilities, 27*(2), 223–233.

Donaldson, A. L., & Olswang, L. B. (2007). Investigating requests for information in children with autism spectrum disorders: Static versus dynamic assessment. *Advances in Speech-Language Pathology, 9*(4), 297–311.

Dunn, L. M., & Dunn, D. M. (1959–2019). *Peabody Picture Vocabulary Test, Fifth Edition* (PPVT-5). Pearson.

Durand, V. M., & Crimmins, D. B. (1992). *The Motivation Assessment Scale (MAS) administration guide.* Monaco and Associates.

Durand, V. M., & Hieneman, M. (2008). *Helping parents with challenging children: Positive family intervention: Facilitator guide.* Oxford University Press.

Eapen, V., Williams, K., Roberts, J., Rinehart, N., & McGillivray, J. (2016). Monitoring progress in autism spectrum disorder. In J. L. Matson (Ed.), *Handbook of assessment and diagnosis of autism spectrum disorder* (pp. 87–115). Springer International Publishing.

Fenson, L., Marchman, V., Thal, D., Reznick, S., & Bates, E. (2007). *MacArthur-Bates Communicative Development Inventories: User's guide and technical manual* (2nd ed.). Paul H. Brookes Publishing Co.

Floyd, R. G., Shands, E. I., Alfonso, V. C., Phillips, J. F., Autry, B. K., Mosteller, J. A., Skinner, M., & Irby, S. (2015). A systematic review of adaptive behavior scales and recommendations for practice. *Journal of Applied School Psychology, 31*(1), 83–113.

Friedman, B. D., & Neuman Allen, K. (2011). Systems theory. In. J. R. Brandell (Ed.), *Theory and practice in clinical social work* (2nd ed., pp. 3–20). Sage Publications.

Frombonne, E. (2003). Epidemiological surveys of autism and other pervasive developmental disorders: An update. *Journal of Autism and Developmental Disorders, 33*(4), 365–382.

Gail-Williams, P., Sears, L. L., & Allard, A. (2004). Sleep problems in children with autism. *Journal of Sleep Research, 13*, 265–268.

Gan, S.-M., Tung, L.-C., Yeh, C.-H., & Wang, C.-H. (2013). ICF-CY based assessment tool for children with autism. *Disability and Rehabilitation, 35*(8), 678–685.

Gardner, L., Erkfritz-Gay, K., Campbell, J. M., Bradley, T., & Murphy, L. (2016). Purposes of assessment. In J. L. Matson (ed.), *Handbook of assessment and diagnosis of autism spectrum disorder* (pp. 27–43). Springer International Publishing.

Gerdts, J., Mancini, J., Fox, E., Rhoads, C., Ward, T., Easley, E., & Bernier, R. (2018). Interdisciplinary Team Evaluation: An effective method for the diagnostic assessment of Autism Spectrum Disorder. *Journal of Developmental and Behavioral Pediatrics, 39*(4), 271–281.

Gillam, S. L., Gillam, R. B., Fargo, J. D., Olszewski, A., & Segura, H. (2017). Monitoring Indicators of Scholarly Language: A progress-monitoring instrument for measuring narrative discourse skills. *Communication Disorders Quarterly, 38*(2), 96–106.

Gillam, R. B., & Pearson, N. (2004–2017). *Test of Narrative Language–Second Edition.* PRO-ED.

Gillam, R. B., Peña, E. D., & Miller, L. (1999). Dynamic assessment of narrative and expository discourse. *Topics in Language Disorders, 20*(1), 33–47.

Glaspey, A. M. (2012). Stimulability measures and dynamic assessment of speech adaptability. *SIG 1. Perspectives, 19*(1), 12–18.

Glaspey, A., & Stoel-Gammon, C. (2007). A dynamic approach to phonological assessment. *Advances in Speech-Language Pathology, 9*(4), 286–296.

Goldman, R., & Fristoe, M. (1969–2015). *Goldman-Fristoe Test of Articulation, Third Edition.* Pearson.

Goldrick, M., & Gerson, B. (1985). *Genograms in family assessment.* W.W. Norton.

Goodluck, C., (1990). *Utilization of genograms and ecomaps to assess American Indian families who have a member with a disability: Making visible the invisible.* Northern Arizona University.

Greenspan, S. (2004). *The social-emotional growth chart.* Pearson.

Greenspan, S. I., De Gangi, G. A., & Wieder, S. (2001). *The Functional Emotional Assessment Scale (FEAS) for Infancy and Early Childhood: Clinical and research applications.* ICDL Press.

Gresham, F., & Elliott, S.N. (2008). *Social Skills Improvement System (SSIS) Rating Scale.* Pearson.

Grzadzinski, R., Carr, T., Colombi, C., McGuire, K., Dufek, S., Pickles, A., & Lord, C. (2016). Measuring changes in social communication behaviors: preliminary development of the Brief Observation of Social Communication Change (BOSCC). *Journal of Autism and Developmental Disorders, 46*, 2464–2479.

Handratty, J., Livingstone, N., Robalino, S., Terwee, C. B., Glod, M., Oono, I. P., Rodgers, J., Macdonald, G., & McConachie, H. (2015). Systematic review of the measurement properties of tools used to measure behavior problems in young children with ASD. *PLoS ONE 10*(12): e0144649.

Hanley, G. P., Iwata, B. A., & McCord, B. E. (2003). Functional analysis of problem behavior: A review. *Journal of Applied Behavior Analysis, 36*, 147–185.

Harris, B., Barton, E. E., & Albert, C. (2014). Evaluating autism diagnostic and screening tools for cultural and linguistic responsiveness. *Journal of Autism and Developmental Disorders, 44*(6), 1275–1287.

Hasson, N., & Joffe, V. (2007). The case for dynamic assessment in speech and language therapy. *Child Language Teaching and Therapy, 23*(1), 9–25.

Heijnen-Kohl, S. M. J., Oude Vashaar, R. C., & van Alphen, S. P. J. (2016). Issues in diagnosis and assessment of autism in later life. In Wright, S. D, (Ed.), *Autism spectrum disorder in mid and later life* (pp. 163–176). Jessica Kingsley Publishers.

Holden, B., & Gitlesen, J. P. (2006). A total population study of challenging behavior in the county of Hedmark, Norway: Prevalence and risk markers. *Research in Developmental Disabilities, 27,* 456–465.

Hutchins, T. L., Lewis, L., & Prelock, P. A. (2020). *Theory of Mind Inventory-Adult Self-Report.* https://www.theoryofmindinventory.com

Hutchins, T. L., & Prelock, P. A. (2016). *Theory of Mind Task Battery (ToMTB).* https://www.theoryofmindinventory.com

Hutchins, T. L., Prelock, P. A., & Bonazinga-Bouyea, L. (2016). *Theory of Mind Inventory-2 (ToMI-2).* https://www.theoryofmindinventory.com

Ikeda, E., Hinckson, E., & Krägeloh, C. (2014). Assessment of quality of life in children and youth with autism spectrum disorder: A critical review. *Quality of Life Research, 23*(4), 1069–1085.

Individuals with Disabilities Education Act (IDEA) of 2004, PL 108-446, 20 U.S.C. §§1400 *et seq.* https://www.congress.gov/105/plaws/publ17/PLAW-105publ17.pdf

Interdisciplinary Council on Developmental and Learning Disorders. (2005). *Diagnostic manual for infancy and early childhood.* ICDL Press.

Kanne, S. M., & Mazurek, M. O. (2011). Aggression in children and adolescents with ASD: Prevalence and risk factors. *Journal of Autism and Developmental Disorders, 41,* 926–937.

Karst, J. S., & Van Hecke, A.V. (2012). Parent and family impact of autism spectrum disorders: A review and proposed model for intervention evaluation. *Clinical Child and Family Psychological Review, 15,* 247–277.

Kasari, C., Brady, N., Lord, C., & Tager-Flusberg, H. (2013). Assessing the minimally verbal school-aged child with autism. *Autism Research, 6,* 479–493.

Kazdin, A. E. (2010). *Single-case research designs: Methods for clinical and applied settings.* Oxford University Press.

Kitzerow, J., Teufel, K., Wilker, C., & Freitag, C. M. (2016). Using the Brief Observation of Social Communication Change (BOSCC) to measure autism-specific development. *Autism Research, 9,* 940–950.

Kjelgaard, M. M., & Tager-Flusberg, H. (2001). An investigation of language impairment in autism: Implications for genetic sub-groups. *Language and Cognitive Processes, 16,* 287–308.

Klaiman, C., Fernandez-Carriba, S., Hall, C., & Saulnier, C. (2015). Assessment of autism across the lifespan: A way forward. *Current Developmental Disorders Reports, 2*(1), 84–92.

Kovach, T. M. (2009). *Augmentative and alternative communication profile: A continuum of learning.* LinguiSystems.

Kroncke, A. P., Willard, M., & Huckabee, H. (Eds.). (2016). *Assessment of autism spectrum disorder.* Springer.

Lecavalier, L., Leone, S., & Wiltz, J. (2006). The impact of behaviour problems on caregiver stress in young people with autism spectrum disorders. *Journal of Intellectual Disability Research, 50*(3), 172–183.

Leitner, Y. (2014). The co-occurrence of autism and attention deficit hyperactivity disorder in children. *Frontiers of Human Neuroscience, 8.*

Lifter, K., Sulzer-Azaroff, B., Anderson, S. R., & Cowdery, G. E. (1993). Teaching play activities to preschool children with disabilities: The importance of developmental considerations. *Journal of Early Intervention, 17*(2), 139–159.

Liu, X., Hubbard, J. A., Fabes, R. A., & Adam, J. B. (2006). Sleep disturbances and correlates of children with autism spectrum disorders. *Child Psychiatry and Human Development, 37,* 179–191.

Lloyd, B. P., & Kennedy, C. H. (2014). Assessment and treatment of challenging behaviour for individuals with intellectual disability: A research review. *Journal of Applied Research in Intellectual Disabilities, 27,* 187–199.

Lord, C., Rutter, M., DiLavore, P. C., Risis, S., Gotham, K., & Bishop, S. L. (2012). *Autism Diagnostic Observation Schedule, Second Edition (ADOS-2).* Western Psychological Services.

Luyster, R. J., Kadlec, M. B., Carter, A., & Tager-Flusberg, H. (2008). Language assessment and development in toddlers with autism spectrum disorders. *Journal of Autism and Developmental Disorders, 38*(8), 1426–1438.

Maddox, B. B., & White, S. W. (2015). Comorbid social anxiety disorder in adults with autism spectrum disorder. *Journal of Autism and Developmental Disorder, 45*, 3949–3960.

Magiati, I. (2016). Assessment in adulthood. In J. L. Matson (Ed.), *Handbook of assessment and diagnosis of autism spectrum disorder* (pp. 191–207). Springer.

Mandell, D. S., Wiggins, L. D., Carpenter, L. A., Daniels, J., DiGuiseppi, C., Durkin, M. S., Giarelli, E., Morrier, M. J., Nicholas, J. S., Pinto-Martin, J. A., Shattuck, P. T., Thomas, K. C., Yeargin-Allsopp, M., & Kirby, R. S. (2009). Racial/ethnic disparities in the identification of children with autism spectrum disorders. *American Journal of Public Health, 99*, 493–498.

Mason, D., McConachie, H., Garland, D., Petrou, A., Rodgers, J., & Paar, J. R. (2018). Predictors of quality of life for autistic adults. *Autism Research, 11*, 1138–1147.

Matson, J. L. (Ed.). (2016). *Handbook of assessment and diagnosis of autism spectrum disorder.* Springer.

Matson, J. L., & Nebel-Schwalm, M. (2007). Assessing challenging behaviors in children with autism spectrum disorders, *Research in Developmental Disabilities, 28*, 567–579.

Matson, J. L., & Shoemaker, M. (2009). Intellectual disability and its relationship to autism spectrum disorders. *Research in Developmental Disabilities, 30*, 1107–1114.

Matson, J. L., Wilkins, J., Boisjoli, J. A., & Smith, K. R. (2008). The validity of the Autism Spectrum Disorders-Diagnosis for intellectually disabled adults (ASD-DA). *Research in Developmental Disabilities, 29*, 537–546.

McCauley, R. J. (1996). Familiar strangers: Criterion-referenced measures in communication disorders. *Language, Speech, and Hearing Services in Schools, 27*, 122–131.

McCauley, R. J. (2001). *Assessment of language disorders in children.* Lawrence Erlbaum Associates.

McClain, M. B., Otero, T. L., Haverkamp, C. R., & Molsberry, F. (2018). Autism spectrum disorder assessment and evaluation research in 10 school psychology journals from 2007 to 2017. *Psychology in the Schools, 55*(6), 661–679.

McConachie, H., Parr, J. R., Glod, M., Hanratty, J., Livingstone, N., Oono, I., Robalino, S., Baird, G., Beresford, B., Charman, T., Garland, D., Green, J., Gringras, P., Jones, G., Law, J., Le Couteur, A. S., Macdonald, G., McColl, E. M., Morris, C., . . . Williams, K. (2015). Systematic review of tools to measure outcomes for young children with autism spectrum disorders. *Health Technology Assessment, 19*(41), 1–506.

McElhanon, B., McCracken, C., Karpen, S., & Sharp, W. (2014). Gastrointestinal symptoms in autism spectrum disorders: A meta-analysis. *Pediatrics, 133*, 872–883.

McWilliam, R.A., Case, A. M., & Sims, J. (2009). The routines-based interview: A method for assessing needs and developing IFSPs. *Infants & Young Children, 22*, 224–233.

Messick, S. (1989). Validity. In R. L. Linn (Ed.), *Educational measurement* (3rd ed., pp. 13–104). American Council on Education and Macmillan.

Miller, J., & Iglesias, A. (2012). Systematic Analysis of Language Transcripts (SALT), Research (Version 2012) [Computer software]. SALT Software, LLC.

Mokkink, L. B., Terwee, C. B., Patrick, D. L., Alonso, J., Stratford, P. W., Knol, D. L., Bouter, L. M., & de Vet, H. C. W. (2010). The COSMIN checklist for assessing the methodological properties of health status measurement instruments: An international Delphi study. *Quality of Life Research, 19*(4), 539–549.

Mundy, P., Delgado, C., Block, J., Venezia, M., Hogan, A., & Seibert, J. (2003). *Early Social Communication Scales (ESCS).* University of Miami.

Murphy, O., Healy, O., & Leader, G. (2009). Risk factors for challenging behaviors among 157 children with autism spectrum disorder in Ireland. *Research in Autism Spectrum Disorders, 3*, 474–482.

Murphy, C. M., Wilson, C. E., Robertson, D. M., Ecker, C., Daly, E. M., Hammond, N., Galanopoulos, A., Dud, I., Murphy, D. C., & McAlonan, G. M. (2016). Autism spectrum disorder in adults: Diagnosis, management and health services development. *Neuropsychiatric Disease and Treatment, 12*, 1669–1686.

Nancarrow, S. A., Booth, A., Ariss, S., Smith, T., Enderby, P., & Roots, A. (2013). Ten principles of good interdisciplinary team work. *Human Resources for Health, 11*, 1–11.

National Autism Center. (2015). *Findings and conclusions: National Standards Project: Phase 2: Addressing the need for evidence-based practice guidelines for autism spectrum disorder.* National Autism Center.

Niehus, R., & Lord, C. (2006). Early medical history of children with autism spectrum disorders. *Journal of Developmental and Behavioral Pediatrics, 27*(2 Suppl.), S120–S127.

Nopprapun, M., & Holloway, J. (2014). A comparison of fluency training and discrete trial instruction to teach letter sounds to children with ASD: Acquisition and learning outcomes. *Research in Autism Spectrum Disorders, 8*(7), 788–802.

Nowell, S. W., Watson, L. R., Faldowski, R. A., & Baranek, G. T. (2018). An initial psychometric evaluation of the Joint Attention Protocol. *Journal of Autism and Developmental Disorders 48*(6), 1932–1944.

Odom, S. L., Collet-Klingenberg, L., Rogers, S. J., & Hatton, D. D. (2010). Evidence-based practices in interventions for children and youth with autism spectrum disorders. *Preventing School Failure, 54*(4), 275–282.

Odom, S. L., Duda, M. A., Kucharczyk, S., Cox, A. W., & Stabel, A. (2014). Applying an implementation science framework for adoption of a comprehensive program for high school students with autism spectrum disorder. *Remedial and Special Education, 35*(2), 123–132.

Olswang, L. B., & Bain, B. A. (1994). Data collection: Monitoring children's treatment progress. *American Journal of Speech-Language Pathology, 3*, 55–66.

O'Neill, D. (2007). The Language Use Inventory for Young Children: A parent-report measure of pragmatic language development for 18- to 47-month-old children. *Journal of Speech, Language, and Hearing Research, 50*, 214–229.

O'Neill, D. (2009). *The Language Use Inventory*. Knowledge in Development.

Paul, R., Landa, R., & Simmons, E. (2014). Communication in Asperger syndrome. In J. McPartland, A. Klin, F. Volkmar, & M. Asperger Felder (Eds.), *Asperger syndrome: Assessing and treating high functioning autism spectrum disorder* (2nd ed., pp. 103–142). Guilford Press.

Peña, E. D., Gillam, R. B., & Bedore, L. M. (2014). Dynamic assessment of narrative ability in English accurately identifies language impairment in English Language Learners. *Journal of Speech, Language, and Hearing Research, 47*, 2208–2220.

Peppé, S., & McCann, J. (2003). Assessing prosodic and pragmatic ability in children with high-functioning autism: The PEPS-C test and the revised version. *Journal of Pragmatics, 38*(10), 1776–1791.

Pijl, M. K., Rommelse, N. N., Hendriks, M., DeKorte, M. W., Buitelaar, J. K., & Oosterling, I. J. (2018). Does the Brief Observation of Social Communication Change help moving forward in measuring change in early autism intervention studies? *Autism, 22*(2) 216–226.

Prelock, P. A. (2019). An interdisciplinary, family-centered, and community-based assessment model for children with ASD. In P. A. Prelock (Ed.), *Autism spectrum disorders: Issues in assessment and intervention* (2nd ed., pp. 81–134). PRO-ED.

Prelock, P. A., & Beatson, J. E. (2019). Learning to work with families to support children with ASD. In P. A. Prelock (Ed.), *Autism spectrum disorders: Issues in assessment and intervention* (2nd ed., pp. 63–79). PRO-ED.

Prelock, P. A., Beatson, J., Bitner, B., Broder, C., & Ducker, A. (2003). Interdisciplinary assessment for young children with Autism Spectrum Disorders. *Language, Speech and Hearing Services in Schools, 34*, 194–202.

Prelock, P. A., Beatson, J., Contompasis, S., & Bishop, K. K. (1999). A model for family-centered interdisciplinary practice. *Topics in Language Disorders, 19*, 36–51.

Prelock, P. A., & McCauley (2021). *Case studies for the treatment of autism spectrum disorder.* Paul H. Brookes Publishing, Inc.

Prizant, B., Wetherby, A., Rubin, E., Laurent, A., & Rydell, P. (2006a). *The SCERTS model: A comprehensive educational approach for children with autism spectrum disorders. Vol. I: Assessment.* Paul H. Brookes Publishing Co.

Prizant, B., Wetherby, A., Rubin, E., Laurent, A., & Rydell, P. (2006b). *The SCERTS model: A comprehensive educational approach for children with autism spectrum disorders. Vol. II: Program planning and intervention.* Paul H. Brookes Publishing Co.

Rempel, G. R., Neufeld, A., & Eastlick Kushner, K. (2007). Interactive use of genograms and ecomaps in family caregiving research, *Journal of Family Nursing, 13*(4), 403–419.

Rice, M., & Wexler, K. (2001). *Rice Wexler Test of Early Grammatical Impairment.* Psychological Corporation.

Rogers, S. J., & Dawson, G. (2009). *Early Start Denver Model Curriculum Checklist for Young Children with Autism.* Guilford Press.

Saulnier, C. A., & Ventola, P. E. (2012). *Essentials of autism spectrum disorders evaluation and assessment.* Wiley.

Schiariti, V., Mahdi, S. H., & Bölte, S. (2018). International Classification of Functioning, Disability and Health Core Sets for cerebral palsy, autism spectrum disorder, and attention-deficit-hyperactivity disorder. *Developmental Medicine and Child Neurology, 60*(9), 933–941.

Shriberg, L. D., Paul, R., Black, L. M., & van Santen, J. P. (2011). The hypothesis of apraxia of speech in children with autism spectrum disorder. *Journal of Autism and Developmental Disorders, 41,* 405–426.

Shire, S. Y., Shih, W., Chang, Y. C., & Kasari, C. (2018). Short Play and Communication Evaluation: Teachers' assessment of core social communication and play skills with young children with autism. *Autism, 22*(3), 299–310.

Sparrow, S. S., Ciccheti, D. V., & Saulnier, C. A., (2005). *Vineland Adaptive Behavior Scales, Second Edition (VABS-II).* Pearson.

Sparrow, S. S., Ciccheti, D. V., & Saulnier, C. A. (2016). *Vineland Adaptive Behavior Scales, Third Edition (Vineland-3).* Pearson.

Sprung, M. (2010). Clinically relevant measures of children's theory of mind and knowledge about thinking: Non-standard and advanced measures. *Child and Adolescent Mental Health, 15*(4), 204–216.

Squires, J., Bricker, D., & Twombly, E. (2003). *The ASQ-SE user's guide for the ages and stages questionnaires: Social-emotional.* Paul H. Brookes Publishing Co.

Suarez, M. A. (2012). Sensory processing children with autism spectrum disorders and impact on functioning. *Pediatric Clinics of North America, 59,* 2013–2014.

Sullivan, A. L. (2013). School-based autism identification: Prevalence, racial disparities, and systematic correlates. *School Psychology Review, 42*(3), 298–316.

Sundberg, M. L. (2008). *VB-MAPP Verbal Behavior Milestones Assessment and Placement Program: A language and social skills assessment program for children with autism or other developmental disabilities: Guide.* AVB Press.

Tager-Flusberg, H., & Kasari, C. (2013). Minimally verbal school-aged children with autism spectrum disorder: The neglected end of the spectrum. *Autism Research, 6*(6).

Tager-Flusberg, H., Paul, R., & Lord, C. E. (2005). Language and communication in autism. In F. Volkmar, R. Paul, A. Klin, & D. J. Cohen (Eds.), *Handbook of autism and pervasive developmental disorder* (Vol 1). Wilcy.

Tager-Flusberg, H., Rogers, R., Cooper, J., Landa, R., Lord, C., Paul, R., Rice, M., Stoel-Gammon, C., Wetherby, A., & Yoder, P. (2009). Defining spoken language benchmarks and selecting measures of expressive language development for young children with autism spectrum disorders. *Journal of Speech-Language, Hearing Research, 52,* 643–652.

Tobias, A. (2018). The use of genograms in educational psychology practice. *Educational Psychology in Practice, 34*(1), 89–104.

Trammel, B., Wilcynski, S. M., Dale, B., & McIntosh, D. E. (2013). Assessment and differential diagnosis of comorbid conditions in adolescents with autism spectrum disorders. *Psychology in the Schools, 50*(9), 936–946.

Ungerer, J. A., & Sigman, M. (1981). Symbolic play and language comprehension in autistic children. *Journal of the American Academy of Child Psychiatry, 20*(2), 318–337.

Varni, J. W., Seid, M., & Kurtin, P. S. (2001). PedsQL™ 4.0: Reliability and validity of the Pediatric Quality of Life Inventory™ Version 4.0 Generic Core Scales in healthy and patient populations. *Medical Care, 39,* 800–812.

Vetter, D. K. (1988). Designing informal assessment procedures. In D. E. Yoder & R. D. Kent (Eds.), *Decision making in speech-language pathology* (pp. 192–193). Paul H. Brookes Publishing Co.

Watson, L. R., Poston, V., & Baranek, G. T. (2003). The attention-following and initiating joint attention protocol (JA protocol). Unpublished manuscript.

Wehman, P., Datlow Smith, M., & Schall, C. (2009). *Autism and the transition to adulthood: Success beyond the classroom.* Paul H. Brookes Publishing Co.

Wetherby, A., & Prizant, B. (2006). *Communication and Symbolic Behavior Scales: Developmental profiles.* Paul H. Brookes Publishing Co.

Wllg, D., & Secord, W. A. (1989). *Test of Language Competence—Expanded Edition.* Pearson.

Wiig, E., Semel, E., & Secord, W. A. (1980–2013). *Clinical Evaluation of Language Fundamentals–Fifth Edition*. Pearson.

Williams, K. T. (1997–2007). *Expressive Vocabulary Test, 2nd edition*. Pearson.

Williams, G. P., Sears, L. L., & Allard, A. (2004). Sleep problems in children with autism. *Journal of Sleep Research, 13*(3), 265–268.

Williams, L., & Matson, J. L. (2016). Current status and future directions. In J. L. Matson (Ed.), *Handbook of assessment and diagnosis of autism spectrum disorder* (pp. 451–462). Springer.

Wilkinson, L. A. (2016). *A best practice guide to assessment and intervention for autism spectrum disorder in schools* (2nd ed.). Jessica Kingsley Publishers.

World Health Organization. (2001). *International classification of functioning, disability, and health*. Author.

World Health Organization Quality of Life (WHOQOL) Group. (1998). Development of the World Health Organization WHOQOL-BREF quality of life assessment. *Psychological Medicine, 28*(3), 551–558.

Yoder, P. J., Lloyd, B. P., & Symons, F. J. (2018). *Observational measurement of behavior* (2nd ed.). Paul H. Brookes Publishing Co.

Zachor, D., & Ben-Itzchak, E. (2019). From toddlerhood to adolescence: Which characteristics among toddlers with autism spectrum disorder predict adolescent attention deficit/hyperactivity symptom severity? A long-term follow-up study. *Journal of Autism and Developmental Disorders, 49*(8), 3191–3202.

Zimmerman, I. L., Steiner, V. G., & Pond, R. E. (2011). *Preschool Language Scales, Fifth Edition* (PLS-5). Pearson.

3

Language and Communication in ASD

Implications for Intervention

Ashley R. Brien and Patricia A. Prelock

INTRODUCTION

With the advancement of diagnostic tools, children with autism spectrum disorder (ASD) are being identified increasingly early in the development process. To date, ASD can be diagnosed with a high degree of certainty by the time a child is 2 years old, but many signs occur before the age of 2 (Barbaro & Dissanayake, 2009; Johnson & Myers, 2007; Shattuck et al., 2009; Wetherby et al., 2007). Infants and toddlers with older siblings who are diagnosed with ASD are at a higher risk for developing autism themselves, with a rate of 2%–32% (Macari et al., 2012). Understanding the early communication challenges in infants and toddlers that may be present in children at risk for ASD will be important in the early detection and treatment of the disorder. Further, because ASD is being diagnosed at such an early age, researchers can develop interventions for parents and clinicians to target early communication challenges in young children with ASD (Harris, 2017). Moreover, addressing communicative deficits in young children with ASD at an early age can have positive effects on a child's nonverbal and verbal communication (Kasari et al., 2012; Vismara et al., 2009), behavior management, play skills, joint attention, and imitation skills (Ingersoll & Schreibman, 2006; Kaale et al., 2014; Rogers & Dawson, 2010).

The goal of this chapter is to highlight the communication challenges often seen in children, adolescents, and adults with ASD, and the chapters that follow offer evidence-based interventions to support these challenges. As you read through the chapters, you will learn about several interventions that address the social-communication impairments characteristic of individuals with ASD, including augmentative and alternative communication approaches, the Early Start Denver Model (Rogers & Dawson, 2010), behavioral intervention strategies, the

Developmental Individual-Differences, Relationship-based model (DIR; Greenspan & Wieder, 1998), functional communication training, joint attention intervention, Enhanced Milieu Teaching, the early social interaction project (Wetherby & Woods, 2006; Woods & Wetherby, 2003), peer-mediated support, Pivotal Response Treatment (Koegel & Koegel, 2006), Social Stories™ (Gray, 2010), video modeling, the social communication, emotional regulation, and transactional supports model (SCERTS®; Prizant et al., 2003; Prizant et al., 2004), and social skills interventions. These interventions have been highlighted by the National Autism Center (2015) as established or emerging evidence-based practices for individuals with ASD.

This chapter reviews the early communication challenges associated with an ASD diagnosis, as well as related deficits in joint attention, play, and theory of mind that impact communication and language development. It also highlights the syntactic, semantic, phonological, and pragmatic impairments that characterize ASD. The chapter closes by discussing the use of a collaborative and family-centered team approach to identify intervention strategies that will bridge the gap between research and intervention for individuals with ASD.

EARLY COMMUNICATION CHALLENGES IN ASD

As described in Chapter 1, individuals with ASD demonstrate challenges with social communication and social interaction. These include difficulties with verbal and nonverbal communication, understanding and using gestures to communicate, engaging in reciprocal conversations about various topics, and using language flexibly. The impact that these communication challenges have on individuals with ASD ultimately affects their development of meaningful social relationships, including friendships and romantic relationships (Müller et al., 2008), as well as educational and community-based opportunities (Horner et al., 2002; Hutchins & Prelock, 2014). An inability to communicate with ease and engage socially may leave individuals with ASD feeling isolated and depressed (Müller et al., 2008) as they enter into adolescence and adulthood.

Understanding the communicative challenges in young children with ASD and how these challenges may present themselves in adolescence and adulthood provides a strong rationale for selecting evidence-based interventions designed to address social communication and social interaction. In this section, impairments in intentional communication, use and understanding of gestures, word learning, and multisensory processing in ASD are discussed. A discussion of how these communication skills develop in children who are typically developing is followed by a description of how these areas might be affected in children, adolescents, and adults with ASD. The implications for interventions given these specific communication challenges are then addressed. Also highlighted are the unconventional verbal behaviors that often characterize the early communication of children with ASD. In addition, because difficulties in joint attention, play, and theory of mind are evident in children with ASD, a description of their development in both typically developing children and children with ASD is provided.

Intentional Communication

Intentional communication is observed early in child development and includes initiating and responding to joint attention through gestures such as pointing, giving, and showing (Bates et al., 1975). These communicative acts occur prior to speech acts in typically developing infants. In this prelinguistic phase of communication, it becomes evident that communication precedes language acquisition and, in fact, may contribute to later language development (Prelock & Nelson, 2012). Intentional communication prior to verbal communication is crucial, as it allows prelinguistic children to express their wants and needs, engage in social interactions with caregivers, and fundamentally display their feelings without words but with intention (Stone et al., 1997). Further, responding to bids of joint attention "permits the child to gain experience sharing a focus on an external object or event with another person and to appreciate the communicative nature of that experience" (Luyster et al., 2008, p. 1435).

Typically Developing Individuals Typically developing infants enter into this intentional communicative phase during the first year of life (Paul et al., 2018) and continue to develop this skill into their second year of life (Shumway & Wetherby, 2009). Infants and caregivers first share attention to a particular object or event by means of mutual gaze. As development continues, infants learn to both respond to joint attention bids from caregivers (i.e., following a caregiver's point to an object and then referencing back to the adult) and initiate joint attention with others (i.e., pointing to an object, referencing back and forth between the object and the adult). This ability to share interest with others through joint attention allows infants to understand communication in a social sense and lays the foundation for language development (Prelock & Nelson, 2012; Wetherby et al., 1998).

Individuals With ASD Young children with ASD often show marked impairments in intentional communication, which is observed through decreased use of responding to and initiating joint attention. Frequently, children with ASD fail to share enjoyment with others during interactions (American Psychiatric Association [APA], 2013), demonstrate challenges shifting their eye gaze between objects and people, and are challenged to coordinate gestures with eye gaze and vocalizations (Shumway & Wetherby, 2009). Retrospective video analyses of children later diagnosed with ASD reveal that by their first birthday, these infants do not engage in intentional communication similarly to the way typically developing 1-year-olds do. Findings indicate impairments in intentional communication, including gesture use (i.e., lack of pointing and showing) and eye gaze (i.e., lack of looking at faces; Osterling & Dawson, 1994; Osterling et al., 2002). As early as 18 months of age, children later diagnosed with ASD perform more poorly than typically developing children on a number of intentional communication measures, including shifting their gaze, following a point, their rate of communication, use of communication for social interaction and joint attention, use of gestures, and use of consonants (Wetherby et al., 2007).

Implications for Intervention As children develop and enter preschool, deficits in intentional communication may appear during peer play. Children with ASD often play by themselves and struggle to engage with others. They may not recognize other children's use of eye gaze as a communicative act. In addition, children with ASD experience impairments associated with integrating and coordinating attention, gesture use, eye gaze, and vocalizations, and these impairments can negatively affect their development of social relationships. Wetherby and colleagues (1998) describe it this way: "Children who displayed a greater capacity to coordinate attention and affect were more likely to communicate for more social reasons, use a larger repertoire of conventional gestures, use a higher rate of communicating" (p. 88).

Joint attention intervention at an early age (described in Chapter 9) as part of intentional communication training should be considered an integral part of treatment for young children with ASD. In addition, Enhanced Milieu Teaching (described in Chapter 10) provides a framework for intervention in which the environment is arranged so that the child can initiate intentional communicative acts, leading to increases in intentional communication.

Gestures

Gestures (e.g., reaching, showing, pointing to request or label, waving hello or goodbye) are used for a number of communicative functions, including to initiate joint attention, regulate behavior, and engage in social interactions (Ellawadi & Weismer, 2014). Gestures begin to develop prior to verbal communication and then contribute, in a coordinated manner, to verbal communication throughout adulthood. The use of gestures allows preverbal infants and toddlers to communicate their thoughts and ideas before language develops (Ellawadi & Weismer, 2014). Over time, children's gesture use becomes integrated with their eye gaze and vocalizations or verbalizations. Gesture use, among other prelinguistic skills, is an important predictor of later language development in children (Crais et al., 2009). Luyster and colleagues (2008) found that gesture use was the best predictor of both receptive and expressive language skills, even more so than initiating or responding to joint attention or imitating.

Typically Developing Individuals   In children who are typically developing, three types of gestures evolve and contribute to language: deictic, symbolic, and representational. Deictic gestures are used when referring to a location and include showing, giving, and pointing. These gestures are the first to emerge in typical development between 10 to 12 months of age (Paul et al., 2018). Another type of deictic gesture, called *ritualized requests*, also develops around this time (between 9 and 13 months of age) and refers to reaching toward objects with an open hand or using an adult's hand to gain an object (Capone & McGregor, 2004). Symbolic gestures, also referred to as *recognitory gestures*, are produced spontaneously on multiple exemplars and are often seen in play schemes in which the child acts on an object to show its function (e.g., using a toy comb on a doll's hair). Symbolic gestures can best be observed during play interactions (Capone & McGregor, 2004). Representational gestures, on the other hand, carry meaning in and of themselves and do not require a referent object. Representational gestures may also be described as *descriptive gestures*, which describe objects, attributes, or actions (Ingersoll et al., 2007). For example, representational gestures include flapping arms to indicate a bird, blowing to indicate that something is hot, or putting a hand near the mouth to indicate eating. Symbolic and representational gestures begin to emerge at approximately 12–13 months of age and, like deictic gestures, continue to develop into toddlerhood (Paul et al., 2018). By roughly 20 months of age, typically developing children are able to use deictic and representational gestures in combination with spoken words and to combine symbolic gestures, resulting in multi-element symbolic play (Capone & McGregor, 2004).

Individuals With ASD   Children with ASD develop gestures differently than do typically developing children. Most notably, children with ASD use fewer deictic gestures to point to or show objects (Osterling & Dawson, 1994; Stone et al., 1997;

Wetherby et al., 2004). Further, use of symbolic gestures is also impaired in children with ASD (Wetherby et al., 1998), whereas use of representational gestures may not be impaired compared to typically developing children (Shumway & Wetherby, 2009). It should be noted, however, that while some researchers have not found a difference in representational gesture use between children with ASD and typically developing children (Shumway & Wetherby, 2009), the communicative function of these gestures was not examined. Of note, children with ASD have been found to use gestures in an unconventional way, including increased use of another person's hand as a tool without acknowledging the other person as a communication partner (Stone et al., 1997; Wetherby et al., 2004). This lack of acknowledging others as potential communication partners is apparent in these children's challenges in coordinating gestures with eye gaze and vocalizations. Children with ASD may use a number of isolated gestures but struggle to link these deictic gestures with gaze and vocalizations (Stone et al., 1997), which presents challenges for communicating intent and establishing a meaningful communicative exchange, including reciprocal communication.

Implications for Intervention   Because of the relationship between gesture use and receptive and expressive language abilities, parents and clinicians working with young children with ASD should consider the underlying social-cognitive skills, including gesture use, associated with later language learning. Gesture imitation intervention has been shown to increase total gesture imitation, combined gesture imitation (i.e., gesture and verbal imitation), spontaneous gesture use, and spontaneous combined gesture use for descriptive gestures (Ingersoll et al., 2007). Imitative gestures provide a social awareness of others, as communicative partners are important for the development of social reciprocity. Nonverbal back-and-forth exchanges via gesture use lay the foundation for later verbal communicative interactions. Capone and McGregor (2004) highlight some of the research that supports the positive role of gesture use in language development. For example, 1) parents' symbolic use of gestures and verbal input influences an infants' gesture use and ability to acquire both gestures and words early in language development (Namy et al., 2000); 2) the modeling of gestures and words for infants supports their early symbol use (Goodwyn & Acredolo, 1993); and 3) infants taught to use gestures will increase their spontaneous gesture use, which does not hinder verbal language development (Goodwyn et al., 2000). In addition, De Giacomo and colleagues (2009) note that the association between nonverbal behaviors and later communication "could be explained by the fact that during the prelinguistic stage of child development, communication is based on nonverbal behavior such as gaze, facial expression and body language (including pointing) to communicate their needs, wishes, and social intentions and gesture often conveys information that is not conveyed in the speaker's words" (p. 360).

Imitation

Imitation skills begin developing in newborn babies and continue to develop during the first 2 years of life. These skills present in a number of different ways, including facial imitation, vocal imitation, gestural imitation, imitation of actions on objects, and imitation with tools. In addition, imitation may occur during turn-taking interactions, such that parents and children imitate one another as a means to share interests and engage in social play (Rogers & Dawson, 2010).

Imitation behaviors often occur automatically and without explicit teaching (Rogers & Dawson, 2010; Waxler & Yarrow, 1970), providing a foundation upon which cultural and social learning can be built (Rogers, Hepburn, Stackhouse, & Wehner, 2003; Tomasello et al., 1993).

Typically Developing Individuals   Infants who are typically developing engage in certain imitative actions as newborns, and these skills continue to develop throughout the child's first and second years of life (Rogers, Hepburn, Stackhouse, & Wehner, 2003). Imitation in typically developing infants and toddlers has been reported to serve a number of functions, including providing a feeling of connectedness, communicating nonverbally with social partners, learning about the physical and social world, and serving as a foundation for peer interactions (Rogers, Hepburn, Stackhouse, & Wehner, 2003).

Individuals With ASD   Infants and toddlers with ASD demonstrate impairments in imitation depending on the nature of the task. Imitation of actions on objects may be less impaired than imitation of facial movements for familiar and simple object manipulations. Novel imitation of actions on objects, however, has been reported to be impaired similarly to impairment of facial/body movement imitation in ASD (Rogers, Hepburn, Stackhouse, & Wehner, 2003). Toddlers with higher verbal skills may have less impaired imitation abilities compared to toddlers with ASD with lower language abilities (De Giacomo et al., 2009). In addition, a child's imitation skills may be associated with joint attention abilities and autism severity (Rogers, Hepburn, Stackhouse, & Wehner, 2003). The challenges associated with imitation in toddlers with ASD may be a key component to the deficits noted in back-and-forth social reciprocity (Rogers, Hepburn, Stackhouse, & Wehner, 2003).

Implications for Intervention   When teaching imitation to children with ASD, it is important to consider the setting for which the skills are taught. Traditional imitation intervention has occurred in a behavioral treatment capacity, which breaks the skills down into individual units. In this way, children are prompted to copy an interventionist with the instructions to "do this." Although children may demonstrate gains in this structured capacity, imitation for communication purposes may not be apparent in this model, and skills may not carry over into spontaneous imitation in multiple settings (Ingersoll et al., 2007; Ingersoll & Schreibman, 2006). Ingersoll and colleagues provide data on reciprocal imitation training that has been shown to be a natural and effective treatment for increasing spontaneous imitation in children (Ingersoll et al., 2007). Because imitation skills have been correlated with later verbal language development, targeting spontaneous imitation in toddlers with ASD may reduce expressive language deficits. Higher imitative skills in ASD have been associated with overall greater communication skills (De Giacomo et al., 2009).

Word Learning

Before a child utters his or her first word, many social-cognitive and social-communicative developments are working behind the scenes. As previously discussed, prelinguistic behaviors (e.g., joint attention, gestures, imitation, symbolic play) contribute to a child's vocabulary and overall language acquisition (Luyster et al., 2008). In typical development, once children demonstrate utility with preverbal behaviors, word learning can occur. A crucial part of language development, word learning can be subdivided into two main facets: receptive word learning and expressive word learning (Chapman, 2000). Receptive word learning considers the vocabulary that a child can understand but not necessarily produce. In contrast, expressive word learning refers to the words that the child is able to express, whether in the form of verbal language, sign language, or augmented language. Typically, receptive language develops before meaningful expressive language; children often have larger receptive vocabularies than expressive vocabularies (Benedict, 1979).

Typically Developing Individuals   The process of word learning occurs early in child development as a continued form of intentional communication (Chapman, 2000). Between 10 and 16 months of age, children begin producing their first words, including words associated with familiar people, pets, objects, recurrence (e.g., *more*), appearance (e.g., *uh-oh*), and disappearance (e.g., *all gone*), as well as words used in communicative games and routines (Chapman, 2000; Kim et al., 2014). During this phase, one-word utterances convey complex and variegated meanings. For example, a child saying "cat" might mean any of the following: *I see a cat; I want the cat; Where is the cat?; Look, a cat!* Between 12 and 18 months of age, children increase their expressive vocabulary to between 50 and 100 words (Paul et al., 2018) and begin combining two words (Roseberry-McKibbin & Hegde, 2011). Between 2 and 3 years of age, a child's expressive vocabulary is typically between 200 and 600 words (Miller, 1981), receptive vocabulary is more than 2,000 words, and children are combining three to four words (Roseberry-McKibbin & Hedge, 2011). During a child's expressive vocabulary spurt, fast-mapping (a mechanism for word learning suggesting a new concept is learned with minimal exposure) occurs during which children acquire new vocabulary after only a few exposures to the words.

Individuals With ASD   Children with ASD are varied in their abilities to learn words, both receptively and expressively. While some children with ASD may be functionally nonverbal and demonstrate marked challenges developing expressive language, others are verbose and word learning is relatively unaffected. Many children with ASD have deficits in both receptive and expressive language abilities, and it has been suggested that children with ASD have stronger expressive language skills than receptive language abilities (Kwok et al., 2015; Luyster et al., 2008; Mitchell et al., 2013). Although children with ASD may demonstrate larger expressive than receptive vocabularies at 30 months of age, this discrepancy does not seem to continue as children reach their preschool years (Davidson & Weismer, 2017). A recent comprehensive literature review study found no clear evidence that expressive language skills are better than receptive language skills in children with ASD (Kwok et al., 2015). Interestingly, Luyster and colleagues (2008) found that preverbal behaviors affect the development of receptive versus expressive language abilities differently in children with ASD. Specifically, receptive language can be predicted by a young child's nonverbal cognitive ability, gesture use, and response to joint attention, whereas later expressive language is related to a child's nonverbal cognitive ability, gesture use, and imitation skills.

Implications for Intervention   Parents and clinicians working with toddlers under the age of 30 months should consider the apparent discrepancy in expressive versus receptive language, which may be age specific. Enhancing a child's receptive language by labeling objects and actions, describing events, and expanding utterances is critical for a child's word learning and understanding of how objects in the world work (Friedlander, 1970). Interpreting a child's prelinguistic behaviors (such as eye gaze, pointing, using an adult's hand as a tool) and modeling simple language provides the child with words to use in future interactions. The following is an example of a 28-month-old child who uses few expressive words; he attempts to communicate to his mother, who is using Enhanced Milieu Teaching (see Chapter 10), that he wants her to retrieve a toy truck from the top shelf.

Child: [takes his mother's hand and reaches it up toward the car on the shelf]

Mother: You're reaching for the car. [takes the car off the shelf]

Mother: Car. [as she hands the car to her child]

Language should be modeled with an utterance length that is one word greater than the child's mean length of utterance (MLU). For example, if the child is not expressively producing any words, adults should emphasize expressive language at the one-word level (as in the preceding example). If the child consistently speaks in one-word utterances, the adult should model utterances that are two words in length, as in this example:

Child: Car. [takes his mother's hand and reaches up toward the car on the shelf]

Mother: Red car. [takes the car off the shelf and hands it to her child]

Using this approach, adult utterances are constantly building upon the child's utterances, fostering the development of children's receptive and expressive word learning skills.

Unconventional Verbal Behavior in Children With ASD

Unconventional verbal behavior describes a variety of nontraditional uses of expressive language, particularly when describing language patterns of individuals with ASD. These verbal behaviors include echolalia, perseverative speech, and excessive questioning (Prizant & Rydell, 1993).

Echolalia, which is the repetition of words, phrases, or sentences, can be immediate (Prizant & Duchan, 1981) or delayed. Immediate echolalia occurs when an individual repeats a word or phrase immediately after hearing it; delayed echolalia occurs when an individual repeats a word or phrase minutes, hours, or even days after hearing it (Prizant & Rydell, 1984). The following is an example of immediate echolalia in a 6-year-old child with ASD:

Teacher: Do you need to go to the bathroom?

Child: Do you need to go to the bathroom?

Children with echolalia may repeat words or phrases spoken by a peer, caregiver, or support person, or they may repeat utterances heard on television or in a movie or video. *Mitigated echolalia*, which can be either immediate or delayed, occurs when a scripted phrase is repeated but is somewhat altered. For example, a phrase can be altered by manipulating the original words, changing the intonation of the phrase, or saying the phrase in a different context. Consider a young child with ASD attending a peer's birthday party with her parents. As the other children begin singing "Happy Birthday," the child with ASD covers her ears and begins crying. Her parents ask, "Do you want to leave?" and then leave the party. Later at school, the child attends a schoolwide assembly with her class. The other children are loud, and the child covers her ears, begins crying, and says, "Do you want to leave!" In this example, the child with ASD may associate the loud noises at the school assembly with the singing of "Happy Birthday" at the party. She repeats the question that her parents asked her at the birthday party that resulted in her being able to leave the situation.

Perseverative speech is also considered an unconventional verbal behavior that children with ASD may exhibit. Perseverative speech may be imitated speech (similar to echolalia) or self-generated speech. The difference between perseverative speech and echolalia is that perseverative scripts are repeated multiple times, seemingly without communicative intent. Anxiety, heightened arousal, or processing challenges may underlie perseverative speech behaviors (Prizant & Rydell, 1993), as seen in the following example of a 7-year-old child with autism.

A child is working with a speech-language pathologist in a room with many desks and bookshelves. The following conversation takes place during the middle of a work session:

Clinician: Cows, pigs, cats, and dogs are all _____.

Child: I like the watch. [without using eye gaze or gesture to indicate the watch]

Clinician: What watch?

Child: I like the watch. [without using eye gaze or gesture to the watch]

Clinician: Do you like my watch or the watch on the table?

Child: I like the watch. [without using eye gaze or gesture to indicate the watch]

Clinician: Hmmm, I don't know which watch you are talking about. It's time to work. Cows, pigs, cats, and dogs are all _____.

Child: I like the watch. [without using eye gaze or gesture to indicate the watch]

Similar to perseverative speech, excessive questioning involves perseverative scripts in the form of questions that continue to be asked after an answer to the question has been provided. When children with ASD use excessive questioning, their questions are often directed to a communication partner, which makes it seem as if the child is expecting an answer. Because children engaging in excessive questioning continue to ask questions even after a response is provided, its function may be similar to that of perseverative speech, such that it occurs as a response to anxiety, heightened arousal, or processing challenges (Prelock, 2019). In the following example, when an 8-year old child with ASD is engaged in excessive questioning with her school aide, the aide first provides the child with the correct answer. When the child continues to ask the same question, the aide allows the child to process her own question by posing the question back to her and providing two possible responses:

Child: Is Mommy coming?

Aide: No, you are riding the bus after school.

Child: Is Mommy coming?

Aide: Is Mommy coming, or are you riding the bus?

Child: Riding the bus.

Aide: You got it. You are riding the bus today.

Child: Is Mommy coming?

Implications for Intervention   Although echolalic and scripted phrases may appear to be nonfunctional forms of verbal communication, researchers are suggesting the opposite. Individuals with ASD may use various forms of echolalia in an attempt to communicate. Specifically, immediate echolalia has been found to be a means of initiating or responding to communication, including requesting, answering questions, declaring statements, and engaging in reciprocal communication. In addition, immediate echolalia has been used to self-regulate in children with ASD (Prizant & Duchan, 1981). Delayed echolalia also has served a number of communicative functions, including conversational turn taking, labeling objects and actions, calling to someone, providing new information, requesting, and protesting (Prizant & Rydell, 1984). The various functions of echolalia, perseverative speech, and excessive questioning should be considered when interacting with individuals with ASD. Communication partners should consider the context in which the unconventional verbal behaviors occur and whether the utterance appears to function as a form of intentional communication, to indicate comprehension difficulties or high arousal/ anxiety, or as a form of cognitive processing.

Multisensory Processing

Today's world stimulates the sensory systems, which then require regulation. These systems (i.e., visual, auditory, tactile, olfactory, taste) work independently, but sensory information gets conveyed to the brain in multiple ways and can be regulated or dysregulated. Baum and colleagues (2015) state that "the integration of information across the different senses is an essential process in the construction of healthy perceptual representations, and can be argued to represent one of the basic building blocks for the construction of cognitive representations and abilities" (p. 141).

Typically Developing Individuals   Children who have intact multisensory processing systems are able to manage variable stimuli in play, communication, and social contexts. In particular, multisensory processing in the area of speech perception allows individuals to rely on visual cues, such as gestures, facial cues, and lipreading, when the auditory stimulus is difficult to process (such as in noisy environments; Schmalenbach et al., 2017).

Individuals With ASD   Challenges in sensory functions have recently been included in the DSM-5 as a core feature of ASD. Individuals with ASD often demonstrate sensitivity to various sensory stimuli, including lights, sounds, smells, and touch (Beker et al., 2018). Sensory processing challenges in individuals with ASD include hypersensitivity (over-sensitivity), hyposensitivity (under-sensitivity), or sensory seeking behaviors (Baum et al., 2015). Individuals with ASD often show hyporesponsiveness to certain stimuli and hyperresponsiveness to other stimuli (Baranek et al., 2008). Research suggests that sensory symptoms might increase as children leave the toddler years and enter into the preschool period (Lord, 1995).

Interestingly, Rogers and colleagues found that sensory impairments are independent of IQ and social-communication skills in young children with ASD. In other words, sensory impairments are not greater in young children with lower IQs or lower social-communication skills (Rogers, Hepburn, & Wehner, 2003).

Individuals with ASD may have a sensory dysfunction that affects any or all of the sensory systems. Although visual processing is often reported as a strength for individuals with ASD, it has been noted to be more challenging when individuals with ASD are viewing more complex visual stimuli. Similarly, individuals with ASD seem to process the details of visual stimuli instead of integrating the details to form a holistic image, or a gestalt (Bertone et al., 2005; Happé & Frith, 2006). Auditory processing in ASD is similar to that of visual processing, such that individuals with ASD seem to process simple auditory information, such as pitch or loudness, with more ease compared to more complex auditory information (e.g., content of a sentence). This has implications for social-communication skills, as language is laden with complex auditory information necessary for successful social interactions (Baum et al., 2015). Tactile processing, although less frequently studied than visual or auditory processing, is often reported to be a sensory challenge in children with ASD (Tomchek & Dunn, 2007). Individuals with ASD may be so hyperresponsive to certain tactile stimuli, such as a tag on a shirt, that they refuse to wear certain clothing. In contrast, individuals with ASD may also be hyporesponsive to tactile stimuli and not be able to feel a light tap on their shoulder (Foss-Feig et al., 2012). Both have implications for positive social connections that often involve physical connections with family members and peers. In addition, olfactory and taste systems are less well studied in ASD, but findings show that individuals with ASD have more food refusals related to texture and consistency, taste and smell, mixtures, brand, and shape than do typically developing individuals (Hubbard et al., 2014) and are less able than typically developing individuals to identify sour and bitter tastes. Individuals with ASD, however, do not seem to demonstrate differences in identifying sweet or salty tastes (Bennetto et al., 2007). In addition to having marked difficulty identifying scents compared to typically developing individuals (Bennetto et al., 2007), persons with ASD find some scents (e.g., cinnamon, pineapple) to be less appealing than do typically developing individuals (Hrdlicka et al., 2010).

Not only do children with ASD demonstrate sensory functioning challenges with the aforementioned senses, but they have difficulty integrating their senses to allow for multisensory processing. Multisensory processing is often found to be impaired even when unisensory performance is intact (Baum et al., 2015). As discussed previously, a process that is inherently multisensory is speech perception. During a conversation, the listener integrates both auditory (speech sounds) and visual information (articulatory movements that accompany the sounds, facial expressions, and gestures) to process speech (Stevenson, Segers, et al., 2014). Whereas simple visual processing is less impaired in children with ASD, during speech perception, there seems to be a disconnect in processing the visual cues associated with sound production. Individuals with ASD may rely on auditory information only and disregard visual information in speech production (Schmalenbach et al., 2017; Stevenson, Siemann, et al., 2014).

Implications for Intervention   Because of the multisensory processing challenges in individuals with ASD, supports should be used that play to the child's intact processing skills and/or areas of strength. Visual skills have been noted to be a strength in individuals with ASD (Grandin, 1995), and supports can be designed that capitalize on these skills. For example, visual supports, including visual schedules, task strips, Social Stories (described in Chapter 16), Comic Strip Conversations (see Gray, 1994, 1998, 2010; Gray & Garand, 1993), and video modeling (described in Chapter 17) offer children with ASD simple visual information to accompany verbal information. Visual supports reduce cognitive overload and can aid in the ability to cognitively and emotionally process events.

CHALLENGES IN JOINT ATTENTION, PLAY, AND THEORY OF MIND

In addition to early communication challenges, children with ASD often demonstrate impairments in joint attention, play, and theory of mind skills. These difficulties also have negative implications for the development and maintenance of social relationships, social connectedness, and educational and community engagement for children with ASD (Hutchins & Prelock, 2014; Müller et al., 2008).

Joint Attention

As mentioned previously and described more fully in Chapter 9, joint attention requires an infant to coordinate attention between an object or event and another person as a means to share interest or awareness of the object (Mundy et al., 1986). Joint attention is more complex than both gaze following and sharing attention (i.e., when an individual references an object and then another person). Joint attention is shared attention in which an individual uses a triadic gaze to first reference an object, then look at another person, and then gaze *back to the object* (Bayliss et al., 2012). For example, when engaging in joint attention, I know that you and I are both looking at and thinking about the same object, and *I know* that *you know* that we are both looking at and thinking about the same object—we are coordinating our attention to an object and to each other (Murray et al., 2008). Joint attention can be present in two ways—initiating joint attention and responding to joint attention bids. *Initiating* joint attention occurs when Individual A directs his gaze to an object as a means to share interest in that object with Individual B. If Individual B notices Individual A's gaze and directs her attention to that object, Individual B has *responded* to a joint attention bid from Individual A (Bayliss et al., 2012; Mundy et al., 2007). Initiating and responding to joint attention typically develop between 6 and 18 months of age (Mundy et al., 2007), and is commonly seen by the time a child is 12 months of age (Dawson et al., 2004; Murray et al., 2008). Joint attention skills provide information on a child's early social cognition skills, including understanding intentionality (Mundy et al., 2007), as well as contribute to a child's concurrent and predictive language abilities, including vocabulary development (McDuffie et al., 2005; Wetherby et al., 2007).

Children with ASD demonstrate impaired joint attention skills and often require explicit teaching in this area (see Chapter 9 on JASPER). Deficits are observed in the ability to both initiate joint attention acts and respond to joint attention bids (Dawson et al., 2004). In preschool-age children, deficits in joint attention often distinguish children with ASD from children with other developmental delays and from their typically developing peers (Dawson et al., 2004). As such, impairments in this area may warrant further assessment of ASD in young children. In addition, children with ASD tend to be more interested in objects than in people, which has implications for the development of joint attention and joint engagement (Adamson et al., 2009). Moreover, deficits in joint attention may contribute to a child's poor receptive and expressive word learning, such that children with ASD may be challenged to follow a communicative partner's attention and thus may "map a novel word to their own focus of attention rather than to the object that is the adult's intended referent" (McDuffie et al., 2005, p. 1081). In other words, children with ASD may learn inappropriate labels of objects because their focus of attention is on something other than what their communication partner is referencing. Murray and colleagues (2008) found that children with ASD who exhibit more responses to an adult's joint attention bids have higher receptive language scores as well as greater utterance lengths.

Play

Play is an integral part of child development that continues throughout one's life. Through play, young children "develop skills, experiment with roles, and interact with others" (Jordan, 2003, p. 349). Although there are many definitions of play, Lifter and colleagues (2011) define play as being spontaneous, naturally occurring, and involving objects of interest. For adults, playing a weekly game of pick-up soccer may be considered play while for adolescents play might involve video games, and for young children, play often occurs with toys. Play can happen in social or solitary settings and may or may not be make-believe (Lifter, Mason, & Barton, 2011). Playing with toys allows children to discover how objects work, both independently and in relation to one another (Lifter et al., 2011), which further provides them with an understanding of their surroundings and insight into how objects in the world work (Prelock, 2006).

In an attempt to fully describe the different aspects of play, researchers have categorized play along 14 levels (Freeman & Kasari, 2013; Kasari et al., 2006; Lifter et al., 1988), which can be divided into four broader phases of play. These types of play skills are considered cognitive play skills in that, as children develop cognitively, their play skills also become more complex. It is important to note that while stages of cognitive play are categorized hierarchically, it is not necessarily the case that once higher levels of cognitive play are achieved, lower levels cease to occur. Depending on the objects, the context, and the individuals' motivation, each level of cognitive play can occur throughout an individual's life (Jordan, 2003). The following list provides the order in which these play skills typically develop:

1. Simple manipulation of objects and relational play

   • Child explores physical properties of object (e.g., bangs a wooden spoon)

2. Combination play

   • Child starts combining objects and using objects with one another (e.g., stacks one block on another)

3. Functional play

   • Child directly acts on objects, dolls, self, or caregivers in play (e.g., hugs a doll)

4. Symbolic/imaginative/pretend play

   • Child uses objects in an imaginative way and in a sequence of events (e.g., pretends to give the baby a bottle and then puts the baby to bed)

Symbolic play has been described as the ability to believe, expect, and manipulate relationships with others (Mastrangelo, 2009). Considering this definition of symbolic play, it is evident that this level of play has implications for children's ability to take perspectives that are different from their own and employ theory of mind skills (theory of mind is discussed in more detail below). As children begin to shift from solitary play to social play, they begin to experience elements that are important in successful social interactions, such as sharing, turn taking, and being a participant in reciprocal conversations.

Social play develops alongside cognitive levels of play, and because play can occur with or without others, social play is a particularly interesting topic when considering children who have challenges with social interactions. Parten (1933) identified stages of social play that are used to describe play interactions, and like cognitive levels of play, each level of social play can occur throughout an individual's life (Jordan, 2003). These types of social play are described below (Gordon Biddle et al., 2014).

1. Solitary play

    • Children play by themselves with their own set of toys without acknowledging others or making any attempts to play with others. Young children engage in this type of play typically until they are 2½ years old.

2. Parallel play

    • Children are still playing by themselves and with their own set of toys but are now sitting near other children who are playing with similar toys. Although children engaged in parallel play are not interacting with others, they are aware of the other children playing around them. This type of play typically occurs between 2½ and 3½ years of age.

3. Associative play

    • At this stage of play, children begin playing with others, including sharing toys. They tend to play in small groups and stick with the group when moving on to other play activities. This type of play typically occurs at approximately 3½ years of age.

4. Cooperative play

    • This is the highest level of social play in which children begin to take on assigned roles in their group to complete a common goal (e.g., when playing house, one child must be the caregiver, one must be the baby, and one must be the big sister or brother). Children engaging in cooperative play often negotiate roles or ideas. This type of play typically emerges at approximately 4½ years of age.

Social play is an important avenue for children to develop friendships. Through this type of play, children learn about developing and maintaining trust, cooperating and negotiating with others, practicing the values of their specific culture and that of their peers, and developing a strong connection to their peers (Jordan, 2003). In essence, play is fundamental to building and maintaining peer relationships as well as to learning how social relationships work in the world.

Young children with ASD experience deficits in many areas of play compared to typically developing children (Mastangelo, 2009). Children with ASD often prefer solitary play over social play or playing near others (Locke et al., 2016). These children have been described as engaging in exploratory play involving the simple manipulation of objects, but they tend to explore the objects to a lesser extent than do typically developing peers. In addition, when children with ASD explore toys, they often engage in behaviors that are restricted and repetitive (e.g., waving a toy back and forth in front of their face; lining up cars in a specific order or by color; Mastrangelo, 2009). Relational play is a challenge, as the restricted and repetitive behaviors of children with ASD may make it difficult for them to learn the appropriate meaning and functions of toys and objects (Mastrangelo, 2009). Because functional play with objects offers an opportunity to learn about a child's surroundings and how objects in the world work, lack of functional play in children with ASD may compromise their ability to understand their environment.

Deficits in social play are widely observed in young children with ASD, and these deficits have implications for functional and symbolic play (Jordan, 2003). Many of the challenges observed in both cognitive and social play can be attributed to impairments in social communication, restricted and/or repetitive behaviors, and social awareness deficits in ASD (APA, 2013). Evidence suggests that children with ASD do engage in symbolic play when they are given appropriate structure and are explicitly taught. Consequently, the symbolic play of children with ASD may appear less "play-like" and less natural compared to children who are typically developing (Jordan, 2003; Manning & Wainwright, 2010). Challenges with more natural and novel symbolic play have been associated with difficulties relating to abstract thinking and expression of symbolic ideas (Mastrangelo, 2009). Because of the limitations in both cognitive and social play, children with ASD frequently avoid certain play scenarios and thus miss out on the social experiences associated with them (Manning & Wainwright, 2010).

Theory of Mind

Defined broadly, **theory of mind** is the ability to understand that others have thoughts, beliefs, feelings, and perspectives that are different from one's own. Traditionally, theory of mind has been measured through standard false-belief tasks. For example, in the classic Sally and Anne task using dolls, puppets, or a visual image, Sally places a marble in a box and then leaves the room. Anne comes in and moves the marble from the box to a basket and then leaves. When Sally returns, the child is asked, "Where will Sally look for her marble?" If the child indicates the box where Sally had put the marble, then he passes the question and it is inferred that the child has taken on Sally's false belief about the marble. If the child indicates that Sally will look for the marble in the basket where Anne put it, the child fails the question and is not able to take Sally's false belief about the marble (Baron-Cohen et al., 1985). While attributing false beliefs to others is certainly an aspect of theory of mind, theory of mind is a complex and multifaceted construct that comprises many social-cognitive skills that vary in developmental level (Hutchins & Prelock, 2016).

A number of approaches have been put forth to describe theory of mind. These include differentiating between cognitive and affective theory of mind (Dvash & Shamay-Tsoory, 2014; Westby & Robinson, 2014); interpersonal and intrapersonal theory of mind (Dvash & Shamay-Tsoory, 2014; Westby & Robinson, 2014); and early, basic, and advanced theory of mind (Hutchins & Prelock, 2014). These approaches are not mutually exclusive but offer a number of ways to think about the complexities associated with theory of mind. Cognitive theory of mind includes "thinking about thoughts, knowledge, beliefs, and intentions of others," whereas affective theory of mind involves "thinking about and experiencing the emotions of others" (Westby & Robinson, 2014, p. 363). Interpersonal theory of mind has been described as thinking about the thoughts of others, whereas intrapersonal theory of mind includes thinking about one's own thoughts or feelings (Westby & Robinson, 2014). Hutchins and colleagues take a developmental approach to understanding theory of mind and consider three distinct levels: early, basic, and advanced theory of mind (Hutchins & Prelock, 2016; Hutchins et al., 2012). This developmental framework was established on the basis of findings from the validation of the Theory of Mind Inventory–2 (Hutchins & Prelock, 2016; Hutchins et al., 2012), which is a caregiver report measure that captures the complexities of theory of mind throughout development. The skills associated with early, basic, and advanced theory of mind are offered in Table 3.1.

It is well established that children with ASD have a core deficit in theory of mind skills. Baron-Cohen and colleagues first described theory of mind challenges in children with ASD using a standard false-belief task (Baron-Cohen et al., 1985). Since then, it has been documented that individuals with ASD show marked impairments in all aspects of theory of mind compared to typically developing children (Hutchins et al., 2012; Hutchins et al., 2016). Challenges employing theory of mind

Table 3.1.   Theory of mind constructs

Early subscale (typically developed in toddlers)	Basic subscale (typically developed in children by age 4)	Advanced subscale (typically developed by age 8)
Early empathy	Physiologically based behavior	Second-order false desire attribution
Discrimination of basic emotions	Emotion-based behavior	Pragmatics: deception by others
Intentionality	Mental state term comprehension: cognitive term (think)	Display rules
Basic positive emotion recognition (happy)	False belief (change location)	Visual perspective-taking (level 2)
Basic negative emotion recognition (sad)	Seeing-leads-to-knowing	Second-order understanding of belief
Basic negative emotion recognition (mad)	Mental state term comprehension: cognitive term (know)	Second-order understanding of emotion
Basic negative emotion recognition (scared)	Appearance–reality distinction	True empathy
Mental state term comprehension: early desire (want)	False belief (unexpected contents)	Interpretive theory of mind: biased cognition
Desire-based emotion	Certainty	Interpretive theory of mind: ambiguous figure perception
	The mental–physical distinction	Mixed emotions
	Counterfactual reasoning	Common sense: social knowledge
	Tactical deception	Complex emotion recognition (embarrassed)
	Cognitive emotion recognition (disgust)	Complex emotion recognition (guilt)
	Promises	Emotional introspection
	Mental state term comprehension: cognitive term (believe)	Situation-based disambiguation of emotion
	Cognitive emotion recognition (surprise)	
	Mental state term comprehension: desire (need)	
	Future thinking	
	Belief-based emotion	

From Hutchins, T. L., & Prelock, P. A. (2016). *Technical Manual for the Theory of Mind Inventory-2.* Adapted by permission.

impact an individual's ability to develop and maintain social relationships. That is, engaging in social relationships requires an individual to possess many theory of mind skills, including (but not limited to) identifying and responding to others' emotions; adjusting behaviors in a given context or experience (i.e., display rules); understanding promises, jokes, and lies; taking others' perspectives; considering others' interests when they differ from one's own; and employing common sense about social experiences. The following are examples of what impairments in theory of mind might look like for a young child with ASD, an older child with ASD, and an adolescent/adult with ASD:

Example for a young child: Jackie, a 4-year-old child with ASD, is in her preschool classroom. All the children are playing. Kameron, a 3-year-old preschooler, is playing with the racetrack and the red race car. Jackie's favorite color is red, and she only plays with the red car. She spots Kameron with the car, runs over, and snatches it out of his hand. She goes back to her spot in the room and rolls the car back and forth by herself. She does not notice that she accidently knocked Sadie over on her way to Kameron or that both Sadie and Kameron are crying.

Analysis: In this example, Jackie does not demonstrate awareness of Kameron's perspective when she takes the car. She does not ask to have a turn or understand that he might be sad if she takes the car. She also does not notice that she knocked Sadie over, nor does she respond to either Sadie's or Kameron's crying. Because she takes the car and plays with it by herself, other children might be discouraged from playing with her. Other children might think that Jackie is mean because she made Kameron and Sadie cry and that she does not seem to care about their feelings. As a result of this and similar recurring behaviors, other children might not invite Jackie to play with them in the future because she only wants to play with the red car and will take it without asking.

Example for an older child: Carlos, a 12-year-old with ASD, is talking to his classmate, Maria, about the newest *Legend of Zelda* video game. He describes in detail how he beat a level last night and goes on to describe each characters' strengths and weaknesses. He does not ask Maria if she has ever played *Zelda* or if she knows the game at all. He is not aware that she looks uninterested in the conversation, and he gets up and walks with her when she starts to walk away from him. Finally, Maria tells Carlos that she has to go because she is getting picked up from school early, which is a lie. Later in the day, at recess time, Carlos sees Maria and reminds her that she was supposed to get picked up early. She responds by saying, "Uhhh . . . my appointment got canceled, so my mom didn't pick me up." Carlos accepts this lie as truth and begins talking about *Zelda* again. He is not aware that Maria is still not interested in talking to him about *Zelda*. He does not ask Maria about her interests and does not leave room in the conversation for her to chime in.

Analysis: In this example, Carlos is unable to read Maria's body cues that portray her disinterest in his topic. His conversation is not reciprocal; he never asks her about her interests or provides her with the opportunity to ask questions about *Zelda*. Carlos does not understand Maria's white lie to remove herself from the conversation, even when he sees Maria later in the day. Because of Carlos's perseverative talk about *Zelda* and his inability to engage Maria in a reciprocal conversation that was of interest to them both, Maria may decide that she does not want to talk to Carlos and may avoid him in the future. Carlos, unaware of Maria's thoughts and feelings, may be left confused about why she seems to leave the area whenever he is present.

Example for an adolescent/adult: Patrick is a 19-year-old college student with ASD. He is majoring in engineering and living in a dorm suite with three other male students. In the shared suite bathroom, Patrick has his toiletries sprawled out on the sink counter and in the shower. There isn't much room for his roommates' toiletries. Patrick studies late into the night in his dorm room, which he shares with Paul. Because Patrick leaves the overhead light on to study, Paul is unable to fall asleep, so he often sleeps on the couch in the common suite area. In the past, when Paul has asked Patrick to use his desk lamp instead of the overhead lamp to study at night, Patrick has indicated that his desk lamp is not strong enough and that he needs the overhead light to really see. In class, Patrick contributes intelligent ideas but often goes off topic. After receiving the midterm test scores, all of the students in the class look disappointed and make comments indicating they did poorly on the test. Patrick, who got an A, exclaims that the test was not hard at all and that he got an A on it. When the professor offers to let the students leave class 30 minutes early on the first nice day of spring, Patrick raises his hand and begins talking about a new topic.

Analysis: In this example, Patrick does not seem to have a social common sense understanding of living in a shared space; he is unaware that his roommates have no space in the bathroom for their toiletries because his belongings are everywhere. Similarly, Patrick is unaware that his late-night study habits are affecting his roommate, Paul. He does not consider Paul's perspective when Paul asks him to use his desk lamp instead of the overhead light, nor does he understand Paul's subtle social cue or make the connection that Paul is sleeping on the couch because he cannot sleep with the overhead light on. In class, Patrick is unable to use appropriate display rules when he exclaims his success on the test while others are disappointed with their grades, nor does he use social common sense when his classmates and professor are ready to leave class early on a nice spring day. These challenges in social common sense, display rules, and perspective taking during adolescent/adult years affect Patrick's ability to develop and maintain true, meaningful peer relationships; Paul may not want to be his roommate in the future, and classmates may become annoyed and frustrated at Patrick's interactions.

These three examples highlight just a few ways in which theory of mind deficits may manifest in individuals with ASD from early childhood to adulthood. For Jackie, her lack of understanding about the social rules for sharing interfere with her ability to develop successful early peer interactions during play. Carlos's tendency to talk about his own ideas and understanding of things he knows interferes with his ability to recognize the perspective of others and how they might be thinking or feeling about a particular topic. Finally, Patrick lacks an ability to recognize the impact of his behavior on others. Each of these examples demonstrates areas of challenge in theory of mind development from joint attention and sharing to perspective taking of self and others and recognizing the impact of one's behavior on another.

SYNTACTIC, SEMANTIC, PHONOLOGICAL, AND PRAGMATIC LANGUAGE DEVELOPMENT

Thus far, the chapter has described the early communication challenges in children with ASD, including prelinguistic skills and word learning. It has also discussed how these challenges contribute to later language and communication skills. Because there is large heterogeneity found across the autism spectrum, and language skills are variable within this population, this section aims to review the syntactic, semantic, phonological, and pragmatic language characteristics that are common in individuals with ASD. Although a portion of individuals with ASD remain nonverbal throughout their life, the majority of children with ASD learn and use at least some verbal speech (Paul et al., 2018). As you read about the syntactic, semantic, phonological, and pragmatic language challenges in children with ASD, you will notice that development of these aspects of language are influenced by the overall language skills of the child, including a comorbid diagnosis of language impairment.

Syntactic and Morphological Skills

Syntax refers to the grammatical arrangement of words in a sentence, while morphology refers to the grammar of individual words. For example, subject–verb agreement or word order in a sentence would be considered syntax, whereas adding /s/ to a word to make it plural or -*ing* to make it present progressive would be considered morphology. Findings indicate that children with ASD tend to produce sentences that are shorter and grammatically simpler compared to typically developing peers (Eigsti et al., 2007; Losh & Capps, 2003). Children with ASD who also have a comorbid language disorder demonstrate difficulties marking third-person regular tense and past-tense verbs, specifically omitting these tense-marking morphemes. Interestingly, children with ASD may use a present-progressive verb (e.g., jump*ing*) when the appropriate verb form is past tense (Roberts et al., 2004). For example, when talking about a visit to camp yesterday, a child with ASD may say, "I playing with the ball," when what he really means to say is, "I played with the ball." Some researchers have found that syntax is not impaired in all individuals with ASD (Colle et al., 2008; Modyanova et al., 2017; Roberts et al., 2004), but some evidence suggests that children with ASD and a comorbid language impairment present with syntactic deficits (Tager-Flusberg, 2015).

Semantic Skills

Semantic skills involve the meaning of words, phrases, and sentences. Many individuals with ASD have atypical semantic skills. Specifically, Happé (1997) found that children with ASD may not use the context of a sentence to determine the appropriate word meaning of a homonym (e.g., there was a *tear* in her eye/there was a *tear* in her dress) when reading. She also found that children with ASD are less likely than typically developing children to self-correct their pronunciation of the homonym after they complete reading the sentence. Studies using electroencephalogram (EEG) provide further information on the semantic skills of individuals with ASD. When typically developing individuals read or are shown a stimulus word, their brains are primed for other words that are related to the target word. Thus, a priming effect occurs when one stimulus (e.g., the word *dog*) influences a response to the second stimulus (e.g., the word *cat*). When shown a stimulus word (e.g., *dog*) followed by a semantically dissimilar word (e.g., *cup;* an unexpected word pair), the brain of a typically developing individual is surprised, and a high N400 response is elicited (Coderre et al., 2017). For the purpose of understanding priming effects, various event-related potentials (ERPs) are associated with cognitive functioning. Specifically, the N400 ERP has been shown to be related to the cognitive function of semantic processing and semantic integration (Lau et al., 2008). Individuals with ASD do not show the same priming effect as those who are typically developing.

When presented with semantically dissimilar words, individuals with ASD do not demonstrate an N400 response, suggesting that the brain is not detecting these semantic incongruities (McCleery et al., 2010). More evidence of semantic challenges occurs with the use of pronouns. Children with ASD tend to produce pronoun reversals more than do typically developing children, and this has been found to occur slightly more in imitative contexts (Naigles et al., 2016). Consider the following example in which a child with ASD and an adult are playing with dolls:

Adult: I want to be the mommy doll. Who do you want to be?

Child: You want the baby doll. [grabs the baby doll for herself]

Phonological Skills

It has been documented that children with ASD generally have intact phonology/ articulation skills (Colle et al., 2008; Kjelgaard & Tager-Flusberg, 2001); however, Shriberg and colleagues (2001) noted residual speech sound errors in adults with ASD at a higher rate than is observed in the typically developing adult population. Deficits in phonological processing have also been observed in ASD. Individuals with ASD have been noted to have challenges in repetition of nonsense words (Kjelgaard & Tager-Flusberg, 2001), blending syllables and phonemes into words, isolating and manipulating phonemes in words (Gabig, 2010), and using voicing patterns (Shriberg et al., 2001).

Pragmatic Language Skills

Pragmatic language is defined as using language in a social manner to communicate (Eigsti et al., 2007). Deficits in pragmatic language are widely documented in individuals with ASD. Specific pragmatic impairments include using fewer communicative functions (Wetherby et al., 1998) and difficulties taking turns during conversations; maintaining topics of conversation; following a communication partner's topic; and providing new information by challenging ideas, expanding upon ideas, or contributing related ideas (Tager-Flusberg & Anderson, 1991).

Another well-documented pragmatic difference in individuals with ASD is their use of prosody (Shriberg et al., 2001). Prosody refers to the intonation, stress, tone, and rhythm of speech. Individuals with ASD often have abnormal prosody and also have challenges interpreting how prosody can affect word meaning (Horie & Okamura, 2017). For example, if I were to say, "Doing the dishes is fun," in a flat and monotonous voice, an individual with ASD may miss my prosodic cues and interpret my message literally. I should not be surprised, then, if the next day, the individual with ASD is dirtying many dishes just so that I can partake in the "fun" task of washing them. Similarly, individuals with ASD have challenges understanding nonliteral language, where the literal meaning of the word or phrase is different from the speaker's intended meaning. Of note, those with ASD may have deficits in understanding the speaker's intent when that person is speaking in hyperbole (extreme exaggeration), using verbal irony, or using metonymy (i.e., a figure of speech in which a part stands for the whole), and difficulty recognizing understatements when dealing with time or quantity (MacKay & Shaw, 2004). Individuals with ASD also have difficulty understanding figurative language, including metaphors and idioms (Norbury, 2010; Whyte et al., 2014), as well as understanding lies, jokes (Leekam & Prior, 1994), and deception (Dennis et al., 2000). Deficits in understanding certain aspects of figurative language, however, may be tied to lower language abilities and may not be ASD specific (Kalandadze et al., 2018; Norbury, 2010; Whyte & Nelson, 2015). Table 3.2 (adapted and expanded upon from MacKay & Shaw, 2004) offers examples of nonliteral language.

Narrative discourse is an important part of pragmatic language in that it is "an essential mechanism for making sense of experiences and relationships" (Losh & Capps, 2003, p. 239). We tell stories to share our experiences with one another as well as to process the world around us. Narrative discourse abilities are impaired in children and adults with ASD. In particular, individuals with ASD tell less organized narratives containing sentences that do not flow well (Colle et al., 2008), understand and use fewer mental-state terms (Barnes & Baron-Cohen, 2012; Whyte & Nelson, 2015), and often do not adjust their speech to the conversation partner (Baron-Cohen, 1988). For example, a child with ASD may not differentiate between the way that he speaks to his little brother and the way he speaks to his teacher, and an adult with ASD may speak to her spouse in the same way that she speaks to her boss. Similarly, when telling personal narratives, children with ASD may make irrelevant comments and require prompts to clarify ambiguous information (Losh & Capps, 2003). In addition, individuals with ASD tend to focus on the details of a story rather than on the bigger picture. Barnes and Baron-Cohen (2012) describe that during a story retelling, typically developing individuals state the specific setting of a story (e.g., in a classroom), whereas individuals with ASD describe the setting more locally, focusing on specific details (e.g., describing the objects on the teacher's desk, what was written on the chalkboard). It has been suggested that this could be due to an inability to take the perspective of a listener who is unfamiliar

Table 3.2. Types of nonliteral language

Type of nonliteral language	Description	Example	Intended meaning
Hyperbole	Extreme exaggeration	"I have a million books."	I have a *lot* of books.
Verbal irony	Literal meaning is opposite of the intended meaning	"I am so excited to do my taxes this year."	I am *not* excited to do my taxes.
Metonymy	Quick and efficient labeling	Waiter 1: "Who ordered the chicken cordon bleu?" Waiter 2: "The yellow shirt at table 5."	Waiter 2: The *woman* in the yellow shirt at table 5.
Understatements	Underplaying an actual event	A person who solely prepared Thanksgiving dinner: "Oh, it was nothing; it didn't take long."	It is no big deal, but it actually took a really long time to prepare.
Metaphors	Comparison of one object or event to another	"She is as beautiful as a rose."	She is *very* beautiful.
Idioms	A phrase whose meaning is not inherent in the individual words	"It's raining cats and dogs."	It's raining really hard.

Source: MacKay & Shaw (2004).

with the story, difficulties planning and organizing the story, or challenges with processing information at a more global level.

Implications for Intervention

As described in the DSM-5, language disorders in ASD are not universal, but language should be assessed in all children with a diagnosis of ASD. Intervention builds on what is learned from assessment, so a comprehensive language evaluation is a critical element of the assessment process. Increasing overall functioning should be a treatment priority. For example, a preschool child with low cognitive skills and high ASD severity may demonstrate challenges in joint attention, using gestures, turn taking, articulation, and syntactic and semantic skills. Certainly, targeting all areas of deficit at one time is unrealistic, and great care should be taken to determine which areas of need are most crucial to the child's current level of functioning. In this example, although addressing articulation skills would increase the child's intelligibility, it may be most functional to work on skills that increase the child's ability to see others as communication partners and/or engage in reciprocal communicative turns with others.

EVIDENCE-BASED PRACTICES: ENGAGING FAMILIES AND TEAMS

The most effective evidence-based practices are those that have a collaborative, interdisciplinary team-based approach that is both family centered and strengths based. The literature tells us that families of children with ASD experience social isolation and chronic stress and are often surrounded by those who have little understanding of autism (Beatson & Prelock, 2002; Dillenburger et al., 2010; Hastings, 2008; Montes et al., 2009; Woodgate et al., 2008). Notably, some families of children with ASD are highly resilient and appear to gain strength from the struggles they experience (King et al., 2009), whereas others describe less positive experiences supporting their children with ASD (Blacher & McIntyre, 2006; Myers et al., 2009). Strong professional–family partnerships, however, where parents have access to needed resources, feel connected, and have social supports in place, can mediate the challenges of raising a child with ASD (Bayat, 2007; Pottie et al., 2008; Twoy et al., 2007). Engaging families in intervention planning and implementation is critical, as they often experience feelings of loss and grief when their child first receives a diagnosis of ASD (Fernández-Alcántara et al., 2016). Further, using a strengths-based approach in which available family resources are considered and built upon will most likely maximize a child's progress (Prelock & Hutchins, 2008). Parent input, knowledge, and ability to foster an environment in which a child can generalize skills is imperative to the child's development of social, emotional, communicative, and daily living skills (Vismara & Rogers, 2010).

Best practices highlight the crucial role families have as members of the intervention team. When providers recognize this priority, goals are more likely to be achieved (Prelock & Hutchins, 2008). Moreover, interdisciplinary teams with professionals from many disciplines who work together, share ideas, and offer support are more likely to include families and ensure a family-centered approach to intervention.

Importantly, parent-mediated instruction and intervention (PMII) has recently been determined to be an evidence-based practice for children with ASD (Oono et al., 2013; Wong et al., 2014). A number of studies report on the positive impacts of parent-mediated intervention, including increases in a child's social engagement (Kasari et al., 2010) and their language and social-communication skills (Coolican et al., 2010; Pickles et al., 2016). As you read the intervention chapters that follow, it will be important to reflect on those interventions that capitalize on the role of the family and the power of working as a collaborative, interdisciplinary team. Several of the interventions discussed (e.g., augmentative and alternative communication, the Early Start Denver Model [Rogers & Dawson, 2010], DIR/Floortime [Greenspan & Wieder, 1998], joint attention training, Enhanced Milieu Teaching, early social interaction project [Wetherby & Woods, 2006; Woods & Wetherby, 2003], Pivotal Response Treatment [Koegel & Koegel, 2006], Social Stories [Gray, 2010], SCERTS [Prizant et al., 2003; Prizant et al., 2004]) highlight the importance of families and working as a team as central to a child's progress.

Also important for consideration is understanding the research that supports the interventions selected to support the language and communication of children with ASD. Chapter authors describe the empirical basis for each intervention and offer the key ingredients or components for the intervention with clear applications to practice. Several interventions have a strong research base for supporting language and communication in ASD (e.g., functional communication training, pivotal response training, video modeling). Notably, however, a variety of established and emerging evidence-based interventions for individuals with ASD are used variably in practice and may not always be appropriately implemented in intervention settings (Dingfelder & Mandell, 2011). Barriers associated with the transition from efficacy intervention research to effective implementation often lies in the discontinuity among terminology, goals, and values of scientists doing the research and providers implementing the intervention. Researchers typically examine functioning in a controlled environment (i.e., efficacy trials), whereas clinicians usually provide services in a more natural real-world environment (i.e., effectiveness trials; Cascio et al., 2016; Dingfelder & Mandell, 2011). Added challenges when implementing evidence-based interventions in educational settings include the complexities of the population of children requiring intervention, funding for the intervention, training for providers, and having clarity on intervention outcomes (Dingfelder & Mandell, 2011).

REFERENCES

Adamson, L., Deckner, D., & Bakeman, R. (2009). Early interests and joint engagement in typical development, autism, and Down syndrome. *Journal of Autism and Developmental Disorders, 40*(6), 665–676.

American Psychiatric Association. (2013). *Diagnostic and statistical manual of mental disorders, 5th edition (DSM-5)*. Author.

Baranek, G., Wakeford, L., & David, F. (2008). Understanding, assessing, and treating sensory-motor issues. In K. Chawarska, A. Klin, & F. R. Volkmar (Eds.), *Autism spectrum disorders in infants and toddlers: Diagnosis, assessment, and treatment* (pp. 104–140). Guilford Press.

Barbaro, J., & Dissanayake, C. (2009). Autism spectrum disorders in infancy and toddlerhood: A review of the evidence on early signs, early identification tools, and early diagnosis. *Journal of Developmental and Behavioral Pediatrics, 30*(5), 447–459.

Barnes, J., & Baron-Cohen, S. (2012). The big picture: Storytelling abilities in adults with autism spectrum conditions. *Journal of Autism and Developmental Disorders, 42*, 1557–1565.

Baron-Cohen, S. (1988). Social and pragmatic deficits in autism: Cognitive or affective? *Journal of Autism and Developmental Disorders, 18*(3), 379–402.

Baron-Cohen, S., Leslie, A., & Frith, U. (1985). Does the autistic child have a "theory of mind"? *Cognition, 21*, 37–46.

Bates, E., Camaioni, L., & Volterra, V. (1975). The acquisition of performatives prior to speech. *Merrill-Palmer Quarterly, 21*, 205–226.

Baum, S., Stevenson, R., & Wallace, M. (2015). Behavioral, perceptual, and neural alterations in sensory and multisensory function in autism spectrum disorder. *Progress in Neurobiology, 134*, 140–160.

Bayat, M. (2007). Evidence of resilience in families of children with autism. *Journal of Intellectual Disability Research, 51*(9), 702–714.

Bayliss, A., Murphy, E., Naughtin, C., Kritikos, A., Schilbach, L., & Beker, S. (2012). "Gaze leading": Initiating simulated joint attention influences eye movements and choice behavior. *Journal of Experimental Psychology: General, 142*(1), 76–92.

Beatson, J. E., & Prelock, P. A. (2002). The Vermont Rural Autism Project: Sharing experiences, shifting attitudes. *Focus on Autism & Other Developmental Disabilities, 17*(1), 48–54.

Beker, S., Foxe, J., & Molholm, S. (2018). Ripe for solution: Delayed development of multisensory processing in autism and its remediation. *Neuroscience and Biobehavioral Reviews, 84*, 182–192.

Benedict, H. (1979). Early lexical development: Comprehension and production. *Journal of Child Language, 6*(2), 183–200.

Bennetto, L., Kuschner, E., & Hyman, S. (2007). Olfaction and taste processing in autism. *Biological Psychiatry, 62*(9), 1051–1021.

Bertone, A., Mottron, L., Jelenic, P., & Faubert, J. (2005). Enhanced and diminished visuospatial information processing in autism depends on stimulus complexity. *Brain, 128*(10), 2430–2441.

Blacher, J., & McIntyre, L. L. (2006). Syndrome specificity and behavioral disorders in young adults with intellectual disability: Cultural differences in family impact. *Journal of Intellectual Disability Research, 50*(3), 184–198.

Capone, N., & McGregor, K. (2004). Gesture development: A review for clinical and research practices. *Journal of Speech, Language, and Hearing Research, 47*, 173–187.

Cascio, C., Woynaroski, T., Baranek, G., & Wallace, M. (2016). Toward an interdisciplinary approach to understanding sensory function in autism spectrum disorder. *Autism Research, 9*(9), 920–925.

Chapman, R. (2000). Children's language learning: An interactionist perspective. *Journal of Child Psychology and Psychiatry, 41*, 33–54.

Coderre, E., Chernenok, M., Gordon, B., & Ledoux, K. (2017). Linguistic and non-linguistic semantic processing in individuals with autism spectrum disorders: An ERP study. *Journal of Autism and Developmental Disabilities, 47*(3), 795–812.

Colle, L., Baron-Cohen, S., Wheelwright, S., & van der Lely, H. (2008). Narrative discourse in adults with high-functioning autism or Asperger syndrome. *Journal of Autism and Developmental Disorders, 38*, 28–40.

Coolican, J., Smith, I., & Bryson, S. (2010). Brief parent training in pivotal response treatment for preschoolers with autism. *Journal of Child Psychology and Psychiatry, 51*(12), 1321–1330.

Crais, E., Watson, L., & Baranek, G. (2009). Use of gesture development in profiling children's prelinguistic communication skills. *American Journal of Speech-Language Pathology, 18*(1), 95–108.

Davidson, M., & Weismer, S. (2017). A discrepancy in comprehension and production in early language development in ASD: Is it clinically relevant? *Journal of Autism and Developmental Disorders, 47*, 2163–2175.

Dawson, G., Toth, K., Abbott, R., Osterling, J., Munson, J., Estes, A., & Liaw, J. (2004). Early social attention impairments in autism: Social orienting, joint attention, and attention to distress. *Developmental Psychology, 40*(2), 271–283.

De Giacomo, A., Portoghese, C., Martinelli, D., Fanizza, I., L'Abate, L., & Margari, L. (2009). Imitation and communication skills development in children with pervasive developmental disorders. *Neuropsychiatric Disease and Treatment, 5*, 355–362.

Dennis, M., Lockyer, L., & Lazenby, A. (2000). How high-functioning children with autism understand real and deceptive emotion. *Autism, 4*(4), 370–381.

Dillenburger, K., Keenan, M., Doherty, A., Byrne, T., & Gallagher, S. (2010). Living with children diagnosed with autistic spectrum disorder: Parental and professional views. *British Journal of Special Education, 37*(1), 13–23.

Dingfelder, H., & Mandell, D. (2011). Bridging the research-to-practice gap in autism intervention: An application of diffusion of innovation theory. *Journal of Autism and Developmental Disabilities, 41,* 597–609.

Dvash, J., & Shamay-Tsoory, S. (2014). Theory of mind and empathy as multidimensional constructs: Neurological foundations. *Topics in Language Disorders, 34*(4), 282–295.

Eigsti, I., Bennotto, L., & Dadlani, M. (2007). Beyond pragmatics: Morphosyntactic development in autism. *Journal of Autism and Developmental Disorders, 37*(6), 1007–1023.

Ellawadi, A., & Weismer, S. (2014). Assessing gestures in young children with autism spectrum disorder. *Journal of Speech, Language, and Hearing Research, 57,* 524–531.

Fernández-Alcántara, M., Garcia-Caro, M., Pérez-Marfil, M., Hueso-Montoro, C., Laynez-Rubio, C., & Cruz-Quintana, F. (2016). Feelings of loss and grief in parents of children diagnosed with autism spectrum disorder (ASD). *Research in Developmental Disabilities, 55,* 312–321.

Foss-Feig, J., Heacock, J., & Cascio, C. (2012). Tactile responsiveness patterns and their association with core features in autism spectrum disorders. *Research in Autism Spectrum Disorders, 6*(1), 337–344.

Freeman, A., & Kasari, C. (2013). Parent-child interactions in autism: Characteristics of play. *Autism, 17*(2), 147–161.

Friedlander, B. (1970). Receptive language development in infancy: Issues and problems. *Merrill-Palmer Quarterly of Behavior and Development, 16*(1), 7–51.

Gabig, C. (2010). Phonological awareness and word recognition in reading by children with autism. *Communication Disorders Quarterly, 31*(2), 67–85.

Goodwyn, S. W., & Acredolo, L. P. (1993). Symbolic gesture versus word: Is there a modality advantage for onset of symbol use. *Child Development, 64*(3), 688–701.

Goodwyn, S. W., Acredolo, L. P., & Brown, C. A. (2000). Impact of symbolic gesturing on early language development. *Journal of Nonverbal Behavior, 24* (2), 81–103.

Gordon Biddle, K., Garcia-Navarez, A., Roundtree Henderson, W., & Valero-Kerrick, A. (2014). *Early childhood education: Becoming a professional* (pp. 256–285). Sage Publications.

Grandin, T. (1995). *Thinking in pictures: My life with autism.* Vintage Books.

Gray, C. (1994). *Comic Strip Conversations.* Future Horizons.

Gray, C. (1998). Social stories and comic strip conversations with students with Asperger syndrome and high-functioning autism. In E. Schopler (Ed.), *Asperger syndrome or high functioning autism?* (pp. 167–194). Plenum Press.

Gray, C. (2010). *The new social story book.* Future Horizons.

Gray, C., & Garand, J. (1993). Social stories: Improving responses of students with autism with inaccurate social information. *Focus Autistic Behavior, 8,* 1–10.

Greenspan, S., & Wieder, S. (1998). *The child with special needs: Encouraging intellectual and emotional growth.* Perseus Books.

Happé, F. (1997). Central coherence and theory of mind in autism: Reading homographs in context. *British Journal of Developmental Psychology, 15,* 1–12.

Happé, F., & Frith, U. (2006). The weak coherence account: Detail-focused cognitive style in autism spectrum disorders. *Journal of Autism and Developmental Disabilities, 36*(1), 5–25.

Harris, S. (2017). Early motor delays as diagnostic clues in autism spectrum disorder. *European Journal of Pediatrics, 176,* 1259–1262.

Hastings, R. P. (2008). Stress in parents of children with autism. In E. McGregor, M. Nunez, K. Cebula, & J. C. Gomez (Eds.), *Autism: An integrated view from neurocognitive, clinical, and intervention research* (pp. 303–324). Blackwell Publishing.

Horie, M., & Okamura, H. (2017). Exploring a method for evaluation of preschool and school children with autism spectrum disorder through checking their understanding of the speaker's emotions with the help of prosody of the voice. *Brain Development, 39*(1), 836–845.

Horner, R., Carr, E., Strain, P., Tood, A., & Reed, H. (2002). Problem behavior interventions for young children with autism: A research synthesis. *Journal of Autism and Developmental Disorders, 32*(5), 423–446.

Hrdlicka, M., Vodicka, J., Havlovicova, M., Urbanek, T., Baltny, M., & Dudova, I. (2010). Brief report: Significant differences in perceived pleasantness found in children with ASD. *Journal of Autism and Developmental Disorders, 41*(4), 524–527.

Hubbard, K., Anderson, S., Curtin, C., Must, A., & Bandini, L. (2014). A comparison of food refusal related to characteristics of food in children with autism spectrum disorder and typically developing children. *Journal of the Academy of Nutrition and Dietetics, 114*(12), 1981–1987.

Hutchins, T. L., & Prelock, P. A. (2016). Technical manual for the Theory of Mind Inventory–2. Copyrighted manuscript. https://www.theoryofmindinventory.com

Hutchins, T., & Prelock, P. (2014). Using communication to reduce challenging behaviors in individuals with autism spectrum disorders and intellectual disability. *Child and Adolescent Psychiatric Clinics of North America, 23*, 41–55.

Hutchins, T., Prelock, P., & Bonazinga, L. (2012). Psychometric evaluation of the Theory of Mind Inventory (ToMI): A study of typically developing children and children with autism spectrum disorder. *Journal of Autism and Developmental Disorders, 42*, 327–341.

Hutchins, T., Prelock, P., Morris, H., Benner, J., LaVigne, T., & Hoza, B. (2016). Explicit vs. applied theory of mind competence: A comparison of typically developing males, males with ASD, and males with ADHD. *Research in Autism Spectrum Disorders, 21*, 94–108.

Ingersoll, B., Lewis, E., & Kroman, E. (2007). Teaching the imitation and spontaneous use of descriptive gestures in young children with autism using a naturalistic behavioral intervention. *Journal of Autism and Developmental Disorders, 37*(8), 1446–1456.

Ingersoll, B., & Schreibman, L. (2006). Teaching reciprocal imitation skills to young children with autism using a naturalistic behavioral approach: Effects on language, pretend play, and joint attention. *Journal of Autism and Developmental Disorders, 36*(4), 487–505.

Johnson, C., & Myers, S. (2007). Identification and evaluation of children with autism spectrum disorders. *Pediatrics, 120*(5), 1183–1215.

Jordan, R. (2003). Social play and autistic spectrum disorders: A perspective on theory, implications and educational approaches. *Autism, 7*(4), 347–360.

Kaale, A., Fagerland, M., Martinsen, E., & Smith, L. (2014). Preschool-based social-communication treatment for children with autism: 12-month follow-up of a randomized trial. *Journal of the American Academy of Child & Adolescent Psychiatry, 53*(2), 188–198.

Kalandadze, T., Norbury, C., Nærland, T., & Næss, K. (2018). Figurative language comprehension in individuals with autism spectrum disorder: A meta-analytic review. *Autism, 22*(2), 99–117.

Kasari, C., Freeman, A., & Paparella, T. (2006). Joint attention and symbolic play in young children with autism: A randomized controlled intervention study. *Journal of Child Psychology and Psychiatry, 47*(6), 611–620.

Kasari, C., Gulsrud, A., Freeman, S., Paparella, T., & Helleman, G. (2012). Longitudinal follow-up of children with autism receiving targeted interventions on joint attention and play. *Journal of the American Academy of Child and Adolescent Psychiatry, 51*(5), 487–495.

Kasari, C., Gulsrud, A., Wong, C., Kwon, S., & Locke, J. (2010). Randomized controlled caregiver mediated joint engagement intervention for toddlers with autism. *Journal of Autism and Developmental Disorders, 40*(9), 1045–1056.

Kjelgaard, M., & Tager-Flusberg, H. (2001). An investigation of language impairment in autism: Implications for genetic subgroups. *Language and Cognitive Processes, 16*(2–3), 287–308.

Kim, S., Paul, R., Tager-Flusberg, H., & Lord, C. (2014). Language and communication in autism. In F. Volkmar, R. Paul, S. Rodgers, & K. Pelphrey (Eds.), *Handbook of autism and pervasive developmental disorders, diagnosis, development, and brain mechanisms* (4th ed., pp. 231–262). Wiley.

King, G., Baxter, D., Rosenbaum, P., Zwaigenbaum, L., & Bates, A. (2009). Belief systems of families of children with autism spectrum disorders or Down syndrome. *Focus on Autism and Other Developmental Disabilities, 24*, 50–64.

Koegel, R., & Koegel, R. (2006). *Pivotal response treatments for autism: Communication, social, and academic development.* Paul H. Brookes Publishing Co.

Kwok, E., Brown, H., Smyth, R., & Cardy, J. (2015). Meta-analysis of receptive and expressive language skills in autism spectrum disorder. *Research in Autism Spectrum Disorders, 9*, 202–222.

Lau, E., Phillips, C., & Poeppel, D. (2008). A cortical network for semantics: (De)constructing the N400. *Nature Reviews Neuroscience, 9*, 920–933.

Leekam, S., & Prior, M. (1994). Can autistic children distinguish lies from jokes? A second look at second-order belief attribution. *Journal of Child Psychology and Psychiatry, 55*(5), 901–915.

Lifter, K., Edwards, G., Avery, D., Anderson, S. R., & Sulzer-Azaroff, B. (1988, November). *The Developmental Play Assessment (DPA) instrument.* Mini seminar presented at the annual convention of the America-Speech-Language-Hearing Association, Boston, MA. Developmental assessment of young children's play: Implications for intervention, revised, July 1994.

Lifter, K., Mason, E., & Barton, E. (2011). Children's play: Where we have been and where we could go. *Journal of Early Intervention, 33*(4), 281–297.

Locke, J., Shih, W., Kretzmann, M., & Kasari, C. (2016). Examining playground engagement between elementary school children with and without autism spectrum disorder. *Autism, 20*(6), 653–662.

Lord, C. (1995). Follow-up of two-year-olds referred for possible autism. *Journal of Child Psychology and Psychiatry, 36*(8), 1365–1382.

Losh, M., & Capps, L. (2003). Narrative ability in high-functioning children with autism or Asperger's syndrome. *Journal of Autism and Developmental Disorders, 33*(3), 239–251.

Luyster, R., Kadlec, M., Carter, A., & Tager-Flusberg, H. (2008). Language assessment and development in toddlers with autism spectrum disorders. *Journal of Autism and Developmental Disorders, 38*, 1426–1438.

Macari, S., Campbell, D., Gengoux, G., Saulnier, C., Klin, A., & Chawarska, K. (2012). Predicting developmental status from 12 to 24 months in infants at risk for autism spectrum disorder: A preliminary report. *Journal of Autism and Developmental Disorders, 42*(12), 2636–2647.

MacKay, G., & Shaw, A. (2004). A comparative study of figurative language in children with autistic spectrum disorders. *Child Language Teaching and Therapy, 20*(1), 13–32.

Manning, M., & Wainwright, L. (2010). The role of high level play as a predictor social functioning in autism. *Journal of Autism and Developmental Disorders, 40*, 523–533.

Mastrangelo, S. (2009). Harnessing the power of play: Opportunities for children with autism spectrum disorders. *TEACHING Exceptional Children, 42*(1), 34–44.

McCleery, J., Ceponiene, R., Burner, K., Townsend, J., Kinnear, M., & Schreibman, L. (2010). Neural correlates of verbal and nonverbal semantic integration in children with autism spectrum disorders. *Journal of Child Psychology and Psychiatry, 51*(3), 277–286.

McDuffic, A., Yoder, P., & Stone, W. (2005). Prelinguistic predictors of vocabulary in young children with autism spectrum disorders. *Journal of Speech, Language, and Hearing Research, 48*, 1080–1097.

Mitchell, S., Cardy, J., & Zwaigenbaum, L. (2013). Differentiating autism spectrum disorder from other developmental delays in the first two years of life. *Developmental Disabilities Research Reviews, 17*(2), 130–140.

Modyanova, N., Perovic, A., & Wexler, K. (2017). Grammar is differentially impaired in subgroups of autism spectrum disorders: Evidence from an investigation of tense marking and morphosyntax. *Frontiers in Psychology, 8*, 1–23.

Montes, G., Halterman, J. S., & Magyar, C. I. (2009). Access to and satisfaction with school and community health services for US children with ASD. *Pediatrics, 124*(4), 407–413.

Miller, J. F. (1981). *Assessing language production in children.* University Park Press.

Müller, E., Schuler, A., & Yates, G. (2008). Social challenges and supports from the perspective of individuals with Asperger syndrome and other autism spectrum disabilities. *Autism, 12*(2), 173–190.

Mundy, P., Block, J., Delgado, C., Pomares, Y., Van Hecke, A., & Parlade, M. (2007). Individual differences and the development of joint attention in infancy. *Child Development, 78*(3), 938–954.

Mundy, P., Sigman, M., Ungerer, J., & Sherman, T. (1986). Defining the social deficits of autism: The contribution of non-verbal communication measures. *Journal of Child Psychology and Psychiatry, 27*(5), 657–669.

Murray, D., Creaghead, N., Manning-Courtney, P., Shear, P., Bean, J., & Prendeville, J. (2008). The relationship between joint attention and language in children with autism spectrum disorders. *Focus on Autism and Other Developmental Disabilities, 23*(1), 5–14.

Myers, B. J., Macintosh, V. H., & Goin-Kochel, R. P. (2009). "My greatest joy and my greatest heart ache": Parents' own words on how having a child in the autism spectrum has affected their lives and their families' lives. *Research in Autism Spectrum Disorders, 3*, 670–684.

Naigles, L., Cheng, M., Rattanasone, N., Tek, S., Khetrapal, N., Fein, D., & Demuth, K. (2016). "You're telling me!" The prevalence and predictors of pronoun reversals in children with autism spectrum disorders and typical development. *Research in Autism Spectrum Disorders, 27*, 11–20.

National Autism Center. (2015). *National Standards Project, Phase 2: Addressing the need for evidence-based practice guidelines for ASD*. https://www.nationalautismcenter .org/national-standards-project/phase-2

Namy, L. L., Acredolo, L. P, & Goodwyn, S. W. (2000). Verbal labels and gestural routines in parental communication with young children. *Journal of Nonverbal Behavior, 24*(2), 63–79.

Norbury, C. (2010). The relationship between theory of mind and metaphor: Evidence from children with language impairment and autistic spectrum disorder. *British Journal of Developmental Psychology, 23*(3), 383–399.

Oono, I. P., Honey, E. J., & McConachie, H. (2013). Parent-mediated early intervention for young children with autism spectrum disorders (ASD). *Evidence-Based Child Health: A Cochrane Review Journal, 8*(6), 2380–2479.

Osterling, J., & Dawson, G. (1994). Early recognition of children with autism: A study of first birthday home videotapes. *Journal of Autism and Developmental Disorders, 24*(3), 247–257.

Osterling, J., Dawson, G., & Munson, J. (2002). Early recognition of 1-year-old infants with autism spectrum disorder versus mental retardation. *Development and Psychopathology, 14*, 239–251.

Parten, M. (1933). Social play among preschool children. *Journal of Abnormal and Social Psychology, 28*(2), 136–147.

Paul, R., Norbury, C., & Gosse, C. (2018). *Language disorders from infancy through adolescence: Listening, speaking, reading, writing, and communicating* (5th ed.). Elsevier.

Pickles, A., Le Couteur, A., Leadbitter, K., Salomone, E., Cole-Fletcher, R., Tobin, H., Gammer, I., Lowry, J., Vamvakas, G., Byford, S., Aldred, C., Slonims, V., McConachie, H., Howlin, P., Parr, J. R., Charman, T., & Green, J. (2016). Parent-mediated social-communication therapy for young children with autism (PACT): Long-term follow-up of a randomised controlled trial. *Lancet, 388*, 2501–2509.

Pottie, C. G., Cohen, J., & Ingram, K. M. (2008). Parenting a child with autism: Contextual factors associated with enhanced daily parental mood. *Journal of Pediatric Psychology*, 1–11.

Prelock, P. A. (2006). *Autism spectrum disorders: Issues in assessment and intervention*. PRO-ED, Inc.

Prelock, P. A. (2019). *Autism spectrum disorders: Issues in assessment and intervention* (2nd ed.). PRO-ED.

Prelock, P., & Hutchins, T. (2008). The role of family-centered care in research: Supporting the social communication of children with autism spectrum disorder. *Topics in Language Disorders, 28*(4), 323–339.

Prelock, P., & Nelson, N. (2012). Language and communication in autism: An integrated view. *Pediatric Clinics of North America, 59*, 129–145.

Prizant, B., & Duchan, J. (1981). The functions of immediate echolalia in autistic children. *Journal of Speech and Hearing Disorders, 46*, 241–249.

Prizant, B., & Rydell, P. (1984). Analysis of functions of delayed echolalia in autistic children. *Journal of Speech, Language, and Hearing, 27*, 183–192.

Prizant, B. M., & Rydell, P. J. (1993). Assessment and intervention considerations for unconventional verbal behavior. In S. F. Warren & J. Reichle (Series Eds.) & J. Reichle & D. Wacker (Vol. Eds.), *Communication and language intervention series: Vol. 3. Communicative alternatives to challenging behavior: Integrating functional assessment and intervention strategies* (pp. 263–297). Paul H. Brookes Publishing Co.

Prizant, B. M., Wetherby, A. M., Rubin, E., & Laurent, A. C. (2003). The SCERTS Model: A Transactional, Family-centered approach to enhancing communication and social emotional abilities of children with autism spectrum disorder. *Infants and Young Children, 16*(4), 296–316.

Prizant, B. M., Wetherby, A., M., Rubin, E., Laurent, A. C., & Rydell, P. (2004). *The SCERTS Model: Enhancing communication and socioemotional abilities of children with autism spectrum disorder.* Paul H. Brookes Publishing Co.

Roberts, J., Rice, M., & Tager-Flusberg, H. (2004). Tense marking in children with autism. *Applied Psycholinguistics, 25,* 429–448.

Rogers, S., & Dawson, G. (2010). *Early Start Denver Model for young children with autism.* Guilford Press.

Rogers, S., Hepburn, S., Stackhouse, T., & Wehner, E. (2003). Imitation performance in toddlers with autism and those with other developmental disorders. *Journal of Child Psychology and Psychiatry, 44*(5), 763–781.

Rogers, S., Hepburn, S., & Wehner, E. (2003). Parent reports of sensory symptoms in toddlers with autism and those with other developmental disorders. *Journal of Autism and Developmental Disorders, 33*(6), 631–642.

Roseberry-McKibbin, C., & Hedge, M. N. (2011). *An advanced review of speech-language pathology* (3rd ed.). PRO-ED.

Schmalenbach, S., Billino, J., Kircher, T., van Kemenade, B., & Straube, B. (2017). Links between gestures and multisensory processing: Individual differences suggest a compensation mechanism. *Frontiers in Psychology, 8,* 1–8.

Shattuck, P. T., Durkin, M., Maenner, M., Newschaffer, C., Mandell, D. S., Wiggins, L., Lee, L.-C., Rice, C., Giarelli, E., Kirby, R., Baio, J., Pinto-Martin, J., & Cuniff, C. (2009). Timing of identification among children with an autism spectrum disorder: Findings from a population-based surveillance study. *Journal of the American Academy of Child and Adolescent Psychiatry, 48*(5), 474–483.

Shriberg, L., Paul, R., McSweeny, J., Klin, A., Cohen, D., & Volkmar, F. (2001). Speech and prosody characteristics of adolescents and adults with high-functioning autism and Asperger syndrome. *Journal of Speech, Language, and Hearing Research, 44,* 1097–1115.

Shumway, S., & Wetherby, A. (2009). Communicative acts of children with autism spectrum disorders in the second year of life. *Journal of Speech, Language, and Hearing Research, 52,* 1139–1156.

Stevenson, R., Segers, M., Ferber, S., Barense, M., & Wallace, M. (2014). The impact of multisensory integration deficits on speech perception in children with autism spectrum disorders. *Frontiers in Psychology, 5*(379), 1–4.

Stevenson, R., Siemann, J., Woynaroski, T., Schneider, B., Eberly, H., Camarata, S., & Wallace, M. (2014). Brief report: Arrested development of audiovisual speech perception in autism spectrum disorders. *Journal of Autism and Developmental Disorders, 44*(6), 1470–1477.

Stone, W., Ousley, O., Yoder, P., Hogan, K., & Hepburn, S. (1997). Nonverbal communication in two- and three-year-old children with autism. *Journal of Autism and Developmental Disorders, 27*(6), 677–696.

Tager-Flusberg, H. (2015). Defining language impairments in a subgroup of children with autism spectrum disorder. *Science China Life Sciences, 58*(10), 1044–1052.

Tager-Flusberg, H., & Anderson, M. (1991). The development of contingent discourse ability in autistic children. *Journal of Child Psychology and Psychiatry, 32*(7), 1123–1134.

Tomasello, M., Savage-Rumbaugh, S., & Kruger, A. (1993). Imitative learning of actions on objects by children, chimpanzees, and encultured chimpanzees. *Child Development, 64*(6), 1688–1705.

Tomchek, S., & Dunn, W. (2007). Sensory processing in children with and without autism: A comparative study using the short sensory profile. *American Journal of Occupational Therapy, 61*(2), 190–200.

Twoy, R., Connolly, P. M., & Novak, J. M. (2007). Coping strategies used by parents of children with autism. *Journal of the American Academy of Nurse Practitioners, 19,* 251–260.

Vismara, L., Colombi, C., & Rogers, S. (2009). Can one hour per week of therapy lead to lasting changes in young children with autism? *Autism, 13*(1), 93–115.

Vismara, L., & Rogers, S. (2010). Behavioral treatments in autism spectrum disorder: What do we know? *Annual Review of Clinical Psychology, 6,* 447.

Waxler, C., & Yarrow, M. (1970). Factors influencing imitative learning in preschool children. *Journal of Experimental Child Psychology, 9,* 115–130.

Westby, C., & Robinson, L. (2014). A developmental perspective for promoting theory of mind. *Topics in Language Disorders, 34*(4), 362–382.

Wetherby, A., Prizant, B., & Hutchinson, T. (1998). Communicative, social/affective, and symbolic profiles of young children with autism and pervasive developmental disorders. *American Journal of Speech-Language Pathology, 7*(2), 79–91.

Wetherby, A., Watt, N., Morgan, L., & Shumway, S. (2007). Social communication profile of children with autism spectrum disorders late in the second year of life. *Journal of Autism and Developmental Disabilities, 37*(5), 960–975.

Wetherby, A., & Woods, J. (2006). Effectiveness of early intervention for children with autism spectrum disorders beginning in the second year of life. *Topics in Early Childhood Special Education, 26*, 67–82.

Wetherby, A., Woods, J., Allen, L., Cleary, J., Dickinson, H., & Lord, C. (2004). Early indicators of autism spectrum disorders in the second year of life. *Journal of Autism and Developmental Disorders, 34*, 473–493.

Whyte, E. M., & Nelson, K. E. (2015). Trajectories of pragmatic and nonliteral language development in children with autism spectrum disorders. *Journal of Communication Disorders, 54*, 2–14.

Whyte, E. M., Nelson, K. E., & Sherf, K. S. (2014). Idiom, syntax, and advanced theory of mind abilities in children with autism spectrum disorders. *Journal of Speech, Language, and Hearing Research, 57*, 120–130.

Wong, C., Odom, S., Hume, K., Cox, A., Fettig, A., Kucharczyk, S., Brock, M. E., Plavnick, J. B., Fleury, V. P., & Schultz, T. (2014). Evidence-based practices for children, youth, and young adults with autism spectrum disorder. *Journal of Autism and Developmental Disorders, 45*(7), 1951–1966.

Woodgate, R. L., Ateah, C., & Secco, L. (2008). Living in a world of our own: The experience of parents who have a child with autism. *Qualitative Health Research, 18*, 1075–1083.

Woods, J., & Wetherby, A. (2003). Early identification and intervention for infants and toddlers at risk for autism spectrum disorders. *Language, Speech, and Hearing Services in Schools, 34*, 180–193.

4

Augmentative and Alternative Communication Strategies

Manual Signs, Picture Communication, and Speech-Generating Devices

Jane R. Wegner

INTRODUCTION

Researchers estimate that one fourth to one half of children and adults with autism spectrum disorder (ASD) do not develop speech sufficiently to meet their daily communication needs (Light et al., 1998; National Research Council [NRC], 2001; Rose et al., 2016; Wendt & Schlosser, 2007). Being able to understand and to be understood are essential to quality of life and participation in activities of one's choice. Because augmentative and alternative communication (AAC) can be any mode of communication that supplements or replaces oral speech (American Speech-Language-Hearing Association [ASHA], n.d.-a), it holds the promise of improving not only the communication but also the lives of many individuals with ASD. The use of AAC has been shown to have positive effects for people with ASD in the areas of behavior (Bopp et al., 2004; Walker & Snell, 2013), social interaction (Garrison-Harrell et al., 1997; Therrien et al., 2016), receptive language and comprehension (Brady, 2000), and speech and expressive language (Millar, 2009; Mirenda, 2003). Cafiero (2001) described the roles AAC can serve for individuals with ASD as enhancing existing communication skills, expanding language, replacing speech, and providing structure to support language development.

As has been pointed out in previous chapters, ASD is thought to be the most common and fastest growing developmental disability in the United States today (Centers for Disease Control and Prevention, n.d.). At the same time, technology and AAC applications are advancing, and researchers are learning more about instruction using AAC. This chapter examines four frequently used AAC strategies: manual signs, the Picture Exchange Communication System (PECS), **graphic symbols,** and **speech-generating devices** (SGDs) for children and adults with ASD.

TARGET POPULATIONS

Deficits in social communication and social interaction, along with restricted, repetitive behaviors, are primary characteristics of ASD (American Psychiatric Association, 2013). Many individuals with ASD who cannot meet their daily needs with speech may benefit from AAC either temporarily or as a lifelong communication mode. Some require AAC for expression, whereas others need it to augment comprehension. Consequently, all individuals with ASD should be considered potential candidates for AAC. That being said, individuals with ASD are a heterogeneous group, and it is not yet possible to predict which forms of AAC will be effective for specific individuals (NRC, 2001). Therefore, according to Mirenda (2009), AAC interventions should always be "made for specific learners, in specific contexts, to meet specific needs" (p. 16).

THEORETICAL BASIS

The underpinnings of AAC use with individuals with ASD include the beliefs that all people have a right to communication (ASHA, 2014; Brady et al., 2016; National Joint Committee for the Communication Needs of Persons with Severe Disabilities [NJC], 1992); that behavior is communicative (Brady et al., 2016; NJC, 1992); that communication is multimodal in nature (Lonke et al., 2006); and that improved communication leads to more participation, increased self-determination, and improved quality of life (Brady et al., 2016; NJC, 1992).

Although individuals with ASD are a heterogeneous group, their learning characteristics are a good match for AAC. Cafiero (2005) delineated the features that characterize AAC and how they correspond to the learning characteristics of individuals with ASD. These are described in Table 4.1.

Assessment and intervention practices with individuals with ASD, and in AAC, are guided by researcher-clinicians' beliefs about development, learning, social interactions, and etiology. Consequently, interventions for individuals with ASD have varied along a continuum, including traditional behavioral, contemporary behavioral, and developmental social-pragmatic approaches (Prizant et al., 2000). AAC is more likely to be used in approaches that have an emphasis on social communication and social interaction (Mirenda & Erickson, 2000). Within a social interactionist or transactional perspective, the individual with ASD, his or her communication partners, and environmental variables are considered within the intervention plan (Wetherby & Prizant, 2000). Prizant and Wetherby (1998) and Woods and Wetherby (2003) describe a social-pragmatic approach as family- or person-centered, occurring in the natural environment, embedded in meaningful contexts, and using transactional communication. Communication, from this transactional perspective, is dynamic and reciprocal; therefore, the intervention strategies to support communication development must be as well.

Initially, AAC was considered primarily for individuals with severe expressive communication challenges but good language comprehension. As the field of AAC has grown and the view of which groups of people can benefit from AAC has

Table 4.1. Autism and augmentative and alternative communication: Factors that make these a good match

Autism	Augmentative and alternative communication (AAC)
Visual learners	Uses visual cues
Interest in inanimate objects	Tools and devices are inanimate
Difficulty with complex cues	Level of complexity can be controlled so AAC grows with individual
Difficulty with change	Is static and predictable
Difficulty with complexities of social interaction	Provides buffer and bridge between communication partners
Difficulty with motor planning	Is motorically easier than speech
Anxiety	AAC interventions do not apply pressure or stress
Behavioral challenges	Provides an instant means to communicate, preempting difficult behaviors
Difficulty with memory	Provides means for language comprehension that relies on recognition rather than memory

From Cafiero, J. M. (2005). *Meaningful exchanges for people with autism: An introduction to augmentative and alternative communication* (p. 26). Bethesda, MD: Woodbine House; Reprinted with permission.

expanded, the understanding of the importance of enhanced input has been realized (ASHA, n.d.-b; Cafiero, 2001; Drager, 2009; Drager et al., 2006; Romski et al., 2006). This is especially important for individuals with ASD because they experience challenges in both generating language and understanding it. Enhanced input has been termed **augmented language input** (Romski & Sevcik, 2003), natural aided language (Cafiero, 2005), aided language stimulation (Goossens' et al., 1992), and aided language modeling (Drager, 2009; Drager et al., 2006). Although slightly different, each of these strategies highlights the importance of communication partners using the AAC system to provide input and a model for use in a meaningful context.

The application of AAC strategies with individuals with ASD is based on the same foundation as AAC strategies for other individuals: maximizing communication. The Participation (Beukelman & Mirenda, 2013), Social Networks (Blackstone & Hunt Berg, 2003), and SCERTS® (Morgan et al., 2018; Prizant et al., 2006b) models all have this focus and include the elements important to social communication intervention: that is, family- or person-centeredness, natural environments, meaningful contexts, and responsive communication partners.

EMPIRICAL BASIS

AAC has been recognized by the National Research Council (2001) and the American Speech-Language-Hearing Association (n.d.-c) as having an important role in supporting the social communication of individuals with ASD. There is a growing body of evidence to support the use of AAC with individuals with ASD (Ganz et al., 2012; Holyfield et al., 2017; Iacono et al., 2016; Logan et al., 2017; Mirenda & Iacono, 2009). Nonetheless, the use of AAC is, at times, not considered for individuals with ASD because families and/or professionals fear that AAC will impede speech development despite the evidence to the contrary (Millar, 2009; Millar et al., 2006). Specifically, this evidence has shown that AAC can be effective in reducing challenging behavior and does not have negative effects on the development of natural speech

Table 4.2. Levels of evidence for studies of treatment efficacy for augmentative and alternative communication

Level	Description	References supporting the intervention	References that do not support the intervention
Ia	Meta-analysis of >1 randomized controlled trial[a]	Holyfield, Drager, Kremkow, & Light, 2017; Ganz et al., 2012; Logan, Iacono, & Trembath, 2017; Sulzer-Azaroff, Hoffman, Horton, Bondy, & Frost, 2009; Iacono, Trembath, & Erickson, 2016; Schlosser, & Koul, 2015; Morin et al., 2018	Swartz & Nye, 2006; Wendt, 2009
Ib	Randomized controlled study	—	—
IIa	Controlled study without randomization (including single case experimental designs)	—	—
IIb	Quasi-experimental study	—	—
III	Nonexperimental studies (i.e., correlational and case studies)	—	—
IV	Expert committee report, consensus conference, clinical experience of respected authorities	National Research Council, 2001; American Speech-Language-Hearing Association, Practice Portal, Autism, www.asha.org/Practice-Portal/Clinical-Topics/Autism	—

Source: ASHA (n.d.) and Scottish Intercollegiate Guideline Network (2001).

[a]Meta-analyses and systematic reviews of controlled, but not randomized, controlled studies are included in Level Ia.

in persons with developmental disabilities including ASD. Much of this evidence can be found in meta-analyses, systematic reviews, and the National Autism Center's National Standards Projects (see Table 4.2).

There are four main AAC approaches that have been used with individuals with ASD. These are manual signs, graphic communication systems, the PECS, and SGDs.

Manual Signs

Manual signing, an **unaided AAC** strategy, has been used with individuals with ASD since the 1970s (Mirenda & Erickson, 2000; Nunes, 2008; Wendt, Schlosser, & Lloyd, 2004). Typically, **manual signs** are used in conjunction with speech, a method that is often referred to as "total" or "simultaneous communication" (Mirenda, 2003; Mirenda & Erickson, 2000; Ogletree & Harn, 2001). Nunes (2008) reports that the use of signs is advantageous because signs are more iconic, easily prompted and shaped, visual, and portable. Wendt (2009) pointed out that the reduced demand on memory and abstract understanding that signs place on the learner may help the individual overcome a negative history related to unsuccessful speech attempts.

There have been several reviews of the research related to the use of manual signs with individuals with ASD (Goldstein, 2002; Mirenda, 2003; Swartz & Nye, 2006; Wendt, 2009). In general, the results of the reviewed studies suggest that manual signing is an effective option for individuals with ASD (Goldstein, 2002; Mirenda, 2003; Wendt, 2009). In contrast, however, Swartz and Nye (2006) noted limited support in the evidence they reviewed and called for high-quality research that includes measures of intervention fidelity, sufficient detail in the description of the interventions for replication, and group studies. The National Standards Project (National Autism Center, 2009–2015) has designated sign instruction as an emerging treatment, indicating that there is some evidence of favorable outcome but citing the need for additional high-quality research with sign instruction.

Most of the research with sign has focused on vocabulary rather than on functional, spontaneous communication, and none has addressed the motor component of signing, two important issues to consider. With respect to functional, spontaneous communication, one disadvantage of manual signs is that communication is limited to partners who know sign and can interpret the signs used, especially for users whose signs are approximations or idiosyncratic in nature (Mirenda & Erickson, 2000). With respect to the motor component of sign, Mirenda (2009) summarized research that suggests that motor impairments are more common in ASD than had been previously thought. If these motor impairments extend to the planning or execution of the movement patterns required for sign, limitations are placed on the persons with ASD who might benefit from their use. In a synthesis of research on AAC interventions for children and youth with ASD, Iacono and colleagues (2016) report that in the studies they reviewed, **aided AAC systems** was favored over unaided forms, such as manual sign. Despite these drawbacks and because some supportive evidence exists (Wendt, Schlosser, & Lloyd, 2004), sign may be part of a multimodal AAC system for some individuals with ASD.

Graphic Communication Systems

Graphic communication systems are aided forms of AAC in that they require something external to the communicator. The use of graphic systems for persons with ASD was introduced in the 1980s, and these systems appear to be a good fit for this population because of the static nature of the symbols and the relative strength of visual processing in people with ASD (NRC, 2001; Wetherby & Prizant, 2000). Graphic communication systems are also described by many authors as visual supports because they can be used for comprehension as well as expression (Dettmer et al., 2000; Hodgdon, 1995; Johnston et al., 2003). Such systems can be used in the form of a communication book, card, wallet, or communication board. The graphics themselves may consist of iconic photographs, line drawings, written words, or other arbitrary symbols that are generated for the user or from commercially available software options, such as Boardmaker Online (Tobii-Dynavox, n.d.).

Graphic communication systems vary in terms of their organization (Beukelman & Mirenda, 2013; Light & Drager, 2007; Porter & Cafiero, 2009). Graphic communication systems include items that are usually arrayed in a grid format. Display options typically include semantic-syntactic, taxonomic, and activity or schematic organizations. *Semantic-syntactic organization* groups vocabulary according to grammatical categories, such as nouns, verbs, adverbs, and so forth. *Taxonomic organization* groups vocabulary items according to categories, such as people, places, and animals. *Schematic organization* groups vocabulary according to activity such as lunch, bath time, or shopping.

The Pragmatic Organization Dynamic Display (PODD; Porter & Cafiero, 2009) combines different vocabulary organizational strategies, such as activity displays and taxonomic category displays, to support differing communicative functions.

The PODD system initially appeared in the form of a communication book but is currently available as software for tablet devices (Tobii Dynavox, n.d.). To date, little research relates to how display organization affects use by individuals with ASD. Some common uses of graphic communication systems with individuals with ASD are visual schedules (Mirenda & Brown, 2009), choice making (Sigafoos et al., 2009), expressive communication (Beukelman & Mirenda, 2013; Cafiero, 2005), and augmented communication input (Cafiero, 2005; Romski & Sevcik, 2003).

Wendt (2009) reviewed research from previous AAC systematic reviews and meta-analyses (Schlosser & Wendt, 2008a, 2008b) focused on graphic symbol and sign use and conducted an additional search relative to AAC and ASD. He found a smaller research base for graphic symbols than manual signs, which he construed was due to the more recent use of graphic symbols than signs with individuals with ASD. Most of the studies related to AAC use focused on teaching their use in requesting. Wendt found the most conclusive and preponderant evidence for the use of graphic symbols to teach requesting. In contrast, he found mixed results for the use of graphic symbols to support transitions within and between activities and places. Wendt concludes that the research base is not sufficient to reliably inform clinical decisions. Not surprisingly, therefore, the National Standards Projects (National Autism Center, 2009–2015) terms **augmentative and alternative communication,** including graphic symbols, an "emerging" treatment.

In their systematic review of AAC intervention research for adolescents and adults with ASD, Holyfield and colleagues (2017) found that picture symbols were used in most of the studies they reviewed. In a meta-analysis of single case studies focused on aided AAC systems, Ganz and colleagues (2012) noted that the effects of PECS and SGDs were larger (improvement rate difference [IRD] = 0.99) than graphic communication systems (IRD = 0.61), where IRD refers to the difference between the improvement during the treatment phase and the improvement rate during baseline (Parker et al., 2009)

Wendt (2009) suggests that practitioners and families consider the advantages and disadvantages of graphic symbols versus signs as well as the universal benefits of each approach. Graphic symbols are easier than signs for partners to interpret and are nontransient, whereas signs are portable and limitless in terms of access to vocabulary.

Picture Exchange Communication System

PECS is a pictorial communication system that was developed by Bondy and Frost in 1985 for children with ASD. PECS incorporates behavioral principles to teach young children with ASD to request and describe what they see during typical activities (Sulzer-Azaroff et al., 2009). Consequently, PECS can be considered a hybrid approach that combines both AAC and behavioral methods—a strategy that is frequently applied in intervention strategies for ASD but that is uniquely manualized in PECS.

Bondy and Frost (2009) have indicated that PECS is beneficial for children who exhibit more limited verbal skills versus those children who have some spoken language and are being taught more complex language skills. PECS consists of six training phases (each preceded by a reinforcer assessment): 1) teaching the communicative exchange, 2) teaching persistence, 3) training discrimination, 4) teaching "I want . . ." sentences, 5) teaching a response to the question "What do you want?" and 6) teaching the use of additional sentence starters, such as "I have . . ." and "I see . . ." (Bondy & Frost, 2009). Researchers have conducted several systematic reviews and meta-analyses of research relative to PECS with positive results (Battaglia & McDonald, 2015; Flippin et al., 2010; Schlosser & Wendt, 2008a; Sulzer-Azaroff et al., 2009). In a meta-analysis including a variety of research designs, Flippin and colleagues (2010) described gains in communication, including increased frequency of exchanges, initiations, and requests. Battaglia and McDonald (2015) conducted a literature review of single subject experimental designs and the effects of PECS on communication and challenging behavior. They reported positive results in that there was an inverse relationship between challenging behavior and use of PECS exchange. Iacono and colleagues (2016) reviewed 17 systematic reviews. The reviews found AAC to be effective with most evidence supporting the use of PECS and SGDs, which are described in some detail in the next section. An SGD well suited for use with PECS is available from LoganTech (https://logantech.com).

Speech-Generating Devices

As technology has advanced, providing more options, and the research base has expanded, SGDs are being considered more often as a viable choice for individuals with ASD (Beukelman & Mirenda, 2013; Cafiero, 2005; Light & McNaughton, 2012; Light et al., 1998; Mirenda, 2009; O'Brien et al., 2016; O'Neill et al., 2017). SGDs are portable, computerized devices that produce synthetic or digitized speech output when graphic symbols are activated. SGDs give a voice to those who use them. SGDs include tablet computers with software that enables them to operate as both SGDs and dedicated devices that serve only communicative functions.

SGDs vary in terms of their output (i.e., synthetic or digitized speech, written language), symbol systems, displays, and language capacity (Beukelman & Mirenda, 2013). Synthetic speech output is probably what most people think of when they think of computerized speech. Synthetic speech is text-to-speech synthesis, text that is converted to wave forms that correspond to spoken output (Beukelman & Mirenda, 2013). In contrast, digitized speech is natural speech that has been recorded and stored for playback once selected by the system user (Beukelman & Mirenda, 2013). Since 2010, the quality and intelligibility of the voices in SGDs have improved greatly, and the devices offer a wider selection of voices as well.

Graphics used in SGDs include photographs, line drawings, and orthography. The organization of the graphics (also called *symbols*) varies in the same way graphic displays vary in visual communication systems. SGDs also vary with respect to the number of symbols available to the user. The displays of the symbols available can be fixed, dynamic, a combination of fixed and dynamic, or a **visual scene display.** Fixed-display selection sets are fixed in that they do not change and are the only symbols available to the user at a particular point in time. Dynamic displays, in contrast, change when activated. Touching one button changes the selection set available to the user. Fixed and dynamic displays are typically in a grid overlay format. A visual scene display is a picture or photograph of an event or experience. In this type of display, messages are programmed onto specific parts of the scene. Drager and colleagues (2009) point to the advantage of visual scene displays over grid displays in that they facilitate an understanding of the concept in context rather than the more isolated presentation associated with fixed and dynamic displays. Use of integrated video visual scene displays have shown potential for improved communication for individuals with ASD (Babb, Gormley, et al., 2018; Babb, McNaughton, et al., 2018; Laubscher et al., 2018; Starr et al., 2018).

Studies examining the use of SGDs with individuals with ASD have increased since 2010. Several systematic reviews have focused solely on SGDs and individuals with ASD, whereas other reviews included individuals with ASD along with other individuals with complex communication needs (Ganz et al., 2012; Morin et al., 2018; Schlosser et al., 2009). Schlosser and colleagues (2009) reviewed research relative to SGD effectiveness for individuals with ASD and concluded, "SGDs are viable options for individuals with ASD who require AAC" (p. 162). Ganz and colleagues (2012) conducted a meta-analysis of single case research on aided AAC systems. They concluded that AAC interventions had large effects on the targeted outcomes with greater effects for communication skills. Morin and colleagues (2018) conducted a systematic review of studies that included high-tech SGDs. They concluded that high-tech AAC is an evidence-based practice to teach social communication skills to individuals with complex communication needs, including individuals with ASD.

Schlosser and Koul (2015) conducted a review of speech output technologies in interventions for individuals with ASD. In terms of effectiveness, the researchers concluded that individuals with ASD can benefit from SGDs in treatments that focus on requesting and challenging behavior.

Other researchers conducted reviews that included SGDs as well as other forms of AAC (Holyfield et al., 2017; Iacono et al., 2016), concluding that AAC was highly effective and beneficial. These researchers suggest that practitioners teach a variety of communicative functions and consider the environments in which research and interventions take place.

In summary, there is accumulating evidence of positive outcomes when manual signs, graphic systems, PECS, and SGDs are used to support the communication of individuals with ASD. The National Standards Project, Phase 1 and 2 (National Autism Center, 2009–2015) considers them emerging treatments because of the quantity and quality of the available research. Given the evidence available, clinicians and families making AAC decisions need to review the current best evidence in light of the goals and outcomes and the needs of the individual with ASD and his or her family.

PRACTICAL REQUIREMENTS

By their nature, AAC interventions are time and labor intensive, are dynamic, and require a collaborative team effort (Beukelman & Mirenda, 2013). Successful AAC intervention requires careful attention to a number of team activities: 1) system selection; 2) system acquisition; 3) system set up and maintenance; 4) instructional strategy selection; 5) training for families and professionals; and 6) ongoing support, collaboration, and monitoring of the AAC intervention.

To address these requirements for AAC assessments and interventions, a successful team approach is imperative. Cumley and Beukelman (1992) have suggested roles and responsibilities for team members based on Light's (1989) definition of communicative competence (linguistic, operational, social, strategic) and areas of support (educational/vocational, home/residence, funding and technical). Cumley and Beukelman propose that once a team has been formed, team members be designated to take the lead in facilitating specific aspects of the AAC intervention.

They suggest that various team members be assigned primary responsibility for the different categories, with assistance and consultation from other team members. For example, the speech-language pathologist (SLP) would take the lead in the area of linguistic competence with assistance from the educator, and the assistive technology specialist would provide technical support with assistance from the paraeducator.

Beukelman and Mirenda (2013) suggest formulating team membership around the expertise needed, individuals who will be affected by team decisions, and those who have an interest in participating. Although the SLP is likely to lead the AAC assessment, a coordinated, explicit effort involving many individuals is needed to initiate, develop, and support AAC strategies for individuals with ASD. Critical components of the coordinated team effort to support AAC users are 1) a shared vision, 2) designated but flexible roles, 3) consistent communication, 4) ways to share information, 5) training communication partners including peers, and 6) a person- or family-centered approach (Downing & Ryndak, 2015).

KEY COMPONENTS

The ultimate goal of AAC is participation in activities important to the person using AAC and his or her family, such as school, work, recreation, and health care. A secondary but equally important goal is meaningful interactions within these activities.

The key components for AAC use include the following: 1) selecting the AAC system, 2) selecting the initial vocabulary and planning for expansion, 3) identifying instructional strategies, 4) training communication partners on the system and strategies, and 5) frequent monitoring and adapting as needed.

Selecting an Augmentative and Alternative Communication System

AAC is best thought of as a system rather than as a single entity (ASHA, n.d.-b; Beukelman & Mirenda, 2013). AAC systems can be aided or unaided. Unaided components are those that do not require a device or equipment external to the user. These include signs, gestures, vocalizations, and speech. Aided AAC components require a device or equipment external to the individual, such as communication books or SGDs (Beukelman & Mirenda, 2013). All AAC systems need a way to represent meaning, a means to select the message, and a way to send the message (McCormick & Wegner, 2003). As an early step, after an assessment, the AAC team needs to reach consensus on the AAC system.

Selecting Vocabulary

An important aspect of an AAC system is the vocabulary initially selected for a system and a plan for expanding it over time. If the appropriate vocabulary is not selected and later expanded, AAC will be ineffective. Beukelman and colleagues (1991) describe vocabulary selection as a dynamic process that reflects "changing experiences, interests, and knowledge" (p. 171). Cafiero (2005) suggests selecting a rich vocabulary and including more vocabulary that the user knows. Several strategies for selecting vocabulary have been documented in the literature. These include ecological inventories, communication diaries, vocabulary word lists, vocabulary generation useful to communicator, word selection from specific categories, preselected vocabulary on devices or symbol sets, and use of informants such as family, peers, and AAC user to generate items to include in the system's vocabulary (Beukelman et al., 1991; Fallon et al., 2001).

Beukelman and Mirenda (2013) describe two types of vocabulary, core and fringe, which are both important to communication. **Core vocabulary** includes words and messages that occur frequently and are used by many individuals across many contexts. **Fringe vocabulary** words and messages are unique to the individual user. They need to be addressed during vocabulary selection in order to provide a fuller means of personal expression in the communication process.

The vocabulary of the system should be reviewed and expanded regularly. Zangari and Van Tatenhove (2009) state that although all students with AAC needs require systematic instruction to learn new vocabulary, there is no research comparing approaches for such semantic instruction. Zangari (2015) describes vocabulary instruction beyond the core as including explicit instruction and continued practice to deepen understanding.

Language expansion is as important as the initial selection and expansion of vocabulary in terms of both expanding language form (word order, use of grammatical markers, etc.) and function (commenting, asking questions to obtain information, etc.). See the discussion of instructional strategies in the next section.

Because communication occurs across environments and with a variety of people, AAC intervention instruction should not occur in just one environment with just one person. AAC intervention is truly a collaborative endeavor. All communication partners who interact with the person who uses AAC need to learn about the AAC system and what strategies to use to support the individual using the AAC system. Although most AAC instruction should be integrated across contexts and people, some individualized instruction may be necessary, indicating that a flexible service delivery model is needed. Alternatives to the traditional model of service delivery for speech-language and perhaps other services include block or cyclical and 3:1 scheduling. In block or cyclical scheduling, direct services are provided for a specific period of time followed by indirect services for that same period of time (ASHA, n.d.-c). The 3:1 schedule involves providing direct services for 3 weeks followed by indirect services for 1 week (ASHA, n.d.-c).

Research provides little guidance as to the cumulative intensity of AAC intervention required for effectiveness as this information is not well defined in the studies reported. Binger and Light (2007) reported using 30 aided input models in a 15-minute session in a study that had positive outcomes using aided AAC modeling to increase multisymbol messages by preschoolers. Goossens' and colleagues (as cited in Smith et al., 2016) suggest that aided language stimulation be provided in 70% of the interactions. Simacek and colleagues (2018) conducted a systematic review of interventions and treatment intensity for aided AAC for people with severe to profound and multiple disabilities, including ASD. They found an underreporting of dosage parameters related to participant outcomes making this an area that requires additional research.

Identifying Instructional Strategies

The instructional strategies selected by the team are important to successful AAC use because providing the AAC system alone is insufficient. The focus of the instructional strategies should be on teaching communication rather than device use given that AAC is the *means* to functional spontaneous communication, not

Table 4.3.   Modeling strategies used in augmentative and alternative communication

Modeling strategy	Description	Reference
Aided Language Stimulation	Communication partners point to graphic symbol while saying the word verbally.	Goossens' et al. (1992)
System for Augmenting Language	Communication partners activate a symbol on a speech-generating device (SGD) while speaking the word in naturally occurring communicative interactions.	Romski & Sevcik (1992, 1996); Romski et al. (2009)
Natural aided language	Communication partners point to or activate symbols on activity- or environment-specific communication boards or technology while speaking key words.	Cafiero (2005)
Aided input	Communication partners incorporate facilitative language strategies such as models, expansion, event casts, or focused contrasts (Bunce & Watkins, 1995) in natural settings with input using the SGD.	Kelpin (1995) Wegner (1995)
Aided language modeling	Communication partner points to the referent while speaking and pointing to the symbol on a board or SGD.	Drager et al. (2006)

an end in itself. Toward that end, instructional strategies that incorporate modeling have been found to be effective with individuals with ASD and can be used by anyone interacting with the individual (Cafiero, 2001; Drager, 2009; Drager et al., 2009; Drager et al., 2006; Romski et al., 2009; Smith et al., 2016). Modeling can help AAC users learn the symbol vocabulary as well as learn how to use them in communicative exchanges that mirrors what occurs when children who are developing typically are learning language and its use. In addition, AAC models may facilitate comprehension (Goossens' et al., as cited in Smith et al., 2016; Wood et al., 1998).

Several modeling strategies are summarized in Table 4.3. Each of these instructional strategies provide input in the mode that the AAC user is expected to use, embed models in meaningful contexts, provide verbal and aided models, and involve communication partners.

Training Communication Partners

Because communication partners are fundamental to social interaction, language learning, and participation, training of these crucial team members is an essential component of AAC interventions. Training is needed in two areas: the AAC system and the strategies used to teach its use. General operation, maintenance, and programming training represent important topics related to the system. Responsibility for the trainings can be assigned through the process described previously. Shire and Jones (2015) conducted a systematic review of 13 studies of AAC partner training programs. They reported positive results in terms of partner skills and improved communication. Kent-Walsh and colleagues (2015) conducted a meta-analysis to investigate the effects of partner interventions on the communication of individuals using AAC. They found the partner interventions to be highly effective. The most frequently taught skills were AAC-aided modeling, open-ended questions, and expectant delay. Several models for partner training in ASD and AAC have been documented and can serve as examples (Culp & Carlisle, 1988; Kent-Walsh &

McNaughton, 2005; Light et al., 1992; McNaughton & Light, 1989; Meehan, 2018). These programs have been used successfully with a variety of participants, including family members, peers, professionals, and students in training.

Frequent Monitoring and Adapting

As individuals who use AAC grow and their needs change, the AAC system must be adapted. For example, as individuals' literacy skills develop, clinicians should introduce spelling options on the AAC device. Consequently, clinicians should frequently monitor device use, vocabulary needs, and changes in environment.

ASSESSMENT FOR TREATMENT PLANNING AND PROGRESS MONITORING

Neither standardized assessments for AAC nor ASD-specific procedures for AAC assessments are yet available. Assessment should be an ongoing process and should be used to help the SLP provide a profile of the individual's social communication skills, identify learning objectives in the natural environment, and examine the influence of the partners and environments on the communication of the individual with ASD (ASHA, n.d.-c). Assessment for AAC should include descriptions of the individual's communicative forms and functions as well as the influence of the communication partners and the learning environment on the individual's communicative competence (ASHA, n.d.). The assessment also should include information about an individual's participation patterns and opportunities as well as the individual's sensory, motor, literacy, and language capabilities. Then, the features of an AAC system that support an individual's strengths, needs, and capabilities can be identified (ASHA, n.d.-c). Important features required for AAC use include symbol representation, lexical organization, and motor skills (Light et al., 1998). The overall goal of assessment is to identify the individual's current and future unmet communication needs along with supports and ways to address those needs (Beukelman & Mirenda, 2013).

To address this overall goal, the SLP collects information using interviews, surveys, and observations of the individual and communication partners in daily activities and conducts assessments of the individual's specific skills. There are several assessment models that include tools useful in meeting AAC assessment goals for individuals with ASD. Among these are several that will be discussed here and are also described in Table 4.4: the Participation Model (Beukelman & Mirenda, 2013), The SCERTS Model (Prizant et al., 2003; Prizant et al., 2006a), the Social Networks: A Communication Inventory for Individuals with Complex Communication Needs and their Communication Partners (Blackstone & Hunt Berg, 2003), and the Augmentative and Alternative Communication Profile: A Continuum of Learning (Kovach, 2009).

The Participation Model (Beukelman & Mirenda, 2013) is focused on AAC as a support to allow the AAC user to participate in daily activities in the same manner as same-age peers without disabilities. Using this model, information is gathered about the individual's current participation and communication patterns, how these differ from that of the individual's peers, as well as barriers to participation, opportunities for communication, and capabilities. The assessment also includes preferences, attitudes, skills, and abilities of communication partners. The Participation Model is a comprehensive guide for assessment over time and across the lifespan.

The SCERTS Model (Prizant et al., 2006a, 2006b) is also a lifespan model, although it has been used more frequently with preschool and elementary age

Table 4.4. Augmentative and alternative communication assessment models and tools

Model/tool	Strategies	Characteristics	Environments	Age
Participation Model (Beukelman & Mirenda, 2005)	Observational data collection, interviews, inventories, specific capabilities assessments, leading to interventions for present and future	Systematic process of assessment based on participation requirements of peers without disabilities	Daily living and learning environments	Lifespan
The SCERTS® Model (Prizant et al., 2006a)	Questionnaires and interviews; observational data collection with person with ASD, the person's environment, and communication partners; quantification of data to generate intervention goals	Focus on the areas of social communication, emotional regulation, and transactional support from partners and environment; multidisciplinary in nature; can be used to measure progress	Social context of daily activities and experiences	Lifespan
Social Networks tool (Blackstone & Hunt Berg, 2003)	Interview by trained professional with expertise in communication; interview augmentative and alternative communication (AAC) user (if possible), family member, and support person	Supports Participation Model, captures multimodal nature of communication, delineates communicative competence (Light, 1989), supports person-centered planning; part of a comprehensive communication assessment; can be used to measure progress	Information obtained in interview reflects daily activities and experiences.	Lifespan
Augmentative and Alternative Communication Profile: A Continuum of Learning tool (Kovach, 2009)	Observation and rating of operational, linguistic, social, and strategic communicative competence (Light, 1989)	Multidisciplinary in nature; can be used to measure progress specific to AAC use	Any environment in which the AAC system is being used	Lifespan

children than with older individuals. SCERTS focuses on both the person with ASD and his or her communication partners as well as on the environment. SCERTS is an acronym for Social Communication, Emotional Regulation, and Transactional Supports, the focus areas of the program (see Chapter 14). The model includes an assessment process, SCERTS Assessment Process (SAP), that is criterion referenced and "designed for profiling relative strengths, needs, and priorities to inform program development and goal setting and to monitor progress" (p. 132). The assessment includes initial determination of a language stage (social partner, language partner, or conversation partner), interviews, observations in daily environments, and behavior sampling. SAP is ongoing with quarterly updates. One important feature of the assessment and SCERTS Model is the inclusion of interpersonal and learning support assessment and goal setting. Rubin and colleagues (2009) point out that relationships between AAC and reductions in challenging behavior, understanding of language, and expressive language can be investigated and monitored with the use of the SAP.

The Social Networks Inventory (Blackstone & Hunt Berg, 2003) is based on the Circle of Friends model (Falvey et al., 1994). The Social Networks tool "helps identify communication goals that lead to successful interactions with diverse partners, across multiple environments, using tools appropriate to the situation" (p. 15). Interviews used in this assessment involve the individual with ASD (when possible), a support person, and a family member. Information in the areas of skills and abilities, circles of communication partners, modes of expression used, representational strategies, and strategies that support interaction and types of communication are gathered. Data gathered with the Social Networks tool supports the Participation Model described earlier (Beukelman & Mirenda, 2013).

The Augmentative and Alternative Communication Profile: A Continuum of Learning (Kovach, 2009) is an observational tool that rates an individual's performance in four areas of learning based on Light's (1989) definition of communicative competence with respect to AAC: operational, linguistic, social, and strategic competence. This tool focuses on assessing individuals who already use AAC. The AAC Profile can be used to compare different AAC modes as well as performance across partners and contexts. Given its descriptive nature, the profile has potential for individuals with ASD.

Decisions about data collection depend on desired outcomes and goals of the AAC users and their family or support system. Outcomes typically articulate the desired result of intervention, whereas goals are more specific steps needed to achieve the outcome. Data related to an individual's specific skills to be an effective communicator can be one focus of data collection and evaluation (Beukelman & Mirenda, 2013). Hill (2009) describes such data as performance data, which typically involves the quantification of usage of specific language targets. Outcome measures include broader concepts such as increased participation, enriched social networks, consumer satisfaction, and quality of life (Beukelman & Mirenda, 2013; Hill 2009). Both types of data are needed to monitor progress and to consider in decision making.

Pretti-Frontczak and Bricker (2004) described guidelines for data collection in activity-based interventions that are applicable to AAC interventions. They suggest that data collection methods should 1) be flexible and applicable across settings, events, and people; 2) yield valid and reliable data; 3) be shared by team members; and 4) be compatible with available resources. Data collection also should not interfere with the intervention process (Arthur-Kelly & Butterfield, 2006). This means that data may not be collected during every session or teaching opportunity but during well-planned probes or videotaped interactions; alternatively, data collected by a third party, such as a paraeducator or teacher, can be used.

Performance data for some AAC users may focus on the use of specific vocabulary or language structure, whereas for others, it may focus on initiations or responses to peers. Data also should be collected on supports provided to the AAC user. For example, a support might be having a partner use aided AAC modeling or providing the AAC user with access to the AAC system across the day. To assure the validity and representativeness of data, it should be obtained from multiple sources in different environments. Data can be collected from live observations, from video recordings, or from data logging on an SGD. Data logging saves words and messages used on an AAC device, similar to a verbal language sample. The data contain a timestamp as well as what was said. Realize Language (https://realizelanguage .com/info) is an online service that analyzes the data that the device has logged. The software can identify words used, when communication occurs, and what parts of speech are being used.

Teams should collaboratively decide what data will be collected, by whom, and when. Collected data should regularly inform team decisions. If teams meet weekly, data collection on at least some targets would be needed on a weekly basis to facilitate meaningful comparison with baseline performance. If a team meets monthly, then monthly data on all targets could help guide decisions. Teams can use cloud storage systems such as Google Docs or OneDrive to share information and data quickly without the need to meet face to face. The assessment tools described previously provide guidance to teams regarding progress monitoring and performance-based decision making as determined by predetermined outcomes measures (Beukelman & Mirenda, 2013; Blackstone & Hunt Berg, 2003; Kovach, 2009; Prizant et al., 2006a).

IMPLICATIONS FOR INCLUSIVE PRACTICE

For children and adults who cannot meet their daily needs through speech, AAC is critical for participation in all of life's events, whether that is school, work, or recreational pursuits. Having a way to communicate and to be communicated with is essential to participation. Not only is communication the gateway to participation, it is critical for self-determination and self-advocacy. For students in school who require AAC, participation in academic and social activities may be possible when the appropriate supports are provided. Downing and Ryndak (2015) point to three necessary components for a student's successful inclusion:

1. Maximizing the student's opportunities to learn and use communication in contexts and during activities that are meaningful to the student and facilitate his or her interactions with classmates throughout the school day

2. Ensuring that communication interventions are implemented with fidelity

3. Monitoring student progress (p. 46)

Successful inclusion and participation are dependent on a student's communication. An AAC system does not guarantee inclusion, but with AAC and appropriate instruction and supports, successful inclusion is more likely.

CONSIDERATIONS FOR CHILDREN FROM CULTURALLY AND LINGUISTICALLY DIVERSE BACKGROUNDS

Considerations for children and adults from culturally and linguistically diverse backgrounds are important because of the shifting U.S. demographics and the growing awareness of cultural diversity and how it affects AAC services. In addition, there is a growing awareness that cultural factors underlie all educational and clinical activities (Soto, 2000). Barrera and Corso (2003) point to the need for cultural competence, which they define as "the ability to craft respectful, reciprocal, and responsive interactions across diverse cultural and linguistic parameters" (p. xx).

Issues that may influence the use of AAC by individuals from culturally and linguistically diverse backgrounds include views of disability, differences in language form and functions, attitudes toward and use of technology, and child rearing practices (Huer, 2008). Thus, cultural differences provide a critically important context for clinicians as they assess and plan for AAC interventions (Soto et al., 1997).

Roseberry-McKibbin (2008) highlighted the following considerations as important when collaborating about AAC with individuals and their families from culturally and linguistically diverse backgrounds: 1) understanding the sociopragmatic rules of a family's culture; 2) recognizing the perceived value of technology use; 3) determining the family's view of AAC use; 4) identifying the family's view of AAC as a priority; and 5) determining the most appropriate ways to teach families to use AAC. Another important consideration is the nature of the graphic elements (symbols) used in the AAC system and the impact on bilingual students.

Roseberry-McKibbin (2008) delineated several aspects to consider with respect to symbols and bilingual students. Do the symbols allow for communication at home and in more mainstream environments? Are the symbols relevant to the cultural experiences of the student? For example, if a written language system is used, is it widely used in the individual's social network? Are the symbols arranged in sequences that are appropriate for the structure of the language? For example, is the array structured so that it conforms to the word order of the language? Is the family involved in vocabulary selection?

Robinson and Solomon-Rice (2009) suggest that the services can be made more culturally responsive by focusing on self-assessment and acquisition of cultural knowledge. Barrera and Corso (2003) propose a particular method for achieving this, which they call *anchored understanding* and *3rd Space*, and describe it as skills needed to attain cultural competence with respect to early childhood education. Specifically, anchored understanding relates to knowing someone at an experiential level rather than just having information about the individual's culture. Similarly, 3rd Space is the ability to take differing perspectives and reframe them to form an additional, third option. For example, if a parent and service providers disagree on use of the device at home, can an option be found (e.g., use the device only to share what happened at school as soon as the child arrives home) that is not the parent or service providers' initial preference?

Providing AAC services for individuals with ASD from culturally and linguistically diverse backgrounds creates complicated demands on service providers and the researchers who support them. Soto (2012) describes culturally competent clinicians as those who "engage in a process by which they identify their own cultural assumptions and the expectations that drive their professional decisions and understand that families may not share those expectations and values" (p. 144). This awareness is particularly relevant to AAC services.

Application to a Child

Tait is a 12-year-old boy who was diagnosed with ASD at age 2. He began receiving speech-language services shortly after his diagnosis and has continued to receive them since that time. Tait is generally healthy, although he has recently been diagnosed with rheumatoid arthritis and is sensitive to pain. He has difficulty with small spaces and bottlenecks where many people are congregated. He has a keen interest in wood and carpentry and an excellent memory. Tait participates in special education at a local elementary school. He has a positive behavior support team (Janney & Snell, 2008) and receives additional speech-language intervention at a university clinic.

Tait's strengths include being curious, social, and visually astute. His challenges include unconventional communication, impulsivity, and challenging behaviors that can consist of tantrums, aggression, and property destruction. These challenges have contributed to making peer interaction difficult for Tait.

Tait began using PECS at age 2 and used it until he was 3½ when he began to prefer using signs. He was introduced to his first SGD when he was 9 years old. He is now a multimodal communicator. He uses a Palm 3 (his second SGD), pictures, idiosyncratic signs, gestures, and some words to communicate. Most of his speech is unintelligible to those who do not know him. Tait can navigate through more than 200 pages and several levels on his SGD. His SGD is programmed with both words and phrases. He uses his PECS materials as a backup when his SGD is not available, and he uses more than 100 signs, though many of them are difficult to read.

Tait's communication was initially assessed with the SCERTS Assessment Process (Prizant et al., 2006a), and he performed at the Language Partner Stage of communication. Goals generated from the assessment addressed increasing Tait's skills related to commenting, expressing his emotions with his SGD, and choosing among offered alternatives needed to calm him when he was upset. Goals for his communication partners included their using augmented input with Tait for purposes of redirection, expansion, and modeling; providing Tait with a binder including a schedule and Social Stories (Gray, 1995; also see Chapter 16) to help him prepare for activities; making the SGD always available; and using an interactive diary for Tait that was developed by his mother.

Since the initial SCERTS assessment, Tait has made many communication gains. He independently expresses his feelings and engages in reciprocal exchanges. He also comments on shared objects or events of interest. To clarify messages, he has started to mark tense using the "later" and "past" icons on his device. He is beginning to combine symbols. His dysregulation has decreased, as has the time it takes him to recoup from a period of dysregulation. He can let his partner know what he needs to calm him when presented with alternatives. He also has more communication partners who are responsive and able to provide him with the learning supports he needs. Current goals focus on increasing his vocabulary, self-regulation, and literacy skills. During a follow-up SCERTS reassessment, Tait's performance was in the Conversational Partner Stage of communication.

Application to an Adult

Joe is a 32-year-old man with a dual diagnosis of Down syndrome and ASD. Joe lives in his own home where he lives with support. Joe is an independent business owner. He owns and operates Poppin' Joe's Kettle Korn. He makes kettle corn to sell at fairs, craft shows, in stores, and online (see http://poppinjoes.org). Joe has made presentations to national organizations about his life and business and testified at a Congressional Briefing using his SGD.

Joe has used an SGD for more than 18 years. He now uses a I 110 (Tobii Dynavox), which is his fourth SGD. Joe uses some speech, but it is difficult to understand him unless you know him well. His speech is less than 50% intelligible. In conversation, he is apt to repeat what his conversational partner is saying.

Joe received speech-language therapy from an early age, with most efforts directed toward improving his speech. Consequently, he did not receive an SGD until he was 14 years old. Joe began receiving speech-language services outside of the school setting when he was 15 years old. At that time, he used his SGD device only rarely and only for specific tasks. Joe received individual intervention focusing on vocabulary, SGD use, and literacy during the academic year and group sessions as part of a summer camp for 5 years. Since then, he has participated in an individual session for an hour and an AAC group for 90 minutes per week. Joe's progress has been slow but steady.

Joe's most recent goals focus on independent and spontaneous communication, as Joe tends to repeat what is said or modeled for him on his SGD. To help Joe be more independent and spontaneous in his communication, he is learning new core vocabulary and how to use those words in three- to five-word spontaneous utterances. New vocabulary is introduced in the individual session and practiced in the group session. One of Joe's support partners observes and participates in his individual and group sessions so that what is taught can be extended to additional environments. The instructional strategies used with Joe are explicit instruction, aided language input, visual supports, and least to most prompting. Joe has made progress in his language development and use. He has increased his use of multiword utterances ("Joe is t-shirt white") with his SGD in conversation. In this instance, Joe was describing what he was wearing in a picture. To address his literacy needs, Joe also participates in the Accessible Literacy Learning curriculum in his individual sessions.

Joe will most likely continue in intervention for the near future. His goals will continue to focus on using longer and more complex novel utterances with support partners, peers, and customers and on improving his literacy skills.

> **To review an extended application and implementation
> of this intervention, see Case 1 about a child with
> ASD and Down syndrome in the companion volume
> *Case Studies for the Treatment of Autism Spectrum Disorder.***

Future Directions

As technology advances, so will the opportunities for people with ASD; yet people with ASD need more information to take full advantage of the opportunities. There are three areas in which future research needs to focus to support the communication needs of individuals with ASD who are using AAC: system design factors, instructional strategies and intensity, and training partners to support AAC learning.

Drager and colleagues (2009) point to the need to investigate the impact of AAC designs on social interaction, language development, and effective communication for individuals with ASD. The effect of different design strategies on partner ability to provide aided language input is also an important area for future investigation

(Porter & Cafiero, 2009). There is a need to investigate which instructional techniques are most effective for individuals with specific characteristics. Given the importance of literacy skills to AAC and quality of life, Light and McNaughton (2009) point to the need to compare the effectiveness of different interventions and instructional approaches to design technology so that communication and curricular content are more integrated and to evaluate different approaches to training parents and support personnel to use evidence-based practices. With the availability of tablet computers and software, research will be needed to provide the advantages and disadvantages of different technologies in relation to individual characteristics.

Although knowledge about AAC and ASD is emerging, there are many unknowns. In the meantime, Cafiero and Delsack (2007) suggest assuming that each "individual with ASD is able to receive and has the potential to generate communication" (p. 25). AAC strategies play an important role in this "least dangerous assumption" (Donnellan, 1984), which proposes that when there is no conclusive evidence, clinicians should make decisions that are likely to have the least harmful effect on the individual if they are wrong.

Suggested Readings

1. American Speech-Language-Hearing Association. (n.d.). *Augmentative and alternative communication* (Practice Portal). https://www.asha.org/Practice -Portal/Professional-Issues/Augmentative-and-Alternative-Communication. The Practice Portal contains information about AAC, including an overview, key issues, resources, and evidence maps. This is a good source for families and professionals.

2. Beukelman, D. R., & Mirenda, P. (2013). *Augmentative and alternative communication: Supporting children and adults with complex communication needs* (4th ed.). Paul H. Brookes Publishing Co. This text provides extensive information about AAC assessment and intervention planning. It describes pertinent information for professionals and students to provide a basic understanding of AAC as well as information about individuals with complex communication needs.

3. Johnston, S., Reichle, J., Feeley, K., & Jones, E. (2012). *AAC strategies for individuals with moderate to severe disabilities.* Paul H. Brookes Publishing Co. This book provides professionals with a variety of evidence-based intervention strategies. The text also comes with a CD containing forms to support the interventions described.

4. Sevcik, R., & Romski, M. (2016). *Communication interventions for individuals with severe disabilities: Exploring research challenges and opportunities.* Paul H. Brookes Publishing Co. This edited text, though not focused on AAC and ASD specifically, presents evidence-based strategies that apply to these populations. In addition to the chapters on intervention strategies and evidence, there are chapters on research design and measuring outcomes for this population. The book contains information for both the practitioner and the researcher.

5. Zangari, C. (n.d.). *Praactical AAC.* https://praacticalaac.org. This daily blog is a good source of information for families and professionals relative to AAC practice. It presents the content in a variety of ways, including videos and written material.

Learning Activities

1. Try out some software. Many manufacturers of SGDs have free downloads of the software that is used in their products. Go to the website of Prentke Romich (https://www.prentrom.com) or Tobii Dynavox (https://www.tobiidynavox.com /en-US/products/mytobiidynavox/tobii-dynavox-for-professionals/?redirect =true) and download software for one of the devices. Try it out on your computer. Explore the software, and then create a context in which you could provide aided input to a child. Script out what you might say during the interaction, and then try it. For example, interactive storybook reading could be the activity. Decide which book you would read, and then try using aided input during the book reading to comment on the book. Reflect on your experience. What was difficult about it? What kind of preparation would you need to actually do this activity with an AAC user?

2. Vocabulary selection. Using the same software as in Question 1, determine what vocabulary is available to use with a fourth or fifth grader with ASD going on a nature hike. First, make a list of the vocabulary that might be needed. Don't forget about peer interactions as well. If, after making your list, you find that the vocabulary needed is not available on the software you have, explore the software to determine if there are other settings with more or different vocabulary. If so, change the settings. If not, try to program a few of the vocabulary words into the software.

3. Interview an AAC user who has ASD or the family of an AAC user who has ASD. Possible questions you could ask to learn about the user's life story include the following:

    a. When did you (your child) obtain an AAC system? What difference has it made in his or her life? In your life?

    b. What do you like and not like about the system?

    c. Describe the AAC system the individual is using. What kind of vocabulary was available? What kind was used?

    d. How effective was the individual's communication? If there were breakdowns in communication, why do you think they occurred? If there were no communication breakdowns, why was the person successful?

Summary of Video Clip

*See the **About the Videos and Downloads** page at the front of the book for directions on how to access and stream the accompanying video to this chapter.*

In this video clip, Tait and his SLP participate in a session focused on the senses. The SLP uses some of the strategies discussed in the chapter. Notice how she provides him with opportunities, uses aided language input, and follows his lead.

REFERENCES

American Psychiatric Association. (2013). *Diagnostic and statistical manual of mental disorders, fifth edition* (DSM-5). Author.

American Speech-Language-Hearing Association (ASHA). (n.d.-a). *Autism* (Practice Portal). Retrieved January 25, 2019, from https://www.asha.org/practice-portal/clinical-topics/autism

American Speech-Language-Hearing Association (ASHA). (n.d.-b). *Augmentative and alternative communication* (Practice Portal). Retrieved January 20, 2019, from https://www.asha.org/Practice-Portal/Professional-Issues/Augmentative-and-Alternative-Communication

American Speech-Language-Hearing Association (ASHA). (n.d.-c). *School-based service delivery in speech-language pathology*. Retrieved January 20, 2019 from https://www.asha.org/slp/schools/school-based-service-delivery-in-speech-language-pathology/#scheduling

American Speech-Language-Hearing Association (ASHA). (2014). International Communication Project 2014. https://leader.pubs.asha.org/doi/10.1044/leader.AN7.19092014.62

Arthur-Kelly, M., & Butterfield, N. (2006). Monitoring progress. In J. Sigafoos, M. Arthur-Kelly, & N. Butterfield (Eds.), *Enhancing everyday communication for children with disabilities* (pp. 107–113). Paul H. Brookes Publishing Co.

Babb, S., Gormley, J., McNaughton, D., & Light, J. (2018). Enhancing independent participation within vocational activities for an adolescent with ASD using AAC video visual scene displays. *Journal of Special Education Technology, 34*(2), 120–132.

Babb, S., McNaughton, D., Light, J., Wydner, K., & Pierce, L. (2018, November). *Enriching communication within vocational tasks for adolescents with CCN using AAC video visual scene displays* [Poster presentation]. American Speech-Language-Hearing Association (ASHA) Conference, Boston, MA, United States.

Battaglia, D., & McDonald, M. (2015). Effects of the Picture Exchange Communication System (PECS) on maladaptive behavior in children with autism spectrum disorders (ASD): A review of the literature. *Journal of the American Academy of Special Education Professions* (Winter), 8–20.

Barrera, I., & Corso, R. M. (2003). *Skilled dialogue: Strategies for responding to cultural diversity in early childhood.* Paul H. Brookes Publishing Co.

Beukelman, D., & Mirenda, P. (2013). *Augmentative and alternative communication: Supporting children and adults with complex communication needs* (4th ed.). Paul H. Brookes Publishing Co.

Beukelman, D. R., McGinnis, J., & Morrow, D. (1991). Vocabulary selection in augmentative and alternative communication. *Augmentative and Alternative Communication, 7,* 171–185.

Binger, C., & Light, J. (2007). The effect of AAC modeling on the expression of multi-symbol messages by preschoolers who use AAC. *Augmentative and Alternative Communication, 23*(1), 30–43.

Blackstone, S., & Hunt Berg, M. (2003). *Social networks: A communication inventory for individuals with complex communication needs and their communication partners.* Augmentative Communication.

Bondy, A., & Frost, L. (2009). The picture exchange system: Clinical and research applications. In P. Mirenda & T. Iacono (Eds.), *Autism spectrum disorders and AAC* (pp. 279–302). Paul H. Brookes Publishing Co.

Bopp, K., Brown, K., & Mirenda, P. (2004). Speech-language pathologists' roles in the delivery of positive behavior support for individuals with developmental disabilities. *American Journal of Speech-Language Pathology, 13,* 5–19.

Brady, N. (2000). Improved comprehension of object names following voice output communication aid use: Two case studies. *Augmentative and Alternative Communication, 16,* 197–204.

Brady, N., Bruce, S., Goldman, A., Erickson, K., Mineo, B., Ogletree, B., Paul, D., Romski, M., Sevcik, R., Siegel, El., Schoonover, J., Snell, M. Sylvester, L., & Wilkinson, K. (2016). Communication services and supports for individuals with severe disabilities: Guidance for assessment and intervention. *American Journal on Intellectual and Developmental Disabilities, 121*(2), 121–138.

Bunce, B. H., & Watkins, R. V. (1995). Language intervention in a preschool classroom: Implementing a language-focused curriculum. In M. Rice & K. Wilcox (Eds.), *Building a language-focused curriculum for the preschool classroom* (pp. 39–72). Paul H. Brookes Publishing Co.

Cafiero, J. M. (2001). The effect of an augmentative communication intervention on the communication, behavior, and academic program of an adolescent with autism. *Focus on Autism and Other Developmental Disabilities, 16*, 179–189.

Cafiero, J. M. (2005). *Meaningful exchanges for people with autism: An introduction to augmentative and alternative communication.* Woodbine House.

Cafiero, J. M., & Delsack, B. S. (2007). AAC and autism: Compelling issues, promising practices and future directions. *Perspectives on AAC, 16*(2), 23–26.

Center for Disease Control Prevention. (n.d.). Autism Data Visualization Tool. Retrieved February 11, 2019 from https://www.cdc.gov/ncbddd/autism/data/index.html

Culp, D., & Carlisle, M. (1988). *PACT: Partners in augmentative communication training.* Communication Skill Builders.

Cumley, G. D., & Beukelman, D. R. (1992). Roles and responsibilities of facilitators in augmentative and alternative communication. *Seminars in Speech and Language, 13*(2), 111–119.

Dettmer, S., Simpson, R., Myles, B., & Ganz, J. (2000). The use of visual supports to facilitate transitions of students with autism. *Focus on Autism and Other Developmental Disabilities, 15*(3), 163–169.

Donnellan, A. (1984). The criterion of the least dangerous assumption. *Behavioral Disorders, 9*, 144–150.

Downing, J., & Ryndak, L. (2015). Integrating team expertise to support communication. In J. Downing, A. Hanreddy, & K. Peckham-Hardin (Eds.), *Teaching communication skills to students with severe disabilities* (3rd ed., pp. 25–50). Paul H. Brookes Publishing Co.

Drager, K. D. (2009). Aided modeling interventions for children with autism spectrum disorders who require AAC. *Perspectives on Augmentative and Alternative Communication, 18*, 114–120.

Drager, K. D., Light, J. C., & Finke, E. H. (2009). Using AAC technologies to build social interaction with young children with autism spectrum disorders. In P. Mirenda & T. Iacono (Eds.), *Autism spectrum disorders and AAC* (pp. 247–278). Paul H. Brookes Publishing Co.

Drager, K. D., Postal, V. J., Carrolus, L., Catellano, M., & Glynn, J. (2006). The effect of aided language modeling on symbol comprehension and production in two preschool children with autism. *American Journal of Speech-Language Pathology, 15*, 112–125.

Fallon, K., Light, J., & Paige, T. (2001). Enhancing vocabulary selection for preschoolers who require augmentative and alternative communication (AAC). *American Journal of Speech-language Pathology, 10*, 81–94.

Falvey, M. A., Forest, M., Pearpoint, J., & Rosenberg, R. L. (1994). *All my life's a circle: Using the tools Circles, Maps and Path.* Inclusion Press.

Flippin, M., Reszka, S., & Watson, L. R. (2010). Effectiveness of the picture exchange communication system (PECS) on communication and speech for children with autism spectrum disorders: A meta-analysis. *American Journal of Speech-Language Pathology, 19*, 178–195.

Ganz, J., Earles-Vollrath, T., Heath, A., Parker, R., Rispoli, M., & Duran, J. (2012). A meta-analysis of single case research studies on aided augmentative and alternative communication systems with individuals with autism spectrum disorders. *Journal of Autism and Developmental Disorders, 42*, 60–74.

Garrison-Harrell, L., Kamps, D., & Kravits, T. (1997). The effects of peer networks on social-communicative behaviors for students with autism. *Focus on Autism and Other Developmental Disabilities, 12*, 241–254.

Goldstein, H. (2002). Communication intervention for children with autism: A review of treatment efficacy. *Journal of Autism and Developmental Disorders, 32*(5), 373–396.

Goossens', C., Crain, S. S., & Elder, P. (1992). *Engineering the preschool environment for interactive, symbolic communication.* Southeast Augmentative Communication Conference Publications.

Gray, C. (1995) Teaching children with autism to "read" social situations. In K. Quill (Ed.), *Teaching children with autism: Strategies to enhance communication and socialization* (pp. 219–241). Delmar Publishers.

Hill, K. (2009). Data collection and monitoring AAC intervention in the school. *Perspectives on Augmentative and Alternative Communication, 18*, 58–64.

Hodgdon, L. (1995). Solving social behavioral problems through the use of visually supported communication. In K. Quill (Ed.), *Teaching children with autism: Strategies to enhance communication and socialization* (pp. 265–286). Delmar Publishers.

Holyfield, C., Drager, K., Kremkow, J., & Light, J. (2017). Systematic review of AAC intervention research for adolescents and adults with autism spectrum disorders. *Augmentative and Alternative Communication, 33*(4), 201–212.

Huer, M. (2008). Toward an understanding of the interplay between culture, language, and augmentative and alternative communication. *Perspectives on Augmentative and Alternative Communication, 17*, 113–119.

Iacono, T., Trembath, D., & Erickson, S. (2016). The role of augmentative and alternative communication for children with autism: current status and future trends. *Neuropsychiatric disease and treatment, 12*, 2349–2361.

Janney, R., & Snell, M. (2008). *Teachers' guides to inclusive practices: Behavioral support* (2nd ed.). Paul H. Brookes Publishing Co.

Johnston, S., Nelson, C., Evans, J., & Palazolo, K. (2003). The use of visual supports in teaching young children with autism spectrum disorder to initiate interactions. *Augmentative and Alternative Communication, 19*, 86–103.

Kelpin, V. C. (1995). *The outcomes of augmented input and facilitative language strategies with children using augmentative communication devices* [Unpublished master's thesis]. University of Kansas.

Kent-Walsh, J., & McNaughton, D. (2005). Communication partner instruction in AAC: Present practices and future directions. *Augmentative and Alternative Communication, 21*(3), 195–204.

Kent-Walsh, J., Murza, K., Malani, M., & Binger, C. (2015). Effects of communication partner instruction on the communication of individuals using AAC: A meta-analysis. *Augmentative and Alternative Communication, 31*(4), 271–284.

Kovach, T. M. (2009). *Augmentative and alternative communication profile: A continuum of learning.* LinguiSystems.

Laubscher, E., Light, J., & McNaughton (2018, November). *Effects of video AAC technology on communication & play in autism: A pilot study* [Poster presentation]. American Speech-Language-Hearing Association (ASHA) Conference, Boston, MA, United States.

Light, J. (1989). Toward a definition of communicative competence for individuals using augmentative and alternative systems. *Augmentative and Alternative Communication, 5*, 137–144.

Light, J., Dattilo, J., English, J., Gutierrez, L., & Hartz, J. (1992). Instructing facilitators to support the communication of people who use augmentative communication systems. *Journal of Speech and Hearing Research, 35*, 865–875.

Light, J., & Drager, K. (2007). AAC technologies for young children with complex communication needs: State of the science and future research directions. *Augmentative and Alternative Communication, 23*, 204–216.

Light, J., & McNaughton, D. (2009). Addressing the literacy demands of the curriculum for conventional and more advanced readers and writers who require AAC. In G. Soto & C. Zangari (Eds.), *Practically speaking: Language, literacy, and academic development for students with AAC needs* (pp. 217–245). Paul H. Brookes Publishing Co.

Light, J., & McNaughton, D. (2012). The changing face of augmentative and alternative communication: Past, present and future challenges. *Augmentative and Alternative Communication, 28*, 197–204.

Light, J., Roberts, B., Dimarco, R., & Greiner, N. (1998). Augmentative and alternative communication to support receptive and expressive communication for people with autism. *Journal of Communication Disorders, 31*, 153–180.

Lonke, F., Campbell, J., England, A., & Haley, T. (2006). Multimodality: A basis for augmentative and alternative communication: Psychological, cognitive, and clinical/educational aspects. *Disability and Rehabilitation, 28*(3), 169–174.

Logan, K., Iacono, T., & Trembath, D. (2017). A systematic review of research into aided AAC to increase social-communication functions in children with autism spectrum disorders. *Augmentative and Alternative Communication, 33*(1), 51–64.

McCormick, L., & Wegner, J. (2003). Supporting augmentative communication. In L. McCormick, D. Loeb, & D. Schiefelbusch (Eds.), *Supporting children with communication difficulties in inclusive settings* (pp. 435–459.). Pearson.

McNaughton, D., & Light, J. (1989). Teaching facilitators to support the communication skills of an adult with severe cognitive disabilities: A case study. *Augmentative and Alternative Communication, 5*, 35–41.

Meehan, S. (2018). *The impact of ImPAACT: Communication partner training for preservice speech-language pathologists* [Unpublished doctoral dissertation]. University of Kansas.

Millar, D. C. (2009). Effects of AAC on the natural speech development of individuals with autism spectrum disorders. In P. Mirenda & T. Iacono (Eds.), *Autism spectrum disorders and AAC* (pp. 171–192). Paul H. Brookes Publishing Co.

Millar, D. C., Light, J. C., & Schlosser, R. W. (2006). The impact of augmentative and alternative communication intervention on the speech production of individuals with developmental disabilities: A research review. *Journal of Speech, Language, and Hearing Research, 49*, 248–269.

Mirenda, P. (2003). Toward functional augmentative and alternative communication: A research review. *Augmentative and Alternative Communication, 16*, 141–151.

Mirenda, P. (2009). Introduction to AAC for individuals with autism spectrum disorders. In P. Mirenda & T. Iacono (Eds.), *Autism spectrum disorders and AAC* (pp. 3–22). Paul H. Brookes Publishing Co.

Mirenda, P., & Brown, K. (2009). A picture is worth a thousand words: Using visual supports for augmented input with individuals with autism spectrum disorders. In P. Mirenda & T. Iacono (Eds.), *Autism spectrum disorders and AAC* (pp. 303–332). Paul H. Brookes Publishing Co.

Mirenda, P., & Erickson, K. (2000). Augmentative communication and literacy. In M. Wetherby & B. Prizant (Eds.), *Autism spectrum disorders: A transactional approach* (pp. 333–369). Paul H. Brookes Publishing Co.

Mirenda, P., & Iacono, T. (2009). *Autism spectrum disorders and AAC.* Paul H. Brookes Publishing Co.

Morgan, L., Hooker, J., Sparapani, N., Reinhardt, V., Schatschneider, C., & Wetherby, A. (2018). Cluster randomized trial of the classroom SCERTS intervention for elementary students with autism spectrum disorder. *Journal of Consulting and Clinical Psychology, 86*(7), 631–644.

Morin, K., Ganz, J., Gregori, E., Foster, M., Gerow, S., Genc-Tosun, D., & Hong, E. (2018). A systematic quality review of high-tech AAC interventions as an evidence-based practice. *Augmentative and Alternative Communication, 34*(2), 104–117.

National Autism Center (2009–2015). *National Standards Projects.* National Autism Center.

National Joint Committee for the Communication Needs of Persons with Severe Disabilities (NJC). (1992). *Guidelines for meeting the communication needs of persons with severe disabilities* [Guidelines]. www.asha.org/policy or www.asha.org/njc

National Research Council (NRC). (2001). *Educating children with autism.* Committee on Education Interventions for Children with Autism, Division of Behavioral and Social Sciences and Education. National Academy Press.

Nunes, D. (2008). AAC interventions for autism: A research summary. *International Journal of Special Education, 23*(2), 17–26.

O'Brien, A., Schlosser, R., Shane, H., Abramson, J., Allen, A., Flynn, S., Yu, C., & Dimery, K. (2016). Brief report: Just-in-time visual supports to children with autism via the Apple Watch®: A pilot feasibility study. *Journal of Autism and Developmental Disorders, 46*, 3818–3823.

Ogletree, B., & Harn, W. (2001). Augmentative and alternative communication for persons with autism: History, issues, and unanswered questions. *Focus on Autism and Other Developmental Disabilities, 16*(3), 138–140.

O'Neill, T., Light, J., & McNaughton, D. (2017). Videos with integrated AAC visual scene displays to enhance participation in community and vocational activities: Pilot case student with an adolescent with autism spectrum disorder. *Perspectives of the ASHA Special Interest Groups, 2*(12), 55–69.

Parker, R., Vannest, K., & Brown, L. (2009). The improvement rate difference for single c-case research. *Exceptional Children, 75*(2), 135–150.

Porter, G., & Cafiero, J. (2009). Pragmatic organization dynamic display (PODD) communication books: A promising practice for individuals with autism spectrum disorders. *Perspectives on Augmentative and Alternative Communication, 18*, 121–129.

Pretti-Frontczak, K., & Bricker, D. (2004). *An activity-based approach to early intervention.* Paul H. Brookes Publishing Co.

Prizant, B., & Wetherby, A. (1998). Understanding the continuum of discrete-trial traditional behavioral to social-pragmatic, developmental approaches in communication enhancement for young children with ASD. *Seminars in Speech and Language, 19*, 329–353.

Prizant, B. M., Wetherby, A. M., Rubin, E., & Laurent, A. C. (2003). The SCERTS model: A transactional, family-centered approach to enhancing communication and socioemotional abilities of children with autism spectrum disorder. *Infants and Young Children, 16*(4), 296–316.

Prizant, B., Wetherby, A., Rubin, E., Laurent, A., & Rydell, P. (2006a). *The SCERTS model: A comprehensive educational approach for children with autism spectrum disorders. Vol. I: Assessment.* Paul H. Brookes Publishing Co.

Prizant, B., Wetherby, A., Rubin, E., Laurent, A., & Rydell, P. (2006b). *The SCERTS model: A comprehensive educational approach for children with autism spectrum disorders. Vol. II: Program planning and intervention.* Paul H. Brookes Publishing Co.

Prizant, B. M., Wetherby, A. M., & Rydell, P. J. (2000). Communication intervention issues for children with autism spectrum disorders. In A. M. Wetherby & B. M. Prizant (Eds.), *Autism spectrum disorders: A transactional developmental perspective* (pp. 193–224). Paul H. Brookes Publishing Co.

Robinson, N. B., & Solomon-Rice, P. L. (2009) Supporting collaborative teams and families in AAC. In G. Soto & C. Zangari (Eds.), *Practically speaking: Language, literacy, and academic development for students with AAC needs* (pp. 289–312). Paul H. Brookes Publishing Co.

Romski, R. A., & Sevcik, R. A. (1992). Developing augmented language in children with severe mental retardation. In. S. F. Warren & J. Reichle (Eds.), *Communication and language intervention series: Vol. 1, Causes and effects in communication and language intervention* (pp. 113–130). Paul H. Brookes Publishing Co.

Romski, R. A., & Sevcik, R. A. (1996). *Breaking the speech barrier: Language development through augmented means.* Paul H. Brookes Publishing Co.

Romski, M. A., & Sevcik, R. A. (2003). Augmented input: Enhancing communication development. In J. C. Light, D. R. Beukelman, & J. Reichle (Eds.), *Augmentative and alternative communication series. Communicative competence for individuals who use AAC: From research to effective practice* (pp. 147–162). Paul H. Brookes Publishing Co.

Romski, M. A., Sevcik, R. A., Cheslock, M., & Barton, A. (2006). The system for Augmenting Language: AAC and emerging language intervention. In R. J. McCauley & M. Fey (Eds.), *Treatment of language disorders in children* (pp. 123–147). Paul H. Brookes Publishing Co.

Romski, M., Sevcik, R. Smith, A., Barker, M., Folan, S., & Barton-Hulsey, A. (2009). The system for augmenting language: Implications for young children with autism spectrum disorders. In P. Mirenda, & T. Iacono (Eds.), *Autism spectrum disorders and AAC* (pp. 219–245). Paul H. Brookes Publishing Co.

Rose, V., Trembath, D., Keen, & Paynter, J. (2016). The proportion of minimally verbal children with autism spectrum disorder in a community-based early intervention programme. *Journal of Intellectual Disability Research, 60*, 464–477.

Roseberry-McKibbin, C. (2008). *Multicultural students with special language needs: practical strategies for assessment and intervention.* Academic Communication Associates.

Rubin, E., Laurent, A., Prizant, B., & Wetherby, A. (2009). AAC and the SCERTS model: Incorporating AAC within a comprehensive, multidisciplinary educational program. In P. Mirenda & T. Iacono (Eds.), *Autism spectrum disorders and AAC* (pp. 195–217). Paul H. Brookes Publishing Co.

Schlosser, R., & Koul, R. (2015). Speech output technologies in intervention for individuals with autism spectrum disorders: A scoping review. *Augmentative and Alternative Communication, 34*(4), 285–309.

Schlosser, R., Sigafoos, J., & Koul, R. (2009). Speech output and speech-generating devices in autism spectrum disorders. In P. Mirenda & T. Iacono (Eds.), *Autism spectrum disorders and AAC* (pp. 141–169). Paul H. Brookes Publishing Co.

Schlosser, R., & Wendt, O. (2008a). Augmentative and alternative communication intervention for children with autism. In J. Luiselli, D. Russo, W. Christian, & S. Wilczynski (Eds.), *Effective practices for children with autism: Educational and behavioral support interventions that work* (pp. 325–389). Oxford University Press.

Schlosser, R., & Wendt, O. (2008b). Effects of augmentative and alternative communication intervention on speech production in children with autism: A systematic review. *American Journal of Speech-Language Pathology, 17*(3), 212–230.

Shire, S. Y., & Jones, N. (2015) Communication partners supporting children with complex communication needs who use AAC: A systematic review. *Communication Disorders Quarterly, 37*(1), 3–15.

Sigafoos, J., O'Reilly, M., & Lancioni, G. (2009). Functional communication training and choice-making interventions for the treatment of problem behavior in individuals with autism spectrum disorders. In P. Mirenda & T. Iacono (Eds.), *Autism spectrum disorders and AAC* (pp. 333–353). Paul H. Brookes Publishing Co.

Simacek, J., Pennington, B., Reichle, J., & Parker-McGowan, Q. (2018). Aided AAC for people with severe to profound multiple disabilities: A systematic review of interventions and treatment intensity. *Advances in Neurodevelopmental Disorders, 2*(1), 100–115.

Smith, A., Barker, M., Barton-Hulsey, A., Romski, M., & Sevcik, R. (2016). Augmented language interventions for children with severe disabilities. In R. Sevcik & M. Romski (Eds.), *Communication interventions for individuals with severe disabilities: Exploring research challenges and opportunities* (pp. 123–146). Paul H. Brookes Publishing Co.

Soto, G. (2000). "We have come a long way . . ." AAC and multiculturalism: From cultural awareness to cultural responsibility. *Perspectives on Augmentative and Alternative Communication, 9*(2), 1–3.

Soto, G. (2012). Training partners in AAC in culturally diverse families. *Perspectives on Augmentative and Alternative Communication, 21*(4), 144.

Soto, G., Huer, M., & Taylor, O. (1997). Multicultural issues. In L. Lloyd, D. Fuller, & H. Arvidson (Eds.), *Augmentative and alternative communication: A handbook of principles and practices* (pp. 407–413). Allyn and Bacon.

Starr, V., Caron, J., Light, J., & McNaughton, D. (2018, November). *Effects of video visual scene display on modes of communication* [Poster presentation]. American Speech-Language-Hearing Association (ASHA) Conference, Boston, MA, United States.

Sulzer-Azaroff, B., Hoffman, A. O., Horton, C. B., Bondy, A., & Frost, L. (2009). The picture exchange communication system (PECS): What do the data say? *Focus on Autism and Other Developmental Disabilities, 24*(2), 89–103.

Swartz, J., & Nye, C. (2006). Improving communication for children with autism: Does sign language work? *EBP Briefs, 1*(2), 1–17.

Therrien, M., Light, J., & Pope, L. (2016). Systematic review of the effects of Interventions to promote peer interactions for children who use aided AAC. *Augmentative and Alternative Communication, 32*(2), 81–93.

Tobii Dynavox (n.d.). *PODD for Compass.* Retrieved January 25, 2019, from https://www.tobiidynavox.com/en-us/software/content/podd-for-compass

Walker, V., & Snell, M. (2013). Effects of augmentative and alternative communication on challenging behavior: A meta-analysis. *Augmentative and Alternative Communication, 29*(2), 117–131.

Wegner, J. R. (1995). *A guide to augmented input and language intervention* [Unpublished paper]. University of Kansas.

Wendt, O. (2009). Research on the use of manual signs and graphic symbols in autism spectrum disorder: A systematic review. In P. Mirenda & T. Iacono (Eds.), *Autism spectrum disorders and AAC* (pp. 83–139). Paul H. Brookes Publishing Co.

Wendt, O., & Schlosser, R. (2007). *The effectiveness of speech-generating devices for children with autism: Results from a systematic research review.* Paper presented at the 27th World Congress of the Association of Logopedics and Phoniatrics, Copenhagen, Denmark.

Wendt, O., Schlosser, R., & Lloyd, L. (2004). *AAC for children with autism: A meta-analysis of intervention outcomes: Preliminary results.* Paper presented at the 2004 Annual Convention of the American Speech-Language-Hearing Association, Philadelphia, PA, United States.

Wetherby, A. M., & Prizant, B. M. (2000). Introduction to autism spectrum disorders. In A. Wetherby & B. Prizant (Eds.), *Autism spectrum disorders: A transactional developmental perspective* (pp. 2–7). Paul H. Brookes Publishing Co.

Wood, L., Lasker, J., Siegel-Causey, E., Beukelman, D., & Ball, L. (1998). Input framework for augmentative and alternative communication. *Augmentative and Communication, 14,* 261–267.

Woods, J. J., & Wetherby, A. M. (2003). Early identification and intervention for infants and toddlers who are at risk for autism spectrum disorder. *Language, Speech, and Hearing Services in Schools, 34,* 180–193.

Zangari, C. (2015, July 13). *Beyond the core: Guide to teaching new words to students using AAC* [Blog post]. https://praacticalaac.org/praactical/beyond-the-core-guide-to-teaching -new-words-for-students-who-use-aac

Zangari, C., & Van Tatenhove, G. (2009). Supporting more advanced linguistic communicators in the classroom. In G. Soto & C. Zangari (Eds.), *Practically speaking: Language, literacy, & academic development for students with AAC needs* (pp. 173–193). Paul H. Brookes Publishing Co.

5

The Early Start Denver Model (ESDM)

Promoting Social Communication in Young Children With ASD

Jill Howard and Geraldine Dawson

INTRODUCTION

The Early Start Denver Model (ESDM) is a comprehensive, empirically tested early intervention for young children with autism spectrum disorder (ASD). The program combines an emphasis on play and relationship building with systematically validated teaching practices of applied behavior analysis (ABA; see Chapter 6 for specific examples and descriptions of ABA strategies, especially discrete trial instruction). In short, according to Rogers and Dawson, the ESDM approach "seeks to empower children with ASD to become active participants in the world, initiating interactions with other people" (2010, p. xi). Broadly, it falls within the category of **Naturalistic Developmental Behavioral Interventions (NDBIs),** which are implemented in the context of naturalistic interactions, involve shared control between child and therapist, employ natural contingencies, and use a variety of behavioral strategies to teach developmentally appropriate and prerequisite skills (Schreibman et al., 2015).

At the core of the ESDM is the child's social interactions with others, which are rich in naturalistic opportunities for learning. ESDM was designed for children who are approximately 12 to 60 months of age and range from having no language to language skills at the 48-month level. The ESDM has the advantage of not being tied to a specific delivery setting, which allows it to reach a wide range of children and families. Caregivers deliver the ESDM at home and in the community (i.e., the child's natural environment), whereas therapists and teachers deliver the intervention in a number of different settings, including the home, clinic, and classroom. An infant version of ESDM has been developed and tested in one small study, which facilitates early intervention for the youngest children with or at risk for ASD (Rogers et al., 2014). Promising outcomes support the need to test treatment efficacy in a larger study.

The program is highly individualized; core features of the model include naturalistic ABA strategies, sensitivity to normal developmental sequences, extensive caregiver involvement, focus on shared positive affect and interaction, shared engagement in activities, and language and communication embedded within a positive, affectively driven relationship. Of note, much of the information in this chapter originates from two key ESDM resources, one written primarily for therapists and professionals (Rogers & Dawson, 2010), and the other primarily for caregivers of young children with ASD (Rogers, Dawson, & Vismara, 2012).

TARGET POPULATIONS

The ESDM is designed for children with ASD between the ages of 12 and 60 months, with developmental skills ranging between 7–9 and 48 months. This can include children with coexisting language and/or intellectual impairments and attention difficulties. The program is meant to serve children with a range of learning styles and abilities.

Children who tend to benefit most from the ESDM generally show some interest in objects and can carry out some one-step actions on objects (e.g., take out/put in) and combine objects in play. However, beyond these basic developmental skills, children with a wide range of developmental profiles may be served effectively through the ESDM. Even those without these skills may benefit; however, this foundation would need to be a primary focus of the earliest phases of the treatment for progress to occur.

Although the teaching strategies may be effective for children beyond the 48-month level of functioning, the curriculum (i.e., set of specific child skills targeted within the program, spanning developmental domains) would not be appropriate. In other words, the teaching strategies are likely relevant to children across a range of ages, though developmental skills targeted in the ESDM reach only approximately the 48-month developmental level.

THEORETICAL BASIS

The theoretical basis for the ESDM is derived from models of child development, behavioral principles, and developmental processes known to be affected in ASD, including social orienting and effects of reduced sensitivity to social stimuli. The ESDM focuses on building the child's social initiative and social engagement, and it seeks to enact positive change on both the child's brain and his or her behavior while targeting a range of developmental domains.

Dominant Theoretical Explanation or Rationale

With regard to predominant models of child development which inform the ESDM, both constructionist (Piaget, 1963) and transactional (Sameroff, 2009) models of child development play important roles. In the constructionist model, young children are viewed as active individuals who create their own social world as a result of motor, sensory, and interpersonal experiences. The child does so by making deliberate decisions regarding with what, with whom, and how they wish to engage. In this way, a child who chooses to engage with other people or in social games constructs a distinctively different world than does a child whose attention is drawn to the nonsocial world or even unusual stimuli, such as fans, lights, or dripping water.

In the transactional model of child development, the world is viewed as a context in which the child and caregiver (as well as other adults) influence one another through exchanging emotions and reacting to each other's temperament and behavior. The way in which the caregiver interacts with the child ultimately affects the way in which the child views the caregiver and behaves, which in turn impacts the caregiver's reaction and behavior, and so on. This cycle continues over the course of an interactive relationship and is thought to contribute in part to the theory and rationale behind the ESDM.

In addition to these broad developmental theories, other approaches influencing the ESDM include the Denver Model, Rogers and Pennington's model relating to interpersonal development in ASD (Rogers & Pennington, 1991); social motivation theory of autism (Chevalier et al., 2012; Dawson, Webb, & McPartland, 2005; Dawson, Webb, Wijsman, et al., 2005); and interventions such as ABA and Pivotal Response Training (PRT; Schreibman et al., 2015). The Denver Model was established as a developmentally based preschool program in 1981 and shares several key tenets with ESDM, including the use of lively, dynamic social interactions; assessing and teaching within all developmental domains; use of an interdisciplinary team; emphasis on both verbal and nonverbal communication; and strong partnership with parents (Rogers et al., 1986). At the core of the Denver Model is a focus on building close relationships between children with ASD and adults as well as other children.

Rogers and Pennington (1991) identified particular areas of need in autism as those involving imitation, sharing of emotion, and theory of mind, which involves the ability to recognize that another person's mental state (e.g., beliefs, intents, emotions) may be different from one's own (Frith & Frith, 2005). All of these skills require the ability to form and coordinate social representations of the self and another person and incorporating representational processes that allow comparisons between oneself and another. The weakness in autism was hypothesized to affect the way in which infants and adults attend to one another, from which cascading impacts on development naturally follow.

Dawson's early work described specific challenges in social attention, characterized by reduced social orienting, shared attention, and attention to others emotions; she and her colleagues described the social motivation hypothesis, which posits that children with ASD demonstrate reduced sensitivity to the reward value of social stimuli and consequently attend less to these stimuli and experience fewer opportunities for learning (Dawson et al., 2002; Dawson et al., 2004). Resulting developmental impacts of this process include impaired social-communication skills.

ABA's influence on the ESDM is primarily in terms of the approach to teaching and the antecedent–behavior–consequence (ABC) model and other related techniques, such as prompting, fading, and shaping. Finally, PRT (see description in Chapter 13) is also based in ABA and shares principles with the ESDM, including a naturalistic and interactive format, maximizing a child's motivation, offering choices, and reinforcing approximations of behavior (Koegel & Koegel, 1988).

Underlying Assumptions

ESDM conveys several assumptions with regard to the nature of the social-communication challenges that it addresses. In particular, it is fundamental to recognize that the nature of autism (i.e., more narrow focus of attention) limits a child's learning opportunities, and as such, one goal of the ESDM is to create and expand opportunities for learning. The more narrow focus of attention in children with autism combined with fewer social initiations results in a limited range of experience with which to construct an understanding of people and events. Beyond its impact on the individual, autism also affects those with whom the child interacts. A caregiver of a child with autism is likely to modify his or her own behavior in response to absent or limited positive feedback during social interactions. In turn, the infant is actively shaping his or her world in terms of the quantity and quality of social exchange with caregivers. This cycle is likely to exert tight control over a child's social world unless steps are taken to actively shift the balance and to teach the child that social interactions can be enjoyable and reinforcing, creating a wider funnel of social attention.

ESDM is rooted in building the child's social initiative and social engagement, similar to other NDBIs (see the Developmental, Individual-Difference, Relationship-Based model in Chapter 7 and Enhanced Milieu Teaching in Chapter 10). Some of the features that distinguish ESDM include use of strategies that promote affective engagement, such as **sensory social routines,** simultaneous targeting of more than own objective at a time, and viewing the caregiver–child relationship as the core of the intervention. Like other empirically validated behavioral interventions, ESDM is based in frequent and thorough data collection, which is used to guide treatment. Finally, the model spans developmental domains (including not only social communication but also motor, personal independence, and cognition) and provides systematic guidance on appropriate modifications in teaching strategies should the child not demonstrate steady progress toward his or her goals.

As mentioned, principles of ABA also contribute to the basis of teaching strategies in ESDM. However, several aspects of the ESDM differentiate it from traditional models of ABA, such as discrete trial instruction. For example, the ESDM curriculum is derived from years of research on children's typical development, and relative to some other ABA approaches, ESDM entails a greater focus on building relationships, exchanging positive affect, and the importance of the adult's sensitivity to the child's preferences and choices. In addition, the tools that facilitate language development are rooted strongly in research on the developmental progression of language learning. One related assumption is that brain systems supporting social and language learning are atypically developing, though modifiable with intervention, in the young child with ASD.

Functional Outcomes Being Addressed

An important expectation of intervention using the ESDM is that it contributes to changes in the brain as well as in the child's behavior. At the core of ESDM is the fundamental need to address challenges in social orienting and social initiation that are characteristic of early autism. Ideally, in developing programmatic objectives, the therapist is writing objectives that are functional—in other words, the goal is to teach children to demonstrate skill use in adaptive, typical situations, not just in the session room. If the child has not yet generalized skills learned in therapy to other real-life settings, then there remains work to be done along the way to confirming mastery.

Target Areas of Treatment

Treatment target areas include a range of developmental domains. Language areas targeted include both receptive and expressive communication, and social skill areas targeted include social skills with both adults and peers, joint attention, imitation, and play. Other areas targeted in the ESDM consist of behavior, cognition, fine motor, gross motor, and personal independence (e.g., hygiene, chores) domains.

EMPIRICAL BASIS

The empirical basis for the ESDM has been examined for several variations of this intervention: the original clinician-implemented version (ESDM), the parent-implemented version (P-ESDM), a version intended for group settings (G-ESDM), a version provided through telehealth, and evidence for international interpretations of the ESDM in China and Italy. Each of these areas is covered briefly in this section. In addition, the chapter presents evidence regarding long-term follow-up and different models of training that have been investigated.

Early Start Denver Model

As mentioned, the ESDM is supported by many years of peer-reviewed, published research, ranging from case studies to randomized controlled trials (RCTs). The first RCT that tested ESDM included 48 children with ASD between the ages of 18 to 30 months, randomly assigned to either 1) an ESDM group, which they received for 2 years (15–20 hours/week of ESDM, plus parent training and 5 or more hours/week of parent-delivered ESDM), or 2) referral to community providers for community treatment as usual (Dawson et al., 2010). Children in the ESDM group showed significant improvements in IQ, adaptive behavior skills, and status of ASD diagnosis 2 years after entering intervention. The average IQ gain was 17 points, greater than 1 standard deviation. The study concluded that the ESDM accelerates rate of development and also generalizes to everyday life. In addition, parents' use of ESDM strategies throughout typical daily routines was acknowledged as likely to be an important ingredient of success.

In addition to generating differences in parent and child behavior, ESDM has also been found to be associated with changes in children's brain activity reflected in normalized brain activity following intervention (Dawson et al., 2012). Specifically, the ESDM group increased cortical activation as measured by electroencephalogram (EEG) when viewing social stimuli. Greater cortical activation while viewing social stimuli was associated with improved social behavior. Other positive effects of ESDM included reduction in maladaptive behaviors, with a Cohen's d of -3.7 (large) for clinician's rating of the child's behavior following approximately 1 year of treatment (Fulton et al., 2014). In the same study, there was also a significant increase to children's overall developmental quotient (Mullen Scales of Early Learning; Mullen, 1995) with an effect size of $d = -0.41$ (approaching medium).

Parent-Delivered Early Start Denver Model (P-ESDM)

An early study investigating the parent-delivered (or **parent-implemented**) ESDM model provided 12 sessions of parent coaching for 1 hour per week (plus four 1-hour follow-up sessions addressing maintenance and generalization) to parents of eight toddlers (36 months of age or younger) diagnosed with ASD (Vismara, Colombi,

& Rogers, 2009). Positive results were found for both parent and child behaviors. Specifically, parents demonstrated fidelity of implementation (mastery of ESDM techniques at or above 85%) at approximately the fifth to sixth intervention session, which was also maintained at follow-up. With regard to child behaviors, at baseline the children produced nearly no social-communicative behaviors, initiation, imitation, or speech. However, over the course of treatment, children demonstrated gradual improvements in all behaviors. One conclusion was that the parent's new skills are the agent of change and that interactions with the parent are the main source of child change. This important conclusion supports the P-ESDM model even in a low-intensity, short-term design.

A case study with a 9-month old infant showing emerging signs of ASD utilized twelve 1.5-hour sessions of **parent coaching** in ESDM (Vismara & Rogers, 2008). Results demonstrated that the parent gained several teaching tactics that were linked to growth in the infant's social-communicative abilities. Researchers also observed improvements in severity of behaviors associated with ASD, indicating support for an intervention model to provide parents with skills needed to engage very young children with or at risk for ASD.

Another study (including seven infants ages 7–15 months with ASD symptoms) piloted a 12-week low-intensity treatment with parents and showed that parents were able to master the intervention and maintain skills postintervention (Rogers et al., 2014). Promising results also emphasized lower rates of ASD at 36 months and lower developmental quotients within the significantly delayed range (<70) relative to a comparison group of children who showed similar symptoms but whose parents elected not to enroll in the treatment study ($n = 4$). At 36 months, the treatment group had significantly higher visual reception scores on the Mullen Scales of Early Learning (Mullen, 1995) than the group who declined enrollment ($d = 2.41$).

Rogers, Estes, and colleagues (2012) conducted the first RCT of P-ESDM, which included 98 children and families. Findings indicated no effect of group assignment on parent–child interaction characteristics or child outcomes. However, children in the P-ESDM group received significantly fewer hours of intervention (and experienced relatively similar outcomes to the community treatment-as-usual group). Overall, younger age at beginning of intervention and number of intervention hours were positively associated with improvement across most variables of interest. When outcomes were compared (children 18–48 versus 48–62 months receiving ESDM for 20 hours per week for 1 year), younger children evidenced superior verbal developmental quotient gains, although groups did not differ on nonverbal developmental quotient, adaptive behavior, or ASD severity (Vivanti, Dissanayake, & The Victorian ASELCC Team, 2016).

To consider how participating in P-ESDM affects aspects of a caregiver's well-being, including parenting-related stress and sense of self-competence, Estes and colleagues (2014) compared 49 parents of children with ASD between 12 and 24 months of age. The participants were randomized to receive either P-ESDM or community treatment-as-usual. Over a 3-month period, those who participated in P-ESDM reported no increase in parenting stress, whereas the community treatment-as-usual group experienced increased stress. However, parental sense of competence was similar between the two groups. This finding suggests that becoming connected with high-quality early intervention may serve to mitigate considerable stress that is otherwise likely to emerge during the period of time following a new diagnosis.

Group Early Start Denver Model

Several studies have demonstrated support for ESDM delivered in a group setting. Eapen and colleagues (2013) evaluated the effectiveness of ESDM for preschoolers with ASD (mean age 49.6 months) using a group-based intervention in a community child care setting. Participants included 26 children with ASD who received 15–20 hours of group-based ESDM and 1 hour of individual ESDM per week for 10 months. Assessment using the Mullen Scales of Early Learning (Mullen, 1995) revealed statistically significant improvements in visual reception ($d = 0.63$), receptive language ($d = 0.48$), and expressive language skills ($d = 0.40$). The Vineland Adaptive Behavior Scales–Second Edition (Sparrow et al., 2005) assessment found statistically significant improvements in receptive communication ($d = 0.49$) and motor skills ($d = 0.45$). A significant decrease in autism-specific features was also observed ($d = -0.39$) (Social Communication Questionnaire; Rutter et al., 2003).

Similarly, in a study by Vivanti and colleagues (2014) investigating feasibility and effectiveness of the ESDM in a group-based community child care setting (27 preschoolers with ASD, 15–25 hours per week of ESDM over 12 months, compared to 30 children with ASD receiving a different intervention), children in both groups developed skills across several domains (cognitive, adaptive, social). In addition, children in the ESDM group evidenced relatively stronger gains in developmental rate (medium effect size) and receptive language skills (large effect size).

In predicting outcomes for children with ASD who received ESDM intervention in a group setting, the greatest developmental gains after 1 year of treatment were associated with those with more advanced skills in the functional use of objects, goal understanding, and imitation at the beginning of the study (Vivanti et al., 2013). A different sample predicted outcomes for preschoolers in group ESDM and found that lower ASD symptomatology (especially higher social affect and play skills) and younger age at beginning of intervention predicted better outcomes (Eapen et al., 2016).

Long-Term Follow-Up

One study has documented the longer-term outcomes of children who received intensive ESDM as toddlers/preschoolers. Estes and colleagues (2015) studied a sample of 39 children with ASD from the original Dawson and colleagues' (2010) RCT of 48 toddlers between 18 and 30 months at the beginning of the program (at long-term follow-up, $n = 21$ for the ESDM group, and $n = 18$ for the treatment-as-usual group). Estes and colleagues evaluated the children 2 years after their 2-year intervention, at age 6, and concluded that the ESDM group maintained gains made in early intervention. An additional finding (not identified immediately post-treatment) was that at 2-year follow-up, the ESDM group showed improved core autism symptoms relative to the community treatment-as-usual group (medium effect size). In addition, the gains evidenced by the ESDM group persisted in response to fewer hours of intervention received during follow-up relative to the community treatment-as-usual group. Importantly, Estes and colleagues were the first to demonstrate the possibility of altering the longer-term developmental course for children with ASD who receive early behavioral intervention.

Furthermore, long-term follow-up of the cost associated with the ESDM has shown that within a few years following the intervention, the cost is completely offset by reductions in service use as a result of reduced need for other services, such as ABA, physical therapy, occupational therapy, and speech language therapy (Cidav et al., 2017).

Training Models of Early Start Denver Model

With regard to empirical studies investigating aspects of training, one study compared distance learning with live instruction for training community therapists in the ESDM (Vismara, Young, et al., 2009). Results indicated that both variants were equally effective for teaching therapists to implement the model and train parents (i.e., there were no differences in therapist fidelity either when working directly with children or when coaching parents). However, one discouraging finding was that at the end of direct intervention, only 50% of the community therapists had achieved a performance level of 85% on the fidelity measure. Didactic workshops and group supervision were deemed necessary for improving therapists' use of ESDM skills. Some positive changes in children's behavior were also observed throughout the course of the program (i.e., number of social initiations and amount of attention to the adult increased significantly between baseline and the beginning of the group supervision phase), with no significant difference between the distance learning and live instruction groups.

In focusing on training through a community implementation lens, preliminary research has investigated the feasibility of using an abbreviated training workshop for community-based providers (Vismara et al., 2013). Practitioners were successful in self-assessing delivery of ESDM strategies. For those who submitted follow-up materials, fidelity of implementation at 85% was also achieved. Additional research is needed to continue to support dissemination work.

Early Start Denver Model and Telehealth

Recently, telehealth has been investigated as a means of making ESDM services more accessible to families (Vismara et al., 2012; Vismara et al., 2018). Preliminary results from a sample of nine families showed that parents learned to use teachable moments to promote children's language and imitation skills, and they expressed satisfaction with the ease and support of learning through telehealth (Vismara et al., 2012). A more recent study involved an RCT for telehealth-delivered P-ESDM (Vismara et al., 2018). Findings supported the feasibility of telehealth training in terms of improving parents' usage of and satisfaction from the program.

International Applications of Early Start Denver Model

In addition to studies in the United States and Australia, research on the ESDM has been conducted in China and Italy. A 26-week, high-intensity P-ESDM program in China showed greater improvements in the P-ESDM group compared to the community treatment-as-usual group for general developmental skill (particularly in the area of language) (Zhou et al., 2018). The groups demonstrated comparable ASD severity post-intervention, although parents in the P-ESDM group showed greater improvements in their report of their child's social communication and symbolic play. Further, children in the P-ESDM group showed more improvement in use of social affect. Parent stress in the P-ESDM group decreased over the course of the intervention, whereas it increased for the community treatment-as-usual group.

Similarly, empirical work in Italy has shown support for the use of the ESDM in a non–English-speaking community. For 22 young children with ASD receiving the ESDM in a center-based setting for 6 hours per week for 6 months, greater gains relative to the community treatment-as-usual group were shown in the areas of cognitive and social skills after 3 and 6 months and in adaptive skills after 3 months (Colombi et al., 2018).

With a strong empirical foundation, continued research on the ESDM should seek to demonstrate active ingredients, compare variations of dosage/intensity, and directly compare the ESDM to other treatments. In addition, future work should determine how to better disseminate the ESDM both in the United States and globally in order to allow more children to access high-quality, evidence-based services.

PRACTICAL REQUIREMENTS

Practically speaking, the ESDM is designed to be implemented and overseen by professionals with training in special education; educational, clinical, or developmental psychology; speech-language pathology, occupational therapy, or ABA. Paraprofessionals often deliver the intervention under the supervision of individuals with advanced training in these disciplines. Regardless of background, it is important for ESDM therapists to possess a strong understanding of child development and behavioral principles in order to most effectively apply therapeutic techniques. A treatment team that represents a number of different disciplines can be helpful for ensuring that all aspects of a child's development (e.g., linguistic, social, motoric, adaptive, cognitive) are fully attended to and for facilitating fidelity of implementation across all skill domains. The ESDM manual (Rogers & Dawson, 2010) has been translated into 16 languages and is used worldwide.

For therapists with backgrounds in child development, ESDM principles of following a child's lead and using play to create learning opportunities tend to come quite naturally, whereas the application of behavioral techniques such as reinforcement, shaping, fading, and prompting may require some additional refinement. Conversely, those with backgrounds in behavior analysis are generally familiar with behavioral teaching strategies for teaching new skills and replacing unwanted behaviors, although the child-directed, affectively based, reciprocal aspects of ESDM may require greater attention in order to attain fidelity to the model.

With regard to training requirements, the ESDM training program (https://www.esdm.co) includes didactic instruction as well as more practical application of the strategies. An individual pursuing certification in ESDM works closely with a certified trainer for supervision and feedback regarding technique. At the end of the training program, the goal is to demonstrate mastery in fidelity of intervention delivery, use of the ESDM Curriculum Checklist for Young Children with Autism (Rogers & Dawson, 2009), writing effective objectives and steps (including task analysis for breaking larger goals into smaller steps), use of a system for taking child data, and fully grasping the ESDM in order to supervise others. The ESDM Curriculum Checklist is a detailed assessment tool for evaluating a child's skills and developing individually tailored objectives and steps. It provides a guide for assessing and tracking individual teaching objectives and skills in all developmental domains at four levels of development.

The ESDM **Teaching Fidelity Rating System** evaluates a therapist's mastery of ESDM principles (e.g., management of child attention, quality of behavioral teaching, quality of dyadic engagement, adult sensitivity and responsivity to child communicative cues), as demonstrated in intervention sessions, and is used to rate skills following each individual play activity (1–5 scale; 1 = very poor usage, 5 = optimal usage). Competence on this scale is defined as 1) achieving an average score of 85% or greater for each play activity, 2) consistent scores of 4 and 5 throughout each activity, and 3) no score lower than 3 for any activity.

For beginner therapists, the expectation is that an overall score of 80%–85% across three or more consecutive administrations is achieved before using ESDM independently. Independent use of ESDM is also contingent upon accurate data collection during a session, with interrater reliability at least 80% with the team leader across three training sessions. For those individuals likely to be involved in leading a team of therapists or supervising others' work, additional training is required, which includes supervised experience with teaching and training others.

Given that ESDM may be delivered in clinic, at school, or at home, a specific set of materials is not required, although recommendations are provided regarding general types of materials. For the curriculum assessment and therapy sessions, the room setup would ideally include a small table, two small chairs, and a bean bag for sitting. For sensory-social routines, materials such as bubbles, balloons, and other sensory toys may be useful. **Object-focused joint activities** generally allow for the demonstration of parallel play, communication, and turn-taking skills with objects; these may include art, cognitive, and play activities. Art activities might involve paper, color markers, and scissors. For activities targeting cognitive skills, materials would likely include puzzles, nesting cups, and objects for matching. For targeting gross and fine motor skills, materials include a set of blocks of different colors and sizes, different-sized balls and bean bags, pegs and pegboard, blocks, pop beads, fat beads to string, ring stacker, toy hammer with balls/pegs, shape sorter, and playdough. In order to target personal independence skills, important items consist of sets of eating objects (i.e., cups, plates, spoons, forks), personal grooming objects (i.e., comb, brush, mirror, hat, necklace), a large doll with clothes, and snacks. For play, useful materials include cars and trucks, sets of farm animals (with identical pictures for matching), and a pop-up toy. Finally, for social goals, photos of the child and important family members are useful.

During an activity, ideally, only one set of materials is available to the child at a given time in order to promote focused attention and eliminate distractions. For materials not in use at the time, adult-level storage cupboards or shelves covered with a sheet can help to keep supplies organized. In general, less complex materials are preferred (i.e., toys with a clear function, as well as materials that allow for simple symbolic play), as are nonelectronic toys.

Central to the treatment team is the parent/caregiver as well as a team leader if multiple therapists collaborate in serving the child. Interdisciplinary treatment teams consist of special educators, child and/or developmental psychologists, speech and occupational therapists, medical providers, and behavior analysts working together to create a treatment plan and to bring it to fruition.

KEY COMPONENTS

As mentioned, goals addressed by ESDM span developmental domains and are addressed simultaneously rather than sequentially. Goals are targeted within typical daily activities such as playtime, mealtime, hygiene, and chore activities. Depending on the mode of delivery, participants beyond the clinician, caregiver, and child might include peers, siblings, teachers, or other individuals in close contact with the child. Roles of these individuals are explained in more detail throughout this section.

Group-Delivered Early Start Denver Model

In group settings such as preschools, peer interactions are the primary vehicle for teaching. The ideal structure in this particular setting consists of peer interaction promoted through activities that elicit engagement in the same physical space. Materials and strategies that tend to facilitate this goal are double sets of toys and face-to-face positioning. Children benefit from the opportunity to practice imitation and parallel play in these settings through increased attention to peers. Although initially the child with ASD may devote greater focus to the activity and materials than to the surrounding peers, the idea is that this is a step along the way to parallel and imitative play.

For a child participating in a group environment, positive results might include the ability to (Rogers & Dawson, 2010)

1. Follow daily routines and transition from one activity to another

2. Participate in activities in dyads or smaller groups, as well as larger (whole class) groups

3. Engage in functional play characterized by appropriate object use

4. Exhibit personal independence related to managing materials (e.g., lunchbox, items needed for activities) and daily living skills (e.g., snack- and lunchtime, clearing dishes and trash after eating, hand washing)

5. Initiate interactions with adults and peers

6. Improve developmental skills across domains

Typical classroom activities are generally designed to achieve these skills, with additional support from the individual child's objectives. An individual child's objectives are addressed on a daily basis as a result of being embedded into classroom activities and also as a result of being targeted in small-group time or during scheduled individual teaching times if needed. Whether in an individual or group setting, the teaching practices remain consistent. Based in ABA principles, teaching procedures begin with setting up an interesting activity and working to keep the child engaged through introducing variation and presenting frequent learning opportunities. When multiple children are involved in one activity, it requires that the teacher shift quickly from one child to the next in order to keep all children engaged and levels of participation high.

One important note about using ESDM in a group setting is that the classroom setup and structure would likely appear similar to those of other toddler or preschool classrooms. Essentially, the techniques geared toward children with ASD can be incorporated into a traditional classroom without significant disruption. It is, however, recommended that additional attention be devoted to sensory aspects of the environment (e.g., reducing distractions) and other learning supports that may be useful (e.g., presenting information visually). With regard to the size of the group, it can be modified according to the needs of individual children so long as the number of staff to children does not fall below a one to four ratio.

In terms of other areas deserving of additional attention, the organization and structure of the classroom are worth noting. Given that children with ASD generally respond well to routine and predictable scheduling, teachers may find that using a consistent, predictable, carefully planned routine allows children with ASD to participate more effectively. Keeping materials in consistent locations and using consistent sequences within activities are other ways in which predictability can be enhanced. This structure helps with promoting independence in navigating the classroom and in organizing goal-directed behavior.

Teachers also conduct the important job of articulating the roles of other staff and members of the support team, both when leading activities and when transitioning between activities. Again, structure can be enhanced through keeping staff in consistent roles from one day to the next. In most group settings, although the majority of the child's time is spent in large- or small-group activities, about 15–20 minutes can be set aside for individual teaching time, occurring either inside or outside of the classroom.

Group activities are constructed according to skills of the group as well as individual objectives. It is possible that, for the same group activity, individual children are participating in varied ways, which allows all children to experience maximum possible benefit from the given activity, due to careful consideration of child variables (e.g., motivation) as well as design of the task (e.g., targeting optimal level of difficulty for the child, likely including practice of new skills just barely outside of the child's skillset, as well as maintenance of recently mastered skills).

Parent-Delivered Early Start Denver Model

For P-ESDM, the relationship between the caregiver and clinician is of utmost importance. The coaching relationship is framed as a partnership in which the caregiver is seen as the expert on the child and the clinician is learning about the child with the help of the caregiver. In contrast with therapist-delivered ESDM, objectives are written in a less technical and scholarly manner and are meant to be more interpretable for someone without formal training in child behavior or behavior analysis. If caregivers can see the objectives as relevant and applicable to everyday life with their child, they may be more likely to appreciate the concept of teaching within daily routines and to build those routines into the typical day. Caregivers are encouraged to capitalize on the time that they already spend with their child rather than to feel they must set aside additional time to "work on ESDM." When the coach strives to be a collaborator and a partner, promoting self-assessment in a nonjudgmental and supportive way, the seed is planted for caregiver self-determinacy and self-evaluation to persist even after the program has formally concluded.

After each activity in P-ESDM sessions, the coach conducts a reflective discussion that encourages caregivers to share what they viewed as their goals within the activity, how the child responded, and what the experience was like for both the caregiver and child. The clinician's role is to comment using descriptive language and to communicate support, acceptance, and respect for the caregiver's efforts. Although P-ESDM sessions are often conducted in clinic or at home, it is possible to conduct coaching sessions in other locations where challenging behaviors are likely to arise, such as grocery stores, restaurants, or other settings that caregivers find particularly challenging.

The P-ESDM is individually tailored to fully incorporate caregivers' preferences on learning styles, strengths, and needs. The primary goal of the program is caregiver behavior change, and the secondary goal is child behavior change. Fidelity of implementation metrics help to identify and track the progression of caregiver behavior change. Caregiver competence and self-efficacy are also directly addressed through hands-on activities and the cycle of live coaching and reflection. To promote dialogue and work on identifying small, actionable steps, motivational interviewing (Miller & Rollnick, 2013) is used to foster productive conversation around challenges, barriers, and successes. Motivational interviewing is a therapeutic technique that assists people in identifying their own intrinsic motivation to change while taking into account readiness to change.

In general, session topics follow the order of the chapters in the book written for caregivers (Rogers, Dawson, & Vismara, 2012), although modifications for the caregiver's needs or child's goals are permitted. Over time, the natural progression of the program is such that once caregivers have started to master ESDM skills, focus begins to shift to child learning and progress through attending more specifically to child objectives.

Depending what is most helpful to the caregiver, the clinician may provide additional supports, such as a written summary of the week's chapter or a cartoon diagram with ideas of daily activities in which ESDM may be utilized. It is recommended that modeling be used only when necessary in order to prevent caregivers from seeing the clinician as the expert and from thinking that a technique should be done in a certain way.

Coaching generally entails a short-term course of treatment. However, in longer-term coaching relationships, the content of sessions may shift once the caregiver reaches fidelity, whereby targeting child objectives becomes a greater focus in relation to targeting ESDM techniques. In addition to generally being short term, P-ESDM is typically low intensity (i.e., one 60- to 90-minute session per week).

Implementation Fidelity

Several methods have been established to measure and track fidelity of implementation. In ESDM training programs, the therapist is deemed to have reached fidelity when no scores fall below 3 on the 5-point Teaching Fidelity Rating System scale (where 1 = very poor usage, 5 = optimal usage), and the mean score is at least 4 on three consecutive joint activity routines, for at least two consecutive children. Items on which fidelity is coded include the following:

- Management of child attention

- ABC format—quality of behavioral teaching

- Instructional techniques application

- Adult ability to modulate child affect and arousal

- Management of unwanted behaviors

- Quality of dyadic engagement

- Adult optimization of child motivation for participating in the activity

- Adult use of positive affect

- Adult sensitivity and responsivity to child communicative cues

- Multiple and varied communicative opportunities occur in the activity

- Appropriateness of adult language for child's language level

- Joint activity structure and elaboration

- Transitions between activities

For assessing a coach's fidelity to the coaching model, a different set of fidelity items were developed. They follow a 1–4 scale, where coaching fidelity is no score under 2 and a mean of 80% or above over three consecutive sessions for the overall performance on the scale. Coaching fidelity items include the following:

- Greeting and checking in

- Warm-up caregiver–child joint activity

- Settling on the topic of the day

- Coaching on the week's topic

- Closing

- Collaborative

- Reflective

- Nonjudgmental

- Conversational and reciprocal

- Ethical conduct

- Organization and management of session

- Managing caregiver implementation and motivational difficulties

ASSESSMENT FOR TREATMENT PLANNING AND PROGRESS MONITORING

The ESDM includes detailed procedures for both treatment planning and progress monitoring. To initially establish the appropriateness of the ESDM for a given child, the first step is to conduct a curriculum assessment using the ESDM Curriculum Checklist for Young Children with Autism (Rogers & Dawson, 2009). This criterion-referenced tool consists of developmental sequences of skills across several domains. The ESDM Curriculum Checklist is organized into four skill levels, corresponding to 12–18, 18–24, 24–36, and 36–48 months of age. Skills within domains were generated from extensive literature reviews on skill progression in typical child development. The ordering of items is a function of both typical developmental progression and common areas of weakness in ASD that may require additional attention in order to achieve optimal progress.

The therapist manual provides specific item descriptions that delineate exactly what is required to be able to score an item as passing. The **Curriculum Checklist** integrates information from therapist observation and caregiver/other report in scoring. When completing the entirety of the Curriculum Checklist, the therapist obtains a comprehensive understanding of the child's working set of skills, including where there might be gaps and what appropriate next steps would be for the child's development.

Following the curriculum assessment, the next step involves generating a set of learning objectives that target growth over the period of the next 12 weeks. For each domain, two or three skills are selected, and learning objectives are written as measurable behaviors, A well-written objective includes four parts: 1) a statement of the antecedent stimulus or event that is meant to elicit the behavior (skill); 2) a description of a measurable, observable behavior to be taught; 3) what defines mastery of the objective (e.g., in 90% of opportunities, three times in a 20-minute period); and 4) how functional, generalized performance of the skill is characterized (often involving skill demonstration across people, settings, and/or materials). For example,

> 1) *When an adult holds up an object and offers it to the child,* 2) *he will **use single words integrated with gaze to request the object if he wants it or to refuse if he does not want it*** 3) *in at least 80% of opportunities, over three consecutive sessions,* 4) *across at least five different objects, with two or more adults and in two or more different settings.*

From the **short-term learning objectives,** each is broken down into small, teachable steps that work toward mastery on the full objective. Smaller steps are generated by conducting a task analysis beginning at the child's baseline level and ending with full mastery and generalization as written in the objective. These smaller steps guide daily teaching plans and behavioral targets for data collection.

The **Daily Data Sheet,** which is used in each session, allows for periodic recordings of child performance and cues the therapist as to which step along the way to mastery is being targeted. The Daily Data Sheet highlights the step on which the child is currently working (which the therapist is currently targeting) for each objective. The therapist gathers data at set intervals throughout the session (e.g., every 15 minutes), and the datasheet both informs the lesson plan for the session and allows for an understanding of how the child is progressing over time.

Should the child not make steady progress toward his or her objectives from week to week, the therapist must determine how to adapt teaching approaches in order to more effectively generate growth. Some options for adjusting the teaching plan include 1) varying reinforcement strength (e.g., by finding a more appealing reinforcer), 2) adding structure to the teaching episode, and 3) adding visual supports (Rogers & Dawson, 2010, p. 131, presents a decision tree that assists with determining what additional support is appropriate). These adjustments are recommended to be implemented only when needed, as they may reduce the naturalistic nature of the intervention.

IMPLICATIONS FOR INCLUSIVE PRACTICE

Group-based ESDM (G-ESDM; Vivanti et al., 2017) is a recently manualized application of the traditional ESDM model. It was designed for the purpose of delivering ESDM in group-based programs, such as existing community programs, and allows for the intervention to be delivered in an environment rich in social interactive opportunities among peers. The ideal environment for promoting social interaction and learning is one that involves children with typical development, and G-ESDM is well suited for fully inclusive programs. The environment may include a combination of children with ASD and peers with typical development.

A previous effectiveness and feasibility study investigated ESDM delivered one to one in the context of a community child care setting and found that participants in the ESDM group showed significantly greater gains in developmental skill acquisition and receptive language relative to those receiving a different intervention (Vivanti et al., 2014). The ideal classroom curriculum for a G-ESDM program is described by Vivanti, Kapes, and colleagues (2016), highlighting the importance of rewarding, meaningful group activities that involve multiple teaching episodes while still targeting individual goals.

Currently, additional research is being conducted to determine the feasibility of establishing inclusion G-ESDM programs in existing community preschools. As for the implications of this mode of delivery, the inclusive classroom setting permits the young child with ASD to participate alongside all other children, and instructors construct small playgroups that facilitate learning opportunities. These playgroups are carefully designed to meet the developmental needs and goals of the child with ASD. As such, this setting is ripe for peer modeling and peer interactions and can be very successful given that sufficient attention is devoted to intervention individualization, rigor and quality, and the caregiver–professional partnership (i.e., involving families in the therapy).

In order for an inclusive setting to convey a positive experience for a child on the spectrum, it is crucial for teachers and other professionals in the classroom to see this arrangement as favorable. With this perspective, the extra effort required to facilitate opportunities for children with ASD to practice social and communication skills in a naturalistic context (with skilled play partners, such as children with typical development) can be viewed as worthwhile, rather than a burden, and this context can be viewed as the ideal one in which to practice, refine, and generalize newly learned skills. The G-ESDM program aligns with the mindset that children with ASD should participate in their social community starting as early as possible and that the lives of children with typical development will also be enriched (e.g., through their gaining a greater appreciation for neurodiversity) as a result of the opportunity to engage with individuals with ASD.

Another implication of using ESDM in an inclusive environment is that it may entail the need for additional training and resources to be made available to teachers, although this is likely to be the case for any inclusive program. Particular attention should be devoted to strategies for facilitating peer interactions. The G-ESDM values transdisciplinary teamwork and finds that teachers who feel empowered with support from the team are more likely to experience success in an inclusive setting than are teachers without support.

With regard to practical implications, the current version of G-ESDM recommends that the staff to child ratio be no lower than one to four. In addition, it is important that a behavioral specialist be available to the team in order to quickly address challenging behavior in terms of both potentially dangerous behavior and behaviors that may disrupt learning.

CONSIDERATIONS FOR CHILDREN FROM
CULTURALLY AND LINGUISTICALLY DIVERSE BACKGROUNDS

Several aspects of the ESDM model facilitate the possibility of its use with children from culturally and linguistically diverse backgrounds. Foremost, the ESDM manual, *The Early Start Denver Model for Young Children with Autism* (Rogers

& Dawson, 2010), and *An Early Start for Your Child with Autism* (written for caregivers, Rogers, Dawson, & Vismara, 2012) have been translated into 16 languages. Furthermore, the focus on following a child's lead and embedding learning into play means that a range of cultural preferences and practices can be accommodated. Also, ESDM allows for flexibility in adapting the intervention to best match an individual family's preferences, customs, and values. Studies are currently underway to adapt the model to community-based settings, such as birth to age 3 centers, and to regions that have fewer resources, such as Africa. Studies have been published utilizing ESDM in the United States, Canada, Italy, Australia, and China.

With that being said, some of the structural features of ESDM (e.g., curriculum assessment content) and teaching practices are derived primarily from studies involving middle-class families from Western cultures. More research with diverse cultures is needed to determine differences in outcomes for those from other backgrounds. Preliminary evidence indicates that in diverse American cultures (varied in both ethnicity and socioeconomic status), no significant differences emerge with regard to parent usage or child outcomes in relation to socioeconomic status or ethnicity (Vismara, Colombi, & Rogers, 2009).

Additional research has explored social and language outcomes in children with ASD from bilingual home environments in order to understand whether children from bilingual home environments experience reduced developmental benefits from early intervention (in particular, ESDM). Results indicate that children from bilingual home environments as well as an age- and nonverbal IQ–matched group from monolingual homes both evidenced significant language growth, with no moderating effect of language environment (monolingual versus bilingual) in the home (Zhou et al., 2019). In conclusion, these findings do not support concern for the potential negative impact of a bilingual home environment on language or social development in young children with ASD receiving early intervention. Future research should consider other aspects of culturally and linguistically diverse environments in order to maximize the benefit that such children receive from ESDM.

Application to a Child

The following section provides a brief description of a child for whom ESDM is considered appropriate and effective. The earlier section on target populations provides additional criteria for determining treatment fit for individual children, as this is just one example of a hypothetical child who would likely benefit from ESDM.

Brooke, a 4-year-old female with ASD, presented to our clinic with her mother. Specifically, her mother expressed interest in receiving parent coaching in ESDM in order to supplement the speech-language therapy and developmental preschool services that were already in place. Given that Brooke's father was not working outside the home and accompanied Brooke to all of her other therapy sessions (obtaining suggestions from therapists along the way about what he could do at home with Brooke), her mother was identified as the primary parent to participate in the live coaching aspects of therapy. However, both parents would have been welcome to attend sessions and participate in discussions that followed the live coaching activities.

Brooke's mother endorsed Brooke's poor eye contact as her family's primary concern. She also described Brooke as being "self-willed," which she indicated made it difficult to socially engage her daughter. However, she also reported that Brooke showed clear affection to family members on her terms. With regard to her language skills, Brooke entered P-ESDM just starting to spontaneously combine words into phrases and with a strong ability to imitate speech. Her mother described her receptive language as stronger than her expressive language and stated that Brooke was following some two-step directions. In the area of personal independence, Brooke was able to participate in bath time by helping to rinse herself with a washcloth and was able to put her shoes on and take her shoes off. With regard to social skills, Brooke tolerated being around other children but showed limited engagement with peers. On the ESDM Curriculum Checklist, most of Brooke's skills clustered near Level 2 (18–24 months developmental level), with the exception of gross motor skills, which emerged at Level 3 (24–36 months).

Brooke and her mother attended twelve 1-hour P-ESDM sessions. Initially, Brooke was able to attend to preferred activities for brief periods of time, although also engaged in some disruptive behavior (e.g., throwing objects). In general, her eye contact was initially reduced, and vocalizations typically consisted of short phrases marked by difficulties with articulation. After just two sessions (including practice at home outside of P-ESDM sessions), Brooke's mother demonstrated improvements in her positioning and commenting and in being less directive in her interactions (following Brooke's lead), which led to longer and less disruptive interactions than before treatment. After three sessions of coaching, Brooke's mother reported that these activities felt good compared to how interactions with Brooke typically felt (e.g., Brooke would push her away or quickly become frustrated). The clinician worked with Brooke's mother on the full set of P-ESDM topics, but devoted particular attention to joint activity routines (emphasizing natural turn-taking as a way of enhancing back-and-forth interactions) and the ABCs of learning, as these were areas in which Brooke's mother expressed less confidence.

By the end of the program, Brooke's mother had identified ways to make activities more varied in order to reduce repetitive play and disruptive behavior, and she showed a good understanding of an appropriate level of prompting when teaching new skills. In addition, she attended more consistently to Brooke's affect and matched her language level most of the time. These changes in interaction style contributed to improvements in Brooke's developmental skills across all domains. At the end of 12 weeks, Brooke had demonstrated mastery of the majority of treatment objectives. If the family were to engage in an additional 12 weeks of intervention, a new set of objectives would be identified and discussed. Although some families elect to continue with P-ESDM sessions following the conclusion of a short-term program, others find that once they have learned the skills, they can continue to implement principles throughout daily routines without the need for weekly sessions.

Application to an Adult

The ESDM is designed for young children (up to 48 months developmental level) and thus is not appropriate for adolescents or adults.

**To review an extended application and
implementation of this intervention, see Case 2 about
a child with ASD in the companion volume
*Case Studies for the Treatment of Autism Spectrum Disorder.***

Future Directions

Several research studies are underway that aim to refine and continue to validate and expand the use of ESDM for treating young children with autism. A National Institutes of Health (NIH)–funded multisite replication study of intensive ESDM in toddlers (replicating Dawson et al., 2010), headed by Sally Rogers, has been completed, and publication of results are anticipated in the near future. Another NIH-funded multisite clinical trial, based at the University of California–Davis, is examining effects of intensity and delivery style for toddlers with ASD (15–30 months). In this study, intervention varies on the basis of two dimensions: dosage (either 15 or 25 hours per week of one to one treatment) and teaching style (discrete trial teaching versus play- and routines-based teaching). The primary outcome consists of overall developmental quotients on the Mullen Scales of Early Learning (Mullen, 1995) at the 2-year time point.

With regard to validating the ESDM approach across diverse populations, another ongoing NIH-funded study, headed by Lauren Franz at Duke University, seeks to improve access to early intervention for autism in settings characterized by low resources and low literacy (specifically, South Africa). Goals of the pilot study address improving access to evidence-based mental health services and developing culturally sensitive early interventions. Primary outcomes include developmental quotient and language subdomain developmental quotient (Griffiths Scales of Mental Development; Griffiths, 1984), caregiver stress, and social affect domain score (Autism Diagnostic Observation Schedule–Second Edition; Lord et al., 2012).

Finally, Sikich, Dawson, Howard, and others at Duke University are conducting an NIH-funded clinical trial investigating the use of ESDM in children with ASD and comorbid behavioral issues, specifically, attention-deficit/hyperactivity disorder (ADHD). The primary goal of the study is to determine whether psychopharmacological treatment augments the efficacy of caregiver-delivered ESDM (P-ESDM), with a primary outcome of social-communication skills as reported by the caregiver.

Other future directions include further research on ESDM in various settings, such as preschools, and in culturally diverse populations (i.e., looking at what adaptations are necessary to make the intervention successful). In addition, follow-up studies continue to examine long-term outcomes of children who received intervention in ESDM as toddlers or preschoolers, as well as other adaptations (e.g., telehealth and other technologically assisted modifications).

Suggested Readings

1. Rogers, S. J., & Dawson, G. (2010). *The Early Start Denver Model for young children with autism: Promoting language, learning, and engagement.* Guilford Press. This book is the primary manual used by therapists learning and delivering the ESDM. It provides hands-on strategies for working with toddlers and preschoolers in both individual and group settings. The manual presents a theoretical basis of infant learning and autism as well as more practical strategies for applying the ESDM. Included in this manual are a nonreproducible checklist of the assessment tool (Early Start Denver Model Curriculum Checklist for Young Children with Autism, which is available for purchase online) and instructions for use as well as detailed item descriptions and the ESDM Teaching Fidelity Rating System (with both administration and coding guidelines).

2. Rogers, S. J., Dawson, G., & Vismara, L. A. (2012). *An early start for your child with autism: Using everyday activities to help kids connect, communicate, and learn.* Guilford Press. This book is written for caregivers with the goal of quickly helping them to empower themselves by providing them with the tools needed to help their child. Specifically, suggestions are provided for how to turn meals, play, and other daily activities into opportunities to promote child development, with a focus on using the caregiver–child relationship to strengthen connection, learning, and communication. Strategies discussed in the book may allow caregivers to augment aspects of a formal early intervention program by promoting communication and learning at home, given that this is the primary setting in which children spend the majority of their time. Although geared for caregivers, the strategies communicated in this book are useful for any individual seeking to learn more about the ESDM model.

3. Dawson, G., Rogers, S. J., Munson, J., Smith, M., Winter, J., Greenson, J., Donaldson, A., & Varley, J. (2010). Randomized, controlled trial of an intervention for toddlers with autism: The Early Start Denver Model. *Pediatrics, 125*(1), e17–e23. This fundamental paper describes results of an RCT investigating the efficacy of the ESDM in children with ASD between 18 and 30 months of age. Results indicated that relative to children who received standard community-based treatments, those who received ESDM (on average, 25 hours of ESDM delivered one to one by parents and trained home therapists) showed significant improvements in IQ, adaptive behavior, and diagnostic status 2 years after entering intervention. The study was the first RCT to investigate the efficacy of a comprehensive developmental behavioral intervention in toddlers with ASD and highlighted the positive impact of the ESDM across a range of developmental skill areas.

Learning Activities

1. Topics for further discussion:

    •   How might learning ESDM strategies create value for a family who is already engaged in an early intervention program of approximately 20 hours per week of non-ESDM interventions?

    •   What are the benefits of constructing an interdisciplinary treatment team for a young child with ASD?

2. Ideas for projects:

    •   List five different toys or sensory social activities that could be used in an ESDM session or during home practice. For each toy or activity, brainstorm a set of skills that could be targeted through play or other daily routines and write an objective for each.

    •   Observe a video of a young child with autism and discuss what would be appropriate teaching objectives for this child.

3. Questions about the reading material:

    •   What aspects of the ESDM lend themselves to use in children who do not yet use verbal language?

    •   Which developmental domains or skill areas are targeted in the ESDM?

- What is the role of the caregiver in ESDM, both for therapist-delivered intervention and for caregiver coaching (P-ESDM)?

- Why is a therapist's understanding of typical development important in implementing the ESDM?

4. Writing assignments:

- Based on Schreibman and colleagues' (2015) paper on NDBI, describe the shared characteristics of the early intervention models that are considered NDBI.

- Explain how principles of ABA are reflected in ESDM teaching strategies.

Summary of Video Clip

*See the **About the Videos and Downloads** page at the front of the book for directions on how to access and stream the accompanying video to this chapter.*

This video clip portrays an interaction between a parent and child during a P-ESDM session. In particular, the child's father uses strategies such as imitating the child's actions, following the child's lead, pausing and waiting for the child to request, and sharing positive affect to facilitate the child's social engagement. Toward the end of the clip, the father targets receptive language objectives.

REFERENCES

Chevalier, C., Kohls, G., Troiani, V., Brodkin, E. S., & Schultz, R. T. (2012). The social motivation theory of autism. *Trends in Cognitive Sciences, 16*(4), 231–239.

Cidav, Z., Munson, J., Estes, A., Dawson, G., Rogers, S., & Mandell, D. (2017). Cost offset associated with Early Start Denver Model for children with autism. *Journal of the American Academy of Child & Adolescent Psychiatry, 56*(9), 777–783.

Colombi, C., Narzisi, A., Ruta, L., Cigala, V., Gagliano, A., Pioggia, G., Siracusano, R., Rogers, S. J., Muratori, F., & Prima Pietra Team. (2018). Implementation of the Early Start Denver Model in an Italian community. *Autism, 22*(2), 126–133.

Dawson, G., Jones, E. J. H., Merkle, K., Venema, K., Lowy, R., Faja, S., Kamara, D., Murias, M., Greenson, J., Winter, J., Smith, M., Rogers, S. J., & Webb, S. J. (2012). Early behavioral intervention is associated with normalized brain activity in young children with autism. *Journal of the American Academy of Child and Adolescent Psychiatry, 51*(11), 1150–1159.

Dawson, G., Rogers, S. J., Munson, J., Smith, M., Winter, J., Greenson, J., Donaldson, A., & Varley, J. (2010). Randomized, controlled trial of an intervention for toddlers with autism: The Early Start Denver Model. *Pediatrics, 125*(1), e17–e23.

Dawson, G., Toth, K., Abbott, R., Osterling, J., Munson, J., Estes, A., & Liaw, J. (2004). Early social attention impairments in autism: Social orienting, joint attention, and attention to distress. *Developmental Psychology, 40*(2), 271–283.

Dawson, G., Webb, S. J., & McPartland, J. (2005). Understanding the nature of face processing impairment in autism: Insights from behavioral and electrophysiological studies. *Developmental Neuropsychology, 27*(3), 403–424.

Dawson, G., Webb, S., Schellenberg, G., Dager, S., Friedman, S., Aylward, E., & Richards, T. (2002). Defining the broader phenotype of autism: Genetic, brain, and behavioral perspectives. *Development and Psychopathology, 14*(3), 581–611.

Dawson, G., Webb, S. J., Wijsman, E., Schellenberg, G., Estes, A., Munson, J., & Faja, S. (2005). Neurocognitive and electrophysiological evidence of altered face processing in parents of children with autism: Implications for a model of abnormal development of social brain circuitry in autism. *Development and Psychopathology, 17*(3), 679–697.

Eapen, V., Črnčec, R., & Walter, A. (2013). Clinical outcomes of an early intervention program for preschool children with autism spectrum disorder in a community group setting. *BMC Pediatrics, 13*(3). https://doi.org/10.1186/1471-2431-13-3

Eapen, V., Črnčec, R., & Walter, A. (2016). There are gains, but can we tell for whom and why? Predictors of treatment response following group Early Start Denver Model intervention in preschool-aged children with autism spectrum disorder. *Autism Open Access, 6*(2). https://doi.org/10.4172/2165-7890.1000168

Estes, A., Munson, J., Rogers, S. J., Greenson, J., Winter, J., & Dawson, G. (2015). Long-term outcomes of early intervention in 6-year-old children with autism spectrum disorder. *Journal of the American Academy of Child and Adolescent Psychiatry, 54*(7), 580–587.

Estes, A., Vismara, L., Mercado, C., Fitzpatrick, A., Elder, E., Greenson, J., Lord, C., Munson, J., Winter, J., Young, G., Dawson, G., & Rogers, S. (2014). The impact of parent-delivered intervention on parents of very young children with autism. *Journal of Autism and Developmental Disorders, 44*(2), 353–365.

Frith, C., & Frith, U. (2005). Theory of mind. *Current Biology, 15*(17), PR644–R645.

Fulton, E., Eapen, V., Črnčec, R., Walter, A., & Rogers, S. (2014). Reducing maladaptive behaviors in preschool-aged children with autism spectrum disorder using the Early Start Denver Model. *Frontiers in Pediatrics, 2*(40). https://doi.org/10.3389/fped.2014.00040

Griffiths, R. (1984). *The abilities of young children*. The Test Agency Ltd.

Koegel, R. L., & Koegel, L. K. (1988). Generalized responsivity and pivotal behavior. In R. H. Horner, G. Dunlap, & R. L. Koegel (Eds.), *Generalization and maintenance: Lifestyle changes in applied settings* (pp. 41–66). Paul H. Brookes Publishing Co.

Lord, C., Rutter, M., DiLavore, P. C., Risi, S., Gotham, K., & Bishop, S. L. (2012). *Autism Diagnostic Observation Schedule* (2nd ed.). Western Psychological Services.

Miller, W., & Rollnick, S. (2013). *Motivational interviewing: Helping people change* (3rd ed.). Guilford Press.

Mullen, E. M. (1995). *Mullen Scales of Early Learning* (AGS ed.). American Guidance Service.

Piaget, J. (1963). *The origins of intelligence in children*. Norton.

Rogers, S. J., & Dawson, G. (2009). *Early Start Denver Model Curriculum Checklist for Young Children with Autism*. Guilford Press.

Rogers, S. J., & Dawson, G. (2010). *The Early Start Denver Model for young children with autism: Promoting language, learning, and engagement*. Guilford Press.

Rogers, S. J., Dawson, G., & Vismara, L. A. (2012). *An early start for your child with autism: Using everyday activities to help kids connect, communicate, and learn*. Guilford Press.

Rogers, S. J., Estes, A., Lord, C., Vismara, L., Winter, J., Fitzpatrick, A., Guo, M., & Dawson, G. (2012). Effects of a brief Early Start Denver Model (ESDM)-based parent intervention on toddlers at risk for autism spectrum disorders: A randomized controlled trial. *Journal of the American Academy of Child and Adolescent Psychiatry, 51*(10), 1052–1065.

Rogers, S. J., Herbison, J. M., Lewis, H. C., Pantone, J., & Reis, K. (1986). An approach for enhancing the symbolic, communicative, and interpersonal functioning of young children with autism or severe emotional handicaps. *Journal of Early Intervention, 10*(2), 135–148.

Rogers, S. J., & Pennington, B. F. (1991). A theoretical approach to the deficits in infantile autism. *Development and Psychopathology, 3*(2), 137–162.

Rogers, S. J., Vismara, L., Wagner, A. L., McCormick, C., Young, G., & Ozonoff, S. (2014). Autism treatment in the first year of life: A pilot study of infant start, a parent-implemented intervention for symptomatic infants. *Journal of Autism and Developmental Disorders, 44*(12), 2981–2995.

Rutter, M., Bailey, A., & Lord, C. (2003). *The Social Communication Questionnaire*. Western Psychological Services.

Sameroff, A. (Ed.). (2009). *The transactional model of development: How children and contexts shape each other*. American Psychological Association.

Schreibman, L., Dawson, G., Stahmer, A. C., Landa, R., Rogers, S. J., McGee, G. G., Kasari, C., Ingersoll, B., Kaiser, A. P., Bruinsma, Y., McNerney, E., Wetherby, A., & Halladay, A. (2015). Naturalistic Developmental Behavioral Interventions: Empirically validated treatments for autism spectrum disorder. *Journal of Autism and Developmental Disorders, 45*(8), 2411–2428.

Sparrow, S., Cicchetti, D., & Balla, D. (2005). *Vineland Adaptive Behavior Scales* (2nd ed.). American Guidance Service.

Vismara, L. A., Colombi, C., & Rogers, S. J. (2009). Can one hour per week of therapy lead to lasting changes in young children with autism? *Autism, 13*(1), 93–115.

Vismara, L. A., McCormick, C. E. B., Wagner, A. L., Monlux, K., Nadhan, A., & Young, G. Y. (2018). Telehealth parent training in the Early Start Denver Model: Results from a randomized controlled study. *Focus on Autism and Other Developmental Disabilities, 33*(2), 67–79.

Vismara, L. A., & Rogers, S. J. (2008). The Early Start Denver Model: A case study of an innovative practice. *Journal of Early Intervention, 31*(1), 91–108.

Vismara, L. A., Young, G. S., & Rogers, S. J. (2012). Telehealth for expanding the reach of early autism training to parents. *Autism Research and Treatment, 2012*, 1–12.

Vismara, L. A., Young, G. S., & Rogers, S. J. (2013). Community dissemination of the Early Start Denver Model: Implications for science and practice. *Topics in Early Childhood Special Education, 32*, 223–233.

Vismara, L. A., Young, G. S., Stahmer, A. C., Griffith, E. M., & Rogers, S. J. (2009). Dissemination of evidence-based practice: Can we train therapists from a distance? *Journal of Autism and Developmental Disorders, 39*(12), 1636–1651.

Vivanti, G., Dissanayake, C., & The Victorian ASELCC Team. (2016). Outcome for children receiving the Early Start Denver Model before and after 48 months. *Journal for Autism and Developmental Disorders, 46*(7), 2441–2449.

Vivanti, G., Dissanayake, C., Zierhut, C., Rogers, S. J., & The Victorian ASELCC Team. (2013). Brief report: Predictors of outcomes in the Early Start Denver Model delivered in a group setting. *Journal of Autism and Developmental Disorders, 43*(7), 1717–1724.

Vivanti, G., Duncan, E., Dawson, G., & Rogers, S. J. (2017). *Implementing the group based Early Start Denver Model for preschoolers with autism.* Springer.

Vivanti, G., Kapes, C., Duncan, E., Dawson, G., & Rogers, S. J. (2016). Development of the G-ESDM classroom curriculum. In G. Vivanti, E. Duncan, G. Dawson, & S. J. Rogers (Eds.), *Implementing the group based Early Start Denver Model for preschoolers with autism* (pp. 59–70). Springer.

Vivanti, G., Paynter, J., Duncan, E., Fothergill, H., Dissanayake, C., Rogers, S. J., & Victorian ASELCC Team. (2014). Effectiveness and feasibility of the Early Start Denver Model implemented in a group-based community childcare setting. *Journal of Autism and Developmental Disorders, 44*(12), 3140–3153.

Zhou, V., Munson, J. A., Greenson, J., Hou, Y., Rogers, S., & Estes, A. M. (2019). An exploratory longitudinal study of social and language outcomes in children with autism in bilingual home environments. *Autism, 23*(2), 394–404.

Zhou, B., Xu, Q., Li, H., Zhang, Y., Wang, Y., Rogers, S. J., & Xu, X. (2018). Effects of parent-implemented Early Start Denver Model intervention on Chinese toddlers with autism spectrum disorder: A non-randomized controlled trial. *Autism Research, 11*, 654–666.

6

Discrete Trial Instruction

Amanda Kazee, Susan M. Wilczynski, Maria Martino,
Shawnna Sundberg, Molly Quinn, and Nicholas L. Mundell

INTRODUCTION

The field of **applied behavior analysis** (ABA) is dedicated to improving the human condition by observing and altering environmental conditions that support optimal outcomes in socially meaningful ways (Steege et al., 2007). **Discrete trial instruction** (DTI) is one of many instructional methods of ABA that can teach learners, regardless of age and developmental delay and/or disability (Lambert et al., 2016; Lerman et al., 2013). Skills addressed using DTI typically range from social-communication initiations and responses to play and daily living skills (e.g., using money). DTI uses individualized instructions and numerous learning opportunities to teach new skills, maintain previously learned skills, generalize behaviors to other relevant situations, and reduce interfering behaviors (Steege et al., 2007). Although DTI can be implemented with any learners, this chapter focuses on learners with autism spectrum disorder (ASD). The goal of DTI is for learners to consistently provide the desired response (i.e., maintenance) in the absence of programmed reinforcement and to generalize the desired response to other environments and variations of the stimuli. DTI comprises four components: 1) **discriminative stimulus (S^D),** 2) **response,** 3) **consequence,** and 4) **intertrial interval** (ITI; Brown-Chidsey & Steege, 2004; Steege et al., 2007). This chapter describes these four key components (see Key Components section) and places particular emphasis on the current literature regarding implementation of DTI. See Figure 6.1 for an example of a DTI implementation fidelity checklist.

Discrete trial instruction implementation steps	Implementation fidelity score		
	Yes	No	N/A
1. Set up instructional space (i.e., stimuli, data collection sheet).			
2. Gain learner's attention.			
3. Deliver discriminative stimulus. (critical item)			
4. Provide appropriate prompt if needed.			
5. Give learner opportunity to respond (1–3 seconds).			
6. Deliver consequence (within 1–3 seconds of response). (critical item)			
7. Use an appropriate intertrial interval (1–5 seconds). (critical item)			
8. Perform error correction procedure (See Table 6.2 for common error correction procedures) if needed.[a]			
Maintenance/Generalization	Implementation fidelity score		
	Yes	No	N/A
1. Mastered skill maintained over time (specify time: _____)			
2. Mastered skill transferred to other people			
3. Mastered skill transferred to other stimuli			
4. Mastered skill transferred to other environments			

Critical item percentage (critical item scored as **Yes**/total critical items): _____

Total implementation percentage (items with **Yes**/8): _____

[a]See Table 6.2 for common error correction procedures.

Notes for use: Items with (critical item) next to them are crucial to the implementation of DTI (i.e., necessary components). Practitioners may use the checklist when implementing DTI to ensure they are including all steps necessary to implement DTI with fidelity, especially critical items.

Scoring: Supervisors can provide practitioners with one of two scores when implementing DTI components (i.e., yes or no). A score of "No" represents practitioners did not implement the step while a score of "Yes" represents practitioners correctly implemented the step. An "N/A" (not applicable) is available for steps that are not applicable to the setting. Each supervisor must determine if a "Yes" requires accurate implementation across all trials or if a lower criterion can be applied. Scoring of Maintenance/Generalization items occurs only if trials to assess maintenance or generalization of a skill are scheduled for review during the DTI session.

Observation: Observe practitioners and learners in person while completing the implementation fidelity checklist. Video recorded sessions may be coded and discussed at a later time.

Figure 6.1.   Implementation fidelity checklist. This checklist includes the steps necessary to implement Discrete trial instruction from beginning to end.

TARGET POPULATIONS

DTI is an instructional approach to teach subcomponents of a skill in manageable units until the behavior of interest is acquired (Taubman et al., 2013). That is, the target behavior is broken down into small instructional units called trials. Of particular relevance for the purposes of this chapter, DTI has been shown to be effective in teaching academic, adaptive, and communication skills to learners diagnosed with ASD (Downs et al., 2007; Geiger et al., 2012; Jones et al., 2007; Smith 2001) and has been used to teach skills to learners with ASD across a wide variety of ages in various settings, including schools, clinics, and homes (Carroll et al., 2015; Dib & Sturmey, 2007; Subramaniam et al., 2017).

THEORETICAL BASIS

This section describes the theoretical framework of DTI, assessment tools that may be beneficial when considering a social-communication curriculum, proposed functional outcomes, and target areas of treatment, including but not limited to expressive and receptive language or social pragmatics.

Theoretical Explanation

The framework of DTI relies heavily on the field of ABA and operant learning. Although many practitioners interchange the terms *ABA* and *DTI*, DTI is one of many instructional methods that relies on behavior analytic principles such as reinforcement. In addition to ABA methods, prompting (i.e., providing an external support that increases the likelihood of correct performance) and **error correction** procedures (i.e., teaching techniques that increase the likelihood of correct future performance when a mistake is made on a given trial) are used to teach learners new skills.

Applied Behavior Analysis   ABA is a science that relies on the application of the principles of behavior to make socially significant and meaningful changes in a learner's life (Steege et al., 2007). The principles of ABA have been beneficial across a variety of targeted areas such as communication, play, social-emotional, and cognitive skills (Klintwall & Eikeseth, 2014). ABA is based on operant conditioning in which new responses (i.e., behaviors) can be strengthened or reinforced on the basis of the outcome delivered immediately following the behavior (i.e., consequences; Skinner, 1981).

DTI is an effective instructional method for teaching new behaviors that integrate the ABC (antecedent–behavior–consequence) of operant conditioning. In the context of DTI, antecedent stimuli are selected by practitioners and presented similarly across trials until mastery of the target behavior occurs (Delprato, 2001). The antecedent (S^D) is commonly presented to learners in the form of an instruction. When programmed effectively, learners are able to distinguish between and respond to different antecedents appropriately. For example, labeling different liquids such as milk, water, and juice when asked, "What is this?" may be the skill learners are addressing in the curriculum. However, they must also be able to respond to the S^Ds, "What do you want to drink?" and "Tell me some things people like to drink," so that they can interact fluently under real world conditions (Klintwall & Eikeseth, 2014).

Responses are typically categorized as correct, incorrect, prompted, or no response. A failure to take any action when presented the S^D is considered an incorrect response and is provided a behavior-altering consequence just as in the case of any other incorrect response. Consequences are any change in the environment following a behavior that either increases or decreases the likelihood the behavior will occur under similar conditions in the future. During skill acquisition, correct responses should result in the immediate delivery of a reinforcer (i.e., a consequence that increases the likelihood that learners will provide the same response in the presence of the S^D in the future). Learners who provide an incorrect response or do not provide responses are not delivered a punishment; instead, an error correction procedure (see Error Correction Procedures section) is used (Klintwall & Eikeseth, 2014). Prompted correct responses should result in reinforcement, and prompted incorrect responses should result in error correction.

Motivating Operations   **Motivating operations** (MOs) have two effects on behavior: they alter the effectiveness of the reinforcer (i.e., value altering) and/or directly change the frequency of the behavior (i.e., behavior altering; Laraway et al., 2003). Even if a reinforcer were unavailable, MOs would still change the value of the reinforcer and could directly alter behaviors. For example, a learner may enter a DTI session after night of poor sleep, so insufficient sleep is the MO. Insufficient sleep changes the value of sleep (i.e., going to sleep is more likely to serve as a reinforcer than when the learner is well rested) because he or she is very tired. With insufficient sleep as the MO, the learner is more likely to take actions (i.e., behavior altering) that have resulted in access to sleep in the past (e.g., yawning loudly led an adult to put the learner to bed, or refusing to complete work resulted in being sent to time-out, where the learner was undisturbed and fell asleep). Practitioners should use knowledge of MOs to anticipate potential challenges that may vary across DTI sessions or even within a given session. For example, knowing insufficient sleep may result in crying by the end of the session, practitioners can prevent escalating fatigue by providing a correct response concurrent with the presentation of the S^D at the beginning of the session. Alteration of the DTI session could include more frequent breaks, presentation of easier tasks if the learner is tired, or discontinuation of the session.

Verbal Behavior   Practitioners using DTI often rely on a curriculum called Verbal Behavior or VB, which is based on Skinner's (1957) behavior analytic description of communication. This curriculum is grounded in the idea that **verbal behavior** is reinforced primarily through the mediation of others. The consequence that maintains different forms of verbal behavior is used to organize the learner's curriculum. For example, learners might be taught to *mand* (i.e., request) for preferred activities, toys, food, or information (e.g., "Where is my truck?"); to *tact* (i.e., label) items according to feature, function, or class; or to engage in intraverbals (i.e., have conversations). The utility of focusing on the consequences of maintaining communicative behaviors lies in connecting inappropriate behaviors (e.g., screaming) to treatment goals (e.g., screaming occurs when toys are unavailable, so a treatment goal of manding for toys can effectively reduce screaming) and guiding individualized treatment goals.

Assessment Tools

The implementation of DTI relies on assessment tools such as the Verbal Behavior Milestones and Placement Program (VB-MAPP; Sundberg, 2008) or the Promoting the Emergence of Advanced Knowledge (PEAK) Relational Training System

(Dixon et al., 2015). The VB-MAPP assesses the learner's verbal repertoire across three developmental levels: 1) requesting basic items; 2) requesting items and conversational exchanges; and 3) expansion of requesting items, conversational exchanges, and advanced language skills. Although the VB-MAPP is commonly used for assessing learners' verbal repertoires to develop treatment plans, little reliability or validity data are available to support it. The VB-MAPP is designed for learners up to the developmental level of a typically developing child of 48 months (Dixon et al., 2015), so this assessment tool is not useful for all learners.

PEAK, also an assessment and curriculum guide, assesses learners' language skill deficits and guides the practitioner in the creation of an individualized curriculum (Dixon et al., 2015). The PEAK Direct Training Module (PEAK-DT) comprises a four-factor model: 1) foundational learning skills; 2) perceptual learning skills; 3) verbal comprehension skills and verbal reasoning; and 4) verbal reasoning, memory, and mathematical skills (Rowsey et al., 2015). The PEAK Generalization Module (PEAK-G) expands on skills in PEAK-DT that apply across people, environments, and other stimuli. PEAK-DT is designed for learners with expected skills consistent with those demonstrated by children 8 years of age or younger, whereas PEAK-G provides targets for children typically 11 years of age or younger (Dixon et al., 2017). Although both the VB-MAPP and PEAK can be useful assessment tools, practitioners should use ongoing progress-monitoring data collection to make timely treatment decisions (see Assessment for Treatment Planning and Progress Monitoring).

Functional Outcomes

Because DTI is an instructional procedure used to teach skills, it is not used to assess functional limitations in learner communication or social interaction skills. Instead, practitioners determine the areas of functional limitation in learners' skills by using assessment tools and observations in real-world contexts, develop an individualized curriculum, *then* consider whether DTI is the appropriate instructional method for each learner. Functionality should be based on the unique context in which the individual learner lives. For example, using the label "snowing" when presented a picture in Alaska can help lead to survival skills, but the same picture in Florida holds little functional utility. To ensure functional outcomes for learners, practitioners should build toward **behavioral cusps** (i.e., a watershed skill) or the integration of subskills that lead to substantial changes in opportunities (e.g., moving from a more restrictive to less restrictive environment). Achievement of behavioral cusps leads to greater access to new reinforcers, contingencies, and environments (Bosch & Fuqua, 2001). For example, learners developing the behavioral cusp of requesting preferred items can now gain access to a variety of new reinforcers, such as a beverage to drink when thirsty or a snack to eat when hungry as well as leisure items, including their preferred toy, by using the previously taught skill (i.e., requesting items). DTI might be deemed an appropriate means of teaching to request preferred stimuli and can thus lead to the acquisition of behavioral cusps.

Target Area of Treatment

The *Diagnostic and Statistical Manual of Mental Disorders, Fifth Edition* (DSM-5; American Psychological Association [APA], 2013) defines ASD on the basis of restricted, repetitive behaviors, interests, or activities (RR-BIA) and persistent deficits in social communication and social interaction across different contexts. These

RR-BIA vary greatly across members of the autism community and can include repetitive motor movements (e.g., rocking, posturing), circumscribed interests (e.g., failure to engage with people unless a keen topic of interest is maintained), or limited pursuit of activities (e.g., preference to repeat the same activity; APA, 2013). Persistent deficits in social communication and social interaction are a core feature of ASD (Volkmar et al., 2004) and are evident across all individuals with ASD regardless of age, ability, or language level (Tager-Flusberg et al., 2001). Thus, programming is needed to support social communication and social interaction skills for all individuals with ASD; however, DTI should be yoked to a comprehensive but individualized curriculum, which can address RR-BIA and social-communication impairments. Although DTI is effective for teaching skills across a variety of domains, the purpose of this chapter is to highlight the effectiveness of DTI with learners diagnosed with ASD.

Expressive and Receptive Language   DTI is an effective instructional method for skills ranging from motor and verbal imitation to receptive and expressive language (Klintwall & Eikeseth, 2014). Expressive language reflects a learner's ability to articulate sounds; use appropriate tone, rhythm, and rate of speech; and use sounds, words, or sentences in a meaningful way. Receptive language is the learner's ability to understand or decode and organize what a speaker says (Prelock et al., 2008). Learners with ASD often have expressive language difficulties such as variable accuracy in speech production, use of verbal scripts, or a mechanical voice quality. Learners may also present with receptive language problems such as difficulty analyzing, integrating, and processing relevant information or misinterpreting social cues (Prelock et al., 2008). DTI may be used as a focused and intensive instructional method to overcome these obstacles (Downs et al., 2008).

Social Pragmatics   Social pragmatics refers to the function of language (Prelock et al., 2008). Learners with ASD have difficulty with functional aspects of language, such as spontaneously initiating interactions, switching topics, talking excessively, or dominating social interactions on focused topics of interest. DTI can be implemented with learners with ASD to teach functional aspects of language (e.g., spontaneous initiation of communication with others). It can be implemented with learners as young as 3 years of age to teach spontaneous communication such as, "Are you okay?" or "Bless you" (Jones et al., 2007).

EMPIRICAL BASIS

Numerous systematic reviews have consistently demonstrated that DTI is an effective intervention (Ospina et al., 2008; Wong et al., 2015). Further study of the intensity, duration, or overall effectiveness of DTI compared to other behavioral interventions is still emerging (Ospina et al., 2008), and researchers continue to investigate refinements in implementation of DTI. This chapter focuses on literature published from 2008 to October 2018 to help readers focus on the common themes emerging on the topic of DTI. We used the keywords *discrete trial instruction, discrete trial training*, and *discrete trial intervention* in the research database PsycINFO. We reviewed the 89 articles identified through this process and deemed 27 directly relevant to the topic of this chapter. We also reviewed one additional relevant article not identified through this process. We excluded articles if they involved "training to implement DTI" or merely mentioned DTI but did not have dependent variables measuring DTI effectiveness.

We evaluated primary quality indicators (i.e., participant characteristics, independent variable, baseline condition, dependent variable, visual analysis, and experimental control) using a high quality, acceptable quality, or unacceptable quality rating developed by Reichow and colleagues (2008). We evaluated secondary quality indicators (i.e., interobserver agreement, kappa, blind raters, fidelity, generalization or maintenance, and social validity) using an evidence or no evidence rating. We determined the strength of evidence for each article by combining the primary and secondary quality indicators.

Common themes emerging in recent literature were **implementation fidelity** (e.g., treatment integrity, implementation integrity), error correction procedures, instructional variables, the role of reinforcement, and DTI compared to other interventions (e.g., fluency training). We primarily highlight research that falls in the adequate strength range for each of these themes but supplement these findings when a treatment was rated in the weak range but the primary indicators related to the quality of the research design and dependent measures allowed us to make useful recommendations to readers.

As depicted in Table 6.1, many studies conducted from 2008 to 2018 did not have adequate strength. Limitations in strength were often due to unacceptable ratings

Table 6.1. Empirical basis articles

Design strength	Description of design level	Studies with strong evidence	Studies with adequate evidence	Studies with weak evidence
IIa	Single-participant experimental designs			
	Nonexperimental studies (i.e., correlational and case studies, single-subject experimental designs)		Carroll et al. (2013; Study 2) Cariveau et al. (2016) Carroll et al. (2016) *Holding et al. (2011)* Majdalany et al. (2014) *Nopprapun & Holloway (2014)* Plaisance et al. (2016)	Carroll et al. (2013; Study 3) Carroll et al. (2015) Carroll et al. (2018) Cook et al. (2015) Dass et al. (2018) DiGennaro Reed et al. (2011) Elliott & Dillenburger (2016) Geiger et al. (2012) Isenhower et al. (2018) Jenkins et al. (2015) *Jennett et al. (2008)* Lambert et al. (2016) Lang et al. (2014) Majdalany et al. (2016) Paden & Kodak (2015) Rispoli et al. (2013) Roxburgh & Carbone (2012) Shillingsburg et al. (2014) Tarbox et al. (2010) Turan et al. (2012; Study 1 and Study 2)

Notes: Unless indicated by italic font, all of the articles provide support for the use of Discrete trial instruction (DTI). Articles in italics demonstrate other instructional methods that were more effective than DTI.

There were no meta-analyses (Level Ia); randomized controlled trials (Level Ib); controlled studies without randomization (Level IIa); quasi-experimental studies (Level IIb); or expert committee reports, consensus conferences, or clinical experience opinions of respected authorities (Level IV) identified for the review for recent research on DTI.

on primary quality variables such as participant characteristics and examination of data through the use of visual analysis. The primary indicator of participant characteristics helps practitioners identify whether each unique learner is reflected in the literature. Reasonable conclusions about overall treatment effectiveness can be gleaned from studies even when they are relatively weak in participant characteristics if the quality of the research design and dependent variables is strong. The primary indicator "examination of data through the use of visual analysis" may be considered a relative weakness in the guidelines of Reichow and colleagues (2008), but this information is immensely useful in helping practitioners make decisions about the utility of a study for each unique learner. For these reasons, this chapter includes articles that were strong in terms of research design and dependent variables but were considered weak based on participant characteristics and/or visual analysis.

Implementation Fidelity

Implementation fidelity refers to the extent to which the independent variable (i.e., intervention) is consistently and accurately applied (Gresham, 1989; Jenkins et al., 2015). Readers cannot draw firm conclusions about treatment effectiveness if an intervention is implemented incorrectly in a study. For example, a treatment could be effective in reality but appear ineffective because of poor implementation fidelity, or poor implementation fidelity could mean a treatment that is truly ineffective could spuriously appear to be effective.

Five studies (one with adequate strength; four with weak strength) focused on the role of implementation fidelity and DTI (Carroll et al., 2013; Cook et al., 2015; DiGennaro Reed et al., 2011; Jenkins et al., 2015). Carroll and colleagues (2013) used an alternating-treatments design (ATD) to compare skill acquisition in high, low, and a control implementation fidelity condition for six learners with ASD. All learners mastered target stimuli with the high-integrity (fidelity) treatment condition. Only one learner mastered targets in the low-integrity treatment condition, and it took twice as long (i.e., 12 high-integrity sessions compared with 24 low-integrity sessions). Efficient mastery of functional skills can change the life trajectory of learners with ASD, so when DTI is used to teach social-communication skills to learners with ASD, implementation fidelity should be assessed not only in research but in real-world adoption of an intervention.

Error Correction Procedures

Six studies (three with adequate strength; three with weak strength) focused on error correction procedures during DTI (Carroll et al., 2015; Carroll et al., 2018; Isenhower et al., 2018; Plaisance et al., 2016; Turan et al., 2012). Although two studies were considered to have weak strength, this chapter discusses their findings because the quality of the research design and dependent variables among the studies allows for expansion and comparison of error correction procedures across disabilities (e.g., ASD and attention-deficit/hyperactivity disorder [ADHD]; Carroll et al., 2015) and implementation or lack thereof of distractor trials (i.e., presentation of a learned response; e.g., Turan et al., 2012).

Error correction is the process of turning a learner's mistake during a discrete trial into a useful learning interaction. See Table 6.2 for a description of common error correction procedures. An ATD (Carroll et al., 2015) compared skill acquisition

Table 6.2.   Error correction procedures

Error correction name	Error correction procedural steps	Example
Single-response repetition	1. Provide vocal model of correct response. 2. If correct, deliver immediate reinforcement. 3. If incorrect or no response, remove target and present next trial.	**Correct response** Practitioner: "Say cracker." Learner: "Cracker." Practitioner: Delivers reinforcer. **Incorrect response** Practitioner: "Say cracker." Learner: "Crrrrr" (incorrect response). Practitioner: "Say cracker." Learner: "Cracker" (correct response). Practitioner: Delivers reinforcer.
Remove and re-present	1. Remove stimuli and turn it away from learner for predetermined time. 2. Re-present stimuli with immediate model. 3. If correct, provide immediate reinforcement. 4. If incorrect or no response, remove target and present next trial.	**Correct response** Practitioner: "Point to the dog." Learner: Correctly points to dog. Practitioner: Delivers reinforcer. **Incorrect response** Practitioner: "Point to dog." Learner: Incorrectly points to horse. Practitioner: Removes stimuli. Re-presents "Point to dog" with model. Learner: Correctly points to dog. Practitioner: Delivers reinforcer.
Re-present until independent	1. Provide vocal model of correct response. 2. Learner responds correctly. 3. Re-present target. 4. If correct, immediate reinforcement. 5. If incorrect or no response, continue until learner delivers correct response up to a predetermined total (i.e., re-present up to 20 times). If still incorrect, remove target and present next trial.	**Correct response** Practitioner: "Find the red square." Learner: Correctly points to red square. Practitioner: Delivers reinforcer. **Incorrect response** Practitioner: "Find the red square." Learner: Points to green square. Practitioner: Provides vocal model of finding red square (e.g., "Here is the red square.") Mixes up stimuli. "Find the red square." Learner: Points to red square (correct response). Practitioner: Mixes up stimuli. "Find the red square." Learner: Points to red square. Practitioner: Mixes up stimuli. "Find the red square." Learner: Points to red square. Practitioner: Delivers reinforcer.
Multiple-response repetition	1. Repeat instruction and model correct response.	**Correct response** Practitioner: "Which one do you drink?" (Correct answer is milk.) Learner: "Milk."

(continued)

Table 6.2.   *(continued)*

Error correction name	Error correction procedural steps	Example	
	2. Continue instruction with immediate model of correct response until learner demonstrates correct response for a predetermined time.	Practitioner:	Praises and delivers reinforcer.
		Incorrect response	
		Practitioner:	"Which one do you drink?"
		Learner:	"Apple."
		Practitioner:	"Which one do you drink?" "Milk." (Correct answer is milk.) "Which one do you drink?"
		Learner:	"Milk."
		Practitioner:	Repeats "Which one do you drink?"
		Learner:	Provides correct answer (e.g., "milk") to predetermined criterion (e.g., five correct).
		Practitioner:	Presents next trial.
Delay	1. Start intertrial interval for predetermined time.	Correct response	
		Practitioner:	"Which one is round?" (Correct response is to point to circle.)
	2. Re-present S^D with most intrusive prompt necessary for correct responding.	Learner:	Points to circle.
		Practitioner:	Delivers reinforcer.
	3. Start new trial with new stimulus.	Incorrect response	
		Practitioner:	"Which one is round?
		Learner:	Points to square.
		Practitioner:	Gives 5-second delay with no feedback. "Which one is round?" with prompt to respond correctly. Starts new trial with new stimulus (i.e., "Which one has five sides?").
Independent probe	1. Start intertrial interval for predetermined time.	Correct response	
		Practitioner:	"Point to the one that barks."
		Learner:	Points to dog.
	2. Re-present S^D with most intrusive prompt necessary for correct responding.	Practitioner:	Delivers reinforcer.
		Incorrect response	
		Practitioner:	"Point to the one that barks."
	3. Respond to distractor trial.	Learner:	Points to dinosaur (incorrect response).
	4. Re-present original S^D.	Practitioner:	Gives predetermined delay time. "Point to the one that barks" and provides most intrusive prompt to get the correct answer. Presents distractor (i.e., mastered task) trial. "Find the one that is red."
		Learner:	Points to apple (correct response).
		Practitioner:	"Point to the one that barks."
		Learner:	Points to dog.
		Practitioner:	Delivers reinforcer.

Sources: Carroll et al. (2015) and Turan et al. (2012).

of stimuli across different error correction procedures and a control condition for five learners with different disabilities (i.e., ADHD, ASD). Three of the five learners acquired skills quickest during the "re-present until independent" error correction procedure; however, the "remove and re-present" and "single-response repetition" error correction procedures were each most effective for one learner. Even for these two learners, the "re-present until independent" error correction procedure was the second-most effective procedure in producing faster acquisition.

Table 6.2 describes error correction procedures practitioners selected on an individual basis to optimize outcomes for each learner. Although error correction always involves delivering another discrete trial targeting the original skill, the timing of the second trial can vary. For example, Turan and colleagues (2012) used delay (i.e., immediate delivery of the same skill) and independent probe error correction procedures (i.e., presentation of a distractor trial followed by delivery of the original skill) to compare three learners with ASD. Both learners acquired receptive skills faster in the delay condition compared to the independent probe condition.

During implementation of error correction procedures, practitioners can decide whether to use maintenance interspersal (i.e., insert a *mastered* target prior to the reintroduction of the original skill); however, the present literature does not provide clear guidance on maintenance interspersal because two studies (rated adequate) provide somewhat different answers. A sequential ATD (Plaisance et al., 2016) across target skill sets compared no task interspersal (i.e., zero mastered-one acquisition task) and task interspersal (e.g., one mastered-one acquisition task) while using error correction procedures for four learners with ASD. There was no difference in the total number of sessions required to reach mastery criteria for two learners. One learner met mastery criterion more quickly in the no task interspersal condition, and the remaining learner took twice as many sessions to meet mastery criterion during the no task interspersal condition. Alternatively, Knutson and colleagues (2018) compared three different task interspersal ratios (i.e., three mastered-one acquisition, one mastered-one acquisition, one mastered-three acquisition, or zero mastered-one acquisition), and the ratio of zero mastered-to-acquisition tasks (i.e., continuously presenting acquisition tasks) was most effective across all learners. Practitioners should know that instructional time allocated to mastered tasks means more time spent away from acquisition tasks (Knutson et al., 2018); thus, we generally recommended erring on the side of low or no mastery interspersal. However, facing only nonmastered tasks for a protracted period of time may yield challenging behavior for some learners, so clinical judgment is required.

Time-Based Instructional Variables and Trial Format

Four DTI studies (three with adequate strength; one with weak strength) focused on time-based instructional variables or trial format (Cariveau et al., 2016; Geiger et al., 2012; Majdalany et al., 2014; Roxburgh & Carbone, 2012). Length of ITI is the period of time between the conclusion of one discrete trial and the presentation of the next trial. Rate of demand delivery reflects how many instructions are delivered during a training session, usually represented by the number of trials per minute. These time-based instructional variables can influence relevant outcomes (e.g., skill acquisition, problem behavior). Trial format involves the presentation of the same target stimulus during each trial (i.e., massed) or the presentation of stimuli in pseudorandom order (i.e., varied), which can also influence learner outcomes.

Intertrial Interval and Presentation   In an extension of Koegel and colleagues (1980), a sequential multiple-probe ATD by Cariveau and colleagues (2016) demonstrated all targets were mastered by the two participant learners with ASD, regardless of ITI duration or trial format. However, learners met the mastery criterion much faster with short ITIs (i.e., roughly 2 seconds) than when other ITIs (i.e., increasing time interval between 2 and 20 seconds; increasing it to 20 seconds) were used. The fastest acquisition occurred when short ITIs were combined with a varied presentation. The implication for real-world contexts is that learners with ASD could more quickly narrow the skill gap between themselves and their typically developing peers when DTI is presented with a very short (2 second) ITI and when treatment targets (i.e., unmastered tasks) are presented in a random order. This outcome is consistent with other research published about ITI length (Majdalany et al., 2014). Both learners also had the fewest number of problem and stereotypic behaviors in the short ITI condition; however, one learner demonstrated low levels of these behaviors across conditions, and the other demonstrated relatively high levels of problem behaviors regardless of the teaching arrangement (Cariveau et al., 2016).

Rate of Demand Delivery   Roxburgh and Carbone (2012) compared the effects of rate of trial delivery (i.e., practitioner instructions) on learner outcomes for two individuals with ASD during DTI. Although the percentage of correct responses per session was not vastly affected by the rate of trial delivery, both learners with ASD exhibited fewer problem behaviors with a faster practitioner rate of presentation (every 1 second) compared to the medium (every 5 seconds) and slow (every 10 seconds) delivery formats. Both learners experienced more positive outcomes (i.e., a larger effects and increased rate of reinforcement) in the fast-rate condition. Although it may seem counterintuitive, practitioners targeting social communication goals using DTI should present instructions, such as "Do this," "Find the one that quacks," "Point to the round one," quickly (i.e., roughly one per second), because it maximizes both the magnitude and rate of reinforcement and effectively reduces problem behaviors. Like shorter ITIs, a faster rate of instruction delivery will also lead to greater skill acquisition, which more expeditiously closes the gap in knowledge and skills between learners with ASD and their neurotypical peers.

Role of Reinforcement

Five studies (two with adequate strength; three with weak strength) focused on the role of reinforcement in DTI (Carroll et al., 2016; Elliott & Dillenburger, 2016; Lang et al., 2014; Majdalany et al., 2016; Paden & Kodak, 2015). One study (Carroll et al., 2016) was considered adequate. Although the Paden and Kodak (2015) study was categorized as weak because of a limited description of learner characteristics (e.g., age/gender or diagnostic information), this chapter includes the findings because the robust dependent variable, experimental design, and visual analysis of data allowed us to draw useful conclusions about the importance, or lack thereof, of considering reinforcer magnitude during implementation of DTI.

Immediacy of Reinforcement Reinforcers should be delivered immediately following a correct response because even a brief delay in reinforcement can interfere with skill acquisition (Carroll et al., 2016; Lovaas, 2003). Skill acquisition with 1) immediate reinforcement (i.e., general praise and 20-second access to preferred item), 2) delayed reinforcement with immediate praise (i.e., general praise, 10 seconds without interaction, and then preferred item for 20 seconds), and 3) delayed reinforcement (i.e., general praise after 10 seconds and then access to preferred item for 20 seconds) was compared for two learners with ASD using an ATD (Carroll et al., 2016). Although one learner mastered targets across all conditions, more training sessions were required to achieve mastery in the delayed reinforcement condition. The second learner mastered targets only in the immediate reinforcement condition. Despite that doing so can be challenging, practitioners should deliver reinforcers immediately after the correct response occurs when teaching new skills. Once a skill has reached mastery criterion established by the treatment team, varying the schedule of reinforcement as well as generalizing that skill to different people, environments, and stimuli can occur.

Magnitude of Reinforcement Paden and Kodak (2015) used a sequential ATD to examine the effects of reinforcer magnitude (small edible, large edible, or praise-only condition) during DTI. A magnitude preference assessment was conducted for four learners with ASD. Small-magnitude reinforcers were sufficient for both maintaining appropriate behavior and producing rapid skill mastery. The praise-only condition also functioned as an effective reinforcer. Clinicians should build a consistent history of pairing praise with edibles or other tangible reinforcers so that praise can be effectively used as a reinforcer during DTI.

Comparing Discrete Trial Intervention to Other Interventions

Two studies with adequate strength compared the effectiveness of fluency training (FT) and DTI on skill acquisition with the ASD population (Holding et al., 2011; Nopprapun & Holloway, 2014). FT is based on precision teaching, which relies on the principles of ABA (e.g., reinforcement, environmental arrangements), uses standardized lesson descriptions, and utilizes self-charting with standardized graphics for monitoring and measuring progress (Holding et al., 2011). Human beings must fluently (i.e., accurately and rapidly) perform functional behaviors (Howell & Lorson-Howell, 1990) to successfully learn and interact under dynamic real-world conditions. Holding and colleagues (2011) compared acquisition, generalization, and retention of noun labels for DTI and FT using an ATD. Four learners with ASD experienced faster acquisition and generalization as well as better retention of labeled nouns with FT. When phonics served as the dependent measure in a second study, FT was more effective in producing acquisition of new letter sounds for half of the learners, but DTI was more effective for the other half. However, FT was more effective across all learners with respect to retention (i.e., 6 weeks of no practice), endurance (i.e., engagement in target skill for increased amount of time without fatigue), stability (i.e., engagement in target response while distracted), and application (e.g., use of mastered single-letter sounds to provide novel consonant-vowel [CV] and consonant-vowel-consonant [CVC] letter combinations; Nopprapun & Holloway, 2014). Because the benefits of FT over DTI have not been consistently demonstrated across multiple relevant treatment targets and dependent measures, practitioners should use their professional judgment to determine which of these instructional strategies will be most effective with each learner with ASD.

PRACTICAL REQUIREMENTS

Once practitioners develop a curriculum, they must consider the practical requirements of DTI, including time and personnel demands, training required, and necessary materials. These practical requirements may influence suitability of DTI. DTI requires a practitioner and one or more learners. Practitioners may include those with advanced degrees and relevant certifications and licensures (e.g., board certified behavior analysts [BCBAs], psychologists, speech-language pathologists), registered behavior technicians (RBTs), teachers, or parents. The time spent on any given skill depends on individual learner characteristics (e.g., the learner's motivation, prior repertoire, ability to perform the skill independently, problem behaviors). DTI is combined with an individualized curriculum that is based on learners' target goals, which means the total time learners spend in treatment can be expected to vary considerably. However, given the number and severity of impairments often associated with ASD, most learners will require a significant number of hours of treatment with DTI in isolation or in combination with other interventions to learn a particular skill.

Because of the highly structured and precise method of instruction, practitioners should obtain training on its basic components and practice with a variety of learners prior to implementing DTI. Behavioral skills training (i.e., instructions, modeling, rehearsal, feedback) can effectively prepare professionals to implement DTI (Sarokoff & Sturmey, 2004). In the absence of significant training for practitioners, which seems destined to result in poor treatment fidelity, learners are likely to make progress at a slow pace, experience frustration leading to problem behavior, and/or experience a greater gap between their skill sets and those of their neurotypical peers.

Materials required during implementation of DTI vary according to the learner's goals, which can be expected to differ across learners. Learners should not have free access to materials during DTI, so practitioners must keep all materials within their own reach. Materials present during DTI include any relevant stimuli (e.g., reinforcers, pictures or physical representations of stimuli to teach concepts) and data collection instruments (e.g., data-collection app, paper and pencil).

KEY COMPONENTS

DTI comprises four components: 1) discriminative stimulus presentation (S^D), 2) response, 3) consequence, and 4) ITI (Brown-Chidsey & Steege, 2004; Steege et al., 2007). DTI breaks skills into manageable chunks, which are taught separately until they can be combined fluently in real-world contexts. Practitioner training and dosage are also key components.

Components of Discrete Trial Instruction

An S^D is a cue or brief instruction provided by the practitioner to initiate a discrete trial (Downs et al., 2008; see Figure 6.1 for a DTI implementation fidelity checklist). S^Ds vary on the basis of the learner's current repertoire and target goals. For example, a practitioner may use the S^D, "What color?" when teaching to label colors with one learner but may use "Tell me what color this is" with another learner. An S[D] does not have to be an instruction. For example, when the target goal is increasing the number of responses to social bids, practitioners may use the S[D] "Hi" to gain a response (e.g., "Hi").

Following the S[D], learners provide a response (correct, incorrect, prompted, or no response). Target responses must be defined at the onset of treatment so each practitioner working with the learner is able to differentiate a correct from an incorrect response. Learners may need a **prompt** (i.e., cue; see Table 6.3) to provide a correct response. Although prompts may be necessary at the onset of teaching a target skill, fading of prompts must occur to ensure learners will independently perform the target skill in response to naturally occurring S[D]s in the real world. For example, Tommy might be able to provide a correct response with a full verbal prompt (i.e., the practitioner states "Tommy, what color? Red," and Tommy repeats back "Red") at the onset of treatment, but the practitioner would still need to fade to the partial verbal prompt, "Tommy, what color? Rrrr," and Tommy would state, "Red." Prompt fading would be complete when Tommy's brother asked him, "What color truck do you have, Tommy?" and Tommy independently responded, "Red."

Two common prompt-fading procedures are most-to-least and least-to-most prompting (Cengher et al., 2016). A most-to-least prompting hierarchy occurs when practitioners use the most intrusive prompt necessary (e.g., full physical) in order to achieve a correct response (Batu et al., 2004) and gradually fade to less intrusive prompts, such as those illustrated previously. For example, learners beginning to initiate social interactions with their peers may not independently orient their bodies to the person with whom they are talking. Although a most-to-least prompting hierarchy beginning with a full physical prompt may be uncommon when working on social-communication goals, an example may include a full physical prompt (i.e., putting hands on the learners' shoulders and physically moving their bodies to the correct orientation) and gradually fade to lesser prompts. A more common

Table 6.3. Prompt hierarchy

Prompt type	Prompt description
Full physical	Practitioner physically guides learner to perform the desired behavior. Examples include hand-over-hand guidance.
Partial physical	Practitioner provides minimal physical guidance in order for the learner to perform the skill. Examples include lightly touching a learner's hand for guidance.
Model	Practitioner demonstrates the desired behavior for the learner. Examples can be live (i.e., practitioner is modeling the behavior in the moment) or video (i.e., learner watches a video of someone performing the skill).
Gestural	Practitioner uses gestures, such as pointing, motioning, or nodding, to indicate the correct response.
Positional	Practitioner positions the target answer closer to the learner than other items.
Visual	Practitioner uses pictures or text to guide the learner through the correct steps. Examples include the learner using a picture visual schedule to learn how to tie his or her shoes.
Verbal	Practitioner verbally states what to do next. Examples of verbal prompts are individual words, instructions, or questions to assist learners to engage in correct responding.

Source: Neitzel & Wolery (2009).

social-communication treatment goal may begin with a most-to-least prompting hierarchy, such as beginning with a more intensive prompt (e.g., pointing to the peer and saying, "Make sure your body is facing Joanna") and gradually fade to a less intrusive prompt, such as "Face Joanna"). A least-to-most prompting hierarchy begins with the least intrusive prompt and gradually progresses to more intrusive prompts, if needed. Both prompting hierarchies effectively teach learners with ASD new skills; therefore, practitioners should consider the type of skill, individual learner, and current environmental conditions when selecting prompts (Cengher et al., 2016).

Learners receive one of two consequences during DTI: a reinforcer or error correction. Practitioners provide reinforcers to increase and maintain correct target responses (Leaf, Cihon et al., 2016). Practitioners should conduct a preference assessment to identify stimuli that might serve as potent reinforcers. Simply asking learners what they want to "work for" is often insufficient. When learners respond incorrectly, error correction procedures are implemented. Table 6.2 discusses a variety of error correction procedures to consider when implementing DTI. Finally, shorter ITIs (i.e., the time between the end of one discrete trial and the beginning of the next) may improve the acquisition, maintenance, and generalization of skills, and reduce problem behaviors (Cariveau et al., 2016; Francisco & Hanley, 2012; Smith, 2001).

Practitioner Training

Extensive training is necessary to ensure accurate practitioner implementation and high rates of learner skill acquisition because of DTI's prescribed and systematic instructional style (Severtson & Carr, 2012; Smith, 2001). Behavioral skills training (i.e., instructions, feedback, rehearsal, modeling; Sarokoff & Sturmey, 2004) is ideally used to teach practitioners to implement DTI; however, a self-instruction manual of implementation may be beneficial (Severtson & Carr, 2012). DTI can be used by diverse professionals (e.g., teachers, behavior analysts, speech-language pathologists), and this teaching method should not be restricted on the basis of specific certifications. However, supervised implementation with feedback from an experienced professional who has successfully supported diverse learners by using DTI is critical. Many decisions must be made when implementing DTI. For example, knowing what types of prompts to deliver, how variable the delivery of the S^D should be, when to rearrange materials, how to identify potent reinforcers, strategies for avoiding prompt dependency, and how to generalize skills to all relevant real-world settings are difficult to determine without sufficient supervised clinical experience. Thus, degree and discipline are useful but insufficient for effectively implementing DTI.

Dosage

The dosage of an intervention may include the number of teaching episodes during a single session, total intervention duration, cumulative intervention intensity, instructional format, and implementation fidelity.

Number of Teaching Episodes During a Single Session   Treatment sessions should be individualized according to strengths and weaknesses so learners will make progress toward treatment goals. DTI is an efficient way to provide a large number of learning opportunities (i.e., roughly 200 per hour; Downs et al., 2008; Smith, 2001). The number of teaching interactions during a session will vary depending on learner motivation, attention span, and other relevant learner variables; however, a

rapid pace as well as an emphasis on shaping (i.e., DTI's use of prompting and error correction procedures) combined with positive reinforcement should provide a positive learning interaction for learners and practitioners (Downs et al., 2008).

Total Intervention Duration   Once a component of a skill is taught to mastery (e.g., learner correctly responds to stimuli 80% of the time across two consecutive sessions; Carroll et al., 2016; Jennett et al., 2008), learners should be taught to use the skill with other stimuli, environments, or people if generalization does not naturally emerge. Alternatively, learners may acquire the next component (e.g., put soap in hands) of the overall skill (e.g., washing hands in the bathroom) until all subcomponents can be fluently used in real-world contexts.

Cumulative Intervention Intensity   There is ongoing debate on the intensity of DTI required to make the most meaningful and beneficial learner improvements (Eikeseth et al., 2014). The best outcomes have occurred in the literature when treatment is intensive (e.g., up to 40 hours of treatment per week). Because of the heterogeneity of learners with ASD, the intensity of DTI will depend on the needs of the individual learner, his or her level of functioning, and his or her overall treatment goals. For example, learners with lower verbal repertoires may need more intensive DTI to build their skills. The time it takes to acquire communicative behavior in the forms of requesting; basic labeling; labeling based on feature, function, and class; conversational usage; and appropriate use in real-world exchanges can be considerable.

Instructional Format   DTI can be implemented in a one-to-one or group instructional format. A one-to-one instructional format consists of the learner and the practitioner. One-to-one DTI has the advantages of minimized distractions and increased number of teaching trials (Leaf et al., 2012). Group instructional format occurs when there are multiple learners and one practitioner, with all learners responding simultaneously (e.g., "Everyone, touch the large circle") or learners taking turns responding (e.g., "Sally, touch the small circle," "Todd, touch the medium circle"). Group instructional DTI mimics a general education classroom, as there will be more than one learner for each practitioner, so skills learned in this format are more likely to generalize to real-world contexts. Group DTI can be a more efficient instructional approach as long as the learners are capable of performing in this format (Leaf et al., 2012).

Implementation Fidelity   *Implementation fidelity, treatment integrity,* and *treatment fidelity* are all terms for the same concept: The degree to which treatments are implemented as planned. Readers are encouraged to examine the National Professional Development Center on Autism Spectrum Disorders to review the extensive description of the components and implementation of DTI (Bogin, 2008). They should be careful when reviewing any ready-made checklists to determine if falsely inflated ratings result from including many noncritical items in the overall implementation fidelity score. For example, many implementation fidelity checklists include the following: 1) set up the instructional space, 2) get the appropriate data collection sheet, 3) determine which target skill to begin with, 4) gain the learner's attention, 5) deliver the S^D, 6) provide reinforcer, and 7) implement error correction procedure if necessary. In this example, practitioners may reach up to 70% implementation fidelity by simply performing Steps 1–5, before implementing core components of DTI. Figure 6.1 describes an implementation fidelity checklist highlighting critical items (i.e., deliver discriminative stimulus, deliver consequence within one to three seconds, and use an appropriate, one to five second, intertrial interval) relevant to the implementation of DTI so practitioners can generate a separate score for critical and helpful items.

ASSESSMENT FOR TREATMENT PLANNING AND PROGRESS MONITORING

Typically, data are collected continuously for all treatment goals using trial-by-trial recording (LeBlanc et al., 2005). Trial-by-trial recording involves documenting correct, incorrect, or prompted responses (Nopprapun & Holloway, 2014) and then calculating the percentage of correct responses by dividing the number of correct responses by the total number of trials in a session (Carroll et al., 2016). If the learner's goal is to increase independent steps completed in a task, percentage of correct responses allows for easier comparison across data sessions and is generally used to guide treatment (Carroll et al., 2015).

In the absence of sufficient progress monitoring, learners may continue with treatment goals even after they have mastered skills or they may continue receiving instructions that are too frustrating, leading to more problem behaviors. Figure 6.2

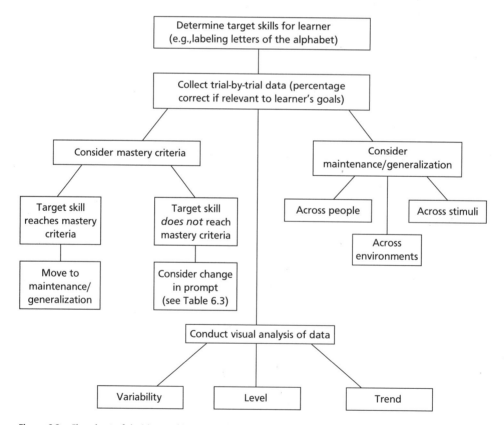

Figure 6.2. Flowchart of decision-making process.

provides a flowchart to aid in the decision-making process when making treatment decisions for learners. Progress monitoring should include 1) evaluating mastery criteria, 2) graphic analysis, and 3) assessment of maintenance and generalization data. Mastery criteria are unique to individual learners and treatment goals. For example, although mastery criteria are commonly set for 80% or higher for correct responses across two consecutive sessions (Carroll et al., 2016; Jennet et al., 2008), criteria could be much higher for dimensions (i.e., percentage correct or number of sessions in which mastery was achieved) if lower criteria was associated with weaker fluency (e.g., the response latency was too slow), safety concerns (e.g., crossing the street), or inconsistent performance in real-world contexts (e.g., classroom, home). Practitioners are also encouraged to collect data on learner affect (i.e., emotional responses; Wilczynski, 2017) to help make decisions about prompting levels, the number of trials until a break is taken, and retaining or rejecting treatment goals.

Clinicians should record responses during DTI, graph them after each session, and visually analyze them (i.e., by examining trend, level, variability). Great tutorials about visual analysis are available through Foxylearning (https://foxylearning .com/tutorials/va). Clinicians should evaluate responses in terms of progress (i.e., increasing, decreasing, stable; little to no change or variable; inconsistent trends; Nopprapun & Holloway, 2014). Maintenance data can be collected to ensure mastered skills are retained. For example, practitioners could assess the learner's performance 6 weeks after targets were considered mastered to evaluate whether high rates of correct responding continue (Nopprapun & Holloway, 2014). Generalization data assess the extent to which learners use mastered skills across different people (i.e., parents and teachers), stimuli (i.e., green versus red apple), and settings (i.e., public bathroom versus bathroom at home). Mastery and generalization data review should be ongoing.

Although DTI can yield skill acquisition, it is often criticized for a lack of skill generalization and rote responding (Steege et al., 2007). Lack of generalization during DTI is primarily a result of the highly structured teaching environment and use of reinforcers that are unrelated to the natural environment or activity (e.g., learners receive an edible reinforcer when they correctly label an animal). Practitioners need to plan for generalization of the target skills from the onset of treatment to overcome this limitation. Termination of a given target skill is based on data collected; continuous progress monitoring, including mastery criteria, generalization, and maintenance; adjustments; and the individual needs of learners.

Practitioners should make adjustments whenever learners are not meeting mastery criteria. Table 6.3 describes different levels of prompting, which represents a common adjustment during DTI. Adjustments are based on learner history (i.e., prompts associated with correct responding for each learner), performance within a session (e.g., if learners respond incorrectly using a partial physical prompt, then a full physical prompt is used), and risk of prompt dependency (i.e., learner waits to respond to tasks until a prompt is offered). Prompting systems (e.g., least-to-most prompting, most-to-least prompting) have been developed to assist practitioners in fading prompts and avoiding possible prompt dependency (Leaf et al., 2014). Strategies such as planned generalization at the onset of treatment and immediately fading prompts once the predetermined criterion for independent mastery occurs allow practitioners to decrease prompt dependency (Hume et al., 2012). When choosing an appropriate prompting system, practitioners should consider the individual needs of the learner as well as the treatment goal being taught (Libby et al., 2008).

IMPLICATIONS FOR INCLUSIVE PRACTICE

DTI is an instructional strategy that can be applied across settings (e.g., schools, homes, and clinics). Too often, DTI is considered an instructional method requiring learners to be seated across from practitioners while seated at a table. In reality, DTI can be implemented anywhere at any time. For example, learners working on social initiations may be prompted at the grocery store to say, "How much is this?" to the cashier. DTI implemented in school settings can increase skills such as self-care (e.g., toileting; Cocchiola et al., 2012) and academics (Carroll et al., 2013). Concerns about generalizability of learned skills can be addressed by training multiple practitioners in the classroom to implement DTI, which could facilitate learners' inclusion (Skokut et al., 2008; Young et al., 2016).

DTI implemented in the home can teach learners with ASD social, cognitive, and behavioral skills to improve their and their family's quality of life (e.g., toileting and self-care; McConnell et al., 2015; Ozonoff & Cathcart, 1998), which can directly impact the likelihood the family will fully participate in their communities. Caregivers and siblings can be trained to effectively administer DTI (Meadan et al., 2009); however, the extent to which home-based DTI results in skill acquisition depends on the family's adherence to treatment, which is historically low (i.e., only 1 in 10 caregivers incorporate all components of a recommended treatment; Barton & Fettig, 2013). Parent training may be an effective method to increase implementation fidelity with DTI. Live or video modeling from the practitioner, guided practice of new skills, review of written materials, and adaptation of DTI for implementation as part of the caregiver's daily routine (Beaudoin et al., 2014; Matson et al., 2009) may increase the overall accuracy of DTI implementation.

DTI is commonly implemented in a clinic setting because practitioners can implement one-to-one intervention with learners in a controlled environment (Leaf et al., 2018; Lovaas, 1987). Clinics should provide practitioners and caregivers with training, support, and supervision, all of which increase implementation fidelity (Brand et al., 2017; Leaf et al., 2018). Group instruction and social opportunities should also be offered in clinic settings, increasing treatment efficiency in a naturalistic environment (Leaf et al., 2012). Some skills are not conducive to learning in a clinic (e.g., changing clothes), and other skills may not generalize to environments outside the clinic. In addition, the cost of clinic-based DTI intervention is often greater than that of home-based treatments (Hay-Hansson & Eldevik, 2013; Leaf et al., 2018). Incorporating DTI into multiple environments (e.g., home and school) is the most effective method to increase generalizability and decrease cost of treatment across relevant settings (Leaf et al., 2018).

CONSIDERATIONS FOR CHILDREN FROM CULTURALLY AND LINGUISTICALLY DIVERSE BACKGROUNDS

DTI should be modified for all learners, and this includes incorporating diverse cultural and linguistic backgrounds into appropriate treatment protocols (Lau, 2006). By considering culture, practitioners can increase implementation fidelity, meaningfulness of the S^D, generalizability of treatment goals, and overall family functioning (Buzhardt et al., 2016; Lang et al., 2011; Leaf, Cihon et al., 2016; Pellecchia et al., 2018). At the onset of treatment (i.e., intervention planning), clinicians should consider the cultural identities of the learner and stakeholders (e.g., family members and any other appropriate community members perspectives; Pellecchia et al., 2018).

Culturally appropriate implementation of DTI includes 1) utilizing the learner's primary language during intervention, 2) selecting culturally sensitive treatment goals, and 3) delivering the S^D in a culturally acceptable manor (Kingsdorf, 2014). When DTI is implemented in languages that are commonly used by the learner's caregivers and community, implementation fidelity increases, problem behavior decreases (DuBay et al., 2018; Lang et al., 2011), and generalization of skills to the natural environment is more attainable (Kingsdorf, 2014). For example, eye contact may not be a beneficial treatment goal if maintaining eye contact with adults is viewed as culturally unacceptable. In addition, effusive praise may actually decrease correct responding if the learner's culture does not encourage exuberant gestures or behaviors. Family functioning is improved when goals and target behaviors that are meaningful to caregivers are targeted as part of the learner's treatment goals (DuBay et al., 2018).

Application to a Child

Penny is a 9-year-old girl diagnosed with Down syndrome and ASD. She attends a life skills classroom at her local elementary school. Penny is nonverbal but uses an augmentative and alternative communication (AAC) device to communicate. She communicates primarily through sequences of three to four words and requests items or activities such as food, preferred toys, and visiting the playground or the sensory room at school.

When Penny was introduced to the AAC device 6 months ago, her classroom teacher, parents, and BCBA used the program Language Acquisition through Motor Planning (LAMP; Center for AAC & Autism, n.d.) to assess Penny's interest for items by observing which toys, activities, and foods Penny reached for, touched, or used. They added Penny's preferred items on the AAC device and used DTI to teach requesting. The adult first gave Penny access to the item after the adult touched the appropriate word (e.g., puppets) on the AAC device while the screen was visible to Penny. After approximately 30 seconds of access to the preferred stimulus, the adult removed the item and repeated the trial, but on this second trial, the adult gave Penny a gestural prompt to push the correct button on the AAC device. The adult gave Penny immediate access to the preferred stimulus once she pressed the button. If Penny was unable to follow the gestural prompt, the adult lightly guided Penny's finger to the button and waited for her to press the item, making the process as errorless as possible while avoiding creating prompt dependency. Once Penny independently and accurately followed gestural prompts for five consecutive trials, the adult systematically faded the prompts, and a natural pause/delay of access to the item or activity acted as the cue for Penny to make the one-word AAC request. This same systematic approach was used to teach requesting with two-word sequences, such as "play puppets."

Application to an Adult

Bryce is a 26-year-old man who is diagnosed with ASD. He is able to communicate vocally, has a vocabulary of a typical fourth grader, has a driver's license, and drives himself to work each day. Bryce works in a factory facility, conducting quality control for tool kits sold by outside distributors. Specifically, he uses a checklist to ensure tool kits are complete. Bryce's boss, Diondreé, reports that Bryce's co-workers treat him as if he were a child. She believes this undermines his chances to fully contribute to the workplace and that it may be due, in part, to his lack of social initiations with co-workers.

Bryce enjoys using his cell phone and having a reason to text his BCBA. Bryce meets with his BCBA once a week, and they incorporate this preference into treatment, including DTI. Bryce was first taught to discriminate between situations in which co-workers are busy with work responsibilities (e.g., in a meeting, working on their computers) and more casual work situations (e.g., lunchtime, having a cup of coffee). Bryce and the BCBA asked Diondreé if they could complete these trials in the workplace to ensure they would be rapidly deployed. Bryce was taught to ask himself, "What is [co-worker's name] doing right now?" Bryce texted one of two answers ("busy working" or "more casual") to his BCBA, who was nearby and therefore aware of the co-worker's status. If Bryce correctly identified the situation, the BCBA texted back and Bryce could send the BCBA another text, with the BCBA sending a response. If Bryce answered incorrectly, the BCBA would say, "Show me some of the work you do around here." This was deemed an appropriate consequence by Bryce and Diondreé because Bryce did have work responsibilities to complete. He momentarily lost the opportunity to send a text to the BCBA, which means his incorrect response was not reinforced but that standard work conditions were followed (i.e., no punishment occurred). At a later time, the BCBA would model correct identification of co-worker status. Once Bryce could make the correct discrimination independently, he was taught to initiate with co-workers when they were "more casual." Specifically, when Bryce texted "more casual," the BCBA prompted him to initiate common social interactions (e.g., "How are you?" "What's up?"). If Bryce initiated the social interaction, the BCBA provided praise via text after the encounter naturally ended. If Bryce did not initiate the social interaction, a more intrusive prompt would occur (e.g., the BCBA would provide a verbal prompt in front of the co-worker). Although Bryce agreed to this procedure, he stated that he did not like being prompted verbally in front of co-workers. However, a verbal prompt was needed on only one occasion because Bryce started independently initiating interactions with co-workers when they were "more casual."

> **To review an extended application and
> implementation of this intervention, see Case 3
> about a child with ASD in the companion volume**
> *Case Studies for the Treatment of Autism Spectrum Disorder.*

Future Directions _____

DTI can be implemented with individuals with various disabilities, including ASD (Thiessen et al., 2009) and other developmental disabilities (Downs et al., 2008), and in a number of settings, including schools, clinics, and homes, with learners in a variety of age groups. Although previous research has demonstrated the usefulness of DTI, most studies have been conducted in a clinical setting (Leaf, Cihon, et al., 2016), where confounding variables can be limited or more easily controlled. Therefore, more research is necessary to evaluate the effectiveness of DTI in real-world settings, allowing practitioners to make in the moment decisions on treatment goals (Leaf, Cihon, et al., 2016).

Suggested Readings

1. Bogin, J. (2008). *Overview of discrete trial training.* National Professional Development Center on Autism Spectrum Disorders, MIND Institute, University of California at Davis Medical School. Bogin (2008) provides readers with a description of DTI, its effectiveness in a variety of settings and age groups, and a detailed implementation fidelity checklist for practitioners to use with learners.

2. Cook, J. E., Subramaniam, S., Brunson, L. Y., Larson, N. A., Poe, S. G., & St. Peter, C. C. (2015). Global measures of treatment integrity may mask important errors in discrete-trial training. *Behavior Analysis in Practice, 8*(1), 37–47. This study assesses implementation fidelity during the implementation of DTI in using both global and individual-component implementation fidelity scores. The way in which practitioners implement DTI can negatively affect learners; therefore, use of implementation fidelity checklists, as well as proper training and supervision of those implementing DTI, are crucial.

3. Radley, K. C., Dart, E. H., Furlow, C. M., & Ness, E. J. (2015). Peer-mediated discrete trial training within a school setting. *Research in Autism Spectrum Disorders, 9*, 53–67. This study evaluates how neurotypical peers can be trained to implement DTI with students with ASD with high levels of implementation fidelity. Although DTI is often seen as a highly structured instructional method, Radley and colleagues demonstrate the flexibility of DTI and how novice individuals (neurotypical fifth-grade students) can be taught to implement this instructional method with a high degree of implementation fidelity.

Learning Activities

DTI is an instructional method that can be implemented with a variety of learners in many different settings (e.g., homes, schools, clinics). Practitioners considering DTI as an instructional method should consider the following learning activities.

Further Discussion

Although DTI has years of research to demonstrate that it can be used to effectively teach learners a variety of skills, further research and discussion are recommended on the varying ways in which DTI can be implemented. For example, elaboration is needed on topics such as the difference in skill acquisition in one-to-one instructional formats versus group formats, the role of motivating operations during the implementation of DTI, and how practitioners can integrate generalization of skills at the onset of treatment. Consider current or past learners you have worked with when answering the following questions.

1. How do you think skill acquisition differs in a one-to-one versus group instructional format?

2. What motivating operations were evident that may have influenced the way in which the treatment session played out? Consider both behavior- and value-altering effects.

3. Consider how generalization of skills from the onset of treatment may have changed the overall look of treatment. Think about what treatments were targeted, why they were chosen, and whether behavioral cusps were considered.

Topics to Discuss

Practitioners are encouraged to discuss the following questions to apply their knowledge of DTI as an evidence-based instructional method.

1. What are the most common challenges that might prevent you from enjoying work with some learners with ASD? How might incorporating DTI on a short-term or long-term basis for these learners help you address this challenge?

2. List advantages and disadvantages of using a rapid pacing of instruction during treatment sessions. Do the advantages outweigh the disadvantages?

3. What do you see as potential barriers to implementation of DTI in your current workplace or in some future workplace you might envisage? Consider the following: staff to implement DTI, training to appropriately implement DTI, data collection procedures, and so on.

4. How would you describe DTI procedures and possible benefits with a learner's family? What about a family from another cultural background that is opposed to DTI and sees this instructional method as "robotic or rote responding"?

Writing Assignment

1. Reflect on learners with ASD for whom you have provided services, both current and past, with a focus on age, developmental ability, and overall goals of therapy. Begin by determining whether DTI would be an appropriate instructional method to teach target skills based on the following questions:

    a. What is the learner's attention span? If he or she has a short attention span, is this something that should be targeted prior to considering DTI as an instructional method?

    b. What does the literature say? Has DTI been effective in increasing the behavior you are targeting?

2. Provide a justification regarding why skills might be appropriately targeted with DTI or why DTI would not be appropriate. Next, identify where the skills identified in Step 1 fit into a larger curriculum.

    a. Are there prerequisite skills that should be taught? Could they lead to a behavioral cusp?

    b. Can the larger skill be broken down and taught in smaller components (i.e., task analysis)?

3. For skills that should *not* be treated with DTI, identify what instructional approach should be considered instead.

    a. Why is DTI not appropriate?

    b. What instructional approaches are more effective, according to the literature?

4. Justify the use of the alternative instructional approach. If there are problems with implementation of this alternative, could a subcomponent (or multiple subcomponents) be taught using DTI to facilitate faster acquisition before using the alternative instructional method?

Summary of Video Clip ──────────────────────────

*See the **About the Videos and Downloads** page at the front of the book for directions on how to access and stream the accompanying video to this chapter.*

The associated video clip for this chapter reflects DTI implemented in the more traditional format (i.e., one-to-one, at a table, with short ITIs). Although this traditional method of DTI is commonly seen in an ABA clinic setting, DTI can be implemented in a more relaxed, less prescriptive manner. An S^D is presented, followed by the learner's response, a consequence (i.e., reinforcer or error correction procedure), and a brief ITI. Short ITI and rapid instruction are demonstrated in the video because they have been shown to promote effectiveness. The practitioner uses a combination of reinforcers, including edibles and praise, to illustrate a variety of reinforcement strategies.

REFERENCES

American Psychiatric Association. (2013). *Diagnostic and statistical manual of mental disorders* (5th ed.). American Psychiatric Publishing.

Barton, E. E., & Fettig, A. (2013). Parent-implemented interventions for young children with disabilities: A review of fidelity features. *Journal of Early Intervention, 35*(2), 194–219.

Batu, S., Ergenekon, Y., Erbas, D., & Akmanoglu, N. (2004). Teaching pedestrian skills to individuals with developmental disabilities. *Journal of Behavioral Education, 13*(3), 147–164.

Beaudoin, A. J., Sébire, G., & Couture, M. (2014). Parent training interventions for toddlers with autism spectrum disorder. *Autism Research and Treatment, 2014,* 1–15.

Bogin, J. (2008). *Overview of discrete trial training.* Sacramento, CA: National Professional Development Center on Autism Spectrum Disorders, MIND Institute, University of California at Davis Medical School.

Bosch, S., & Fuqua, R. W. (2001). Behavioral cusps: A model for selecting target behaviors. *Journal of Applied Behavior Analysis, 34,* 123–125.

Brand, D., Mudford, O. C., Arnold-Saritepe, A., & Elliffe, D. (2017). Assessing the within-trial treatment integrity of discrete trial teaching programs using sequential analysis. *Behavioral Interventions, 32*(1), 54–69.

Brown-Chidsey, R., & Steege, M. W. (2004). Discrete trial teaching. *Encyclopedia of School Psychology,* 96–97.

Buzhardt, J., Rusinko, L., Heitzman-Powell, L., Trevino-Maack, S., & McGrath, A. (2016). Exploratory evaluation and initial adaptation of a parent training program for Hispanic families of children with autism. *Family Process, 55*(1), 107–122.

Cariveau, T., Kodak, T., & Campbell, V. (2016). The effects of intertrial interval and instructional format on skill acquisition and maintenance for children with autism spectrum disorders: Intertrial interval and instructional format. *Journal of Applied Behavior Analysis, 49*(4), 809–825.

Carroll, R. A., Joachim, B. T., St. Peter, C. C., & Robinson, N. (2015). A comparison of error-correction procedures on skill acquisition during discrete-trial instruction. *Journal of Applied Behavior Analysis, 48*(2), 257–273.

Carroll, R. A., Kodak, T., & Adolf, K. J. (2016). Effect of delayed reinforcement on skill acquisition during discrete-trial instruction: Implications for treatment-integrity errors in academic settings. *Journal of Applied Behavior Analysis, 49*(1), 176–181.

Carroll, R. A., Kodak, T., & Fisher, W. W. (2013). An evaluation of programmed treatment-integrity errors during discrete-trial instruction. *Journal of Applied Behavior Analysis, 46*(2), 379–394.

Carroll, R. A., Owsiany, J., & Cheatham, J. M. (2018). Using an abbreviated assessment to identify effective error-correction procedures for individual learners during discrete-trial instruction. *Journal of Applied Behavior Analysis, 51*(3), 482–501.

Cengher, M., Shamoun, K., Moss, P., Roll, D., Feliciano, G., & Fienup, D. M. (2016). A comparison of the effects of two prompt-fading strategies on skill acquisition in children with autism spectrum disorders. *Behavior Analysis in Practice, 9*(2), 115–125.

Center for AAC and Autism. (n.d.). *What Is LAMP?* Retrieved on September 6, 2018 from https://www.aacandautism.com/lamp

Cocchiola, M. A., Martino, G. M., Dwyer, L. J., & Demezzo, K. (2012). Toilet training children with autism and developmental delays: An effective program for school settings. *Behavior Analysis in Practice, 5*(2), 60–64.

Cook, J. E., Subramaniam, S., Brunson, L. Y., Larson, N. A., Poe, S. G., & St. Peter, C. C. (2015). Global measures of treatment integrity may mask important errors in discrete-trial training. *Behavior Analysis in Practice, 8*(1), 37–47.

Dass, T. K., Kisamore, A. N., Vladescu, J. C., Reeve, K. F., Reeve, S. A., & Taylor-Santa, C. (2018). Teaching children with autism spectrum disorder to tact olfactory stimuli. *Journal of Applied Behavior Analysis, 51*(3), 538–552.

Delprato, D. J. (2001). Comparisons of discrete-trial and normalized behavioral language intervention for young children with autism. *Journal of Autism and Developmental Disorders, 31*(3), 315–325.

Dib, N., & Sturmey, P. (2007). Reducing student stereotypy by improving teachers' implementation of discrete-trial teaching. *Journal of Applied Behavior Analysis, 40*(2), 339–343.

DiGennaro Reed, F. D., Reed, D. D., Baez, C. N., & Maguire, H. (2011). A parametric analysis of errors of commission during discrete-trial training. *Journal of Behavior Analysis, 44*(3), 611–615.

Dixon, M. R., Belisle, J., Stanley, C., Rowsey, K., Daar, J. H., & Szekely, S. (2015). Toward a behavior analysis of complex language for children with autism: Evaluating the relationship between PEAK and VB-MAPP. *Journal of Developmental and Physical Disabilities, 27*(2), 223–233.

Dixon, M. R., Belisle, J., McKeel, A., Whiting, S., Speelman, R., Daar, J. H., & Rowsey, K. (2017). An internal and critical review of the PEAK relational training system for children with autism and related intellectual disabilities: 2014–2017. *The Behavior Analyst, 40,* 493–521.

Downs, A., Downs, R. C., Fossum, M., & Rau, K. (2008). Effectiveness of discrete trial teaching with preschool students with developmental disabilities. *Education and Training in Developmental Disabilities, 43*(4), 443–453.

Downs, A., Downs, R. C., Johansen, M., & Fossum, M. (2007). Using discrete trial teaching within a public preschool program to facilitate skill development in students with developmental disabilities. *Education and Treatment of Children, 30*(3), 1–27.

DuBay, M., Watson, L. R., & Zhang, W. (2018). In search of culturally appropriate autism interventions: Perspectives of Latino caregivers. *Journal of Autism and Developmental Disorders, 48*(5), 1623–1639.

Eikeseth, S., Smith, D. P., & Klintwall, L. (2014). Discrete trial teaching and discrimination training. In J. Tarbox, D. R. Dixon, P. Sturmey, & J. L. Matson (Eds.), *Handbook of early intervention for autism spectrum disorders: Research, policy, and practice* (pp. 293–324). Springer.

Elliott, C., & Dillenburger, K. (2016). The effect of choice on motivation for young children on the autism spectrum during discrete trial teaching. *Journal of Research in Special Educational Needs, 16*(3), 187–198.

Francisco, M. T., & Hanley, G. P. (2012). An evaluation of progressively increasing intertrial intervals on the acquisition and generalization of three social skills. *Journal of Applied Behavior Analysis, 45*(1), 137–142.

Geiger, K. B., Carr, J. E., LeBlanc, L. A., Hanney, N. M., Polick, A. S., & Heinicke, M. R. (2012). Teaching receptive discriminations to children with autism: A comparison of traditional and embedded discrete trial teaching. *Behavior Analysis in Practice, 5*(2), 49–59.

Gresham, F. M. (1989). Assessment of treatment integrity in school consultation and prereferral intervention. *School Psychology Review, 18,* 37–50.

Hay-Hansson, A. W., & Eldevik, S. (2013). Training discrete trials teaching skills using videoconference. *Research in Autism Spectrum Disorders, 7*(11), 1300–1309.

Holding, E., Bray, M. A., & Kehle, T. J. (2011). Does speed matter? A comparison of the effectiveness of fluency and discrete trial training for teaching noun labels to children with autism. *Psychology in the Schools, 48*(2), 166–183.

Howell, K. W., & Lorson-Howell, K. A. (1990). What's the hurry? Fluency in the classroom. *Teaching Exceptional Children, 22*(3), 20–23.

Hume, K., Plavnick, J., & Odom, S. L. (2012). Promoting task accuracy and independence in students with autism across educational setting through the use of individual work systems. *Journal of Autism and Developmental Disorders, 42*(10), 2084–2099.

Isenhower, R. W., Delmolino, L., Fiske, K. E., Bamond, M., & Leaf, J. B. (2018). Assessing the role of active student response during error correction in discrete trial instruction. *Journal of Behavioral Education*, 1–17.

Jenkins, S. R., Hirst, J. M., & DiGennaro-Reed, F. D. D. (2015). The effects of discrete-trial training commission errors on learner outcomes: An extension. *Journal of Behavioral Education, 24*(2), 196–209.

Jennett, H. K., Harris, S. L., & Delmolino, L. (2008). Discrete trial instruction vs. mand training for teaching children with autism to make requests. *The Analysis of Verbal Behavior, 24*(1), 69–85.

Jones, E. A., Feeley, K. M., & Takacs, J. (2007). Teaching spontaneous responses to young children with autism. *Journal of Applied Behavior Analysis, 40*(3), 565–570.

Kingsdorf, S. (2014). Review of research: Do you speak my language? Are behavior analysts considering the needs of learners on the autism spectrum? *Childhood Education, 90*(2), 143–147.

Klintwall, L., & Eikeseth, S. (2014). Early and Intensive Behavioral Intervention (EIBI) in autism. In V. B. Patel, V. R. Preedy, & C. R. Martin (Eds.), *Comprehensive guide to autism: Vol. 1* (pp. 117–137). Springer.

Koegel, R. L., Dunlap, G., & Dyer, K. (1980). Intertrial interval duration and learning in autistic children. *Journal of Applied Behavior Analysis, 13*, 91–99.

Knutson, S. C., Kodak, T., Costello, D. R., & Cliett, T. (2018). Comparison of task interspersal ratios on efficiency of learning and problem behavior for children with autism spectrum disorder. *Journal of Applied Behavior Analysis*, 1–15.

Lambert, J. M., Copeland, B. A., Karp, E. L., Finley, C. I., Houchins-Juarez, N. J., & Ledford, J. R. (2016). Chaining functional basketball sequences (with embedded conditional discriminations) in an adolescent with autism. *Behavior Analysis in Practice, 9*(3), 199–210.

Lang, R., Rispoli, M., Sigafoos, J., Lancioni, G., Andrews, A., & Ortega, L. (2011). Effects of language of instruction on response accuracy and challenging behavior in a child with autism. *Journal of Behavioral Education, 20*(4), 252–259.

Lang, R., van der Werff, M., Verbeek, K., Didden, R., Davenport, K., Moore, M., Lee, A., Rispoli, M., Machalicek, W. A., O'Reilly, M. F., Sigafoos, J., & Lancioni, G. (2014). Comparison of high and low preferred topographies of contingent attention during discrete trial training. *Research in Autism Spectrum Disorders, 8*(10), 1279–1286.

Laraway, S., Snycerski, S., Michael, J., & Poling, A. (2003). Motivating operations and terms to describe them: Some further refinements. *Journal of Applied Behavior Analysis, 36*(3), 407–414.

Lau, A. S. (2006). Making the case for selective and directed cultural adaptations of evidence-based treatments: Examples from parent training. *Clinical Psychology: Science and Practice, 13*(4), 295–310.

Leaf, J. B., Leaf, R., McEachin, J., Taubman, M., Ala'i-Rosales, S., Ross, R. K., Smith, T., & Weiss, M. J. (2016). Applied behavior analysis is a science and, therefore, progressive. *Journal of Autism and Developmental Disorders, 46*(2), 720–731.

Leaf, J. B., Cihon, J. H., Leaf, R., McEachin, J., & Taubman, M. (2016). A progressive approach to discrete trial teaching: Some current guidelines. *International Electronic Journal of Elementary Education, 9*(2), 361–372.

Leaf, J. B., Leaf, R., McEachin, J., Cihon, J. H., & Ferguson, J. L. (2018). Advantages and challenges of a home-and clinic-based model of behavioral intervention for individuals diagnosed with autism spectrum disorder. *Journal of Autism and Developmental Disorders, 48*(6), 2258–2266.

Leaf, J. B., Leaf, R., Taubman, M., McEachin, J., & Delmolino, L. (2014). Comparison of flexible prompt fading to error correction for children with autism spectrum disorder. *Journal of Developmental and Physical Disabilities, 26*(2), 203–224.

Leaf, J. B., Tsuji, K. H., Lentell, A. E., Dale, S. E., Kassardjian, A., Taubman, M., McEachin, J., Leaf, R., & Oppenheim-Leaf, M. L. (2012). A comparison of discrete trial teaching implemented in a one-to-one instructional format and in a group instructional format. *Behavioral Interventions, 28*(1), 82–106.

LeBlanc, M. P., Ricciardi, J. N., & Luiselli, J. K. (2005). Improving discrete trial instruction by paraprofessional staff through an abbreviated performance feedback intervention. *Education & Treatment of Children, 28*(1), 76–82.

Lerman, D. C., Hawkins, L., Hoffman, R., & Caccavale, M. (2013). Training adults with an autism spectrum disorder to conduct discrete-trial training for young children with autism: A pilot study. *Journal of Applied Behavior Analysis, 46*(2), 465–478.

Libby, M. E., Weiss, J. S., Bancroft, S., & Ahearn, W. H. (2008). A comparison of most-to-least and least-to-most prompting on the acquisition of solitary play skills. *Behavior Analysis in Practice, 1*(1), 37–43.

Lovaas, O. I. (1987). Behavioral treatment and normal educational and intellectual functioning in young autistic children. *Journal of Consulting and Clinical Psychology, 55*(1), 3–9.

Lovaas, O. I. (2003). *Teaching individuals with developmental delays: Basic intervention techniques.* PRO-ED.

Majdalany, L. M., Wilder, D. A., Greif, A., Mathisen, D., & Saini, V. (2014). Comparing massed-trial instruction, distributed-trial instruction, and task interspersal to teach tacts to children with autism spectrum disorders. *Journal of Applied Behavior Analysis, 47*(3), 657–662.

Majdalany, L., Wilder, D. A., Smeltz, L., & Lipschultz, J. (2016). The effect of brief delays to reinforcement on the acquisition of tacts in children with autism. *Journal of Applied Behavior Analysis, 49*(2), 411–415.

Matson, M. L., Mahan, S., & Matson, J. L. (2009). Parent training: A review of methods for children with autism spectrum disorders. *Research in Autism Spectrum Disorders, 3*(4), 868–875.

McConnell, D., Parakkal, M., Savage, A., & Rempel, G. (2015). Parent-mediated intervention: Adherence and adverse effects. *Disability and Rehabilitation, 37*(10), 864–872.

Meadan, H., Ostrosky, M. M., Zaghlawan, H. Y., & Yu, S. (2009). Promoting the social and communicative behavior of young children with autism spectrum disorders: A review of parent-implemented intervention studies. *Topics in Early Childhood Special Education, 29*(2), 90–104.

Neitzel, J., & Wolery, M. (2009). *Overview of prompting.* National Professional Development Center on Autism Spectrum Disorders, Frank Porter Graham Child Development Institute, University of North Carolina.

Nopprapun, M., & Holloway, J. (2014). A comparison of fluency training and discrete trial instruction to teach letter sounds to children with ASD: Acquisition and learning outcomes. *Research in Autism Spectrum Disorders, 8*(7), 788–802.

Ospina, M. B., Seida, J. K., Clark, B., Karkhaneh, M., Hartling, L., Tjosvold, L., Vandermeer, B., & Smith, V. (2008). Behavioural and developmental interventions for autism spectrum disorder: A clinical systematic review. *PLoS ONE, 3*(11), 1–32.

Ozonoff, S., & Cathcart, K. (1998). Effectiveness of a home program intervention for young children with autism. *Journal of Autism and Developmental Disorders, 28*(1), 25–32.

Paden, A. R., & Kodak, T. (2015). The effects of reinforcement magnitude on skill acquisition for children with autism. *Journal of Applied Behavior Analysis, 48*(4), 924–929.

Pellecchia, M., Nuske, H. J., Straiton, D., Hassrick, E. M., Gulsrud, A., Iadarola, S., Vejnoska, S. F., Bullen, B., Haine-Schlagel, R., Kasari, C., Mandell, D. S., Smith, T., & Stahmer, A. C. (2018). Strategies to engage underrepresented parents in child intervention services: A review of effectiveness and co-occurring use. *Journal of Child and Family Studies,* 1–14.

Plaisance, L., Lerman, D. C., Laudont, C., & Wu, W. (2016). Inserting mastered targets during error correction when teaching skills to children with autism. *Journal of Applied Behavior Analysis, 49*(2), 251–264.

Prelock, P. A., Hutchins, T., & Glascoe, F. P. (2008). Speech-language impairment: How to identify the most common and least diagnosed disability of childhood. *Medscape Journal of Medicine, 10*(6), 136.

Radley, K. C., Dart, E. H., Furlow, C. M., & Ness, E. J. (2015). Peer-mediated discrete trial training within a school setting. *Research in Autism Spectrum Disorders, 9*, 53–67.

Reichow, B., Volkmar, F. R., & Cicchetti, D. V. (2008). Development of the evaluative method for evaluating and determining evidence-based practices in autism. *Journal of Autism and Developmental Disorders, 38*, 1311–1319.

Rispoli, M., Ganz, J., Neely, L., & Goodwyn, F. (2013). The effect of noncontingent positive versus negative reinforcement on multiply controlled behavior during discrete trial training. *Journal of Developmental and Physical Disabilities, 25*(1), 135–148.

Rowsey, K. E., Belisle, J., & Dixon, M. R. (2015). Principal component analysis of the peak relational training system. *Journal of Developmental and Physical Disabilties, 27*(1), 15–23.

Roxburgh, C. A., & Carbone, V. J. (2012). The effect of varying teacher presentation rates on responding during discrete trial training for two children with autism. *Behavior Modification, 37*(3), 298–323.

Sarokoff, R. A., & Sturmey, P. (2004). The effects of behavioral skills training on staff implementation of discrete-trial teaching. *Journal of Applied Behavior Analysis, 37*(4), 535–538.

Severtson, J. M., & Carr, J. E. (2012). Training novice instructors to implement errorless discrete-trial teaching: A sequential analysis. *Behavior Analysis in Practice, 5*(2), 13–23.

Shillingsburg, M. A., Bowen, C. N., & Shapiro, S. K. (2014). Increasing social approach and decreasing social avoidance in children with autism spectrum disorder during discrete trial training. *Research in Autism Spectrum Disorders, 8*(11), 1443–1453.

Skinner, B. F. (1957). *Verbal behavior.* Prentice Hall.

Skinner, B. F. (1981). Selection by consequences. *Science, 213*(4507), 501–504.

Skokut, M., Robinson, S., Openden, D., & Jimerson, S. R. (2008). Promoting the social and cognitive competence of children with autism: Interventions at school. *The California School Psychologist, 13*(1), 93–108.

Smith, T. (2001). Discrete trial training in the treatment of autism. *Focus on Autism and Other Developmental Disabilities, 16*(2), 86–92.

Steege, M. W., Mace, F. C., Perry, L., & Longenecker, H. (2007). Applied behavior analysis: Beyond discrete trial teaching. *Psychology in the Schools, 44*(1), 91–99.

Subramaniam, S., Brunson, L. Y., Cook, J. E., Larson, N. A., Poe, S. G., & St. Peter, C. C. (2017). Maintenance of parent-implemented discrete trial instruction during videoconferencing. *Journal of Behavioral Education, 26*, 1–26.

Sundberg, M. L. (2008). *VB-MAPP Verbal Behavior Milestones Assessment and Placement Program: A language and social skills assessment program for children with autism or other developmental disabilities: Guide.* AVB Press.

Tager-Flusberg, H., Joseph, R., & Folstein, S. (2001). Current direction in research on autism. *Mental Retardation and Developmental Disabilities Research Reviews, 7*, 21–29.

Tarbox, J., Wilke, A. E., Findel-Pyles, R. S., Bergstrom, R. M., & Granpeesheh, D. (2010). A comparison of electronic to traditional pen-and-paper data collection in discrete trial training for children with autism. *Research in Autism Spectrum Disorders, 4*(1), 65–75.

Taubman, M. T., Leaf, R. B., McEachin, J. J., Papovich, S., & Leaf, J. B. (2013). A comparison of data collection techniques used with discrete trial teaching. *Research in Autism Spectrum Disorders, 7*, 1026–1034.

Thiessen, C., Fazzio, D., Arnal, L., Martin, G. L., Yu, C. T., & Keilback, L. (2009). Evaluation of a self-instructional manual for conducting discrete-trials teaching with children with autism. *Behavior Modification, 33*(3), 360–373.

Turan, M. K., Moroz, L., & Paquet Croteau, N. (2012). Comparing the effectiveness of error-correction strategies in discrete trial training. *Behavior Modification, 36*(2), 218–234.

Volkmar, F., Lord, C., Bailey, A., Schultz, R., & Klin, A (2004). Autism and pervasive developmental disorders. *Journal of Child Psychology and Psychiatry, 45*, 135–170.

Young, K. R., Radley, K. C., Jenson, W. R., West, R. P., & Clare, S. K. (2016). Peer-facilitated discrete trial training for children with autism spectrum disorder. *School Psychology Quarterly, 31*(4), 507.

Wilczynski, S. M. (2017). *A practical guide to finding treatments that work for people with autism.* Academic Press.

Wong, C., Odom, S. L., Hume, K. A., Cox, A. W., Fettig, A., Kucharczyk, S., Brock, M. E, Plavnick, J. B., Fleury, V. P., & Schultz, T. R. (2015). Evidence-based practices for children, youth, and young adults with autism spectrum disorder: A comprehensive review. *Journal of Autism and Developmental Disorders, 45*(7), 1951–1966.

7

The Developmental, Individual-Difference, Relationship-Based (DIR) Model and Its Application to Children With ASD

Sima Gerber

INTRODUCTION

In their book *The Child with Special Needs*, Stanley Greenspan, a child psychiatrist, and Serena Wieder, a child psychologist, introduced the **Developmental, Individual-Difference, Relationship-Based (DIR) model** to the world of child development (Greenspan & Wieder, 1998). This model presents a comprehensive developmental approach to assessment and intervention for children with developmental disorders, particularly those with autism spectrum disorder (ASD). The approach is rooted in theoretical foundations and empirical research from child development, neuroscience, autism, and early intervention. The DIR model is distinguished from many other contemporary approaches by its scope and its integration of developmental, interpersonal, biological, and contextual components into the assessment and intervention process. Notably, the term *DIR* is often mistakenly used interchangeably with the term *Floortime*. Whereas DIR is the comprehensive model of assessment and intervention just described, **Floortime** is a therapeutic strategy that is specific to the DIR approach. Floortime describes the spontaneous, developmentally appropriate, one-to-one interactions during which the six **functional emotional developmental levels (FEDLs)** are mobilized.

Three components are addressed in the DIR paradigm: the child's FEDL, the child's **individual processing profile**, and the relationship between the child and his or her caregivers. The model reflects the breadth of child and interpersonal development and the complexity of addressing the challenges faced by children and their families when development is derailed. Educators and clinicians who embrace the DIR model adopt the view that a number of areas of development are often affected in children with challenges and that developmental problems in one domain (e.g., sensory processing) can significantly impact others (e.g., social interaction), all of which affect the family's life and dynamics.

A primary goal of the DIR practitioner is to develop a profile of the child and his or her family based on the three major components of the model: *D*, the functional emotional *developmental* levels, which encompass the child's social-emotional-symbolic development (see Table 7.1); *I*, the profile of *individual* differences in sensory, motor, and language abilities (see Table 7.2); and *R*, the caregiver–child *relationships.*

The central innovation and foundation of the DIR approach is its attention to the FEDLs that characterize typical development in the early years of life (described later in the chapter). Greenspan and colleagues (2001) explained,

> The functional emotional developmental approach provides a way of characterizing emotional *functioning* and, at the same time, a way of looking at how all the

Table 7.1. Functional emotional developmental levels and ages at which these levels are achieved in children with typical development

Level	Age	Emotional abilities
1. Shared attention and regulation	Birth–3 months	The child can attend to multisensory affective experience and at the same time organize a calm, regulated state (e.g., looking at, listening to, and following the movement of a caregiver).
2. Engagement and relating	2–6 months	The child can engage with and evidence affective preference and pleasure for a caregiver or caregivers (e.g., showing joyful smiles and affection with a caregiver).
3. Two-way intentional communication	4–9 months	The child can initiate and respond to two-way presymbolic gestural communication (e.g., engaging in the back-and-forth use of smiles and vocalizations).
4. Complex problem solving	9–18 months	The child can organize chains of two-way social problem-solving communications (opening and closing many circles of communication), maintain communication across space, integrate affective polarities, and synthesize an emerging pre-representational organization of self and others (e.g., taking Dad by the hand to get a toy from the shelf).
5. Creative representations (ideas) and elaboration	18–30 months	The child can create and functionally use ideas as a basis for creative or imaginative thinking and for giving meaning to symbols (e.g., engaging in pretend play, using words).
6. Representational differentiation and emotional thinking	30–48 months	The child can build bridges between ideas as a basis for logic, reality testing, thinking, and judgment. The child can elaborate in both make-believe and dialogues and can plan "how, what, and why" elaborations that give depth to the make-believe dramas or reality-based dialogues (e.g., engaging in opinion-oriented conversations and elaborate planned pretend dramas).

Sources: Greenspan (2004); Greenspan and Wieder (1998).

Table 7.2. Elements of the individual processing profile

Sensory modulation	Includes hyporeactivity and hyperreactivity in each sensory modality (e.g., touch, sound, smell, vision, movement in space)
Sensory processing	Includes the capacity to register, decode, and comprehend sequences and abstract patterns in each sensory modality (e.g., auditory processing, visual-spatial processing)
Sensory-affective processing	Includes the ability to process and react to affect in each modality and the capacity to connect intent or affect to motor planning and sequencing, language, and symbols
Motor planning and sequencing	Includes the capacity to sequence actions, behaviors, and symbols, such as thoughts, words, visual images, and spatial concepts

Source: Interdisciplinary Council on Developmental and Learning Disorders (2005).

components of development (cognition, language, and motor skills) work together (as a mental team) organized by the designated emotional goals. In this model, therefore, emotional capacities serve as the orchestra leader that enables all the developmental components to work together in a *functional* manner. (p. xiii)

The first six levels of the FEDLs are shared attention and **regulation,** engagement and relating, two-way intentional communication, complex problem solving, creative representations and elaboration, and representational differentiation and emotional thinking (see Table 7.1). An understanding of the child's FEDLs anchors the DIR assessment and intervention for the clinician, educator, and parents. The goal of the intervention is to facilitate development at and above the child's FEDLs within the context of the child's individual processing profile (sensory modulation, sensory processing, sensory-affective processing, motor planning and sequencing; see Table 7.2). For example, some children will be able to achieve their highest level of social-emotional engagement while they are moving on a swing, whereas others will be most interactive when motor-planning demands are minimal. In addition, parent–child interaction patterns are central to the DIR model, theoretically and clinically. In fact, **parent coaching,** that is, guiding the parents' understanding of how best to help their child move to higher FEDLs in light of his or her individual processing patterns becomes a primary goal of the DIR clinician or educator.

TARGET POPULATIONS

Although DIR is often identified with the assessment of and intervention for children on the autism spectrum, a range of children with developmental disabilities can benefit from the integrated perspective on development inherent in the model, including children with sensory-processing and regulatory disorders, language delays and disorders, cognitive delays, and attachment disorders. Because of the broad age span across which emotional development occurs, and because children with developmental delays are often functioning at earlier developmental levels, the approach is appropriate for infants, toddlers, young children, school-age children, and teens. Similarly, children at all stages of language and communication can be treated using this paradigm. The choice of this approach over others has more to do with the practitioner's view of human development and developmental difficulties than with the relevance of the approach for particular etiological categories or developmental language levels.

THEORETICAL BASIS

The DIR model is based on an interdisciplinary developmental model that integrates information from cognitive, language, social, emotional, sensory, motor, and interpersonal paradigms of development. Like cognitive and social interaction models of language acquisition (Bates, 1975; Bloom & Lahey, 1978; Bloom & Tinker, 2001; Piaget, 1955), the DIR model prioritizes the role of the child's stage of development and agency in the child's development. An innovation in the model was the emphasis on the parent–child interaction as key to understanding the developmental process. Unlike these models, DIR considers the child's emotional experiences as foundational, with emotional exchanges leading to symbol formation and intelligence.

In addressing the question of how children learn to think and use symbols, Greenspan and Shanker (2004) proposed that the capacity of humans to exchange emotional signals with each other, which begins early in life, leads to symbols, abstract thinking, language, and a variety of complex emotional and social skills that enable social groups to function. Research (Seigel, 1999; Tronick, 2007) suggests that the development of specific areas of the brain may be significantly affected by these exchanges of emotional signals. The areas most likely affected include the higher cortical centers dealing with language and thinking, the prefrontal cortex dealing with planning and problem solving, and the integrating pathways that connect subsymbolic systems, which process basic emotions such as fear and anxiety, with cortical symbolic capacities.

According to Greenspan and Shanker,

> Through their progressive transformations, emotions, which can be experienced in an almost infinite number of subtle variations, and can organize and give meaning to experience. They can therefore serve as the architect or orchestra leader for the mind's many functions. At each stage in the pathway to intelligence, emotions orchestrate cognitive, language, motor, sensory, and social experience. (2004, p. 51)

Greenspan and Shanker (2004) suggested that through the interactive experiences between the child and his or her caregivers, emotions, first experienced in the baby's physiologic-sensory system, become the vehicles of interpersonal and intrapersonal development.

Underlying Assumptions

The assumptions of the DIR model address the nature of typical and atypical development; the role of affect in the development of relating, thinking, and communicating; the role of the parent–child interaction; and the nature of assessment and intervention. More specifically, the assumptions are as follows:

1. Early typical development can be described in terms of six FEDLs and the child's individual processing profile.

2. The emotional signaling and interaction that occurs between the baby and his or her caregiver paves the way for functional developmental capacities.

3. Impairments in the child's functional emotional development may be related to the child's individual processing profile.

4. Disruptions in the development of the functional emotional levels lead to the increased occurrence of developmental disorders.

5. Affect (emotion) is the anchor in the development of thinking, relating, and communicating.

6. Assessment involves a broad range of observations by professionals from different disciplines who can assess the child's capacities in functional emotional development, individual processing patterns, and caregiver–child interactions.

7. Intervention involves an interdisciplinary program that serves to move the child through the functional emotional levels, address the child's individual processing needs therapeutically and biomedically, coach parent interactions, and develop home and school programs.

Functional Outcomes

Because the DIR model is interdisciplinary, the target areas encompass all of the developmental domains of early childhood, such as affective, social, cognitive, language, sensory, and motor domains. The priority of intervention is to facilitate the child's capacity to move from shared attention to engagement, to two-way communication, to complex problem solving, to the use of symbols and ideas, and finally, to building logical connections between symbols and ideas. Intervention outcomes are measured by assessing the child's stage of development throughout the treatment process.

Professionals from different disciplines working within a DIR model will have, in addition to the FEDLs and individual processing targets, functional outcomes based on models from their own disciplines. For example, the language paradigm of the ***Interdisciplinary Council on Developmental Learning Disorders— Diagnostic Manual for Infants and Young Children*** (**ICDL-DMIC;** ICDL, 2005) includes an assessment that leads to determining intervention targets in speech, language, and communication. The *Affect-Based Language Curriculum* (Lewis & Greenspan, 2005), based on a somewhat different conceptualization of language development and intervention than that presented here, was developed to serve as a more structured adjunct to DIR intervention, providing parents with a detailed list of speech and language goals to be addressed using a combination of Floortime and semi-structured interactions.

Target Area of Treatment

Speech, language, and communication constitute one of the many developmental areas that are considered in the DIR model. In an effort to more fully describe the language acquisition process and to provide an assessment and intervention protocol consistent with the most contemporary thinking about typical language acquisition and with the interdisciplinary broad thinking of the DIR model, a task force of clinicians (Cawn et al., 2005) developed a paradigm that provides a perspective on typical and atypical development (ICDL, 2005). This paradigm reflects a reexamination of the developmental areas that are frequently impaired in children on the autism spectrum and offers a complementary approach to existing protocols and language assessments.

Development of the Language Paradigm of the DIR Model   The ICDL (2005) speech, language, and communication framework is distinguished from similar conceptualizations by its connection to the DIR model and its emphasis on particular *developmental language levels* and *modalities*, such as shared attention and affective engagement, that typically are not addressed in more traditional speech and language assessments.

In reference to the developmental language levels, subsequent to the review and organization of information from the research literature on typical language acquisition, the clinical task force (Cawn et al., 2005) outlined six levels of speech, language, and communication development (ICDL, 2005). Although chronological ages are aligned with the language levels, in practice, the description of any particular child depends on the composite of his or her developmental profile across the modalities, regardless of the child's age. The descriptors of the early language levels are similar to those of the FEDLs, although the language paradigm was developed independently. The similarity in perspectives on the fundamental capacities typical of early development accounts for the overlap in terminology. The six developmental language levels described in the ICDL-DMIC (2005) are as follows:

1. Self-regulation and interest in the world (birth though 3 months of age)

2. Forming relationships and affective vocal synchrony (2–7 months)

3. Intentional two-way communication (8–12 months)

4. First words: Sharing meaning in gestures and words (12–18 months)

5. Word combinations: Sharing experiences symbolically (18–24 months)

6. Early discourse: Reciprocal symbolic interactions with others (24–36 months)

At each language level, development that is typical of selected modalities is considered. Each of these modalities represents an aspect of development that is considered central to the process of acquiring language and being a successful communicator. The behaviors noted at each of the language levels provide the basis for what will be addressed during assessment and intervention. The modalities are as follows:

• Shared attention

• Affective engagement

• Reciprocity

• Shared intentions

• Shared forms and meanings

• Emerging discourse

• Sensory processing and audition

• Motor planning

An example of the format of the language paradigm for Language Level 2, forming relationships and affective vocal synchrony, can be found in Table 7.3. The table lists selected behaviors for each of the modalities. By observing the child during natural interactions with a caregiver, the clinician determines whether the child is demonstrating each behavior (e.g., uses eye gaze with gestures and sounds to coordinate attention; tunes into the affective state of others using smiles, frowns, etc.; incorporates vocalizations into two-way affective exchanges). Those behaviors that have not yet been achieved would become goals for language intervention.

Table 7.3.   Language Level 2: Forming relationships and affective vocal synchrony (2–7 months)

Shared attention	Uses eye gaze with gestures and sounds to coordinate attention
	Shifts gaze between people and objects
Affective engagement	Tunes into the affective state of others using affect cues (e.g., smiles, frowns)
	Participates in affective exchanges with caregiver
Reciprocity	Includes vocalizations as components of two-way affective exchanges
	Initiates interaction with others using early gestures (reaching), babbling, or cooing
Shared intentions	Responds to others' intentions to regulate behavior and turns to caregiver for comfort
	Begins to respond to others' intentions to draw attention to objects
Shared forms and meanings	Discriminates affective state of caregiver
	Vocalizes pleasure and displeasure
	Varies volume and pitch of vocalizations
Sensory processing and audition	Localizes sounds from a distance
	Engages caregiver across space
	Is comforted by some sounds, distressed by others
Motor planning	Participates with caregiver in rhythmic movement through touch, looking, listening
	Initiates gestures, such as beginning to reach, grab, lift arms up, to indicate communicative intentions

Source: Interdisciplinary Council on Developmental and Learning Disorders (2005).

Use of the Language Paradigm   The use of this paradigm involves determining the level at which the child is functioning in each of the modalities. The primary context for assessment is observation of the child during interactions with his or her caregiver and/or clinician. The analysis is clearly a qualitative rather than a quantitative one. The goal is to generate a dynamic description of the child's capacities at each level in each modality, which will then allow the clinician to identify intervention goals for the comprehension and production of language. When using this paradigm, the clinician must be flexible in determining goals, because observation may show the child to be at different levels depending on the modality. For children who are at the higher levels of the paradigm, additional assessment through language sampling to determine the child's phase of **form–content relations** (Lahey, 1988) and formal testing would be necessary to complete the child's profile of strengths and impairments in speech, language, and communication.

It should be noted that several existing speech-language-communication assessments and interventions target similar areas of language and communication development. These include the Communication and Symbolic Behavior Scales™ (CSBS™; Wetherby & Prizant, 2002), The SCERTS® (Social Communication, Emotional Regulation, and Transactional Supports) Model (Prizant et al., 2006), and parent training programs such as More Than Words (Sussman, 1999) and Responsivity Teaching (Mahoney & Perales, 2005). Clearly, the programs mentioned here are more fully developed and comprehensive than the ICDL-DMIC (ICDL, 2005), which is not a standardized clinical tool. Nonetheless, the consideration of modalities such as shared attention, affective engagement, and reciprocity not only bridges the language paradigm to the DIR early functional emotional levels but also provides the practitioner with a way to operationalize the origins of language development. Further, the language paradigm of the ICDL-DMIC points out that even when a child uses verbal language, he or she may still be working to achieve the basic foundations of language.

EMPIRICAL BASIS

Several studies and reviews support the DIR approach to working with children with developmental impairments. The first study that provided evidence for the DIRFloortime model was a retrospective chart review of 200 children (Greenspan & Wieder, 1997). The children, who ranged in age from 22 months to 4 years at the time of diagnosis, 1) met the criteria for autism or pervasive developmental disorder-not otherwise specified (PDD-NOS) as described in the American Psychiatric Association (APA)'s *Diagnostic and statistical manual of mental disorders* (3rd ed., rev., and 4th ed.; APA, 1987, 1994); 2) scored in the autistic range on the Childhood Autism Rating Scale (CARS; Schopler et al., 1988), with scores ranging from 30 to 52; and, 3) participated in evaluations and interventions for 2 or more years. The children had received at least 2 years of a DIR approach to intervention and were followed over a period of 8 years. The results suggested that after 2 years of intervention using the DIR approach, 58% of the children were described as being in the "good to outstanding" outcome group based on their ability to relate, affectively engage with others, participate in circles of spontaneous verbal communication, and so forth. The children in this outcome group shifted into the non-autistic range on the CARS (Schopler et al., 1988).

In 2005, Wieder and Greenspan published a 10- to 15-year follow-up study of 16 boys with ASD who had shown significant improvements in the original group. Their mean age at follow-up was 13.9 years. Between the ages of 2 and 8.5 years, these children received a comprehensive intervention program for a minimum of 2 years and a maximum of 5 years, which included Floortime and DIR consultation. The authors described these adolescent boys as empathetic, creative, and reflective and noted that they were experiencing good peer relationships and academic achievement.

In 2007, Solomon and colleagues reported on the results of the PLAY (Play and Language for Autistic Youngsters) Project Home Consultation, a program that trained parents of children with ASD in the DIRFloortime model. Sixty-eight children participated in this study, completing an 8- to 12-month program in which parents were encouraged to do 15 hours per week of one-to-one interaction. The results of ratings on the **Functional Emotional Assessment Scale** (FEAS; Greenspan et al., 2001) pretraining and posttraining revealed that 45.5% of the children made good to very good functional developmental progress. The parents' overall satisfaction with the program was 90%.

The first randomized controlled trial study on the DIRFloortime-based treatment approach was conducted by Casenhiser and colleagues (2010). The study included two groups of 51 children who were stratified by age and language functioning and randomly assigned to one of two groups. One group received DIR-based treatment, and the other group received community treatment, which was primarily behaviorally based. The DIR treatment involved 2 hours per week with the clinicians; in addition, as is typical in the DIR paradigm, parents were asked to spend 20 hours per week with their children in Floortime intervention. The community treatment group received an average of 4 hours per week of other behavioral interventions, chiefly speech therapy, applied behavior analysis (ABA), and occupational therapy.

Clinicians used a modified version of Mahoney's Child Behavior Rating Scale (Kim & Mahoney, 2004) to code the following five variables from a videotaped parent–child play interaction: initiation of joint attention, attention to activity, involvement, enjoyment in interaction, and compliance. The children in the DIR group did significantly better than the children in the community treatment group on all the scales except compliance. A regression analysis was performed to see if improvements in the social-interaction behaviors predicted language improvements. This relationship was found for the scale overall, with the strongest predictors being involvement and initiation of joint attention. Effect sizes (Cohen's d) ranged from 0.51 to 1.02. As might be expected, intervention directed toward improving various aspects of social interaction clearly has an impact on language development (see Kasari et al., 2008).

Two studies have reported results that further support the positive effects of using a DIR approach. Pajareya and Nopmaneejumruslers (2011) conducted a pilot study with children with mild to severe ASD. The parents of these children received home-based training in the overarching themes of DIR, including observing the child's cues, following the child's lead, and implementing the Floortime techniques that were appropriate for their child's particular FEDL. The parents added an average of 15.2 hours per week of the DIRFloortime intervention to their typical schedules for 3 months. Results indicated that the intervention group improved significantly in engagement, relating, and communicating, as measured by the FEAS (Greenspan et al., 2001).

A single-case design was used in a study reported by Dionne and Martini (2011). A DIR-trained occupational therapist taught the mother of a 3.5-year-old child with ASD Floortime strategies, including extending circles of communication using playful obstruction; joining the child's play, such as pretending to sleep; and identifying sensory overload. The occupational therapist noticed a significant increase in the number of circles of communication in the intervention phase of the study as compared with the observation phase. In addition, the mother reported that she was enjoying the experience of interacting with her child in more typical play situations.

Finally, Mercer (2017) reviewed DIRFloortime as a treatment for children with ASD in the field of social work. She concluded that the foundations of DIRFloortime were consistent with contemporary thinking about early child development and that its congruence with other child psychotherapies lent support to its effectiveness.

Although the number of randomized controlled studies supporting DIRFloortime is limited and the approach is not rated positively in the National Standards Project (NSP) Phase 2, professionals and parents should consider the overlap between DIRFloortime and other categories of intervention studies that were rated favorably in the report. The NSP Phase 2 (National Autism Center, 2015) extended the initial NSP report (National Autism Center, 2009) to include studies up to 2012. The goal of the report was again to disseminate the results of a review of existing education and behavioral research in autism interventions. The 2015 report categorizes treatments as *established, emerging*, or *unestablished.*

Two categories of intervention discussed in the NSP Phase 2, Developmental-Relationship Based Intervention (DRBI) and parent training packages, indirectly support the efficacy of the DIRFloortime model. These intervention approaches clearly share a commonality in foundational principles and strategies with DIRFloortime. For example, developmental approaches, as distinguished from behavioral approaches, prioritize the relationship between the child and caregiver, address foundational developmental capacities, and focus on opportunities for pleasurable shared affective experiences between parent and child. These goals lay the groundwork for achieving more complex levels of interaction (Cullinane et. al., 2017). In the NSP 2 report, intervention approaches grouped under DRBI are considered emerging.

According to the National Autism Center (2015), the parent training package category is

> New to NSP. NSP1 focused on the elements of the interventions used in studies in which parents acted as the therapist or received training to implement various strategies. NSP2 made the change to highlight parents' and caregivers' integral role in providing a therapeutic environment for their family members with autism spectrum disorder (ASD). (p. 55)

Here again, the resonance to DIRFloortime is apparent. Parent training approaches are categorized as established in the NSP 2 report.

The addition of the parent training category reflects the growing number of intervention studies that address the feasibility and impact of teaching parents to use responsive social interaction strategies in playful exchanges with their children. McConachie and colleagues (2005) and Girolametto and colleagues (2007) found that the children whose parents improved in their responsiveness made gains in vocabulary, frequency of communication, and/or participation in turn-taking routines. Other studies have reported increases in joint attention, initiation of communication, periods of engagement, and expressive language in children whose parents were taught how to change their interaction styles to facilitate relationships and responsiveness with their children (Aldred et al., 2004; Mahoney & Perales, 2005; Siller & Sigman, 2002).

Most recently, a number of studies by Pickles and colleagues (2016) have reported the positive results of a parent training approach referred to as PACT, Preschool Autism Communication Trial. The series of studies explored the outcomes of children and families who participated in a randomized controlled trial of a parent-mediated social-communication intervention for children 2–4 years of age with core autism. Perhaps the strongest support for parent-mediated training comes from the follow-up studies done by Pickles and colleagues (2016), which showed long-term symptom reduction for children with autism after implementation of PACT. Specifically, the results indicated that a 12-month parent-mediated preschool intervention resulted in "sustained improvement in child autism symptoms and social communication with parents, which remained at nearly 6 years after the end of treatment. These findings support the potential long-term effects and value of early parent-mediated interventions for autism" (Pickles et al., 2016, p. 2502).

Historically, DIRFloortime was one of the first intervention approaches to prioritize parent–child interaction. This component of the paradigm, the R for relationship, was one of three anchors of the model and, as discussed earlier in this chapter, parent coaching was considered central to the therapeutic process. Although the parent training in DIRFloortime was not manualized as it is in some of the research studies mentioned previously, the centrality of this aspect of the child's and family's intervention program was clearly delineated.

The National Standards Project report (National Autism Center, 2009) encourages parents, educators, and service providers to consider factors in addition to treatment effectiveness when making decisions about intervention options. That is, parents and service providers should consider the judgment and data-based clinical recommendations of professionals as well as the values and preferences of the person with ASD and his or her family and caregivers.

Finally, one of the major contributions of the DIRFloortime approach to the world of ASD is that the model encompasses an interprofessional, multidisciplinary approach to service delivery. The complex conceptualization of development, unique to DIRFloortime, has been a roadblock to accumulating evidence to support its use. The practitioners who embrace the model as a paradigm for intervention programming have acknowledged this duality for many years. For children with complex challenges across developmental domains, the need to address various areas of functioning simultaneously makes for best practices relative to assessment and intervention and, at the same time, translates poorly to the rigors of randomized controlled studies.

PRACTICAL REQUIREMENTS

The practical demands of the DIR model can be thought of in terms of the personnel needs, that is, the number of different professionals working with the family, the number of hours of intervention provided by these professionals, and the parents' commitment of time and energy.

Each child involved in a DIR program receives individual therapy sessions many times—optimally, six to eight 20-minute sessions—throughout the day. If the child is very young, spending most of the day at home, the Floortime interactions are facilitated by the parent who is being coached by a DIR professional (e.g., psychologist, speech-language pathologist [SLP], occupational therapist, educator). Similar to other comprehensive programs, the child's individual processing needs (e.g., occupational therapy, visual-spatial training) are a key component of a DIR program and often become a priority in the treatment. Older children involved in a school program participate in individual, small-group, and large-group interactions throughout the day, led by professionals from a variety of disciplines who share a DIR perspective. In the best-case scenario, the team of professionals working with the child coordinates its efforts by meeting and discussing roadblocks and progress on a regular basis.

Optimally, the primary DIR professionals working with the child are certified in DIR or are in the process of being certified. The certification process requires participating in online training with DIR faculty members in interdisciplinary approaches to working with children and families with special needs. Ongoing individual and small-group clinical supervision from a DIR faculty member is a critical component of the training (see http://www.ICDL.org and http://www.Profectum.org).

KEY COMPONENTS

As suggested by Figure 7.1, DIR clinicians set goals across developmental capacities for an interdisciplinary team of professionals and for the family. DIR goals address skills in several domains—including social-emotional, affective, language, sensory, regulatory, motor planning, and visual-spatial—as well as patterns of family interaction. The philosophical perspectives discussed throughout this chapter lead to this kind of big-picture thinking relative to DIR intervention. Furthermore, although DIR is often thought of as individually based treatment, a number of schools have adopted the principles of DIRFloortime and translated them into group contexts within academic programs.

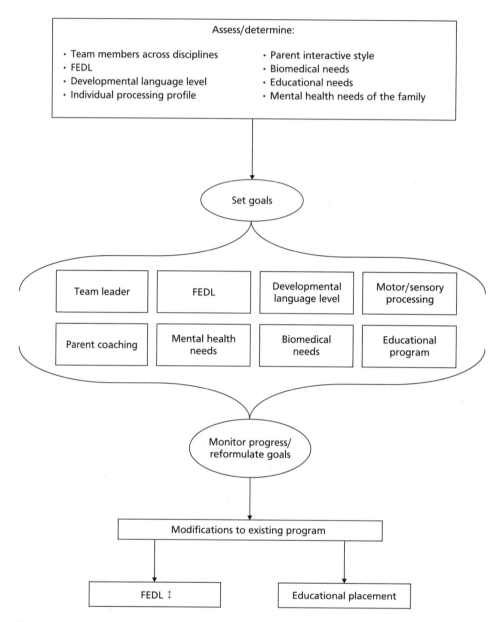

Figure 7.1. DIR assessment process. *Key:* FEDL, functional emotional developmental level.

Goals and Activities

In a DIR program, interdisciplinary goals are targeted simultaneously, although at any point in time, priorities will be based on the child's needs and the family's resources and preferences. Families choosing this approach may have to take an active role in enlisting DIR-trained clinicians and educators for their child's program or, in some cases, support the training of the educators and clinicians working with their child.

Each of the six FEDLs can be thought of in terms of the specific behaviors targeted by that level (see Table 7.1). In fact, similar to individualized education programs (IEPs), goals can be operationalized to ensure that the levels are easily translatable into educational or clinical paradigms (Wieder & Kalmanson, 2000). For example, at Level 1 of the FEDLs for shared attention and regulation, a typical goal might be, "The child will sustain shared attention with a special adult in sensorimotor interactive play using the child's preferred and pleasurable sensory and motor modalities" (Wieder & Kalmanson, 2000, p. 299); at a later stage, a goal might be, "The child will sustain shared attention with a peer in interaction" (p. 299). At Level 3, two-way intentional communication, a typical goal might be, "The child will initiate purposeful interactions around desires (open circles) and will close circles following an adult's response to her initiative" (p. 299); and at a later stage, the goal might be, "The child will sustain engagement with a peer with adult mediation (p. 299)." At Level 6, representational differentiation and emotional thinking, a typical goal might be, "The child will close all symbolic circles in both pretend play and reality-based dialogues" (p. 300); at a later stage, the goal might be, "The child will identify motives of other people or characters' actions and understand different points of view and feelings" (p. 300).

The notion of opening and closing circles of communication is a central construct in the model. In this approach, where the child's ideas and interests are used as the basis of the adult's interaction, the child opens a circle by initiating or showing interest in something or someone. The caregiver follows this initiation by joining and expanding the interaction. The child then closes the circle if he or she responds to the adult or perhaps begins a new circle with a new initiation or interest. In this exchange, the child becomes more aware of his or her actions, and the caregiver can become more aware of the child's sense of self and interests. By respecting these interests and following the child's lead, the adult can then set the stage for expanding the child's ideas and challenging him or her to move up the developmental ladder (Breinbauer, 2010). Greenspan and Wieder (1998) explained,

> When a child reaches out—with a look, for example—he opens the circle. When the parent responds—by looking back—he builds on the child's action. When the child in turn responds to the parent—by smiling, vocalizing, reaching, or even turning away—he is closing the circle. When the parent responds to the child's response—by holding out a toy, by saying, "Don't you want to play?", by echoing the child's vocalization—and the child responds with another gesture (a look, smile, or hand movement) they have opened and closed another circle. (pp. 76–77)

In educational settings, three types of DIR activities are used to support the child's development (ICDL, 2005): 1) Floortime, or spontaneous interactions during which the adult or peer follows the child's lead and facilitates the child's expansion of his or her ideas and intentions; 2) semistructured problem-solving interactions during which specific learning objectives are addressed through dynamic interactions in which the child is encouraged to problem-solve and think creatively; and 3) motor, sensory, perceptual-motor, and visual-spatial activities to address processing challenges.

Because the DIR goals cross developmental disciplines, activities may be specific to particular disciplines. For example, the occupational therapist will see the child in a sensory gym with activities geared toward addressing the child's sensory profile. For speech and language goals, the clinician may engage in spontaneous play-based interactions with the child and parent as well as in more semistructured activities to address the child's language comprehension issues. For the educator, goals will be incorporated into group learning activities in the classroom. The mental health professional on the team may meet weekly with the parents to discuss their reactions and responses to their child's challenges, the impact on the child's siblings, and any issues in the couple's marriage.

Finally, the goal of moving the child up through the developmental levels is addressed by embracing Floortime strategies. These strategies include working within the context of play and/or other natural interactions; enacting a vivid range of affective states to woo the child into interpersonal interactions; following the child's lead and ideas, no matter how primitive or perseverative; scaffolding the expansion of ideas and/or interaction; facilitating responsiveness by pursuing the child in a playful way; facilitating initiation by responding to all of the child's nonintentional as well as intentional behaviors; coaching the parent to develop interactive strategies; and considering the child's sensory and regulatory needs when planning activities (Wieder, 2004). For examples, see the video that accompanies this chapter.

Parent Coaching

Programs that prioritize the parent–child relationship in the therapeutic process do so because they believe that the parent–child relationship is the key to healthy development and that parents are the most emotionally invested agents of their child's growth. As noted previously, there is a growing body of research that supports the positive impact of parent-mediated therapy for young children with ASD. Parents not only are seen as the best facilitators of development but also are recognized as the ones who can offer the intensity of intervention recommended by the National Research Council (Lord & McGee, 2001). As such, parents are seen as indispensable to their child's progress in learning to interact and communicate. The DIR approach seeks to empower parents to become their child's primary language and social-emotional facilitator through natural interactions that take place during everyday events, such as mealtime, bath time, or when looking at books. The role of the clinician is seen as providing a collaborative, respectful partnership with the parents, who clearly know their child best (Longtin & Gerber, 2008) but who may need specific instruction in how to help their child climb the social-emotional-symbolic ladder.

In a typical DIR session, the therapist asks the parent to play with the child while he or she provides suggestions as to how to use the DIR principles. The therapist encourages the parent to promote circles of communication, or continuous back-and-forth exchanges between the child and the parent, by following the child's lead, joining the focus of the child's interest, using high affect and playfulness, and enjoying the interaction. The clinician reflects with the parent, addressing questions and concerns relative to the roadblocks to achieving interactive flow and higher symbolic capacity. The clinician also guides the parent's understanding of the child's sensory and regulatory challenges and models how the parent might work around and with them. For example, the parent might help the child stay regulated (i.e., calm, alert, attentive) and thereby increase affective interactions, opportunities for face-to-face interactions, and vocalizations by bouncing the child on a large therapy ball.

Although parent involvement in programs for children on the autism spectrum is often pro forma, dynamic parent coaching that has an interdisciplinary base may be a less familiar part of the intervention process for many SLPs. Because the parent–child relationship is the preferred intervention context in this approach, the DIR clinician is encouraged to embrace his or her own learning about parent training, perhaps through reflective supervision, in order to assume the role of coach during the treatment. A webcast series created specifically for parents and that will also be helpful for clinicians is now available from Profectum (https://profectum .org/free-parent-program).

The possibility that any particular child will benefit from alternative treatments—for example, nutritional supplements—is considered by a DIR physician (Robinson, 2011). The changing needs of the child and family and the realities of the highs and lows of atypical development suggest that the educator and clinician working with the child should keep an open mind about the possible pathways to development. In this sense, the fact that the DIR professional is encouraged to receive reflective supervision increases the chances that the therapist will remain sensitive to how his or her own perspectives, prejudices, and emotional reactions may influence treatment decisions.

ASSESSMENT FOR TREATMENT PLANNING AND PROGRESS MONITORING

The DIR approach provides a model of assessment for any child experiencing developmental delays and disorders, regardless of the child's diagnosis, chronological age, or functioning level.

Based on a DIR assessment (described next), children are described as functioning within one of four types of neurodevelopmental disorders of relating and communicating that are set forth in the ICDL-DMIC (ICDL, 2005). The four types (see Table 7.4) refer to levels of functioning within and across developmental domains and individual differences. The range includes the child who shows intermittent capacities for relating, reciprocity, and shared problem solving, as well as the child who shows fleeting capacities for engagement and reciprocity and may experience multiple regressions.

Because of its comprehensive nature, the DIR functional developmental evaluation involves an interdisciplinary team of professionals, including a physician, a mental health professional, an SLP, an occupational therapist, and an educator. The DIR assessment paradigm consists of the three key components previously mentioned: the FEDLs, the individual differences profile, and the caregiver–child relationships. Each of these is described in the remainder of this section.

Table 7.4. Neurodevelopmental disorders of relating and communicating

Type	Description
Type I: Early symbolic with constrictions	Children in this group show intermittent capacities for attending, relating, reciprocal interactions, shared social problem solving (with support), and the beginning use of meaningful ideas. Children in this group typically show rapid progress.
Type II: Purposeful problem solving with constrictions	Children in this group show intermittent capacities for attention, relating, and a few back-and-forth reciprocal interactions, with only fleeting capacities for shared social problem solving and imitation of words. Children in this group tend to make steady progress.
Type III: Intermittently engaged and purposeful	Children in this group show fleeting capacities for attention and engagement and can engage in a few back-and-forth reciprocal interactions (with considerable support). Often, the children in this group show no capacity for using words and ideas, although they may be able to repeat a few words in a memory-based manner. Children with this pattern often make slow but steady progress.
Type IV: Aimless and not purposeful	Children in this group are similar to children in Type III but with a pattern of multiple regressions. These children may also evidence a greater number of neurological challenges, such as seizures. Children with this pattern often make very slow progress.

Source: Interdisciplinary Council on Developmental and Learning Disorders (2005).

Determining where the child is relative to the FEDLs is the hallmark of the assessment. Assessment tools such as the FEAS (Greenspan et al., 2001) and Social-Emotional Growth Charts (Greenspan, 2004) can be used to determine the child's FEDL. Although, as in all developmental assessments, chronological ages are associated with each level, in DIR, a composite of the child's strengths and challenges rather than age is used to determine functioning level and intervention targets. The levels are as follows (see Table 7.1 for a more detailed description of each level):

1. Shared attention and regulation (birth through 3 months)

2. Engagement and relating (2–6 months)

3. Two-way intentional communication (4–9 months)

4. Complex problem solving (9–18 months)

5. Creative representations (ideas) and elaboration (18–30 months)

6. Representational differentiation and emotional thinking (30–48 months)

For many children on the autism spectrum, intervention will focus on the early levels of development, as these are the foundations for further emotional, social, cognitive, and language abilities (Gerber, 2003, 2017).

The second component of the DIR model, assessment of the child's individual processing, is critical to determining the goals for intervention as well as the optimal learning contexts for the child. For example, if the child needs to be moving to know where he or she is in space, the SLP would not expect the child to sit at a table when engaging in activities. Greater understanding of such individual differences underscores how the interdisciplinary orientation of the DIR model influences all aspects of the child's therapeutic and educational experience. The four areas of individual processing assessed in the DIR model are sensory modulation, sensory processing, sensory-affective processing, and motor planning and sequencing (see Table 7.2).

The third component of the DIR model, a description of caregiver–child interactions and family patterns, also is integral to the assessment paradigm and to the intervention. The child is observed while interacting with his or her parent in order to help the clinician understand what patterns are typical of the dyad—for example, whether the parent is more or less directive in his or her interactions with the child, how well the parent is reading the child's cues and signals, and whether the parent is finding the appropriate level of stimulation to support engagement. Once these patterns are identified, the parent is guided in understanding the child's developmental stage; how the child's individual differences are affecting his or her ability to learn, engage, and function in the world; and how best to modify their interactive styles to enhance development.

The following outline delineates the steps of a DIR assessment (see Figure 7.1), some of which will be specific to the individual child's and family's needs (ICDL, 2005):

1. Prenatal and developmental history

2. Two or more observational sessions of child–caregiver interactions to develop hypotheses about

   • The child's FEDLs

   • The individual processing profile

   • Caregiver interactions and family patterns

3. Evaluation of motor and regulatory-sensory processing, including

   - Sensory modulation
   - Sensory processing
   - Sensory-affective processing
   - Motor planning and sequencing

4. Biomedical evaluations (e.g., nutritional needs, pharmacological interventions, environmental interventions to reduce exposure to allergens in the home)

5. Speech and language evaluation

6. Evaluation of cognitive functions, including neuropsychological and educational assessments

7. Mental health evaluations of family members, family patterns, and family needs

The FEAS (Greenspan et al., 2001) is considered the primary assessment tool in the DIR process. The FEAS is used to determine the child's FEDLs as well as the nature of the interactions between the child and his or her caregivers. This determination leads, in turn, to creating a treatment plan based on the child's individual profile and provides a baseline for measuring his or her progress.

Professionals working within a DIR approach will use, in addition to the FEAS, the ICDL-DMIC (ICDL, 2005) as a guide for assessing functioning in a range of developmental areas. Each section of the diagnostic manual is intended for several audiences. For example, SLPs will base their assessment in part on the manual's section on language acquisition and language disorders, whereas non-SLPs will read that section to get an overview of typical preschool speech and language development. The DIR professional is obliged to understand many areas of development, and the ICDL-DMIC provides an orientation to all disciplines.

Initial and ongoing assessments of the child's strengths and challenges that take place within the DIR model are based on various paradigms of typical development, such as the FEAS (Greenspan et al., 2001), the ICDL-DMIC (ICDL, 2005) language model, and the individual processing profile. The evaluation of progress will be discipline specific relative to the frequency of assessment and the identification of measures to be used for assessing change. For example, SLPs may use language sampling (Lahey, 1988; Systematic Analysis of Language Transcripts [SALT], Miller, 2010) as a measure of the child's progress in language development. In DIR school programs, as in all school programs, data must be collected to chart the child's progress over time and to determine the efficacy of the strategies being used. The procedures noted in Table 7.5 are some of those used in DIR educational settings.

Clinicians working in a DIR model will consider all developmental domains if the child is not progressing so that they can determine where roadblocks to further progress may lie. One could say that the beauty of the DIR approach is its developmental breadth, which expands the range of interdisciplinary thinking and in that way comes closer to a true, integrated understanding of the child's capacities. However, this breadth also obligates the clinician and educator to be versed in a range of possibilities when changes are needed in the child's individual intervention program. Simply put, the DIR professional has to be informed enough in all areas of development to know when and with whom to consult in order to gain a deeper understanding of the child's developmental delays.

Table 7.5. Developmental, Individual-Difference, Relationship-Based (DIR) model data collection procedures and options

Indicate change in the percentage of response. For example, for a child who may be closing circles of communication 30% of the time, the specific goal would be to close circles 50% of the time at the next time interval.

Indicate change in the number of responses. For example, if a child is opening and closing 20 circles per time spent on the goal, the next goal would be 50 circles or that the child will respond three out of five times.

Indicate the time interval designated for the goal—for example, over a 1-week time period or during the next 3 months.

Indicate the amount of time to be spent on the goal, such as 10-minute periods eight times a day.

Consider the use of the Functional Emotional Assessment Scale (FEAS), which has established reliability and provides specific examples for each level. The FEAS could be scored at preintervention and postintervention intervals.

Indicate the context in which the child will demonstrate each developmental capacity, such as at school, on the playground, or at home.

Indicate whether the child will demonstrate the developmental capacity spontaneously or with natural prompts, such as questions during interactions.

Indicate whether the child will demonstrate the developmental capacity independently.

Source: Wieder and Kalmanson (2000).

IMPLICATIONS FOR INCLUSIVE PRACTICE

The service delivery model is as broad as the theoretical-clinical framework. Therefore, a home program that incorporates the goals and strategies developed by the DIR team, a school program, specific therapies, biomedical intervention, and family support via counseling are all incorporated into the intervention plan. The team working with the child includes professionals from many disciplines who are asked to collaborate closely to ensure that the child's program is an integrated one.

Although spontaneous interactions are the hallmark of the DIR approach, both semistructured and structured learning activities are also included in each child's program. The use of these alternatives depends on the child's developmental capacities, the priorities for intervention, the contexts of learning in which the child is engaged, and the child's processing profile.

The intervention strategies of DIR can be adapted to the various learning environments that the child experiences throughout his or her day, such as dyadic, small-group, and large-group interactions. In the child's school program, individual spontaneous interactions will be supplemented with semistructured problem-solving interactions. However, even within these more structured interactions, Floortime principles, such as prioritizing the child's intentions and ideas, using supportive rather than directive teaching, and addressing the child's individual sensory processing needs, must be central to the educational approach.

CONSIDERATIONS FOR CHILDREN FROM CULTURALLY AND LINGUISTICALLY DIVERSE BACKGROUNDS

Given the individualized nature of the DIR approach, practitioners working with children from all cultural and linguistic backgrounds can feel comfortable using the model. In fact, DIR-certified clinicians are now practicing in many countries, including Argentina, Australia, China, Colombia, Georgia, Ireland, Israel, Italy,

South Africa, Spain, Turkey, and the United Kingdom. DIR faculty from the United States are frequently invited to do training in countries where a core of professionals, including psychiatrists, SLPs, occupational therapists, educators, and/or mental health practitioners, are making inroads in their communities and bringing DIR thinking to the work they do with children and families.

Application to a Child

To illustrate how the DIR model can be integrated with developmental language goals, consider Mark, a child who received speech and language therapy at the Queens College Speech-Language-Hearing Center over a 4-year period. The following case study discusses two points in the DIR intervention he received—at 5 years of age, when he first began the intervention, and at 9 years.

Mark had been diagnosed with ASD at the age of 3 years and had received intensive ABA intervention between the ages of 3 and 5, before beginning DIR intervention. The shift to the DIR intervention occurred because Mark's mother, Ms. Z., was concerned about the nature of ABA treatment and the lack of skill generalization to everyday life. In addition, she noted the lack of improvement in Mark's engagement and his limited capacity for shared emotion. Ms. Z. also worried about the system of reinforcement being used because Mark's preoccupations—for example, watching a video—were used as rewards. Finally, Ms. Z. questioned why certain behaviors, such as attention, were tied to receiving rewards. Ms. Z. was referred to the Queens College clinic because she was interested in speech and language intervention that was more deeply rooted in DIR and in coaching in DIR principles.

DIR and Language Assessment: Mark at Age 5

To introduce Mark from a DIR perspective, consider Mark's FEDLs and individual sensory profile. At age 5, Mark had islands of capacity at the first four FEDLs when given persistent and predictable support (see Figure 7.2). He had not yet reached the higher levels, including creating representations and ideas and representational differentiation and emotional thinking. In reference to his individual sensory-processing profile, specifically, sensory modulation and regulation, Mark was hyperreactive to auditory, tactile, and taste sensations. In terms of sensory processing, Mark could observe and focus on desired objects and differentiate salient visual stimuli; however, he demonstrated challenges in initiating and responding to joint attention through gaze. In the area of sensory-affective processing, Mark demonstrated challenges in the ability to connect intent or affect to the use of symbols, including language. Finally, in reference to motor planning and sequencing, Mark could initiate ideas in play with clear goals and purposes with a few preferred toys but had difficulties developing a play plan and enacting steps of a play sequence across a range of play themes.

When DIR clinicians analyze caregiver patterns, they address six areas of interaction and rate them on a 1 (low = less skilled) to 5 (high = more skilled) scale (FEAS; Greenspan et al., 2001). The purpose of this assessment is to help parents discover those areas of interaction where they need support to further enhance their child's availability for deepening relationships and learning. In each of the areas, comforting, finding an appropriate level of stimulation, engaging in the relationship, reading cues and signals, maintaining

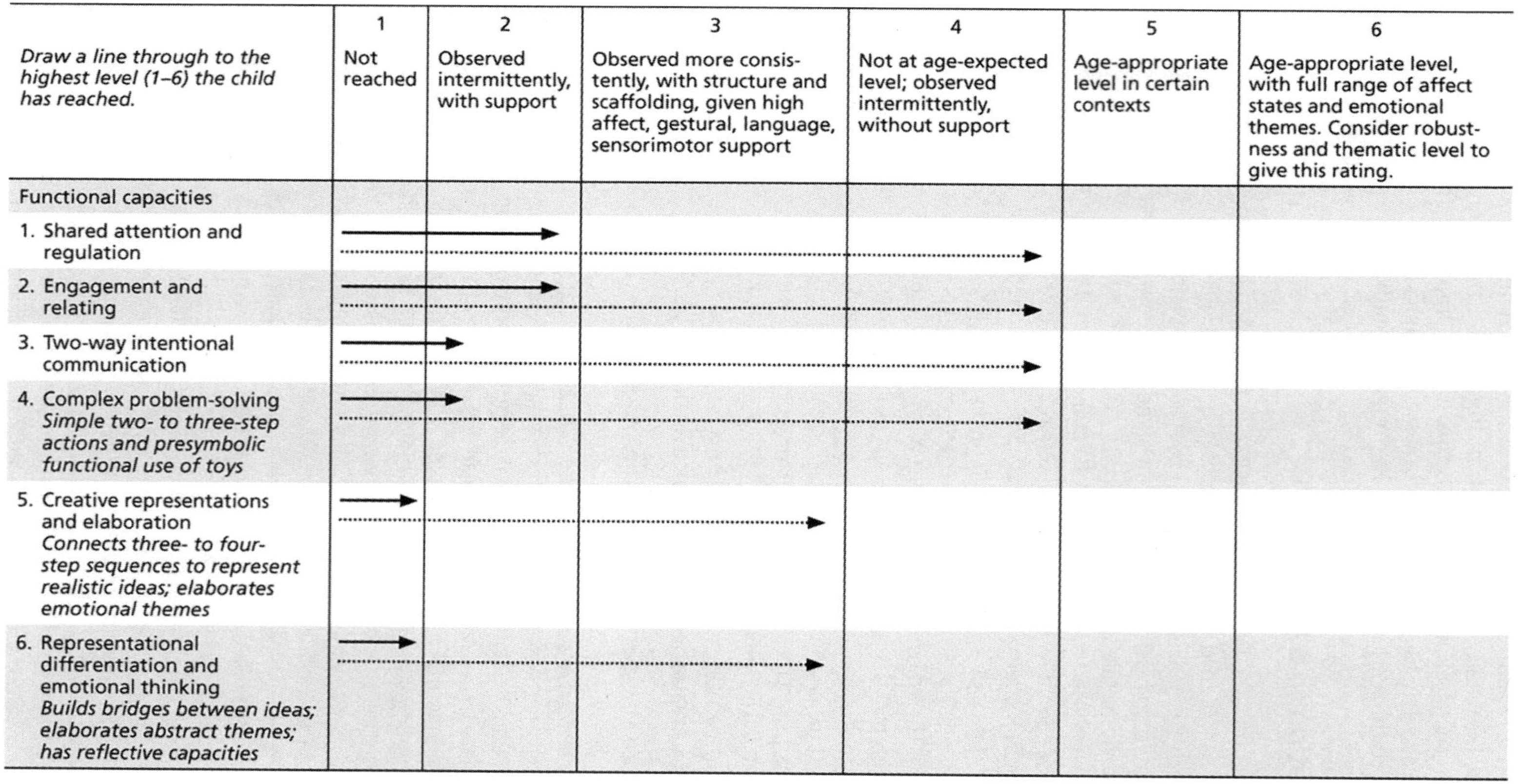

Draw a line through to the highest level (1–6) the child has reached.	1 Not reached	2 Observed intermittently, with support	3 Observed more consistently, with structure and scaffolding, given high affect, gestural, language, sensorimotor support	4 Not at age-expected level; observed intermittently, without support	5 Age-appropriate level in certain contexts	6 Age-appropriate level, with full range of affect states and emotional themes. Consider robustness and thematic level to give this rating.
Functional capacities						
1. Shared attention and regulation						
2. Engagement and relating						
3. Two-way intentional communication						
4. Complex problem-solving *Simple two- to three-step actions and presymbolic functional use of toys*						
5. Creative representations and elaboration *Connects three- to four-step sequences to represent realistic ideas; elaborates emotional themes*						
6. Representational differentiation and emotional thinking *Builds bridges between ideas; elaborates abstract themes; has reflective capacities*						

Figure 7.2. Assessment of functional emotional developmental levels for Mark at ages 5 (⟶) and 9 (⤑). (*Source:* Greenspan & Wieder, 1998.)

affective flow for coregulation, and encouraging development, Mark's mother received high ratings. Although this is obviously not typical of all parents or professionals, Ms. Z. was simply a natural in DIR. Her intuitive skill enabled Ms. Z. to collaborate with the clinician in determining intervention goals and strategies, and the therapy process was enhanced by her interpretations of her son's behaviors, such as the origins of Mark's **scripted language**. The term *scripted language* (or *scripts*) refers to the use of phrases, sentences, and longer strings of language that are repeated, often verbatim, from movies, books, television shows, and so forth.

When Mark was 5 years old, the clinician assessed his language on the basis of the language paradigm of the ICDL-DMIC (ICDL, 2005). At age 5, Mark's shared attention, affective engagement, and reciprocity did not meet the expectations of typically developing 24-month-olds (see Figure 7.3). These capacities were seen only intermittently in interactions with his mother. Mark's language comprehension and production were compromised, with some strengths in production, including self-generated language, delayed echolalia, and scripts. Mark used scripts frequently to communicate his ideas and feelings. Mark's symbolic play skills were below those for a 24-month-old level, with the majority of his play at the level of exploratory and cause-and-effect play. He did not engage in peer interactions.

Language Intervention Goals and Strategies

The intervention goals developed for Mark were rooted in the DIR paradigm and developmental language models. The focus of Mark's intervention at 5 years was to increase his shared attention, affective engagement, reciprocity, and shared intentions with adults, primarily his mother; to expand his expression of affective states, including frustration, anger, and delight; to facilitate emotional regulation to help him deal with extreme upset and aggression when his wishes could not be met; to facilitate the development of contingent schemas in play related to favorite activities, such as playing with trains, playing circus, and watering plants; and to coach Ms. Z. in Floortime techniques that could be used to address the goals at home.

During early stages of Mark's language intervention, clinicians considered comprehension and production of language secondary goals. Mark's capacities for shared attention, engagement, reciprocity, shared intentions, regulation, expression of affect, and play were the priorities, as these foundations for language were significantly compromised. Given the primary goals and that the capacities they addressed typically develop in a child's interactions with his or her caregivers, Ms. Z. was often the primary interactant during therapy sessions.

Intervention strategies included following Mark's lead and joining his play contingently, regardless of the focus of the play or the frequency with which the play theme was introduced (e.g., train play); following preferred play scenarios and taking a role in them, including scripted ideas (e.g., circus themes); modeling early form–content relations to code his ideas; and coaching facilitation of goals in mother–child interactions.

Process and Progress

Mark's relatedness with the therapist and the graduate clinicians who were working with him developed well over the course of the first year. Many of the play interactions used during intervention centered around scripted schemas that Mark introduced in the play,

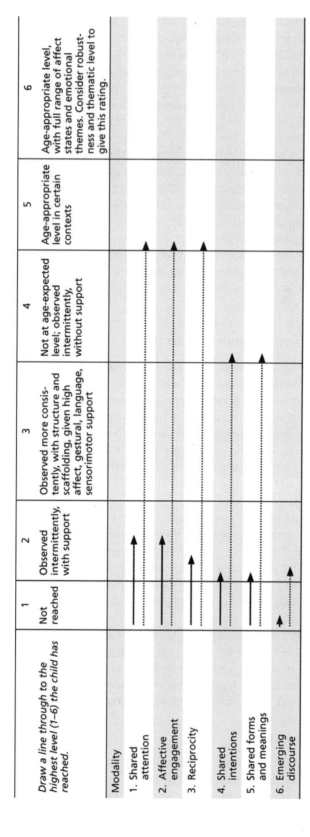

Figure 7.3.   Assessment of speech-language-communication for Mark at age 5 (⟶) and age 9 (⋯⋯▶). (*Source:* Interdisciplinary Council on Developmental and Learning Disorders, 2005.)

such as watering plants or playing circus. The clinicians expanded these scripts by gradually adding to the scenarios (e.g., having dolls perform in the circus; adding an audience, including adult turns in the performance) and then returning to Mark's interest in the scheme. Although the clinicians introduced many different play schemas, Mark had his favorites, and the play often returned to these scenarios.

Mark's persistent interests, such as playing with a train, were not discouraged. Rather, these interests were used to encourage interactions, such as finding the train together, locating the missing pieces, adding figurines to the play theme, and taking the train to Mark's favorite places (e.g., McDonald's restaurants). Consistent with DIR thinking, joining the child in his or her strongest interests generally leads to greater engagement, affective expression, and continuity of the story line. Over time, Mark stopped requesting the train and went on to explore other play possibilities. To address his sensory-processing and regulatory needs Mark's exploration of what he could do with his body was also encouraged.

By the end of the first year of DIR-based language intervention, Mark's level of engagement ranged from many circles of affective interactions around simple pretend games (e.g., playing monster) to shorter, more fragmented interactions. Mark's widest range of affect was seen in his interactions with his mother, where high positive affect, humor, frustration, and anger were expressed.

Although not addressed directly, Mark's language production increased both quantitatively and qualitatively. Greater diversity was seen in his vocabulary, word combinations, and early semantic-syntactic relations. Mark began to code a range of ideas (Lahey, 1988) using the basic constituent structure (subject plus verb plus complement) and also demonstrated the beginnings of semantic-syntactic complexity ("I want to go on the bolster"). Despite this progress, Mark's formulation difficulties were apparent, as can be seen in the following utterances: "Can I make a plant some seeds?"; "Put in the more"; "Can I water pour?" More important, Mark's comprehension of decontextualized language continued to be limited.

As previously mentioned, Mark's use of repetitive language and play was considered an opportunity to facilitate both of these domains of development. For example, in the monster game, Mark turned off the lights, went out of the room, waited until the clinicians were pretending to sleep and to snore, and then scared us when he came back in. Soon, Mark was one of the sleepers, joining the others in the room and trying to catch the monster when he returned. These shifts in the play schemas allowed for facilitation and expansion of the language and affect associated with this script.

DIR and Language Assessment: Mark at Age 9

Selected components of Mark's profile at 9 years illustrate how a child's intervention program might change over time using the DIR paradigm. In terms of the FEDLs (see Figure 7.2), Mark had achieved the first four levels in certain contexts, although his emotional range continued to be somewhat restricted. His capacity for creating representations and elaboration had expanded, with continuing constriction in his symbolic play abilities. Finally, with persistent and predictable support, Mark demonstrated islands of capacity in representational differentiation and emotional thinking.

In terms of the ICDL-DMIC (ICDL, 2005), at 9 years, Mark was a spontaneous and frequent communicator. In certain contexts, he had achieved the shared attention, affective engagement, and reciprocity that are seen in 36-month-old typically developing children (see Figure 7.3). Mark's language comprehension and production were similar to a 36-month-old's level in some ways, below this level in other ways (e.g., difficulty understanding and responding to why questions), and above typical developments of 36-month-olds in certain skills (e.g., ability to read). Mark continued to use scripts frequently to communicate his ideas and feelings, and his symbolic play skills were beginning to reach the 36-month-old level. Mark was interested in peer interactions but had difficulty joining and sustaining them.

Language Intervention Goals and Strategies

Intervention goals continued to focus on facilitating shared attention, affective engagement, reciprocity, shared intentions, and emotional regulation. Newer goals included expanding understanding of others' emotional states; facilitating the expansion of new schemas and stories within play scenarios; improving the comprehension of language, specifically, the response to why questions; expanding the capacity for symbolic play—decontextualization, themes, organization, and roles (Westby, 2000); supporting problem solving and flexibility; and enhancing theory of mind perspectives (Howlin et al., 1999).

In terms of intervention strategies, the integration of DIR thinking and developmental language models dictated the procedures that were used. At this point in the therapy, the clinician used Mark's interest in books to address the expression and understanding of emotional themes, the expansion of symbolic play, and the comprehension of language. The clinicians continued to use Mark's scripts as a context for the intervention as they joined in the meaning and affective tone of the script; developed an interaction within the context of the script by taking a role in the play; and changed or added to the characters, problems, outcomes, and roles while staying within the story line. Scripts were played out many times, and novel form—content relations were modeled to accompany the action.

Process and Progress

One of the most significant signs of progress noted when Mark was 9 was the depth of the relationship that he developed with the graduate clinicians who were working with him. Mark's connection to the students represented a qualitative change in his capacity for relating to people and his capacity for engagement.

Mark's use of spontaneous language and social language with the adults ("Hi guys. What are you doing?") continued to increase and become a more natural part of his repertoire. Mark's interest in reading books led to acting out a story—for example, Mercer Mayer's *Hansel and Gretel* (1989)—at first in a prescribed way, and then with changes within the roles and, eventually, in the story's ending. Mark was quite clever about using different props for the reenactment and easily accepted the clinician's suggestions—for example, a basket for the dungeon. The day that Mark announced that he was going to be Gretel after many times of being Hansel, pride in his accomplishment was obvious. The clinicians saw Mark's spontaneous, self-initiated role change from Hansel to Gretel as an example of the benefits of replaying the story many times rather than prematurely moving him on or directing the play.

Although the clinicians have been delighted with the role Mark's scripts have played in his language development, they are aware that the scripts continue to reflect Mark's challenges in the comprehension and production of language. For example, based on an assessment of Mark's comprehension at 9 years of age, although he has mastered the earlier occurring *wh* forms, such as *what, who, where,* later developing ones, such as *why* and *how* are a challenge for him. In his responses, Mark displayed comprehension patterns characteristic of earlier typical development, such as answering later occurring question forms with earlier occurring interpretations (e.g., answering why questions as if they were who questions).

In terms of production, although Mark continues to expand his use of spontaneous self-generated language, he continues to use scripts to communicate ideas and feelings. Because the author had the opportunity to study Mark's language development over time, she has come to a deeper appreciation of the ongoing role scripts may play in a child's expression of intention and meaning. Although not always apparent to a more naïve listener, a connection can be made between Mark's use of a script and the affect or idea he was trying to communicate. For example, when Mark was feeling nervous during one of his therapy sessions, he borrowed a script used by a character in the movie *Cars* to refer to anxiety.

Before ending this section, it is important to mention how a DIR–developmental language approach to scripting differs from more familiar intervention approaches to this form of communication. In more traditional approaches, clinicians and educators often address a child's scripting by ignoring it and redirecting the child to activities proposed by the adult, by modeling language that relates to the adult-determined activity, and by telling the child, "We're not talking about that now," when he or she returns to the scripts. These strategies are obviously generated from very different thinking about the origins of language, the reasons that a child might be using scripts, and the interpersonal and intrapersonal functions of the scripts. The principles of intervention shared by a DIR approach and a developmental language approach speak to the theoretical foundations for generating the intervention goals and strategies, which were used to address Mark's scripting. These include prioritizing affective engagement and reciprocal interaction, following the contents of the child's mind, treating all behaviors as intentional and meaningful, acknowledging that the child's idea is always better than yours, and joining first and then gently expanding the child's affect, ideas, and/or language.

Application to an Adolescent

Although the topic is not specifically discussed in this chapter, the DIR model does address higher levels of functional emotional development (Levels 7, 8, and 9), which would be appropriate to consider for older children, adolescents, and adults (Greenspan & Mann, 2001). For example, Level 8 is referred to as *Emotionally Differentiated Gray-Area Thinking*, which would be seen typically in grade school children. This capacity refers to the ability to understand and describe graduations of feelings such as anger, love, excitement, and disappointment. The child also begins to assess his or her status relative to a peer group and expands his or her ability to solve problems. The child's understanding of shades of gray thinking represents a significant step in emotional development ("I am a little disappointed" versus "I am very disappointed").

To review an extended application and implementation of this intervention, see Case 4 about a child with ASD in the companion volume *Case Studies for the Treatment of Autism Spectrum Disorder*.

Future Directions

Needless to say, clinicians working with children with ASD and with their families understand the importance of improving the quantity and quality of intervention research to assure improved outcomes. Not only is the quality of service dependent on more and better research, but many families need such data to access a greater range of treatment options. Because insurance reimbursement and school districts look to the research findings to support and develop programs, moving forward in this regard needs to be one of our highest priorities.

Nevertheless, it is clear that research findings for groups of children will always have to be viewed through the lens of real individual differences. The individual complexity of the challenges faced by children with ASD and their parents necessitates a clear conviction regarding individually designed intervention programs. This, in turn, leads to the recommendation that various types of research, including individual case studies, must be considered seriously for these children and no doubt for all children who have atypical developmental trajectories.

Suggested Readings

1. Gerber, S. (2017). Embracing the potential of play for children on the autism spectrum facilitating the earliest stages of developmental integration. *Topics in Language Disorders, 37(3), 229–240.* This article explores the importance of the foundations of development as key to a child's progress in language and integral to an intervention program. Contemporary models of child development and language acquisition are used to generate a therapy program for a child with significant regulatory and play challenges. The role of parent training is highlighted.

2. Interdisciplinary Council on Developmental and Learning Disorders. (2005). *Interdisciplinary Council on Developmental Learning Disorders— Diagnostic manual for infancy and early childhood.* ICDL Press. The ICDL-DMIC presents a developmentally based classification system for infants and young children with developmental disorders. The comprehensive classification system can be used to describe challenges in emotional, speech-language, cognitive, regulatory-sensory, and motor capacities.

3. Interdisciplinary Council on Developmental and Learning Disorders. (2000). *Clinical practice guidelines: Redefining the standards of care for infants, children, and families with special needs.* ICDL Press. The clinical practice guidelines, which are based on research and clinical experience, address the identification, assessment, and treatment of all relevant areas of developmental functioning in childhood. These include child–caregiver relationships, speech and language, motor functioning, visual-spatial processing, sensory modulation, the functional emotional developmental capacities, cognitive functioning, social skills, family patterns, and peer relationships. The guidelines embrace a functional developmental approach and can serve as the basis for recommenda-

tions for changes in screening, assessment, and intervention services and in local, state, and federal policies.

Learning Activities

1. Topics for further discussion

   - Compare and contrast the similarities and differences in the role of the parent between the DIR model and other intervention approaches that focus on incorporating the parent into the intervention process (e.g., the Hanen program More Than Words [Sussman, 1999]):

   - Identify the areas of developmental functioning embraced in the DIR model that will be familiar to SLPs and those that will require further exposure and learning.

2. Ideas for projects

   - Interview the parent of a child with autism who has had experience with both adult-directed approaches to intervention, such as ABA, and child-directed approaches, such as DIR. Ask the parent to discuss the pros and cons of each treatment approach for the child and family.

   - Interview an SLP who uses primarily behavioral interactions in intervention, such as ABA, and one who uses primarily spontaneous interactions, such as DIRFloortime. Ask the clinicians to explain what theories and clinical findings have motivated their decisions.

   - Interview an occupational therapist and ask him or her to give examples of sensory and regulatory problems that children on the autism spectrum might experience that would affect their ability to develop nonverbal forms of communication.

3. Writing assignments

   - Using the information discussed in this chapter on the FEDLs, the individual sensory profile, and caregiver patterns, write an assessment of a child with whom you are working.

   - Based on your assessment described in the preceding assignment, generate goals relative to the FEDLs, sensory profile, and caregiver–child interactions.

Summary of Video Clip

*See the **About the Videos and Downloads** page at the front of the book for directions on how to access and stream the accompanying video to this chapter.*

This three-part video segment shows language intervention goals and strategies based on the principles of the DIR approach in combination with a developmental language model. Emma, a 2-year-old child who had a history of challenges in relating and communicating, was seen for a period of 1 year at our clinic. The duration of time between the first segment and the last was approximately 2 months. Although Emma was capable of producing words, assessment of her speech, language, and

communication suggested that her challenges in shared attention, affective engagement, reciprocity, and shared intentionality (ICDL-DMIC, Interdisciplinary Council
on Developmental and Learning Disorders, 2005) should be considered the priority
goals of intervention.

The strategies that were used with Emma were also derived from a DIR–
developmental language perspective. They included the following:

- Sharing the focus of the child's attention.

- Maintaining the child-directed focus by treating all behaviors as communicative.

- Interpreting all of the child's behaviors as intentional.

- Using exaggeration and easily readable affective range.

- Maintaining a reciprocal flow by consistently giving the child a turn in the interaction and then taking yours—keeping the interaction going!

By the third segment, you can see the increase in Emma's engagement with her
communication partner, the more robust reciprocity and turn-taking in the
exchange, and the use of intentional communication with gestures, eye contact, and
words.

REFERENCES

Aldred, C., Green, J., & Adams, C. (2004). A new social communication intervention for children with autism: Pilot randomized controlled treatment study suggesting effectiveness.
Journal of Child Psychology and Psychiatry, 45, 1420–1430.

American Psychiatric Association. (1987). *Diagnostic and statistical manual of mental
disorders, third edition, revised* (DSM-III-R). Author.

American Psychiatric Association. (1994). *Diagnostic and statistical manual of mental
disorders, fourth edition* (DSM-IV). Author.

Bates, E. (1975). *Language and context: The acquisition of pragmatics.* Academic Press.

Bloom, L., & Lahey, M. (1978). *Language development and language disorders.* Wiley.

Bloom, L., & Tinker, E. (2001). The intentionality model and language acquisition. *Monographs of the Society for Research in Child Development, 66*(4, Serial No. 267), 1–91.

Breinbauer, C. (2010). *Circles of Communication.* Lecture presented at the ICDL Graduate
School, Functional Emotional Assessment Scale Reliability Training (IMH 401), Interdisciplinary Council on Developmental and Learning Disorders, Bethesda, MD, United States.

Casenhiser, D., Shanker, S., & Stieben, J. (2010, May). *Learning through interaction in
children with autism.* Paper presented at the International Meeting for Autism Research,
Philadelphia, PA, United States.

Cawn, S., Gerber, S., Greenspan, S., Harrison, C., Lewis, D., Madell, J., & Wetherby, A. (2005).
Language disorders. In Interdisciplinary Council on Developmental and Learning Disorders (ICDL) (Ed.), *Diagnostic manual for infancy and early childhood: Mental health,
developmental, regulatory-sensory processing, language and learning disorders*
(pp. 129–166). ICDL Press.

Cullinane, D., Gurry, S., & Solomon, R. (2017). *Research evidence re: Developmental-
relationship based interventions for autism.* https://affectautism.com/wp-content
/uploads/2020/10/Research-evidence-for-DRBI-by-Diane-Cullinane.pdf

Dionne, M., & Martini, R. (2011). Floortime play with a child with autism: A single-subject
study. *Canadian Journal of Occupational Therapy, 78*, 196–203.

Gerber, S. (2017). Embracing the potential of play for children on the autism spectrum: Facilitating the earliest stages of developmental integration. *Topics in Language Disorders,
37*, 229–240.

Gerber, S. (2003). A developmental perspective on language assessment and intervention for
children on the autistic spectrum. *Topics in Language Disorders, 23*(2), 74–95.

Girolametto, L., Sussman, F., & Weitzman, E. (2007). Using case study methods to investigate the effects of interactive intervention for children with autism spectrum disorders. *Journal of Communication Disorders, 40*, 470–492.

Greenspan, S. I. (2004). *The social-emotional growth charts.* Pearson.

Greenspan, S. I., De Gangi, G. A., & Wieder, S. (2001). *The Functional Emotional Assessment Scale (FEAS) for infancy and early childhood: Clinical and research applications.* ICDL Press.

Greenspan, S. I., & Mann, H. (2001). Adolescents and adults with special needs: The Developmental Individual differences, Relationship-based (DIR) approach to intervention. In Interdisciplinary Council on Developmental and Learning Disorders, *ICDL clinical practice guidelines: Redefining the standards of care for infants, children, and families with special needs* (pp. 639–656). ICDL Press.

Greenspan, S. I., & Shanker, S. G. (2004). *The first idea: How symbols, language, and intelligence evolved from our primate ancestors to modern humans.* Da Capo Press.

Greenspan, S. I., & Wieder, S. (1997). Developmental patterns and outcomes in infants and children with disorders in relating and communicating: A chart review of 200 cases of children with autistic spectrum disorder. *Journal of Developmental and Learning Disorders, 1*, 87–141.

Greenspan, S. I., & Wieder, S. (1998). *The child with special needs: Encouraging intellectual and emotional growth.* Perseus Books.

Greenspan, S. I., & Wieder, S. (2001). Developmentally appropriate interactions and practices. In Interdisciplinary Council on Developmental and Learning Disorders, *ICDL clinical practice guidelines: Redefining the standards of care for infants, children, and families with special needs* (pp. 261–281). ICDL Press.

Howlin, P., Baron-Cohen, S., Hadwin, J., & Swettenham, J. (1999). *Teaching children with autism to mind-read.* Wiley.

Interdisciplinary Council on Developmental and Learning Disorders (ICDL). (2005). *Diagnostic manual for infancy and early childhood: Mental health, developmental, regulatory-sensory processing, language and learning disorders.* ICDL Press.

Kasari, C., Paparella, T., Freeman, S. N., & Jahromi, L. (2008). Language outcome in autism: Randomized comparison of joint attention and play interventions. *Journal of Consulting and Clinical Psychology, 76*, 125–137.

Kim, J. M., & Mahoney, G. (2004). The effects of mother's style of interaction on children's engagement: Implications for using responsive interventions with parents. *Topics in Early Childhood Special Education, 24*(1), 31–38.

Lahey, M. (1988). *Language disorders and language development.* Wiley.

Lewis, D., & Greenspan, S. I. (2005). *The affect-based language curriculum (ABLC): An intensive program for families, therapists, and teachers* (2nd ed.). ICDL Press.

Longtin, S., & Gerber, S. (2008). Contemporary perspectives on facilitating language acquisition for children on the autistic spectrum: Engaging the parent and the child. *Journal of Developmental and Learning Disorders, 3*, 38–51.

Lord, C., & McGee, J. P. (Eds.). (2001). *Educating children with autism.* Committee on Educational Interventions for Children with Autism, Commission on Behavioral and Social Sciences and Education, National Research Council. National Academy Press.

Mahoney, G., & Perales, F. (2005). Relationship-focused early intervention with children with pervasive developmental disorders and other disabilities: A comparative study. *Journal of Developmental and Behavioral Pediatrics, 26*, 77–85.

McConachie, H., Randle, V., & Le Couteur, A. (2005). A controlled trial of a training course for parents of children with suspected autism spectrum disorder. *Journal of Pediatrics, 147*, 335–340.

Mercer, J. (2017). Examining DIRFloortime as a treatment for children with autism spectrum disorders: A review of research and theory. *Research on Social Work Practice, 27*, 625-635.

Mercer, M. (1989). *Little critter Hansel and Gretel.* Western Publishing Co.

Miller, J. (2010). Systematic Analysis of Language Transcripts (SALT), English (Version 2010) [Computer software]. SALT Software, LLC.

National Autism Center. (2009). *National Standards Project—Findings and conclusions Phase 1: Addressing the needs for evidence-based practice guidelines for autism spectrum disorders.* Author.

National Autism Center. (2015). *National Standards Project—Findings and conclusions Phase 2: Addressing the needs for evidence-based practice guidelines for autism spectrum disorders.* Author.

Pajareya, K., & Nopmaneejumruslers, K. (2011). A pilot randomized controlled trial of DIR/Floortime™ parent training intervention for pre-school children with autistic spectrum disorders. *Autism, 15*(5), 563–577.

Piaget, J. (1955). *The language and thought of the child.* Meridian.

Pickles, A., Le Couteur, A., Leadbitter, K., Salomone, E., Cole-Flectcher, R., Tobin, H., Gammer, I., Lowry, J., Vamvakas, G., Byford, S., Aldred, C., Slonims, V., McConachie, H., Howlin, P., Parr, J., Charman, T., & Green, J. (2016). Parent-mediated social communication therapy for young children with autism (PACT): Long-term follow-up of a randomised controlled trial. *Lancet, 388*, 2501–2509.

Prizant, B., Wetherby, A., Rubin, E., Laurent, A., & Rydell, P. (2006). *The SCERTS® Model: A comprehensive educational approach for children with autism spectrum disorders.* Paul H. Brookes Publishing Co.

Robinson, R. (2011). *Autism solutions: How to create a meaningful life for your child.* Harlequin.

Schopler, E., Reichler, R., & Rochen-Renner, B. (1988). *Childhood Autism Rating Scale (CARS).* Western Psychological Services.

Seigel, D. (1999). *The developing mind: How relationships and the brain interact to shape who we are.* Guilford Press.

Shonkoff, J. P., & Phillips, D. A. (Eds.). (2000). *From neurons to neighborhoods: The science of early childhood development.* National Academy Press.

Siller, M., & Sigman, M. (2002). The behaviors of parents of children with autism predict the subsequent development of their children's communication. *Journal of Autism and Developmental Disorders, 32*, 77–89.

Solomon, R., Necheles, J., Ferch, C., & Bruckman, D. (2007). Pilot study of a parent training program for young children with autism: The PLAY Project Home Consultation model. *Autism, 11*, 205–224.

Sussman, F. (1999). *More Than Words: Helping parents promote communication and social skills in children with autism spectrum disorders.* The Hanen Centre.

Tronick, E. (2007). *The neurobehavioral and social-emotional development of infants and children.* W.W. Norton.

Westby, C. (2000). A scale for assessing development of children's play. In K. Gitlin-Weiner, A. Sandgrund, & C. Schaefer (Eds.), *Play diagnosis and assessment* (2nd ed., pp. 15–58). Wiley.

Wetherby, A., & Prizant, B. (2002). *Communication and Symbolic Behavior Scales™ (CSBS™).* Paul H. Brookes Publishing Co.

Wieder, S. (2004, June). *Building foundations for children and families.* Seminar presented in Tarrytown, NY, United States.

Wieder, S., & Greenspan, S. I. (2005). Can children with autism master core deficits and become empathetic, creative, and reflective? *Journal of Developmental and Learning Disorders, 9*, 39–61.

Wieder, S., & Kalmanson, B. (2000). Educational guidelines for preschool children with difficulties in relating and communicating. In S. I. Greenspan & S. Wieder (Eds.), *ICDL clinical practice guidelines: Redefining the standards of care for infants, children and families with special needs* (pp. 283–333). ICDL Press.

8

Functional Communication Training

Treating Challenging Behavior

V. Mark Durand and Lauren J. Moskowitz

INTRODUCTION

Challenging behaviors such as **aggression,** self-injury, stereotyped behaviors, and **tantrums** are highly prevalent among children and adults with autism spectrum disorder (ASD). (This chapter uses the terms *challenging behavior* and other variations to indicate those difficulties presented by individuals that interfere with educational, vocational, and family activities. It is also referred to as *problem behavior* in the research literature.) Research suggests that challenging behavior is three to four times more frequent in individuals with ASD than in individuals without disabilities. In addition, between 10% and 40% of children with disabilities display frequent and severe challenging behaviors (Einfeld & Tonge, 1996; Lowe et al., 2007). Along with frequency, the stability of these behaviors is also of serious concern (Totsika et al., 2008). Several studies document that, even with treatment, these behaviors may still be problematic a decade later (Einfeld & Tonge, 1996; Einfeld et al., 2001; Emerson et al., 2001; Green et al., 2005; Jones, 1999).

It is difficult to estimate the impact of challenging behaviors on the lives of people with ASD and their families. These behaviors are among the most frequently cited obstacles to placing students in community settings (Eyman & Call, 1977; Hodgetts et al., 2013; Jacobson, 1982; Myers et al., 2009). Further, their presence is associated with significantly increased recidivism among those individuals referred to crisis intervention programs from community placements (Shoham-Vardi et al., 1996). Challenging behavior interferes with such essential activities as family life (Cole & Meyer, 1989), educational activities (Koegel & Covert, 1972), and employment (Hayes, 1987). Parental stress is shown to significantly increase when caring for a child with challenging behavior (Floyd & Gallagher, 1997; Hastings, 2002;

Saloviita et al., 2003). Mothers of children with disabilities tend to have higher rates of depression, and depressed parents are more likely to have a child with behavior problems (Feldman et al., 2007). In addition, in one of the largest studies of its kind, researchers examined almost 10,000 children and found that the single best predictor of early school failure was the presence of behavior problems (Byrd & Weitzman, 1994). In fact, the presence of behavior problems was a better predictor of school difficulties than factors such as poverty, speech and hearing impairments, and low birth weight. One study found that almost 40% of preschool teachers reported expelling a child each year because of behavior problems (Gilliam & Shahar, 2006). Such behaviors also can pose a physical threat to these individuals and those who work with them.

One of the most frequently used approaches to reduce challenging behaviors in people with ASD involves replacing the behavior with an alternative behavior—a technique known as **functional communication training (FCT)** (Carr & Durand, 1985; Durand, 1990; Durand & Moskowitz, 2015). FCT entails a multi-step process to 1) assess the function of the challenging behavior to be targeted, 2) select an appropriate alternative behavior, and 3) teach the alternative and fade out prompts to fit the current environment. The types of challenging behaviors that appear to be appropriate targets for FCT run the behavioral gamut, from aggression and self-injury to elopement (Lang et al., 2009) and inappropriate sexual behavior (Fyffe et al., 2004). Family members and a range of professionals use FCT in homes, schools and in the community (Dunlap et al., 2006; Durand, 1999). Research on FCT targets individuals across all ages (from infants and toddlers to older adults), developmental levels (from those with pervasive needs for support to those with average or above average cognitive abilities), and language abilities (Petscher et al., 2009; Snell et al., 2006). FCT is one of the few skill-focused behavioral interventions cited as having extensive support from initial efficacy studies (Smith et al., 2007).

TARGET POPULATIONS

Research on a broad range of individuals with ASD as well as a variety of other disorders (e.g., attention-deficit/hyperactivity disorder [ADHD], schizophrenia, traumatic brain injury) supports the wide-ranging applicability of this approach (Durand & Merges, 2009). In addition, research demonstrates that this approach to reducing challenging behavior can be adapted to individuals with a range of abilities, from those needing the most intensive levels of support (Bird et al., 1989) to individuals who have no educational or clinical diagnosis and who have typical verbal and cognitive abilities (Petscher et al., 2009).

Functional Behavioral Assessment

Functional behavioral assessment is at the core of the process used in FCT (Durand, 1990). The function or functions of challenging behavior are determined, and this information is used to select the alternative communication behavior (i.e. the alternative form of communication, also referred to as the *communicative response* or *functional communication response*) that is taught to replace the behavior. The primary goal is to identify an appropriate behavior that serves the same function as the challenging behavior and that therefore can serve as a replacement. To assess the function of a behavior, the antecedents that lead to the behavior and consequences that follow the behavior need to be identified, which can be accomplished in a number of ways (Matson & Minshawi, 2007; Matson & Nebel-Schwalm, 2007). In order to improve the accuracy of assessment results, it is typically recommended that multiple forms of assessment be used.

A number of functional assessment strategies can be useful for determining the function of behavior—including the use of informal observations, antecedent–behavior–consequence (ABC) charts, a variety of rating scales, and functional analyses. An experimental **functional analysis**—manipulating aspects of the environment to assess behavior change—is frequently cited as the most accurate method of determining the function of a behavior (Hanley et al., 2003).

Informal Observation and Interviews

Typically, the assessment process begins with informal observations and interviews of significant others. Once a broad range of information is collected and hypotheses about the function(s) of the behaviors are developed, more formal assessments are used to validate these hypotheses. A number of assessment instruments are available to provide additional information about the functions of behavior, including the **Motivation Assessment Scale** (Durand & Crimmins, 1992), the Functional Analysis Interview Form (O'Neill et al., 1990), and the Questions About Behavioral Function (Paclawskyj et al., 2000). These types of instruments can be used to provide additional and convergent information about behavioral functions. This information is then used to help select the alternative communication to be taught.

THEORETICAL BASIS

It is valuable to understand the theoretical foundation of several aspects of FCT in order to adapt this procedure to diverse individuals and settings. Described next are the concepts behind why challenging behavior is reduced with FCT (**functional equivalence**), why the effects of FCT generalize to new people and settings (**natural communities of reinforcement**), and how these concepts lead to understanding the conditions under which FCT is most effective (features of the alternative response).

Functional Equivalence

The mechanism of behavior change that underlies the reduction of challenging behavior using FCT is the concept of functional equivalence (Carr, 1988; Durand, 1987; Durand & Moskowitz, 2015). The assumption is that challenging behaviors are maintained by a particular reinforcer or reinforcers (e.g., attention from others, escape from work). Theoretically, then, these challenging behaviors can be replaced by other behaviors if these new behaviors serve the same function and are more efficient at gaining the desired reinforcers (See Table 8.1 for examples of common functions for challenging behavior). For example, if a girl hits herself to get attention from her parent, then teaching her a different, more effective way to get this attention (e.g., saying, "Come here, please") should serve the same function for the girl. This alternative behavior then would result in a decrease in the frequency of her self-injury as she becomes successful in gaining attention in this new way. FCT is presumed to reduce challenging behavior because it involves teaching and reinforcing a replacement behavior that serves the same function.

Table 8.1. Common behavioral functions

Behavioral function	Description
Attention	Behaviors that occur to obtain social attention from others (which can include interactions such as praising, spending time together, comforting, but for some children it can also include yelling or providing explanations). Being left alone can trigger these behaviors.
Tangible	Behaviors that occur to obtain desired things (e.g., toys, foods) or activities. These behaviors can be triggered by a request to end an activity (e.g., stop watching a movie) or to give up a desired item (e.g., a toy picked up at a store).
Escape	Behaviors that occur to remove undesired requests or activities. This can include actions that may appear to be punitive (e.g., sending children to their room) that to the children may instead actually be desired (e.g., sending children to their room results in ending a request to brush their teeth). These behaviors can be triggered by requests to perform some undesired activity.
Sensory	Behaviors that occur to obtain the sensory feedback provided by the behavior itself. This can include behaviors that may feel good (e.g., face rubbing, twirling in circles), look good (e.g., waving hands in front of eyes), taste good (e.g., eating things off of the floor), or sound good (e.g., making unusual noises). Being left alone or overstimulation can trigger these behaviors.

Natural Communities of Reinforcement

In the special case of FCT as an intervention strategy, using communication as the replacement behavior provides an added benefit because of its unique ability to recruit natural communities of desired reinforcers (Durand, 1990). In other words, if a child learns to ask or otherwise solicit the reinforcers from others, then the child is able to recruit these reinforcers without an interventionist having to specifically train other people how to respond. For example, one study examined whether nonverbal children would be able to recruit reinforcers from community members, thereby resulting in a reduction of their challenging behaviors (Durand, 1999). Five students were identified who 1) exhibited severe and frequent behavior problems and 2) were unable to communicate verbally with others. Their teachers were shown how to assess the functions of the students' behaviors and select more appropriate alternatives for them to use. Then the teachers were instructed in how to assist their students to use vocal output communication devices to request things such as assistance or attention from others. The teachers were successful in teaching their students to use their devices to gain access to the stimuli previously maintaining their challenging behaviors, and they observed significant reductions in such behavior in the classroom. Next, the teachers took their students out into typical community settings and observed that the students used their devices to appropriately solicit attention and help from untrained people in settings such as the library and stores at the local shopping mall. Again, challenging behavior was significantly reduced in the community settings once the students were able to recruit reinforcers from others. Importantly, this success was achieved without specifically instructing community members how to respond to the students. The librarians or store clerks responded naturally to the requests made by the students through their devices and this, in turn, resulted in reduced challenging behavior in the community (Durand, 1999).

The concept of recruiting natural communities of reinforcement (Stokes et al., 1978) is central to the success of FCT outside of structured environments staffed with highly trained individuals (Durand, 1990). This is a particularly important aspect of FCT when comparing the outcomes of FCT to other intervention strategies. Typically, with other interventions, once a behavioral plan is developed, training ensues for all individuals who come in contact with the person who exhibits the challenging behavior. If people do not follow the behavioral procedures, it is expected that regression will occur and behavior problems will increase. In contrast, rather than trying to train each person a child encounters on a daily basis to implement a formal behavioral program, FCT essentially allows the child to actively solicit from others the reinforcers that have previously maintained their challenging behavior. In effect, the child becomes his or her own intervention agent.

An experimental analysis of this bootstrapping aspect of FCT was examined in a study comparing this treatment approach with another, common approach to reacting to challenging behavior—time-out from positive reinforcement (TO; Durand & Carr, 1992). In this study, the researchers selected 12 school-age students, all of whom engaged in a variety of challenging behaviors (e.g., tantrums, self-injury, and aggression). In addition, the students were screened to identify those whose challenging behaviors were being maintained by attention from others. The rationale for selecting students who had only attention-maintained problem behavior was to ensure that they would be appropriate for using TO. Selecting TO as an intervention for challenging behavior involves the assumption that the targeted behavior is reinforced by attention and that removing attention would put the problem behavior under extinction. The six students were randomly assigned to one of the two treatment conditions—FCT or TO. Just prior to introducing the treatments, the students were individually placed with teachers who had no knowledge of the study and who were instructed to work with the student on a task. The teachers received no instructions about how to react to behavior problems. Treatment was then introduced by other teachers and was successful in reducing challenging behaviors for each child. Thus, the first finding was that both FCT and TO could successfully reduce challenging behavior. Next, the students were placed back with the teachers who were naïve to the treatment program. For the students who had received TO as a treatment, their challenging behaviors resumed almost immediately. The students quickly realized that TO as a consequence would not occur in this setting, and they resumed their behavior problems. In contrast, the students who received FCT as a treatment used their communication responses to request attention, and the naïve teachers responded appropriately, maintaining the reduction of the challenging behavior. In short, the advantage of FCT was not solely in the initial reduction in challenging behavior—which both treatments could produce—but also in its ability to recruit natural communities of reinforcement, in this case, teacher attention (Durand & Carr, 1992). This aspect of FCT is examined more fully in subsequent discussions of the effectiveness of this approach.

One consequence of viewing behavior problems as functionally equivalent to other forms of communication is the idea that these behaviors are not just responses that need to be reduced or eliminated. In the past, the de facto view of challenging behaviors was that they were excesses to be reduced. However, a functional view of challenging behavior suggests that they are just less acceptable (and sometimes much less acceptable) forms of reasonable requests for reinforcers (e.g., attention from others, help with difficult tasks). This perspective is a reminder that attempting to eliminate these behaviors through some reductive technique would leave these individuals with no way of accessing their desired reinforcers and therefore other inappropriate behaviors would likely take their place (also called *symptom substitution* or *response covariation*).

Features of the Alternative Response

Although functional equivalence and recruiting natural communities of reinforcement are the major underlying conceptual underpinnings for the effectiveness of FCT, other components of FCT become important for the ultimate success of the intervention in typical settings (Durand & Merges, 2009). These components offer an alternative response that is a functional equivalent and include response match, response success, response efficiency, response acceptability, response recognizability, and response milieu (see Table 8.2 and Figure 8.1 for an illustration of the steps to implementing FCT).

Response Match   Response match refers to matching the communication behavior to the function of the challenging behavior; thus, it is closely related to functional equivalence. In the initial study of FCT, students with challenging behavior were taught two different communication responses—one phrase designed to elicit adult attention and another phrase designed to request assistance (Carr & Durand, 1985). The rationale behind the design of this study was to determine if just teaching a form of communication that elicited a response from others would be sufficient to reduce challenging behavior. It is sometimes speculated that challenging behavior is used to control one's environment generically. If this were the case, then simply teaching a response that changed the behaviors of others should replace the challenging behavior. However, this was not the case; the study found that if students had attention-maintained challenging behavior, the teaching and reinforcing requests for assistance had no impact on their behavior. Similarly, teaching and reinforcing responses for attention to students with escape-maintained challenging

Table 8.2.   Step-by-step instructions for functional communication training

Steps	Description
1. Assess the function of behavior.	Use two or more functional assessment techniques to determine what variables are maintaining the problem behavior.
2. Select the communication modality.	Identify how you want the individual to communicate with others (e.g., verbally, through alternative communication strategies).
3. Create teaching situations.	Identify situations in the environment that are triggers for problem behavior (e.g., difficult tasks), and use these as the settings for teaching the alternative responses.
4. Prompt communication.	Prompt the alternative communication in the setting where you want it to occur. Use the least intrusive prompt necessary.
5. Fade prompts.	Quickly fade the prompts, ensuring that no problem behaviors occur during training.
6. Teach new communicative responses.	When possible, teach a variety of alternative communication responses that can serve the same function (e.g., saying "Help me" or "I don't understand").
7. Modify the environment.	When appropriate, implement changes in the environment, such as improving student–task match in school.

From Durand, V. M., & Merges, E. (2008). Functional communication training to treat challenging behavior. In W. O'Donohue, & J. E. Fisher (Eds.), *Cognitive behavior therapy: Applying empirically supported techniques in your practice* (2nd ed., pp. 222–229). New York, NY: Wiley; reprinted by permission.

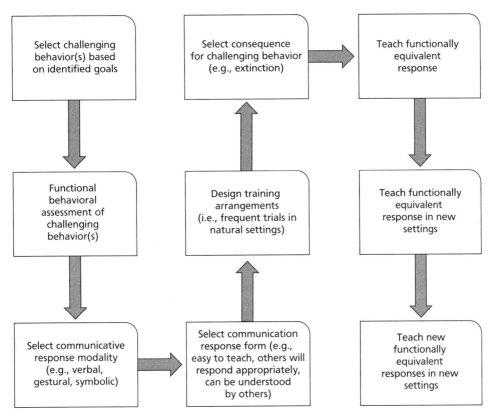

Figure 8.1.   Functional communication training flowchart. *Source:* Durand & Merges (2009).

behavior produced no behavior change. Only when students were taught responses that matched the function of challenging behavior did the behavior problems reduce in frequency (Carr & Durand, 1985).

Response Success   To be successful, use of a conventional behavior as an alternative to a challenging behavior must be followed by a reinforcer that serves the same function as that served by the challenging behavior (e.g., attention or escape). For example, simply saying "Help me" without having someone respond with assistance is not likely to result in a reduction in escape-maintained behaviors. Other people must take action in response to these communication efforts—a concept referred to as *response success.* In one study, FCT was used to reduce the chronic and severe challenging behaviors exhibited by three students with ASD (Durand & Carr, 1991). When these students were followed across several years, two of the three students continued to use the new communication responses they had been taught, and their challenging behaviors remained at low levels. However, the behaviors of one of the students had returned to prior high levels a year after our initial intervention. Observing him in his classroom, the authors reported that although he was attempting to request assistance from his new teacher by saying, "I don't understand," when he was asked a question (the strategy he had been taught previously), his teacher was not responding. The teacher did not seem to know what he was saying because of his articulation and therefore did not respond by prompting him or clarifying the questions she directed to him. As a result, he returned to hitting himself and screaming, which usually resulted in the termination of the teaching session—the same pattern that occurred prior to our intervening with FCT.

Intervention was reinstated so that the student was taught to articulate his request for assistance more clearly (saying, "I don't understand"). Typically, in these cases, one would inform the teacher of his articulation difficulties, and the teacher would adapt his or her teaching style to accommodate the student's unclear speech. However, because the goal was for the student to be able to solicit assistance not only from this teacher but also from a variety of other people, articulation training was conducted. Once he was able to more clearly make his request known, his teacher responded as expected—providing him with prompts when he said he did not understand the question—and his challenging behaviors again were reduced. This study and others highlight the importance of the communication response resulting in an appropriate reaction from others in the environment (e.g., Durand & Carr, 1991; Volkert et al., 2009).

Response Efficiency   Research on FCT suggests that the approach is most effective when the new communication response is more efficient at eliciting the desired reinforcers than the challenging behavior. In other words, if it is easier to say, "Help me," to get assistance than it is to scream or hit, FCT will be successful. A number of studies directly examine this aspect of FCT (Fisher et al., 2000; Horner & Day, 1991; Horner et al., 1990; Reed Schindler & Horner, 2005; Richman et al., 2001). For example, in a series of studies, Horner and his colleagues examined this aspect of functional communication training (Horner & Day, 1991; Horner et al., 1990). In one study, for example, the researchers examined the aggression of one 12-year old boy (Horner & Day, 1991). They found that his aggressive behavior was maintained by escape from demands and decided to use FCT to teach him how to appropriately request a break from work. The researchers systematically examined the effects of teaching him to sign I WANT TO GO, PLEASE on aggression. They observed no significant reduction in aggression with this strategy. They then taught him to sign BREAK—a much easier way to communicate for escape—and this resulted in significant reductions in his challenging behavior. They hypothesized that effort impacts the outcome of FCT such that if the new communication response requires more effort than the challenging behavior, individuals will choose to continue using their challenging behavior. Similarly, they examined the impact of delay in gaining reinforcement and schedule of reinforcement and saw that individuals choose the most efficient means of gaining their preferred reinforcers—whether it be through communication or challenging behavior. These types of studies demonstrate that response efficiency is an important consideration in predicting the success of FCT (Fisher et al., 2000; Horner & Day, 1991; Horner et al., 1990; Reed Schindler & Horner, 2005; Richman et al., 2001).

Response Acceptability   Clinical experience with FCT suggests that another important consideration in the success of FCT involves whether or not the response is acceptable to significant others (Durand & Merges, 2009). If the new communication response is seen as unacceptable in community settings, then others will not respond appropriately and the desired consequences will not be obtained.

Response acceptability can be viewed as a cultural consideration—making sure that the relevant local culture will respond appropriately to the communication requests. For example, in one case that the coauthors of this chapter observed, a young woman who was living in a group home would scream and remove her clothing, both extremely disruptive to the other residents (Durand, 1990). Her challenging behavior was assessed as being maintained by the attention she subsequently received by staff when she was disruptive. Given her limited communication repertoire (she had no conventional communication skills), we taught her to raise her hand to signal to the group home staff that she was requesting some of their attention. Although this strategy was initially successful in reducing her disruptive behavior, over the course of several weeks, the frequency of behavior problems returned to pretreatment levels. We revisited her in her group home and conducted a series of observations to see why FCT was no longer successful. It quickly became clear that the staff was only occasionally responding to her hand raising, and she was gradually shifting from raising her hand to gain attention back to using her disruptive behavior. Staff interviews revealed that although they initially agreed to respond to her request for attention through hand raising, they were too busy with their other tasks and found her constant requests for attention annoying. Subsequently, efforts involved trying to change their local culture, namely, to educate the staff on the basic need of all people to get attention from others and how this was part of their role as staff working in a group home. Unfortunately, this strategy was not successful, and the staff continued to view her requests for attention as problematic.

At this point, abandoning efforts and assigning blame to the staff were a clear possibility. Instead, the communication behavior was assigned a different function. Now, rather than hand raising signifying the young woman's request for the staff to stop their other tasks to spend time with her, it was used to signal her request to help the staff with their work. For example, if they were emptying the dishwasher and she raised her hand, they were to go get her and have her help them empty the dishwasher. This minor change was extremely successful in changing whether or not they responded to her and resulted in a significant reduction in the young woman's challenging behavior. Hand raising still resulted in attention from staff, but now it was in a form that was more acceptable to them. They could continue with their tasks, she could get attention from them, and the bonus was that she was now engaged in more functional activities during the day.

This case highlights a dilemma when trying to intervene with individuals who engage in challenging behavior. There are times when the response clinicians select as alternatives may not be perceived as acceptable to others in the person's immediate community. For example, a clinician once relayed how he used FCT to reduce challenging behavior of an adult in the community. This person's challenging behavior appeared to be maintained by attention, and the clinician taught the man how to request attention from others. The clinician reported that although this strategy (requesting a hug) was successful at his prevocational work environment, it was not successful out in the general community. Perhaps the world would be a better place if strangers were more open to hugs, but realistically, requesting hugs is not acceptable in most cases. This cultural consideration—making sure that the forms of communication we teach are acceptable to others—is an essential concern for the ultimate success of FCT in reducing challenging behavior (Durand, 1990; Durand & Merges, 2009).

Response Recognizability   An important consideration for individuals with significant communication needs is teaching them a response that can be recognized, especially by others who may not be highly trained, so that it can effectively replace the challenging behavior. To date, much of the research on FCT has used verbal and signed speech as the means of communication. Unfortunately, spoken speech can often be misunderstood, and signed speech can be so idiosyncratic that few can understand the message being relayed. Several studies have addressed the issue of the recognizability of the communication response as it relates to FCT—for example, in the case involving the young boy returning to serious self-injury because poorly intelligible speech did not provide a realistic functional alternative (Durand & Carr, 1991). This study found that when the boy's articulation skills improved, the teacher responded appropriately. Following the improvement in the student–teacher interaction, the boy's challenging behavior was again reduced, which generalized to a new teacher and was maintained 1 year later.

Response recognizability is of particular importance for students with the most severe disabilities. This issue has led to a growing number of studies with students who have severe communication disabilities that demonstrate success using augmentative and alternative strategies as the means of communication with FCT (Bingham et al., 2007; Durand, 1993, 1999; Durand & Berotti, 1991; Franco et al., 2009; Mirenda, 1997, 2003; Olive et al., 2008; Schepis et al., 1996; Wacker et al., 1990). The presumed rationale is to improve the recognizability of the communication requests being made by these individuals.

Use of augmentative and alternative communication (AAC) improves recognizability of responses not only for students with severe disabilities and their trained communication partners but also for untrained communication partners in the community who understand the requests and respond appropriately (Durand, 1999; Durand & Berotti, 1991). In addition, the devices have at times been programmed to speak in both English and other languages when a student's family does not speak English at home and the teacher speaks only English at school. In essence, students with severe and multiple disabilities are taught to be bilingual. These devices have permitted the teaching of making relatively simple responses (pressing a pad on the machine) that can result in successful interchanges. Again, because the output can be recognized by anyone, the success of the communication training can be extended into the community. A recent meta-analysis found that FCT involving AAC was effective in reducing challenging behavior and improving aided or unaided AAC use among students with disabilities (most of whom were diagnosed with intellectual disability [ID] or ASD) in school settings (Walker et al., 2018).

Response Milieu   What are the characteristics of the optimal environment in which FCT should take place? Can clinicians describe, and therefore design, settings that will facilitate the success, generalization, and maintenance of reductions in challenging behavior using FCT? Unfortunately, research has not specifically focused on environmental or contextual influences as they relate to this intervention approach. To our knowledge, no research has yet systematically explored the types of environmental variables that would positively or negatively impact on these outcomes. However, based on our extensive experience using FCT in a wide variety of environments, we offer some of our observations on the role of the environment in the success of FCT.

One factor that appears to influence the outcome of efforts to implement functional communication training is the participant's degree of control or choice. The availability of choice-making opportunities has received considerable attention and has been implicated in the success of various educational activities (Carlson et al., 2008; Dyer et al., 1990; Watanabe & Sturmey, 2003). Special attention has been paid to communication training that allows individuals to make choices in their day-to-day activities (e.g., choosing when to take a break, have a drink, get social attention). We have observed that in those settings where choice making is encouraged, FCT is more likely to succeed. Conversely, where choice making is discouraged, FCT often has had limited success. FCT in these settings sometimes has been described as giving in and has been received with some reticence. Again, this aspect of the intervention environment seems to offer a fruitful avenue for further empirical attention.

A second environmental factor that seems to be implicated in outcomes of FCT involves the ways that participants are grouped. Despite initiatives to include all students in regular classrooms and community settings, environments still exist where students are grouped together because of their challenging behavior. Historically, the logic behind such groupings has been that they facilitate students' access to staff who are specially trained to deal with challenging behavior. In addition, such groupings allow for groupwide programs and contingencies and minimize disruptions of other students.

Space does not permit a full discussion of the anticipated as opposed to the actual results of such homogeneous groupings. However, we have had the opportunity to compare and contrast the ability of these different settings to support efforts at FCT. Our observation has been that staff who work in such behavior classes are at particular risk of being overtaxed by the demands of the classroom and may find it especially difficult to be responsive to all of their students. Staff members in more heterogeneous groupings appear to have more flexibility. They are able to shift priorities toward activities that may require more intensive yet temporary effort (e.g., FCT). This flexibility may be attributable to the other students in these classrooms who can benefit from periods of independent work. In such a setting, the teacher is more available to be responsive to the children receiving FCT than is a teacher in a behavior class.

EMPIRICAL BASIS

There is an extensive literature on the outcomes of using FCT to treat and reduce challenging behavior. This section selectively reviews the substantial body of research in this area. To date, nearly 200 published studies document the successful use of FCT with a range of individuals and their challenging behaviors. Fortunately, several published reviews document the depth and breadth of research studies that examine the outcomes of FCT across populations, behavior topographies, and variations in the methods for using this approach (e.g., Bambara et al., 1994; Durand & Merges, 2009; Halle et al., 2006; Mancil, 2006; Matson et al., 2005; Mirenda, 1997; Petscher et al., 2009). For example, Mirenda (1997) reviewed research that used AAC strategies (e.g., manual signing, communication books, voice output communication aids) as the method for communicating with FCT. A review by Matson and colleagues (2005) evaluated the literature on a number of techniques used to treat aggression and found that FCT was one of the most heavily researched approaches. Petscher and colleagues (2009) broadly reviewed research using differential reinforcement of alternative behavior, which includes variations of FCT. In fact, FCT is frequently cited as one of the few behavioral interventions having extensive support from initial efficacy studies (Smith et al., 2007).

In their review of research on differential reinforcement of alternative behavior, Petscher and colleagues (2009) identified more than 80 studies that used FCT to treat challenging behavior, met specific criteria such as being published in peer-reviewed outlets, and reported behavioral data. Those authors used the standards set by the American Psychological Association's Division 12 Task Force on the Promotion and Dissemination of Psychological Procedures to determine if FCT or its variations met the task force's criteria for interventions that are "well established," "probably efficacious," or "experimental" (Chambless et al., 1996; Task Force Promoting Dissemination of Psychological Procedures, 1995). The task force provides criteria for judging the quality of single subject design research (see Table 8.3).

Petscher and colleagues (2009) reviewed the studies meeting the task force criteria as they pertain to the demonstrated efficacy of FCT. Given the diverse nature of the behavior topographies examined, the authors decided to combine aggression, **self-injurious behavior,** property destruction, and other disruptive behaviors into a category they labeled "destructive behavior." Overall, they found that differential reinforcement of alternative behavior (DRA) in general, and FCT in specific, met the criteria for being well-established treatments for destructive behavior. This level of evidence was present whether or not extinction for challenging behavior was added as a component of the treatment (Petscher et al., 2009). They also noted that these results were obtained with few unwanted side effects across children and adults with a range of disorders. Similarly, results of a review by Kurtz and colleagues (2011) that evaluated FCT studies (using APA Division 12 and Division 16 criteria) demonstrated that FCT far exceeds criteria to be designated as a well-established treatment for a range of problem behaviors displayed by children and adolescents with ID and with ASD and can be classified as probably efficacious with adults. In addition, a meta-analysis of 36 single-case FCT studies found that FCT is highly effective in reducing challenging behavior, with verbal modes of communication appearing to be the most effective mode of communication, followed by aided AAC, and with stronger effects for children than adults (Heath et al., 2015). Moreover, in a comprehensive systematic review of evidence-based, focused intervention practices for youth with ASD, FCT was classified as an evidence-based

Table 8.3.   Criteria for empirically validated treatments using single-subject designs

Well-established treatments	I. A large series of single-case design experiments ($n > 9$) must demonstrate efficacy. These experiments must have
	  a. Used good experimental designs
	  b. Compared the intervention to another treatment and been found superior to a placebo or to the other treatment

	II. Experiments must be conducted with treatment manuals.
	III. Characteristics of the client samples must be clearly specified.
	IV. Effects must have been demonstrated by at least two different investigators or investigating teams.
Probably efficacious treatments	I. A small series of single-case design experiments ($n > 3$) must otherwise meet well-established treatment.

Source: Chambless et al. (1996).

practice (Wong et al., 2015). The results of these reviews attest to the robust nature of FCT as a treatment for a range of challenging behaviors across a number of different populations (Bambara et al., 1994; Durand & Merges, 2009; Halle et al., 2006; Heath et al., 2015; Kurtz et al., 2011; Mancil, 2006; Matson et al., 2005; Mirenda, 1997; Petscher et al., 2009; Walker et al., 2018; Wong et al., 2015). Occasional reports of unwanted effects—including using the new communication response too often—have been the focus of component analyses of FCT; the next section reviews some of this research next.

Resurgence

Although FCT has been shown to be highly effective, challenging behavior has been found to relapse in some cases, particularly when FCT is implemented by caregivers in the natural environment (e.g., Reed Schindler & Horner, 2005). If the communication response that is taught in FCT does not produce reinforcement (i.e., extinction) or is less efficient or requires more effort than the challenging behavior, then the challenging behavior will often reappear or show a resurgence (Volkert et al., 2009). Resurgence is the reemergence of a previously reinforced response (e.g., the challenging behavior) that occurs after the elimination or reduction of reinforcement for an alternative response (e.g., communication; Kimball et al., 2018). Thus, in addition to addressing response effort and efficiency, an important issue to address when using FCT is the reinforcement schedule for the alternative communication being used to replace challenging behavior. Initially, a rich schedule of reinforcement is typically recommended to ensure that acquisition of the functional communication response (FCR) occurs quickly (Durand, 1990). As we have seen, if reinforcement is delayed too long or is otherwise not sufficient, the individual will return to using challenging behavior to gain access to preferred reinforcers (e.g., escape from demands, attention from others) at an acceptable rate (Horner & Day, 1991). However, continued reinforcement of the new communication response at high rates (e.g., every time someone makes a request) can itself be viewed as problematic. Constant requests for attention, for example, can be annoying to teachers or family members, regardless of the form they take. In addition, requesting escape from work on a continual basis can seriously interfere with educational and vocational goals. These practical issues may lead teachers or parents or other intervention agents to stop reinforcing the FCR (i.e., extinction) or thin the schedule of reinforcement for the FCR too quickly, either of which may lead to a resurgence of challenging behavior. For example, Wacker and colleagues (2011) found that, following FCT, which successfully reduced problem behavior by replacing it with a request, even brief periods of extinction led to resurgence of problem behavior.

Although some studies have approached schedule thinning by removing the alternative response (e.g., an exchangeable FCT card) during periods in which reinforcement is unavailable (e.g., Fisher et al., 2014; Roane et al., 2004), results from a study by Kimball and colleagues (2018) suggest that higher levels of resurgence may actually occur during response restriction than when the alternative response is available. Specifically, they found that resurgence may occur at higher rates if the alternative response is absent (e.g., if a picture card is lost or an AAC device is broken) compared to if the recently reinforced alternative response is present but placed on extinction (e.g., a parent or teacher stops responding to a functional communication response). This finding suggests that special consideration should be given to the topography of the FCR that is selected in order to prevent or mitigate resurgence.

In addition to altering reinforcement schedules, Saini and colleagues (2018) proposed several suggestions for avoiding or mitigating resurgence when FCT is introduced into the natural environment, including the following:

- Using noticeable discriminative stimuli (e.g., wristbands) to establish stimulus control over FCRs (e.g., green wristband signals availability of reinforcement for FCR, red wristband signals unavailability of reinforcement) and transferring those stimuli to generalization contexts (Fisher et al., 2015)

- Making the FCT training environment more similar to the natural environment by transferring treatment stimuli (e.g., classroom curricular materials) across contexts

- Using multiple FCT trainers and/or introducing FCT into multiple contexts before implementing FCT in the generalization context

- Having caregivers implement FCT alongside therapists

- Introducing FCT directly into the context in which the problem behavior generally occurs, such as the parent implementing FCT at home

Almost all of these strategies suggest that, in some cases, it may be necessary to explicitly program for maintenance and generalization of the FCR (Ringdahl & St. Peter, 2017), which has received scant attention in the literature. A review by Neely and colleagues (2018) synthesized 37 studies evaluating the maintenance and generalization of behavioral change achieved through FCT for individuals with developmental disability; of the six studies that met all maintenance and generalization standards that also met What Works Clearinghouse design standards, five did not implement any additional strategies beyond contacting natural contingencies (which is inherent in FCT). This suggests that, although there is substantial research on the acquisition of FCRs, there is a lack of research that focuses on the maintenance and generalization of learned communication skills. Explicitly programming for generalization and maintenance (i.e., Stokes & Baer, 1977) could make it less likely that problem behavior will resurge or reappear following successful FCT. At the same time, it is important to consider what the prevailing environment can support. As we discussed in the previous section on response milieu, some environments can support relatively high rates of requests and others cannot. Research on contextual fit with regard to requests for reinforcement and the environment's ability to maintain responses should be an important next step in researching the nature of responses to appropriate requests for reinforcement in FCT.

Consequences for Challenging Behavior

A somewhat controversial concern related to FCT use involves the issue of how to respond to the challenging behavior itself. As noted previously, evidence suggests that FCT is effective with or without extinction for the challenging behavior (Petscher et al., 2009). In work with FCT strategy (Durand, 1990), response-independent consequences have been used as the primary reactive. In other words, communication partners try (as much as possible) to continue to behave with the person as if the challenging behavior did not occur. The goal is to make the challenging behavior nonfunctional in the environment. For example, a therapist working with the person who screams tries to continue working. If the person is alone and starts to have a tantrum, intervention is resisted. Also avoided are what might be perceived as negative consequences, such as reprimands or withdrawing attention, because these may also serve as reinforcers for some individuals. At the same time that an alternative communication behavior is taught, the therapist should try to make the challenging behavior less efficient (nonfunctional) as a strategy for obtaining reinforcers.

A caveat is in order when using response-independent consequences. The protection of individuals demonstrating challenge behavior and those around them remain the most important priority. In other words, although altering the therapist's behaviors as a function of the person's challenging behavior is generally to be avoided, steps to protect all involved are taken when the behaviors are dangerous to the individual or others. Such intervention is always conducted in as neutral a manner as possible to limit the changes in the environment.

Several studies have directly examined the issue of continuing reinforcement for the challenging behavior. One study looked at whether FCT would be an effective approach if the challenging behavior continued to be reinforced while an alternative response was being taught (Shirley et al., 1997). For three individuals who engaged in self-injurious behavior, manual signing was used as the alternative communication response. The researchers found that self-injury was not initially reduced if it continued to be reinforced concurrently with the new alternative. However, once extinction was initiated for the challenging behaviors, these behaviors were reduced and signing was increased. Even when extinction was suspended for self-injury, the behavior problems remained at low levels for two of the three individuals (Shirley et al., 1997). Wacker and colleagues (1990) described the use of FCT with three individuals and the use of specific consequences with two of these people. It was observed that hand biting and aggression in these two individuals were significantly reduced with a package of procedures including FCT and negative consequences (TO for one person, graduated guidance for a second participant). The authors observed that when they attempted to remove the negative consequences as part of the package, the challenging behaviors increased. It was concluded that some individuals may require mild forms of negative consequences, at least initially.

It is difficult to interpret why individuals in the previous research and the third participant in this study did not require negative consequences to reduce their challenging behavior (Wacker et al., 1990). One interpretation mentioned by the authors is that introducing the negative consequences from the beginning of their treatment may have affected their later behavior. It is possible that if the negative consequences were never introduced concurrently with FCT, these consequences may not have been required to reduce their challenging behavior. These data suggest that behavioral contrast (the tendency to evaluate situations compared to how these situations have been presented previously) may have been at work in this study—with the effectiveness of FCT alone influenced by the removal of the contingencies for challenging behavior (i.e., TO and graduated guidance). For example, if a student is used to getting reinforced frequently and the reinforcement is abruptly ended when starting FCT, the success of this approach might initially be limited, because the reinforcers expected might be reduced when compared to before FCT. This issue points to the need to be cautious in implementing and interpreting such intervention packages.

One goal in FCT is to make the new communication response more efficient than the challenging behavior at receiving reinforcers. As discussed previously, one way to accomplish this goal is to teach a response that is, right from the start, *more* efficient than the challenging behavior. However, as this section suggests, another avenue to pursue is to make the challenging behavior *less* efficient than the communicative response. Work such as that of Durand (1990) has been aimed at accomplishing this by removing the contingency between the challenging behavior and the therapist's behavior using response-independent consequences.

Outcome Research

Although there is an extensive body of published research assessing the effectiveness of FCT, the vast majority of these studies employ single-case designs with a small number of participants in each study. Although several larger studies exist (e.g., Durand & Carr, 1992; Hagopian et al., 1998; Kurtz et al., 2003; Wacker et al., 1998), there are to date no randomized clinical trials comparing outcomes of FCT to no treatment, treatment as usual, or other traditional techniques. This reliance on a single category of research design may limit understanding of FCT as an intervention.

Several potential limitations on the generalizability of single-subject design results relate to descriptive information about methods that are routinely described in randomized clinical trials but are rarely included in single-subject design studies. For instance, how individuals are selected for participation in treatment studies can potentially have a significant impact on the interpretation of the results. For example, selecting for parent training only families who will pay clinical fees out of pocket and who will faithfully attend numerous and long training sessions may limit the extent to which the results can be generalized to families of low socioeconomic status and families who are less involved. Similarly, including only those individuals referred to a clinic known for working with young children with mild behavior problems may limit the study's usefulness with older individuals with more severe challenges. Selection bias—systematically including certain participants in research (and therefore excluding others)—can artificially influence the results in a positive or negative way. One method for reducing selection bias that is used in group experimental research studies involves random assignment to treatment groups. Randomization helps improve internal validity by reducing systematic bias in assignment, although it does not necessarily eliminate all bias in the groups, especially if they are small (Barlow & Hersen, 1984). How do researchers using single-subject designs select the participants for their research studies?

To attempt to answer this question, a review of the behavioral intervention literature was conducted to more accurately gauge these rates (Durand & Rost, 2005). The review of 149 research articles published in the *Journal of Applied Behavior Analysis* from 1968 to 2001 found that only 26.04% (44 out of 169) indicated any selection criteria, and the percentage of experiments addressing selection bias was 8.28% (14 out of 169). The percentage of experiments that noted attrition was 2.37% (4 out of 169), and the percentage of experiments that addressed attrition bias was 0%. There were no trends suggesting a significant increase in reporting this information in more contemporary research studies.

Overall, a relatively low number of these single-subject design studies mentioned how studies were selected for inclusion (26%), and fewer still mentioned whether procedures to reduce selection bias were used. Almost none of the studies published over the past three decades indicated whether participants dropped out of treatment prematurely (3%), and of those few studies that did so, none assessed for any potential subject characteristics that would predict differential attrition. In addition, none of the articles reported whether potential participants and/or guardians refused to be included in their treatment studies. This relative lack of information on potential selection bias and attrition calls into question the generalizability of otherwise positive outcome data on the treatment of challenging behavior.

The culture in single-subject design research rarely addresses population issues, an essential concern for issues of clinical efficacy and utility (Smith et al., 2007). For example, one handbook on single-subject research methods recommends that researchers select only those participants who will reliably show up for sessions (Bailey & Burch, 2002). Although this is a practical suggestion, its consequences—studying only highly motivated and reliable people—limits conclusions about the larger population of people who request our help. The report from the National Institutes of Health (NIH)–sponsored meeting on methodological challenges in psychosocial interventions in ASD (Lord et al., 2005) addresses this issue and lists the need for additional randomized clinical trials in this area as the highest priority.

An important caveat involves representativeness of the treatment literature. The lack of information in these areas cannot be interpreted to suggest that there are significant biases in selection and attrition. We do not know, for example, if the intervention research systematically excludes certain individuals, which in turn improperly influences the results and leaves the research literature open to substantial criticism. To address these serious concerns, research on FCT and other behavioral interventions for challenging behavior must be subjected to scrutiny that examines these population-related questions (Durand & Rost, 2005).

PRACTICAL REQUIREMENTS

There are a number of reasons why the act of teaching communication to individuals with severe challenging behavior is difficult—the most obvious of which is the challenging behavior itself. Trying to teach someone who is hitting the teacher, is hitting him- or herself, or is generally disruptive in the teaching situation is, at best, very frustrating and provides a rationale for using restrictive procedures: On the assumption that no teaching can take place while the person continues to engage in disruptive behavior, a temporary program is recommended using some form of aversive consequence to reduce the frequency of the challenging behavior. The reasoning continues that once the rate of such behavior is reduced, teaching can finally be carried out.

Efforts at teaching communication strategies to individuals exhibiting challenging behavior can begin prior to reductions in these behavior problems, using teaching efforts adapted so they can continue despite the behavior problems. When possible, therapists should set up the teaching situation so that behavior problems are minimized. Challenging behavior should not be viewed as a major barrier to teaching communication.

A second obstacle to teaching communication lies in the training of those who work daily with individuals with ASD, many of whom do not have extensive training in how to teach communication skills. It is common, for example, that relatively few training resources are available to teach how to properly fade a prompt or to set up the environment to encourage communication interactions (Durand,

1987). Extraordinary effort is required to successfully intervene with severe behavior problems. This is true whether it involves training and safeguards in the use of restrictive procedures, which will be an ongoing, disheartening task, or training and monitoring of programs involving teaching alternative skills, which can often yield more satisfying interactions for all of those involved.

Scheduling Teaching Opportunities

Once the function of the challenging behavior and an appropriate replacement communication skill are determined, one person typically takes responsibility for initial communication training. Time commitments can be as short as 30–60 minutes per day several days per week. However, an ideal teaching strategy creates numerous teaching opportunities throughout the day in typical settings. For example, if a student in a classroom screams in response to frustrating situations, one strategy is to program minor frustrating situations throughout the student's day. Specifically, clinicians might plan to have his or her typical routines interrupted in order to create teaching opportunities. For example, the student would be prompted to open a desk drawer to take out his or her favorite toy. However, the clinician would have taped the drawer closed, making it difficult to open. As soon as the student found he or she could not open the drawer, the clinician would prompt him or her to request assistance ("Say, 'help me'"). Similar scenarios would be repeated in multiple situations and settings (e.g., putting on his or her coat, opening the door to go outside, tying his or her shoes), and all of the adults who came in contact with the child would be taught how to prompt him or her. As important, moreover, they would also be taught how to fade their prompts.

Training throughout the day is referred to as *distributed practice* (Gaylord-Ross & Holvoet, 1985). Distributed practice allows students to engage in other activities between teaching trials. This method is in contrast to *massed practice*, which involves presenting teaching trials one after another, with limited interruptions. Most teaching occurs somewhere along a continuum from highly massed practice (very little time between teaching trials) to highly distributed practice (long delays between trials). Because opportunities to make requests occur at varying times throughout the day, distributed practice more closely resembles these interactions and is therefore preferred when possible.

Despite these advantages, initial use of highly distributed practice with some students may be problematic. Because distributed practice may involve fewer trials (although it does not have to), the opportunities to learn the skill may be sporadic. Acquisition may be slow, creating problems for students who may become disruptive to avoid such training situations. In addition, training for staff in how to identify and use intermittent teaching opportunities may be unavailable in many settings.

Because of these limitations, we have often begun training using more frequent teaching trials in a concentrated period of time. We use this approach to ensure rapid acquisition and because we are often faced with situations in which skilled trainers are available for a limited period of time during the day. For example, there may be one work supervisor who knows the learner best and who is most capable of carrying out training. However, this person may be available for only 30 minutes each day to conduct teaching sessions. In these situations, the training should be set up so that the supervisor could conduct a number of trials during that 30-minute period. Trials typically would be interspersed with breaks, opportunities to manipulate requested objects, or time for access to social interactions. The environment is arranged to create opportunities for communication (e.g., putting an obstacle in the path of a student's wheelchair and prompting him or her to ask for assistance). However, distributing sessions across the day would not occur until there was some initial communication success for the student. At that point, the training arrangements might lie somewhere in the middle of the massed practice or distributed practice continuum. As soon as possible, however, training trials should be interspersed throughout the student's day (Durand, 1990).

Choosing Contexts for Teaching

The settings or contexts in which such teaching takes place can also be viewed on a continuum from highly artificial contexts (e.g., teaching social interactions with peers in a therapist's office) to more natural contexts (e.g., teaching social interactions with peers at a party). The naturalness of the setting depends largely on where clinicians want the student to use the new communication response. Using the criterion environment (i.e., where clinicians want the student to communicate) as the training environment may facilitate generalization and maintenance of intervention effects. With the typical model of teaching skills in a separate setting (e.g., in the speech therapist's office), once the response is learned, clinicians need to encourage the performance of that behavior in settings where they want it to occur (e.g., in the cafeteria). By beginning training in the natural or criterion setting, extensive programming for generalization is not necessary because it will be occurring where clinicians want it to occur. In addition, obstacles to maintenance can be immediately identified when teaching in the criterion environment (e.g., are the consequences being provided in that setting going to maintain the new response?).

KEY COMPONENTS

Table 8.2 and Figure 8.1 illustrate the key components used to assess behavior and conduct FCT. These steps can often be complicated. Refer to the Suggested Readings for more detailed instructions.

Step 1. Assess the Function of Behavior

To assess the function of a challenging behavior, clinicians must first identify the antecedents and consequences of that behavior. Once clinicians understand the purpose of a targeted behavior, they can teach individuals to request the variables previously obtained by the challenging behavior. The previous section on assessment provides recommendations for conducting this important aspect of FCT.

Step 2. Select the Communication Modality

Once clinicians identify the function of the challenging behavior, they need to determine the type of response to encourage from the individual. If the individual already has some facility in a mode of communication (e.g., verbal, signing), clinicians should consider that mode for FCT. Usually, if an individual has been unsuccessful in learning to communicate effectively after extensive verbal language training, clinicians should use an alternative signing or symbolic mode. If the person has also been unsuccessful with sign language training (e.g., has not learned to sign or uses poorly demonstrated or incomprehensible signs), clinicians should try graphic symbolic communication training, at least initially. Symbolic communication training can involve the use of picture books, tokens with messages written on them, or other assistive devices in which symbol selection occurs visually (e.g., vocal output devices). This form of communication training has the advantage of being relatively easy to teach and is universally recognizable to potential communication partners.

Step 3. Create Teaching Situations

As a next step, clinicians arrange the environment to create opportunities for communication (e.g., putting an obstacle in the way of a person trying to open a door and prompting him or her to ask for assistance). This use of incidental teaching (Hart & Risley, 1975; McGee et al., 1999; McGee & Daly, 2007)—that is, arranging the environment to establish situations that elicit interest and that are used as teaching opportunities—is an important part of successful communication training. Using the person's interest in some interaction, whether it be a desire to stop working on a difficult task or to elicit the attention of an adult, is a powerful tool in teaching generalized communication.

As soon as possible and where appropriate, clinicians intersperse training trials throughout the individual's day. Using the criterion environment (i.e., where clinicians want the person to communicate) as the training environment facilitates generalization and maintenance of intervention effects. In addition, clinicians can immediately identify obstacles to maintenance when teaching in the criterion environment (e.g., the interventionist can determine whether the consequences being provided in that setting are going to maintain the new response).

Step 4. Prompt Communication

Teaching individuals to communicate, as a replacement for their challenging behavior, requires a range of sophisticated language training techniques (Durand et al., 1999). Clinicians use a multiphase prompting and prompt-fading procedure to teach the new communication response. They introduce prompts as necessary, then fade them as quickly as possible. Some learners negatively resist attempts to be taught important skills (e.g., the individual screams and kicks), others positively resist (e.g., the individual laughs and giggles instead of working), and still others passively resist (e.g., the individual does not look at materials, makes no response). When an individual kicks, screams, and rips up work materials whenever they are presented or passively ignores efforts to get him or her to attend to a task, teaching becomes a difficult challenge and learning becomes highly unlikely.

One procedure is to teach the individual to request assistance (e.g., "Help me") or a brief break from work. Often, the challenging behaviors appear to be attempts to avoid or escape from unpleasant situations. It makes sense, then, that if the clinician teaches the individual to appropriately request assistance and then the individual receives it, the task will seem easier and challenging behaviors should be reduced. Similarly, if an individual has been working for some time on a task and is allowed to ask for a break and receives it, this individual's challenging behavior should also be reduced.

Step 5. Fade Prompts

Clinicians begin pulling back their prompts by fading them as soon as possible. When necessary, fading can involve going from a full physical prompt to partial prompts (e.g., just touching the hand), to gestural prompts (e.g., motioning to encourage use of the hands), to finally, only the verbal prompt (e.g., "Say 'break'" or just "Break") (see Figure 8.2). Throughout training, clinicians rely heavily on delayed prompting as another method of fading (Halle et al., 1981; Kratzer & Spooner, 1993; Schwartz et al., 1989; Walker, 2008). After several trials, clinicians can intersperse a trial with a delayed prompt (e.g., wait approximately 5 seconds) to see if the person will respond without the next level of prompt. For example, if a boy had been responding to just a touch of his hand to prompt the use of sign, clinicians would make a gesture as if they were going to prompt him, then wait 5 seconds. If he made the sign for BREAK, then clinicians would let him go on the break.

Clinicians do not wait until responding is extremely stable to move on to the next level of prompting. In other words, someone does not have to be correctly responding to, say, 9 out of 10 prompts for 2 weeks for us to move to the next step. Clinicians would attempt to move to the next step if a person is successful at a step for three to five consecutive response opportunities. Clinicians do this in order to prevent individuals from becoming prompt dependent (i.e., too reliant on prompts to respond). Challenging behavior typically improves most dramatically as soon as the person begins to make requests without prompts.

Step 6. Teach New Communication Responses

Once successful, intervention continues by introducing new forms of communication (e.g., requests for food, music, work) while at the same time reintroducing work demands or expanding the settings in which requests are made and introducing new staff into the training program.

Step 7. Modify the Environment

Recommendations are often made concerning environmental and curricula changes. Several authors have described scenarios in which an individual was found to engage in challenging behavior in the presence of certain stimuli, such as certain

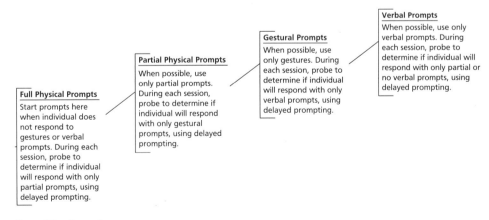

Full Physical Prompts
Start prompts here when individual does not respond to gestures or verbal prompts. During each session, probe to determine if individual will respond with only partial prompts, using delayed prompting.

Partial Physical Prompts
When possible, use only partial prompts. During each session, probe to determine if individual will respond with only gestural prompts, using delayed prompting.

Gestural Prompts
When possible, use only gestures. During each session, probe to determine if individual will respond with only verbal prompts, using delayed prompting.

Verbal Prompts
When possible, use only verbal prompts. During each session, probe to determine if individual will respond with only partial or no verbal prompts, using delayed prompting.

Figure 8.2. Prompting sequence.

instructional programs or certain staff (e.g., Barratt et al., 2012; Blakeley-Smith & Carr, 2009; Carr et al., 1997; Dunlap et al., 1991; Kennedy & Itkonen, 1993). Therefore, when students who participate in this program are observed to engage in challenging behavior when directed to participate in nonfunctional or age-inappropriate activities (e.g., stringing beads), we recommend that they no longer be required to work on these tasks. Instead, we suggest alternatives that might be more useful and engaging.

ASSESSMENT FOR TREATMENT PLANNING AND PROGRESS MONITORING

Data collection within FCT is conducted to serve four phases associated with successful intervention (Durand & Hieneman, 2008a, 2008b): establishing goals, analyzing patterns of behavior, assessing obstacles in the environment, and monitoring results (see Figure 8.1).

The establishing goals phase involves collecting sufficient information to define the problem, including the person's behaviors of concern and specific changes that are desired at home, at school, or in the community. During the beginning stages of program planning, we typically employ the use of interviews and formal checklists (e.g., the Scales of Independent Behavior–Revised [SIB-R]; Bruininks et al., 1996) to determine the nature and extent of the problems.

The analyzing patterns phase involves using various forms of functional assessment to understand why the person is behaving in this manner (see previous section describing functional assessments).

Concurrent with assessing the behavior of the targeted person, in the assessing obstacles phase, we informally assess the learning environment to determine if it will support the new communication responses (see Response Milieu section). In addition, we assess attitudinal obstacles that may be present in family members or educators that can interfere with successful intervention (see Future Directions section; Durand & Hieneman, 2008a, 2008b).

During the monitoring results phase, we train responsible individuals (e.g., instructional aides, interventionists) to collect data on challenging behavior, communication, and educational progress to ensure that the strategies are working. Data collection continues in order to assess whether changes in the plan are needed (see Durand & Hieneman [2008a] for an extensive discussion and sample data forms).

IMPLICATIONS FOR INCLUSIVE PRACTICE

There are numerous studies in which parents implement FCT at home (e.g., Berg et al., 2007; Derby et al., 1997; Dunlap et al., 2006; Harding et al., 2009; Moes & Frea, 2002; Schieltz et al., 2011; Wacker et al., 2005; Wacker et al., 2008; Wacker et al., 2011) and teachers implement FCT in special education classrooms (e.g., Davis et al., 2012; Durand, 1993, 1999; Flynn & Lo, 2016; Lambert et al., 2012; O'Neill & Sweetland-Baker, 2001). In addition, several studies have evaluated FCT in an inclusive school setting (e.g., Casey & Merical, 2006; Gibson et al., 2010; Mildon et. al., 2004; O'Neill & Sweetland-Baker, 2001; Umbreit, 1996).

In illustration, Casey and Merical (2006) implemented FCT with Karl, an 11-year-old boy with autism and average intelligence who was in the sixth grade at a rural middle school. Karl received instruction in a resource room for two class periods and for the rest of the day was integrated into general education classes with a full-time aide. All assessments and treatment conditions were conducted in Karl's general education classrooms. A brief functional analysis indicated that Karl's self-injury served the function of escaping or avoiding demands. During treatment, Karl was taught to ask for a break using either the verbal response "I would like a break, please," or the gestural response of a sticky note with the same written phrase. A preference assessment revealed that Karl preferred using the gestural response to the verbal response, likely because of his apprehensiveness about public speaking. Of note, Karl's aide initially provided verbal prompts every 1 to 5 minutes, although the aide discontinued prompts 3 days into intervention at Karl's request (because he understood what he needed to do if he wanted a break). This is noteworthy because it is possible that prompts from an aide might be more stigmatizing in an inclusive setting than in a special education setting.

It is also important to note that, during FCT, Casey and Merical (2006) did not use extinction, meaning that a brief escape (45–60 seconds) was allowed after self-injury in intervention just as in baseline. A multiple baseline (across classrooms) design was used to evaluate the effects of the FCT intervention. Results indicated that Karl's self-injury was ameliorated with FCT alone, without any augmentative procedures, providing evidence that FCT can be successful without using extinction or punishment, even though Karl could still obtain escape through self-injury. This is important, given that it is particularly critical to use the least intrusive intervention (without sacrificing effectiveness) in inclusive classroom settings. Further, whereas most studies using FCT in inclusive school environments do not provide long-term follow-up results, Casey and Merical observed no occurrences of self-injury at 5-, 12-, and 24-month follow-ups, supporting the durability of the effects of FCT.

One promising direction in terms of facilitating the use of FCT in inclusive settings and other natural environments is the use of telehealth to train parents or teachers to implement FCT. For families or teachers or other providers who live far away from behavior analysts who can train them in FCT, or who encounter transportation or other logistical barriers to receiving training in FCT, being trained by a professional via the Internet in their own homes or classrooms can promote the use of FCT in formerly difficult-to-reach settings and populations. Wacker and colleagues have successfully conducted FCT via telehealth with parents of children with ASD (Suess et al., 2014; Wacker et al., 2013), and Gibson and colleagues (2010) demonstrated the effectiveness of FCT delivered via distance videoconference for a boy with autism in an inclusive preschool program. On a positive note, Wacker and colleagues (2013) reported that very similar effects of FCT occur when it is delivered via telehealth as when it is delivered in vivo. Although there were many instances of fidelity problems (with the most typical being parents not reinforcing appropriate behavior), the fidelity problems did not appear to have a detrimental effect on treatment outcome (Suess et al., 2014). That said, Wacker and colleagues (2017) cautioned that these fidelity problems should still be cause for concern regarding the long-term maintenance of the effects of FCT.

CONSIDERATIONS FOR CHILDREN FROM CULTURALLY AND LINGUISTICALLY DIVERSE BACKGROUNDS

Treating challenging behavior in children from culturally and linguistically diverse backgrounds can pose unique challenges when using FCT. Cultural and linguistic factors might affect the outcomes of FCT as a result of response effort, the child's preference for specific types of communication, and the quality of attention provided by the parent (Padilla Dalmau et al., 2011) as well as affect the types of communication responses that parents consider to be acceptable. In addition to influencing *how* FCT is implemented, cultural variables may also impact *whether* parents choose to implement FCT in the first place. Mandell and Novak (2005) noted that culture influences parents' beliefs about the causes of their children's problem behavior, their choice of possible intervention strategies, and prognosis of the intervention effectiveness. For example, if parents of children with ASD are more likely to believe their child cannot control his or her challenging behavior, they may be more likely to engage in lax parenting (e.g., backing down and giving in when their child gets upset; Berliner et al., 2020) rather than trying to teach their child a functional communication response or any other skill.

In terms of linguistic diversity, if, for example, a child's teacher speaks only English at school and the family speaks only Spanish at home, home–school communication may be affected and teaching the student a communication strategy that will be successful in both environments can be difficult, if not impossible. One strategy to use in cases of a mismatch between home and school languages is to rely on augmentative and alternative communication strategies, such as picture books or vocal output devices. In past research, we used vocal output devices programmed in both languages to teach students functionally equivalent responses (e.g., "help me") (Durand, 1999; Durand & Berotti, 1991). We have, in essence, taught students with severe and multiple disabilities to be bilingual—making a single selection that is realized in the language appropriate to the language context. These devices have permitted us to teach students to make relatively simple responses (pressing a pad on the machine) that can result in sophisticated output (full sentences) in clear, spoken English and Spanish. Again, because the output can be recognized by anyone within a particular language community, the success of the communication training has been extended more broadly into the community.

Application to a Child

Hal was a 9-year-old boy who was attending a school for students with developmental disabilities (Durand & Carr, 1991). Teachers reported that Hal frequently became upset at varying times during the day, typically in response to requests he found difficult to respond to and when he could not answer a question presented to him. He would violently slap his face and scream, ultimately falling to the floor. He had some verbal ability, although he would frequently talk rapidly and unclearly.

As a first step, clinicians decided to teach Hal to say, "I don't understand," in response to questions for which he didn't have an answer. After several weeks of this training, he would reliably and spontaneously use this communication strategy, and the frequency of face slapping and screaming was substantially reduced. A follow-up observation of Hal several months later in a new classroom and with a different teacher, however, revealed that he was again slapping his face and screaming and rarely using the trained phrase.

Clinicians observed Hal with his new teacher and clearly saw what was wrong. His teacher would ask a question such as "Hal, what's your address?" At times, Hal would say, "I don't understand," but very quickly and unintelligibly. Because the teacher didn't understand what he was saying, she did not provide him with sufficient prompts. After several interactions like this, Hal would eventually get upset, hit himself, and begin screaming. His teacher would respond by leaving him, saying she would return when he calmed down. In short, the teacher not only failed to respond to his statement but also appeared to be reinforcing his behavior by ending the task (negative reinforcement).

The intervention involved working to help Hal slow down and better articulate the phrase "I don't understand." Clinicians did this without informing his teacher to see if she would respond appropriately to his phrase when it was intelligible. After the training, clinicians again observed Hal in the classroom. They found that his speech was more understandable and that the teacher would now provide prompts for him (e.g., "Say, 'I live at 25 Smith Street'") when he said he did not understand. In addition, his self-injury and screaming was reduced. An additional follow-up observation 12 months later found that Hal was using the phrase and behaving appropriately in the classroom.

Application to an Adult

Bill, who was 32 years old, was engaging in severe aggression (punching and grabbing others), self-injurious behavior (hand and arm biting), and other disruptive behaviors (throwing work materials, knocking over tables and chairs). He had lived most of his life in a large institution. Bill had recently moved from the institution to a group home and was attending a vocational education program through a local agency.

The vocational program was concerned because Bill was making minimal progress and, on occasion, would seriously hurt staff members. An analysis of ABC charts along with administrations of the Motivation Assessment Scale indicated that his aggression and self-injury may have been maintained by both escape from demands and access to tangibles (e.g., favorite foods). Clinicians decided to begin by teaching him the sign for BREAK and allowing him to take time away from work if he asked. A request to leave work was selected as opposed to a request for tangibles because the work demands appeared to evoke the most frequent and severe outbursts. A request for a break was chosen over a request for assistance because he had no difficulty completing the work (i.e., it wasn't difficult) and because, at a job site, it was more appropriate to request a period of time away from work than to request help.

Bill's response to initial training efforts was characteristic of many individuals. He was fine during the prompting and while he was taking a break (see Figure 8.2). However, when clinicians attempted to bring him back to work, he resisted. Occasionally, he would hit the trainer or passively resist efforts to get back to the work table. During these times, the trainer firmly led Bill back to work in a neutral manner, with no reprimands or lengthy explanations. Bill's resistance quickly abated over several sessions. It appeared as though Bill learned that if he went right back to work, he could escape it within a short amount of time.

Clinicians did not wait until Bill's responding was extremely stable to move on to the next level of prompting. In other words, Bill did not have to be correctly responding to 9 out of 10 prompts for 2 weeks, for example, for clinicians to move to the next step. They would attempt to move to the next step if he was successful at a step for three to five consecutive responses. Clinicians did this to prevent him from becoming prompt dependent (i.e., too reliant on prompts to respond).

Training progressed quickly over several weeks to the point that Bill would sign for a break with only the pulling back of the work as a prompt. This too was faded, and within 3 months, he was requesting a break without any cues by the trainer. As is typical, his behavior improved most dramatically as soon as he began to make requests without prompts.

Once successful, intervention continued by introducing new signs (e.g., food, music, work), reintroducing work demands, expanding the settings in which his signs were encouraged to include his whole day, and introducing new staff into the training program. These latter steps were introduced systematically to avoid having Bill become disruptive. Nine months after initial intervention, the number of episodes of aggression and self-injury was significantly decreased, Bill was using a large number of signs spontaneously throughout the day, and he was working at a level that exceeded his preintervention performance.

> **To review an extended application and implementation of this intervention, see Case 5 about a child with ASD in the companion volume *Case Studies for the Treatment of Autism Spectrum Disorder*.**

Future Directions

The extensive body of evidence accumulated over the past 30 plus years since we first introduced FCT as an intervention (Carr & Durand, 1985; Durand & Moskowitz, 2015) points to its success in reducing challenging behavior. However, we are finding that up to 50% of the families and teachers with whom we work are not able to fully carry out this (or any other) intervention. Evidence is growing that parents differ in their perceptions of themselves (e.g., feeling out of control or inadequate as a parent), their child with a disability (e.g., whether their child is capable of making behavioral improvements), and their degree of optimism about future prospects for change. Their perceptions, in turn, influence their ability to implement the interventions professionals design for them. And professionals know this. Most have worked with families who willingly do anything asked of them and other families who actively resist their suggestions (e.g., "That won't work with my child," "We've tried that already") or passively (e.g., not completing assessments, missing multiple training sessions). Yet, rather than view the unsuccessful families as needing a different approach, many clinicians eventually write off those families as being uncooperative or noncompliant (or worse, as bad parents).

Typically, the fallback assumption for families who struggle with intervention plans is that they need additional support. There is a long history of recommending support for families in the form of financial assistance, respite services, and parent support groups to help reduce some of the obstacles to successful intervention. Although these are important considerations, our experience is that these efforts are less effective with families who are highly pessimistic—perhaps 50% of the families with whom we work (Durand, 2007). Respite, for example, is used as a temporary reprieve for these families rather than an opportunity to learn new skills or prepare them to become reinvolved with their children. Parent support groups are often viewed as negative experiences. For family members who already feel guilty about their performance as parents, being in the company of parents perceived as more successful—for example, those who seem unmoved by people in the supermarket who comment on their misbehaving child—results in even more negative self-talk and pessimism. Families with pessimistic views need very specific intervention to assist them to become engaged in behavioral parent training.

Our recent work addresses the needs of these families by integrating cognitive behavioral interventions (optimism training) with behavioral parent training (positive behavioral support)—a new treatment approach referred to as *Positive Family Intervention* (Durand & Hieneman, 2008a). In this approach, parents are not only taught to better understand and treat their child's challenging behavior, but to become aware of their thoughts and feelings about themselves and their child and how these might interfere with success. Tailoring behavioral parent training to meet the particular needs of the family as well as the child leads to highly successful child behavior outcomes (Durand et al., 2009). Continuing research in this area promises to broaden the benefits associated with FCT to a larger group of individuals and families involved with FCT and over a longer period of time.

In addition to research on those who implement FCT, continuing research is needed in other aspects of FCT. For example, the issue of response acceptability (how individuals in the student's environment respond to new communication forms) is a potentially fruitful and important research topic. A related topic is the aspect of FCT referred to as response milieu (the nature of the environment in which the student is communicating). Both of these areas lack any systematic study, yet they are essential to the success of this treatment approach. To guide intervention efforts in this area, more research is needed to assess environments (e.g., how others will respond to a request for assistance) and whether and when to change the communication form or the environment itself (e.g., switching classrooms to one that is more accepting of requests for choices). Answers to these types of questions will likely result in even more successful outcomes for individuals with challenging behavior.

Suggested Readings

1. Durand, V. M. (1990). *Severe behavior problems: A functional communication training approach.* Guilford Press. This is the first book to describe functional communication training. It includes extensive case examples that illustrate how to assess and intervene with significant challenging behaviors in individuals with a broad range of abilities (from those who are very verbal to individuals with no functional communication skills). Step-by-step instructions are included for all assessment and intervention activities.

2. Durand, V. M., & Hieneman, M. (2008). *Helping parents with challenging children: Positive family intervention: Facilitator guide* and *Helping parents with challenging children: Positive family intervention: Parent workbook.* Oxford University Press. These books are the treatment protocols used to help families with their challenging child—one designed for therapists and the other for parents. Behavioral interventions (including FCT) are outlined along with how to change attitudes to assist with implementing these procedures (optimism training).

3. Reichle, J., & Wacker, D. P. (2017). *Functional communication training for problem behavior.* Guilford Press. This book provides a comprehensive approach to using FCT. Geared especially to professionals, it provides complete step-by-step instructions on how to conduct functional assessments and how to develop behavior intervention plans with FCT.

Learning Activities

1. Topics for further discussion

    • Discuss when you would not recommend using FCT for the treatment of challenging behaviors.

    • How would you address the following comment shared by a teacher or family member: "This will not work for my student/child!"

    • What does the information about functional equivalence suggest about programs that rely primarily on punishment to reduce the frequency of challenging behaviors?

2. Ideas for projects

    • Select an individual who is engaging in problem behavior and try to determine why these problems are occurring, including identifying the situations that seem to trigger outbursts.

    • Make a list of how family members and/or friends deal with frustrating situations (both the positive strategies, e.g., asking for help, and the unproductive strategies, e.g., yelling, blaming others), and describe how their positive strategies could be modified for individuals with ASD.

3. Questions about the reading material

    • What are the functional categories specifically covered on the Motivation Assessment Scale?

    • Regarding challenging behavior, the current emphasis is on _____ (i.e., what motivates the behavior) rather than on _____ (i.e., what the behavior looks like).

    • Julie continues to scream at home because her parents spend time with her during these outbursts (i.e., they sit beside her and try to calm her). What appears to be a factor in maintaining Julie's screaming behavior?

    • Angela's teacher keeps Angela close by her side throughout the day as Angela participates in her school tasks and activities. She finds that Angela seldom engages in problem behavior. Given this information, what would be your best guess of the function of Angela's behavior?

    • What are the steps used in functional communication training?

4. Writing assignments

    • Write a paper on the controversy over the use of punishment, especially for those individuals with ASD. Be sure to include issues of ethics as well as evidence for effectiveness.

    • FCT was described as a well-established treatment. Write a paper describing the issue of using only evidence-based treatments. Include a discussion about when it might be appropriate to use techniques that currently lack empirical support but may be useful for an individual with ASD.

REFERENCES

Bailey, J. S., & Burch, M. R. (2002). *Research methods in applied behavior analysis*. Sage Publications.

Bambara, L. M., Mitchell-Kvacky, N. A., & Iacobelli, S. (1994). Positive behavioral support for students with severe disabilities—an emerging multicomponent approach for addressing challenging behaviors. *School Psychology Review, 23*(2), 263–278.

Barlow, D. H., & Hersen, M. (1984). *Single case experimental design: Strategies for studying behavior change* (2nd ed.). Pergamon Press.

Barratt, N., McGill, P., & Hughes, C. (2012). Antecedent influences on challenging behaviour: A preliminary assessment of the reliability, generalisability and validity of the Ecological Interview. *International Journal of Positive Behavioural Support, 2*(2), 31–41.

Berg, W. K., Wacker, D. P., Harding, J. W., Ganzer, J., & Barretto, A. (2007). An evaluation of multiple dependent variables across distinct classes of antecedent stimuli pre and post functional communication training. *Journal of Early and Intensive Behavior Intervention, 4*(1), 305–333.

Berliner, S., Moskowitz, L. J., Braconnier, M., & Chaplin, W. F. (2020). The role of parental attributions and discipline in predicting child problem behavior in preschoolers with and without Autism Spectrum Disorder. *Journal of Developmental & Physical Disabilities, 32*(5), 695–717.

Bingham, M. A., Spooner, F., & Browder, D. (2007). Training paraeducators to promote the use of augmentative and alternative communication by students with significant disabilities. *Education and Training in Developmental Disabilities, 42*(3), 339–352.

Bird, F., Dores, P. A., Moniz, D., & Robinson, J. (1989). Reducing severe aggressive and self-injurious behaviors with functional communication training. *American Journal on Mental Retardation, 94*(1), 37–48.

Blakeley-Smith, A., & Carr, E. G. (2009). Environmental fit: A model for assessing and treating problem behavior associated with curricular difficulties in children with autism spectrum disorders. *Focus on Autism & Developmental Disabilities, 24*, 131–145.

Bruininks, R. H., Woodcock, R. W., Weatherman, R. F., & Hill, B. K. (1996). *Scales of independent behavior- revised*. Riverside.

Byrd, R. S., & Weitzman, M. L. (1994). Predictors of early grade retention among children in the United States. *Pediatrics, 93*, 481–487.

Carlson, J. I., Luiselli, J. K., Slyman, A., & Markowski, A. (2008). Choice-making as intervention for public disrobing in children with developmental disabilities. *Journal of Positive Behavior Interventions, 10*(2), 86–90.

Carr, E. G. (1988). Functional equivalence as a mechanism of response generalization. In R. H. Horner, G. Dunlap & R. L. Koegel (Eds.), *Generalization and maintenance: Lifestyle changes in applied settings* (pp. 194–219). Paul H. Brookes Publishing Co.

Carr, E. G., & Durand, V. M. (1985). Reducing behavior problems through functional communication training. *Journal of Applied Behavior Analysis, 18*(2), 111–126.

Carr, E. G., Yarbrough, S. C., & Langdon, N. A. (1997). Effects of idiosyncratic stimulus variables on functional analysis outcomes. *Journal of Applied Behavior Analysis, 30*, 673–686.

Casey, S. D., & Merical, C. L. (2006). The use of functional communication training without additional treatment procedures in an inclusive school setting. *Behavioral Disorders, 32*, 46–54.

Chambless, D. L., Sanderson, W. C., Shoham, V., Bennett Johnson, S., Pope, K. S., Crits-Christoph, P., Baker-Ericzen, M., Baucom, D. H., Beutler, L. E., Calhoun, K. S., Daiuto, A., DeRubeis, R. J., Detweiler, J., Haaga, D., McCurry, S. M., Mueser, K., Stickle, T., Williams, D. A., & Woody, S. R. (1996). An update on empirically validated therapies. *The Clinical Psychologist, 49*, 5–18.

Cole, D. A., & Meyer, L. H. (1989). Impact of needs and resources on family plans to seek out-of-home placement. *American Journal on Mental Retardation, 93*, 380–387.

Davis, D. H., Fredrick, L. D., Alberto, P. A., & Gama, R. (2012). Functional communication training without extinction using concurrent schedules of differing magnitudes of reinforcement in classrooms. *Journal of Positive Behavior Interventions, 14*(3), 162–172.

Derby, K. M., Wacker, D. P., Berg, W., Deraad, A., Ulrich, S., Asmus, J., Harding, J., Prouty, A., Laffey, P., & Stoner, E. A. (1997). The long-term effects of functional communication training in home settings. *Journal of Applied Behavior Analysis, 30*(3), 507–531.

Dunlap, G., Ester, T., Langhans, S., & Fox, L. (2006). Functional communication training with toddlers in home environments. *Journal of Early Intervention, 28*(2), 81–96.

Dunlap, G., Kern-Dunlap, L., Clarke, S., & Robbins, F. R. (1991). Functional assessment, curricular revision, and severe behavior problems. *Journal of Applied Behavior Analysis, 24*, 387–397.

Durand, V. M. (1987). "Look homeward angel": A call to return to our (functional) roots. *The Behavior Analyst, 10*, 299–302.

Durand, V. M. (1990). *Severe behavior problems: A functional communication training approach.* Guilford Press.

Durand, V. M. (1993). Functional communication training using assistive devices: Effects on challenging behavior and affect. *AAC: Augmentative and Alternative Communication, 9*, 168–176.

Durand, V. M. (1999). Functional communication training using assistive devices: Recruiting natural communities of reinforcement. *Journal of Applied Behavior Analysis, 32*(3), 247–267.

Durand, V. M. (2007). Positive family intervention: Hope and help for parents with challenging children. *Psychology in Mental Retardation and Developmental Disabilities, 32*(3), 9–13.

Durand, V. M., & Berotti, D. (1991). Treating behavior problems with communication. *ASHA, 33*, 37–39.

Durand, V. M., & Carr, E. G. (1991). Functional communication training to reduce challenging behavior: Maintenance and application in new settings. *Journal of Applied Behavior Analysis, 24*(2), 251–264.

Durand, V. M., & Carr, E. G. (1992). An analysis of maintenance following functional communication training. *Journal of Applied Behavior Analysis, 25*(4), 777–794.

Durand, V. M., & Crimmins, D. B. (1992). *The Motivation Assessment Scale (MAS) administration guide.* Monaco and Associates.

Durand, V. M., & Hieneman, M. (2008a). *Helping parents with challenging children: Positive family intervention: Facilitator guide.* Oxford University Press.

Durand, V. M., & Hieneman, M. (2008b). *Helping parents with challenging children: Positive family intervention, workbook.* Oxford University Press.

Durand, V. M., Hieneman, M., Clarke, S., & Zona, M. (2009). Optimistic parenting: Hope and help for parents with challenging children. In G. D. W. Sailor, G. Sugai, & R. Horner (Eds.), *Handbook of positive behavior support* (pp. 233–256). Springer.

Durand, V. M., Mapstone, E., & Youngblade, L. (1999). The role of communicative partners. In J. Downing (Ed.), *Teaching communication skills to students with severe disabilities within general education classrooms* (pp. 139–155). Paul H. Brookes Publishing Co.

Durand, V. M., & Merges, E. (2009). Functional communication training to treat challenging behavior. In W. O'Donohue & J. E. Fisher (Eds.), *General principles and empirically supported techniques of cognitive behavior therapy* (pp. 320–327). Wiley.

Durand, V. M., & Moskowitz, L. (2015). Functional communication training: Thirty years of treating challenging behavior. *Topics in Early Childhood Special Education, 35*(2), 116–126.

Durand, V. M., & Rost, N. (2005). Does it matter who participates in our studies? A caution when interpreting the research on positive behavioral support. *Journal of Positive Behavior Interventions, 7*, 186–188.

Dyer, K., Dunlap, G., & Winterling, V. (1990). Effects of choice making on the serious problem behaviors of students with severe handicaps. *Journal of Applied Behavior Analysis, 23*(4), 515–524.

Einfeld, S. E., & Tonge, B. J. (1996). Population prevalence of psychopathology in children and adolescents with mental retardation: II epidemiological findings. *Journal of Intellectual Disability Research, 40*, 99–109.

Einfeld, S. E., Tonge, B. J., & Rees, V. W. (2001). Longitudinal course of behavioral and emotional problems in Williams syndrome. *American Journal on Mental Retardation, 106*, 73–81.

Emerson, E., Kiernan, C., Alborz, A., Reeves, D., Mason, H., Swarbrick, R., Mason, L., & Hatton, C. (2001). Predicting the persistence of severe self-injurious behavior. *Research in Developmental Disabilities, 22*, 67–75.

Eyman, R. K., & Call, T. (1977). Maladaptive behavior and community placement of mentally retarded persons. *American Journal of Mental Deficiency, 82*, 137–144.

Feldman, M., McDonald, L., Serbin, L., Stack, D., Secco, M. L., & Yu, C. T. (2007). Predictors of depressive symptoms in primary caregivers of young children with or at risk for developmental delay. *Journal of Intellectual Disability Research, 51*(8), 606–619.

Fisher, W. W., Greer, B. D., Fuhrman, A. M., & Querim, A. C. (2015). Using multiple schedules during functional communication training to promote rapid transfer of treatment effects. *Journal of Applied Behavior Analysis, 48*, 713–733.

Fisher, W. W., Greer, B. D., Querim, A. C., & DeRosa, N. (2014). Decreasing excessive functional communication responses while treating destructive behavior using response restriction. *Research in Developmental Disabilities, 35*, 2614–2623.

Fisher, W. W., Thompson, R. H., Hagopian, L. P., Bowman, L. G., & Krug, A. (2000). Facilitating tolerance of delayed reinforcement during functional communication training. *Behavior Modification, 24*(1), 3–29.

Floyd, F. J., & Gallagher, E. M. (1997). Parental stress, care demands and use of support services for school age children with disabilities and behavior problems. *Family Relations, 46*(4), 359–371.

Flynn, S. D., & Lo, Y. (2016). Teacher implementation of trial-based functional analysis and differential reinforcement of alternative behavior for students with challenging behavior. *Journal of Behavioral Education, 25*(1), 1–31.

Franco, J. H., Lang, R. L., O'Reilly, M. F., Chan, J. M., Sigafoos, J., & Rispoli, M. (2009). Functional analysis and treatment of inappropriate vocalizations using a speech-generating device for a child with autism. *Focus on Autism and Other Developmental Disabilities, 24*(3), 146–155.

Fyffe, C. E., Kahng, S., Fittro, E., & Russell, D. (2004). Functional analysis and treatment of inappropriate sexual behavior. *Journal of Applied Behavior Analysis, 37*(3), 401–404.

Gaylord-Ross, R. J., & Holvoet, J. F. (1985). *Strategies for educating students with severe handicaps*. Little, Brown & Company.

Gibson, J. L., Pennington, R. C., Stenhoff, D. M., & Hopper, J. S. (2010). Using desktop videoconferencing to deliver interventions to a preschool student with autism. *Topics in Early Childhood Special Education, 29*, 214–225.

Gilliam, W. S., & Shahar, G. (2006). Preschool and child care expulsion and suspension: Rates and predictors in one state. *Infants & Young Children, 19*(3), 228–245.

Green, V. A., O'Reilly, M., Itchon, J., & Sigafoos, J. (2005). Persistence of early emerging aberrant behavior in children with developmental disabilities. *Research in Developmental Disabilities, 26*(1), 47–55.

Hagopian, L. P., Fisher, W. W., Sullivan, M. T., Acquisto, J., & LeBlanc, L. A. (1998). Effectiveness of functional communication training with and without extinction and punishment: A summary of 21 inpatient cases. *Journal of Applied Behavior Analysis, 31*(2), 211–235.

Halle, J. W., Baer, D., & Spradlin, J. (1981). Teachers' generalized use of delay as a stimulus control procedure to increase language use in handicapped children. *Journal of Applied Behavior Analysis, 14*, 389–409.

Halle, J. W., Ostrosky, M. M., & Hemmeter, M. L. (2006). Functional communication training: A strategy for ameliorating challenging behavior. In R. J. McCauley & M. E. Fey (Eds.), *Treatment of language disorders in children* (pp. 509–548). Paul H. Brookes Publishing Co.

Hanley, G. P., Iwata, B. A., & McCord, B. E. (2003). Functional analysis of problem behavior: A review. *Journal of Applied Behavior Analysis, 36*, 147–185.

Harding, J. W., Wacker, D. P., Berg, W. K., Lee, J. F., & Dolezal, D. (2009). Conducting functional communication training in home settings: A case study and recommendations for practitioners. *Behavior Analysis in Practice, 2*(1), 21–33.

Hart, B., & Risley, T. R. (1975). Incidental teaching of language in preschool. *Journal of Applied Behavior Analysis, 8*, 411–420.

Hastings, R. P. (2002). Parental stress and behavior problems of children with developmental disability. *Journal of Intellectual and Developmental Disability, 27*(3), 149–160.

Hayes, R. P. (1987). Training for work. In D. C. Cohen & A. M. Donellan (Eds.), *Handbook of autism and pervasive developmental disorders* (pp. 360–370). Wiley.

Heath, A. K., Ganz, J. B., Parker, R., Burke, M., & Ninci, J. (2015). A meta-analytic review of functional communication training across mode of communication, age, and disability. *Review Journal of Autism and Developmental Disorders, 2*, 155–166.

Hodgetts, S., Nicholas, D., & Zwaigenbaum (2013). Home sweet home? Families' experiences with aggression in children with autism spectrum disorders. *Focus on Autism and Other Developmental Disabilities, 28*, 166–174.

Horner, R. H., & Day, H. M. (1991). The effects of response efficiency on functionally equivalent competing behaviors. *Journal of Applied Behavior Analysis, 24*(4), 719–732.

Horner, R. H., Sprague, J. R., O'Brien, M., & Heathfield, L. T. (1990). The role of response efficiency in the reduction of problem behaviors through functional equivalence training: A case-study. *Journal of the Association for Persons with Severe Handicaps, 15*(2), 91–97.

Jacobson, J. W. (1982). Problem behavior and psychiatric impairment within a developmentally disabled population. I: Behavior frequency. *Applied Research in Mental Retardation, 3*, 121–139.

Jones, R. S. P. (1999). A 10 year follow-up of stereotypic behavior with eight participants. *Behavioral Intervention, 14*, 45–54.

Kennedy, C. H., & Itkonen, T. (1993). Effects of setting events on the problem behavior of students with severe disabilities. *Journal of Applied Behavior Analysis, 26*, 321–328.

Kimball, R. T., Kelley, M. E., Podlesnik, C. A., Forton, A., & Hinkle, B. (2018). Resurgence with and without an alternative response. *Journal of Applied Behavior Analysis, 51*(40), 854–865.

Koegel, R. L., & Covert, A. (1972). The relationship of self-stimulation to learning in autistic children. *Journal of Applied Behavior Analysis, 5*, 381–387.

Kratzer, D. A., & Spooner, F. (1993). Extending the application of constant delay prompting: Teaching a requesting skill to students with severe multiple disabilities. *Education and Treatment of Children, 16*(3), 235–253.

Kurtz, P. F., Boelter, E. W., Jarmolowicz, D. P., Chin, M. D., & Hagopian, L. P. (2011). An analysis of functional communication training as an empirically supported treatment for problem behavior displayed by individuals with intellectual disabilities. *Research in Developmental Disabilities, 32*, 2935–2942.

Kurtz, P. F., Chin, M. D., Huete, J. M., Tarbox, R. S. F., O'Connor, J. T., Paclawskyj, T. R., & Rush, K. S. (2003). Functional analysis and treatment of self-injurious behavior in young children: A summary of 30 cases. *Journal of Applied Behavior Analysis, 36*(2), 205–219.

Lambert, J. M., Bloom, S. E., & Irvin, J. (2012). Trial-based functional analysis and functional communication training in an early childhood setting. *Journal of Applied Behavior Analysis, 45*(3), 579–584.

Lang, R., Rispoli, M., Machalicek, W., White, P. J., Kang, S., Pierce, N., Mulloy, A., Fragale, T., O'Reilly, M., Sigafoos, J., & Lancioni, G. (2009). Treatment of elopement in individuals with developmental disabilities: A systematic review. *Research in Developmental Disabilities, 30*(4), 670–681.

Lord, C., Wagner, A., Rogers, S., Szatmari, P., Aman, M., Charman, T., Dawson, G., Durand, V. M., Grossman, L., Guthrie, D., Harris, S., Kasari, C., Marcus, L., Murphy, S., Odom, S., Pickles, A., Scahill, L., Shaw, E., Siegel, B., . . . Yoder, P. (2005). Challenges in evaluating psychosocial interventions for autistic spectrum disorders. *Journal of Autism and Developmental Disorders, 35*(6), 695–708.

Lowe, K., Allen, D., Jones, E., Brophy, S., Moore, K., & James, W. (2007). Challenging behaviours: Prevalence and topographies. *Journal of Intellectual Disability Research, 51*(8), 625–636.

Mancil, G. R. (2006). Functional communication training: A review of the literature related to children with autism. *Education and Training in Developmental Disabilities, 41*(3), 213–224.

Mandell, D., & Novak, M. A. M. (2005). The role of culture in families' treatment decisions for children with autism spectrum disorders. *Mental Retardation and Developmental Disabilities Research Reviews, 11*, 110–115.

Matson, J. L., Dixon, D. R., & Matson, M. L. (2005). Assessing and treating aggression in children and adolescents with developmental disabilities: A 20-year overview. *Educational Psychology, 25*(2), 151–181.

Matson, J. L., & Minshawi, N. F. (2007). Functional assessment of challenging behavior: Toward a strategy for applied settings. *Research in Developmental Disabilities, 28*(4), 353–361.

Matson, J. L., & Nebel-Schwalm, M. (2007). Assessing challenging behaviors in children with autism spectrum disorders: A review. *Research in Developmental Disabilities, 28*(6), 567–579.

McGee, G. G., & Daly, T. (2007). Incidental teaching of age-appropriate social phrases to children with autism. *Research and Practice for Children with Severe Disabilities, 32*, 112–123.

McGee, G. G., Morrier, M. J., & Daly, T. (1999). An incidental teaching approach to early intervention for toddlers with autism. *Journal of the Association for Persons with Severe Handicaps, 24*, 133–146.

Mildon, R. L., Moore, D. W., & Dixon, R. S. (2004). Combining noncontingent escape and functional communication training as a treatment for negatively reinforced disruptive behavior. *Journal of Positive Behavior Interventions, 6*(2), 92–102.

Mirenda, P. (1997). Supporting individuals with challenging behavior through functional communication training and AAC: Research review. *AAC: Augmentative and Alternative Communication, 13*, 207–225.

Mirenda, P. (2003). Toward functional augmentative and alternative communication for students with autism: Manual signs, graphic symbols, and voice output communication aids. *Language Speech and Hearing Services in Schools, 34*(3), 203–216.

Moes, D. R., & Frea, W. D. (2002). Contextualized behavioral support in early intervention for children with autism and their families. *Journal of Autism and Developmental Disorders, 32*(6), 519–533.

Myers, B. J., Mackintosh, V. H., & Goin-Kochel, R. P. (2009). "My greatest joy and my greatest heart ache." Parents' own words on how having a child in the autism spectrum has affected their lives and their families' lives. *Research in Autism Spectrum Disorders, 3*(3), 670–684.

Neely, L., Garcia, E., Bankston, B., & Green, A. (2018). Generalization and maintenance of functional communication raining for individuals with developmental disabilities: A systematic and quality review. *Research in Developmental Disabilities, 79*, 116–129.

Olive, M. L., Lang, R. B., & Davis, T. N. (2008). An analysis of the effects of functional communication and a voice output communication aid for a child with autism spectrum disorder. *Research in Autism Spectrum Disorders, 2*(2), 223–236.

O'Neill, R. E., Horner, R. H., Albin, R. W., Storey, K., & Sprague, J. R. (1990). *Functional analysis of problem behavior: A practical assessment guide.* Sycamore.

O'Neill, R. E., & Sweetland-Baker, M. (2001). Brief report: An assessment of stimulus generalization and contingency effects in functional communication training with two students with autism. *Journal of Autism and Developmental Disorders, 31*, 235–240.

Paclawskyj, T. R., Matson, J. L., Rush, K. S., Smalls, Y., & Vollmer, T. R. (2000). Questions about behavioral function (QABF): A behavioral checklist for functional assessment of aberrant behavior. *Research in Developmental Disabilities, 21*(3), 223–229.

Padilla Dalamau, Y. C., Wacker, D. P., Harding, J. W., Berg, W. K., & Schiettz, K. M. (2011). A preliminary evaluation of functional communication training effectiveness and language preference when Spanish and English are manipulated. *Journal of Behavioral Education, 20*, 233–251.

Petscher, E. S., Rey, C., & Bailey, J. S. (2009). A review of empirical support for differential reinforcement of alternative behavior. *Research in Developmental Disabilities, 30*(3), 409–425.

Reed Schindler, H., & Horner, R. H. (2005). Generalized reduction of problem behavior of young children with autism: Building trans-situational interventions. *American Journal on Mental Retardation, 110*(1), 36–47.

Richman, D. M., Wacker, D. P., & Winborn, L. (2001). Response efficiency during functional communication training: Effects of effort on response allocation. *Journal of Applied Behavior Analysis, 34*(1), 73–76.

Ringdahl, J. E., & St. Peter, C. (2017). Resurgence: The unintended maintenance of problem behavior. *Education and Treatment of Children, 40*, 7–26.

Roane, H. S., Fisher, W. W., Sgro, G. M., Falcomata, T. S., & Pabico, R. R. (2004). An alternative method of thinning reinforcer delivery during differential reinforcement. *Journal of Applied Behavior Analysis, 37*, 213–218.

Saini, V., Sullivan, W. E., Baxter, E. L., DeRosa, N. M., & Roane, H. S. (2018). Renewal during functional communication training. *Journal of Applied Behavior Analysis, 51*(3), 603–619.

Saloviita, T., Italinna, M., & Leinonen, E. (2003). Explaining the parental stress of fathers and mothers caring for a child with intellectual disability: A double ABCX model. *Journal of Intellectual Disability Research, 47*(Pt. 4–5), 300–312.

Schepis, M. M., Reid, D. H., & Behrman, M. M. (1996). Acquisition and functional use of voice output communication by persons with profound multiple disabilities. *Behavior Modification, 20*(4), 451–468.

Schieltz, K. M., Wacker, D. P., Harding, J. W., Berg, W. K., Lee, J. F., Padilla Dalmau, Y. C., Mews, J., & Ibrahimović, M. (2011). Indirect effects of functional communication training on non-targeted disruptive behavior. *Journal of Behavioral Education, 20*(1), 15–32.

Schwartz, I. S., Anderson, S. R., & Halle, J. W. (1989). Training teachers to use naturalistic time delay: Effects on teacher behavior and on the language use of students. *Journal of the Association for Persons with Severe Handicaps, 14*(1), 48–57.

Shirley, M. J., Iwata, B. A., Kahng, S. W., Mazaleski, J. L., & Lerman, D. C. (1997). Does functional communication training compete with ongoing contingencies of reinforcement? An analysis during response acquisition and maintenance. *Journal of Applied Behavior Analysis, 30*(1), 93–104.

Shoham-Vardi, I., Davidson, P. W., Cain, N. N., Sloane-Reeves, J. E., Giesow, V. E., Quijano, L. E., & Hauser, K. D. (1996). Factors predicting re-referral following crisis intervention for community-based persons with developmental disabilities and behavioral and psychiatric disorders. *American Journal on Mental Retardation, 101*, 109–117.

Smith, T., Scahill, L., Dawson, G., Guthrie, D., Lord, C., Odom, S., Rogers, S., & Wagner, A. (2007). Designing research studies on psychosocial interventions in autism. *Journal of Autism and Developmental Disorders, 37*(2), 354–366.

Snell, M. E., Chen, L. Y., & Hoover, K. (2006). Teaching augmentative and alternative communication to students with severe disabilities: A review of intervention research 1997–2003. *Research and Practice for Persons with Severe Disabilities, 31*(3), 203–214.

Stokes, T. F., & Baer, D. M. (1977). An implicit technology of generalization. *Journal of Applied Behavior Analysis, 10*, 349–367.

Stokes, T. F., Fowler, S. A., & Baer, D. M. (1978). Training preschool children to recruit natural communities of reinforcement. *Journal of Applied Behavior Analysis, 11*, 285–303.

Suess, A. N., Romani, P. W., Wacker, D. P., Dyson, S. M., Kuhle, J. L., Lee, J. F., Lindgren, S. D., Kopelman, T. G., Pelzel, K. E., & Waldron, D. B. (2014). Evaluating the treatment fidelity of parents who conduct in-home functional communication training with coaching via telehealth. *Journal of Behavioral Education, 23*(1), 34–59.

Task Force Promoting Dissemination of Psychological Procedures. (1995). Training in and dissemination of empirically-validated psychological treatments: Report and recommendations. *Clinical Psychology: Science and Practice, 48*, 3–23.

Totsika, V., Toogood, S., Hastings, R. P., & Lewis, S. (2008). Persistence of challenging behaviours in adults with intellectual disability over a period of 11 years. *Journal of Intellectual Disability Research, 52*(5), 446–457.

Umbreit, J. (1996). Functional analysis of disruptive behavior in an inclusive classroom. *Journal of Early Intervention, 20*(1), 18–29.

Volkert, V. M., Lerman, D. C., Call, N. A., & Trosclair-Lasserre, N. (2009). An evaluation of resurgence during treatment with functional communication training. *Journal of Applied Behavior Analysis, 42*(1), 145–160.

Wacker, D. P., Berg, W. K., Harding, J. W., Barretto, A., Rankin, B., & Ganzer, J. (2005). Treatment effectiveness, stimulus generalization, and acceptability to parents of functional communication training. *Educational Psychology, 25*(2), 233–256.

Wacker, D. P., Berg, W. K., Harding, J. W., Derby, K. M., Asmus, J. M., & Healy, A. (1998). Evaluation and long-term treatment of aberrant behavior displayed by young children with disabilities. *Journal of Developmental and Behavioral Pediatrics, 19*(4), 260–266.

Wacker, D. P., Harding, J. W., & Berg, W. K. (2008). Evaluation of mand-reinforcer relations following long-term functional communication training. *Journal of Speech and Language Pathology–Applied Behavior Analysis, 3*(1), 25–35.

Wacker, D. P., Harding, J. W., Berg, W. K., Lee, J. F., Schieltz, K. M., Padilla Dalmau, Y. C., Nevin, J. A., & Strahan, T. A. (2011). An evaluation of persistence of treatment effects during long-term treatment of destructive behavior. *Journal of the Experimental Analysis of Behavior, 96*(2), 261–282.

Wacker, D. P., Lee, J. F., Padilla Dalmau, Y. C., Kopelman, T. G., Lindgren, S. D., Kuhle, J., Pelzel, K. E., Dyson, S., Schieltz, K. M., & Waldron, D. B. (2013). Conducting functional communication training via telehealth to reduce the problem behavior of young children with autism. *Journal of Developmental and Physical Disabilities, 25*(1), 35–48.

Wacker, D. P., Schieltz, K. M., Berg, W. K., Harding, J. W., Dalmau, Y. C. P., & Lee, J. F. (2017). The long-term effects of Functional Communication Training conducted in young children's home settings. *Education and Treatment of Children, 40*, 43–56.

Wacker, D. P., Steege, M. W., Northup, J., Sasso, G., Berg, W., Reimers, T., Cooper, L., Cigrand, K., & Donn, L. (1990). A component analysis of functional communication training across 3 topographies of severe behavior problems. *Journal of Applied Behavior Analysis, 23*(4), 417–429.

Walker G. (2008). Constant and progressive time delay procedures for teaching children with autism: A literature review. *Journal of Autism and Developmental Disorders, 38*(2), 261–275.

Walker, V. L., Lyon, K. J., Loman, S. L., & Sennott, S. (2018). A systematic review of Functional Communication Training (FCT) interventions involving augmentative and alternative communication in school settings. *Augmentative and Alternative Communication, 34*(2), 118–129.

Watanabe, M., & Sturmey, P. (2003). The effect of choice-making opportunities during activity schedules on task engagement of adults with autism. *Journal of Autism and Developmental Disorders, 33*(5), 535–538.

Wong, C., Odom, S. L., Hume, K. A., Cox, C., Fettig, A., Brock, M. E., Plavnick, J. B., Fleury, V. P., & Schultz, T. R. (2015). Evidence-based practices for children, youth, and young adults with autism spectrum disorder: A comprehensive review. *Journal of Autism and Developmental Disorders, 45*(7), 1951–1966.

9

The JASPER Model for Children With Autism

Improving Play,
Social Communication, and Engagement

Connie Kasari[1] and Kyle Sterrett

INTRODUCTION

Joint Attention, Symbolic Play, Engagement, and Regulation (JASPER) is a targeted, social-communication intervention that is included in the broader category of **Naturalistic Developmental Behavioral Interventions** (**NDBIs**; Schreibman et al., 2015). Rooted in developmental theory, the approach pays homage to the idea that children learn to communicate in the context of social interactions with more sophisticated partners. Within JASPER, these partners use both developmental and behavioral strategies to teach children the building blocks of communication and language skills. Interventionists assess the child to identify developmentally appropriate social communication and play-level targets, then select motivating toys that match the child's skill level. Sessions are densely packed with targeted, systematic instruction designed to engage the child in the development of **play routines** for the purpose of teaching children to communicate. The goal of JASPER is to support children's social-communication skills, including spontaneous initiations of both nonverbal communication and spoken (and/or augmented) language for the purpose of joint attention (socially sharing with others by pointing at, showing, or giving objects and/or commenting on the object) and requesting. Play routines within JASPER also provide opportunities to advance children's play skills (both flexibility and level of play).

---

[1]*Acknowledgements:* This work was supported by National Institutes of Health Grants R01HD073975, P50HD055784, and R01HD095973 to C. Kasari.

The JASPER approach has been tested in more than 10 randomized controlled trials (RCTs) involving more than 500 children. Trials have varied in who implements the intervention (therapists, teachers, parents, paraprofessionals), the setting (clinic, home, school), the age of the child (age 12 months to 9 years), the developmental level of the child (children who have intellectual disabilities to neurotypical children), and the length of intervention (typically 20–48 sessions over 6 weeks to 6 months). In general, JASPER is appropriate for young children who are learning language, for older children who are considered **minimally verbal** (Tager-Flusberg & Kasari, 2013), and for children who have fluent language skills but need support to engage and play with others.

Outcomes of the JASPER intervention have focused on measures that index the core social-communication impairment of ASD. These core social-communication skills include joint attention, requesting, social play skills, **engagement,** and **regulation** of behaviors and emotions. Increased **joint engagement** between the child and a social partner, a proximal outcome that is directly related to the intervention, is a consistent and replicable finding. Joint engagement also has been found to generalize to an untrained partner (Kaale et al., 2012; Kasari et al., 2006). Outcomes also include increases in social-communication skills, particularly the spontaneous initiation of joint attention skills and requesting skills as well as increased play diversity, and play level. More distal outcomes include cognitive and language skill improvements as examined through standardized assessments (Chang et al., 2016; Kasari et al., 2012).

Importantly, JASPER is considered a social-communication module that can be added to any other intervention services the child receives, thus providing maximum benefit for child outcomes. A single intervention will not be effective for all children. Even if one intervention is effective now, it may not be effective later, and similarly, an intervention not effective now may become effective later. **Modular** approaches to intervention allow one to build the most flexible and effective comprehensive intervention package for individual children (Kasari et al., 2018).

Interventions can also be blended together for some children, as demonstrated by Kasari, Kaiser, and colleagues (2014) with older children who are minimally verbal; the study delivered JASPER with the addition of Enhanced Milieu Training (EMT), a targeted spoken language intervention with a focus on word choice and prompting strategies (milieu-teaching prompts). Future trials involve the addition of more structured, discrete applied behavior analysis (ABA), programs such as discrete trial instruction, and the addition of an oral-motor intervention, Prompts for Restructuring Oral Muscular Phonetic Targets (PROMPT), with JASPER for children who are minimally verbal.

TARGET POPULATIONS

Because JASPER is based heavily in play and activity, it is appropriate for children learning language (including children up to approximately 9 years of age who are minimally verbal) or younger children (preschoolers). Some of the strategies may be useful to individuals older than 10 who are minimally verbal if clinicians use appropriate materials and activities; however, it has not been tested with individuals older than age 9.

JASPER has been tested primarily with children with ASD, but it is currently being tested with children with Down syndrome and children with tuberous sclerosis complex (TSC). The JASPER intervention has been used by therapists (with many different backgrounds, including speech-language therapists and occupational therapists) and has been taught to parents, paraprofessionals, and teachers. In each published study, researchers examined fidelity of implementation with generally high levels of fidelity reported (above 75%–80% for fidelity ratings that involve the execution and quality of strategy use). Researchers examined the fidelity ratings of parents and paraprofessionals specifically for their effects on child outcomes. Shire, Shih, Chang, and Kasari (2018) noted that parents who implemented the strategies at 75% fidelity got better results with their children than parents who implemented the strategies below 70% fidelity. Similar results were found for paraprofessional use of strategies, and more important, results showed that implementing these strategies was sustainable after support from the study team was removed (Shire et al., 2019).

THEORETICAL BASIS

JASPER was derived from both developmental and behavioral theoretical perspectives. It is widely recognized that children learn from repeated social interactions with a more sophisticated other such as the parent (Vygotsky, 1978). Theoretically, and more broadly, JASPER draws from the social-interactionist theory of development that keys in on the concept of the zone of proximal development (ZPD). The ZPD concept represents the difference between what a child can currently do independently and what the child cannot do without guidance and support. The ZPD provides the more sophisticated partner the opportunity to scaffold the child's learning and development by operating within that child's ZPD. The child's ZPD becomes a moving target as the child masters new skills.

Similarly, and more specifically relevant to language development, social-pragmatic theory recognizes that language development is an inherently social process (Tomasello, 2000). Within this theory, children's language development is supported through periods of joint engagement, that is, a shared state of attention between two people around an object or activity (Tomasello, 2000; Tomasello & Farrar, 1986). Joint engagement provides a referential context for children during social interactions to determine their partner's communicative intentions and to learn meaningful language.

Although these two theories—one more broadly focused on development and the other more specific to language learning—provide a theoretical framework for JASPER, JASPER also draws from behavioral theory. Providing a context for learning is critical, but context alone is not sufficient to teach children meaningful social and communication skills. Clinicians must select developmentally appropriate targets and scaffold within children's ZPD as well as explicitly teach strategies drawn from behavioral theory (Skinner, 1957). The strength of behavioral theories lies in their focus on the use of simplified and direct teaching of socially meaningful behaviors that are appropriately reinforced. Behavioral teaching methods codified through the principles of ABA (Cooper et al., 2007) have consistently shown to be effective for children with ASD, albeit mostly for increasing preacademic skills and decreasing behavioral challenges.

Underlying Assumptions

Based on early experimental studies of the social communication, language, and cognitive abilities of young children with ASD, JASPER makes several assumptions about the core deficits of ASD and the modifiability of these deficits. First, the delay in language often prompts parents to seek developmental help for their children (De Giacomo & Fombonne, 1998), but these delays in language are generally the downstream sequelae of earlier developing difficulties in social-communication skills. Early studies by Marian Sigman and colleagues demonstrated the specific differences in early social-communication abilities between children with ASD and matched samples of children with developmental delays and typical development (Mundy et al., 1990; Mundy et al., 1986; Sigman et al., 1986). These early skills, which develop before children have spoken language, included initiating and responding to joint attention and diversity in use of functional and symbolic play skills. Controlling for cognitive and language levels, the deficits in these skills were specific to children with ASD when compared to children with developmental delay and typical development.

Second, the social-communication difficulties that children with ASD demonstrate are related to their development of language. In a series of early studies, responding to and initiating joint attention were specifically associated with later language abilities in children with ASD (Mundy et al., 1986; Sigman et al., 1999). Thus, a reasonable assumption would be that teaching joint attention skills may lead to better language outcomes. This assumption was borne out in later clinical trials of JASPER that linked improvements in joint attention to later expressive language abilities (Kasari et al., 2008).

Teaching children with ASD to develop spontaneous initiations of joint attention or to have imagination in their play requires the integration of teaching approaches drawn from both developmental and behavioral theories of learning. The necessity of both developmental and behavioral strategies is attributable not only to the delays in development observed in children with ASD but also to interfering behaviors, including rigidity and resistance to change, that often can limit their learning.

Functional Outcomes

Early interventions vary in what they measure as an outcome of the intervention. Interventions of a year or more typically examine changes in standardized developmental tests, such as a cognitive or language test. Most NDBI are shorter term, usually 12–24 weeks, and typically examine outcomes that are considered proximal (i.e., directly targeted in the intervention) instead of distal (i.e., downstream effects of the intervention). In line with other NDBI, JASPER studies are short term and examine the proximal outcomes directly targeted by the intervention—joint attention, play, and joint engagement. Distal outcomes have been reported in studies that follow children after 6, 12, and 48 months. For example, increases in joint attention have predicted later expressive language, and play skills have predicted later cognitive levels (Gulsrud et al., 2014; Kasari et al., 2012).

Proximal Outcomes   A main outcome of JASPER trials has been child-initiated joint engagement between a social partner and the child. Engagement generally is an attentional state of being with objects and/or people, with higher states of engagement involving more coordination of attention between objects and people. JASPER follows the developmental model of engagement that Adamson and colleagues (2004) described for typically developing children. In interactions with others, children can cycle through different states of engagement, ranging from unengaged to onlooking to person or object engagement to supported or coordinated joint engagement. Being jointly engaged (i.e., supported or coordinated joint engagement) is an important domain in JASPER, given that children must be engaged in order to learn and that children with ASD spend significantly less time jointly engaged than do their typically developing peers (Adamson et al., 2009). In typical development, children's language tends to increase as they spend more time in supported joint engagement (between 18 and 36 months of age). They also begin coordinating the attention of social partners over this time period; that is, they actively use eye contact, gestures, and vocalizations/words to direct the partner's attention and behaviors within the interaction.

For most JASPER trials, joint engagement is reported as a duration measure and has been collapsed across the coded categories of supported joint engagement and coordinated joint engagement. Decreases in unengaged, onlooking, and object engagement are also important outcomes as children begin to increase periods of joint engagement. In addition to total time in joint engagement, the longest duration of a joint engagement episode can be an important outcome, demonstrating the child's stamina and maintenance of engagement with a social partner at any one time during the interaction. Improvements in the quality and quantity of engagement are crucial to make sustained and generalized progress across the other domains. Spending more time in this high-quality social context with adults has been shown to mediate joint attention outcomes (Shih et al., 2017).

Joint Attention JASPER places an emphasis on child spontaneous initiations of joint attention. Joint attention involves the use of gesture and spoken words to share an event or topic of conversation. Joint attention can also be coded as initiated by the child or in response to another person. Gestures include showing, pointing to share, giving to share, and coordinating joint looks between objects and people for the purpose of sharing. Joint attention language includes commenting on a topic for the purpose of sharing. The measures used for joint attention include an assessment of social-communication skills; the Early Social-Communication Scales (ESCS; Mundy et al., 2003); and observed, coded behaviors during social interactions of children with adults or peers. For JASPER's published studies, both administration of the ESCS and coding of joint attention behaviors from interactions have been conducted by independent, blinded, and trained assessors.

Although joint attention behavior has been a critical outcome measure of JASPER, other communication functions have also been targeted in intervention and coded from the assessments. These include requesting or behavior regulation behaviors. The gestures of pointing, reaching, and giving to request or using language to request (e.g., "I want ball") are important for children to use as well as joint attention. Requesting behaviors are generally more concrete and easier to teach than joint attention behaviors. In trials of JASPER, joint attention and requesting behaviors are coded and analyzed separately.

Play Clinicians have assessed play from a developmental assessment of play, the Structured Play Assessment (SPA; (Ungerer & Sigman, 1981), and coded observations of the child's play in interactions with others. Two variables are important. One is play diversity (or types), which reflects the child's ability to demonstrate several different play acts at the same level of play, such as feeding the doll, brushing the doll's hair, and wiping the doll's nose, all different play types within the child-as-agent level of play. Children must demonstrate multiple types within a play level to achieve mastery of a particular play level.

The second variable is **play level.** Play levels range from indiscriminate acts (mouthing, dropping toys) to simple play levels (discriminate acts, which are simple actions such as pushing a button on a pop-up toy or banging a drum, and take apart actions, such as pulling apart pop-together beads). Children then progress to combination play behaviors involving putting puzzle pieces into a form board, completing a shape sorter, or placing rings on a ring stacker (presentation combination) and next to general combinations. The final category of functional play involves actions deemed to be presymbolic play, that is, not yet symbolic but having some qualities of pretend, such as when the child pretends to feed him- or herself or pretends to feed dolls. Finally, symbolic play commences with substitutions, as when a child pretends one object is really something else (a block is a hat) and progresses further as the child begins to give life to dolls and to engage in dress-up and thematic play actions. Altogether, clinicians code 17 levels of play (Lifter et al., 1993; Ungerer & Sigman, 1981), and one goal of JASPER is to move children along the developmental continuum of play skills.

Target Areas of Treatment

The target areas of treatment align closely with the functional outcomes measured, which, for JASPER, include joint attention (the *JA* in JASPER), symbolic play (the *SP* in JASPER), engagement (the *E* in JASPER), and regulation (the *R* in JASPER).

Joint Attention   Joint attention is one of the core domains of JASPER. Although there is explicit focus and teaching of joint attention skills (pointing, showing, and giving to share), clinicians teach other social-communication skills, including requesting skills (giving, reaching, and pointing to request). Clinicians code separately responding to versus initiating joint attention and requesting. Further joint attention and requesting language are also taught via modeling as well as direct language prompting.

Play   Another primary goal of JASPER is to teach play. Children with ASD often have delays and differences in play, and their skills tend to be more functional and concrete than symbolic and abstract. To teach play, clinicians start at the child's current play level and systematically work toward the higher, more symbolic levels of play. The intervention follows a hierarchy of play skills (adapted from Lifter et al., 1993; Ungerer & Sigman, 1981), from the lowest level of play (simple play) to the highest (symbolic). In addition to teaching play skills, clinicians focus on the social aspects of play as a developmentally appropriate context for learning.

Engagement   JASPER uses specific strategies to help children extend joint engagement between themselves and the social partner. Joint engagement is the context for interactions, and play provides the topic. A goal is to increase joint engagement while decreasing the child's time unengaged, onlooking, and object engaged. Person engaged time is a strategy used to reengage children with objects, activities, and the social partner.

Regulation   JASPER stresses the importance of emotion and behavior regulation, as children with ASD have greater difficulty regulating compared to their typically developing peers (Konstantareas & Stewart, 2006). A child's behavior is regulated if he or she is calm, attentive, and amenable to learning. Many of the

JASPER strategies are directed specifically at helping children regulate their behaviors, first with adult support and coregulation strategies and later independently.

EMPIRICAL BASIS

JASPER is evidence based and has been rigorously tested through RCTs, which are considered the gold standard for determining efficacy (Kasari & Smith, 2016). These studies are summarized in Table 9.1. Altogether, these trials demonstrate gains in children's time jointly engaged in play activities with others (noticing both the partner and the shared activity), initiations of joint attention (e.g., Kasari et al., 2010; Kasari, Lawton, et al., 2014), language (e.g., Kasari et al., 2008; Kasari, Kaiser, et al., 2014), play diversity (e.g., Kasari et al., 2010), and play level (e.g., Kasari, Kaiser, et al., 2014). Short-term longitudinal follow-up studies find that children maintain these skills, and long-term follow-up finds maintenance of social-communication skills and gains in language and cognitive skills (Kasari et al., 2012).

Evolution of the JASPER Model

JASPER grew out of an experimental study comparing the addition of two content-based modules, one on **joint attention (JA)** and the other on **symbolic play (SP)**, to best-informed current treatment at that time, an ABA approach called discrete trial instruction (DTI). Researchers compared outcomes for three groups of children: a joint attention group, a play group, and a comparison group of general ABA practice only (Kasari et al., 2006).

This study had several important controls. One was that all children came from the same early intervention program, ensuring that dose of intervention was controlled. All children received the base ABA program of 30 hours per week of DTI programming, an intensive program. The children who entered the program were randomized (randomly assigned to one of the three groups)—the ABA program alone or ABA plus one-to-one teaching in joint attention or ABA plus one-to-one teaching in symbolic play skills during the morning period of free play just prior to the program start. For the children in the ABA program, child care workers provided one-to-one therapy during this 30-minute period so that all children had a similar amount of adult attention. Children receiving the joint attention or symbolic play conditions received their intervention in small intervention rooms (Kasari et al., 2006).

The main question in this study was whether clinicians could teach joint attention to children with autism, and if they could, would improving joint attention skills result in better expressive language skills? Researchers were uncertain at the time which methods would best improve these targets. While the premise of the intervention they developed was rooted in developmental principles of early prelinguistic behaviors, researchers recognized the important role of behavioral strategies based on ABA, an approach that had gained a lot of traction after the Lovaas (1987) data were published. Although DTI effects on social communication had not been reported, researchers decided to prime children to learn the particular target of joint attention or play skills with a few discrete trials at the table prior to generalizing these skills through play on the floor (Kasari et al., 2006).

The study's results found that both the joint attention and the play interventions improved language significantly more than the ABA program alone. The joint attention intervention also improved joint attention skills more than did the other

Table 9.1. Summary of effects and quality of evidence of JASPER intervention trials based on Reichow and colleagues (2008) criteria

Authors	Quality of evidence	Age (months)	N	Proximal effect (Cohen's *d*, unless specified)	Distal effect (Cohen's *d*)
Chang et al. (2016)	Strong	36–60	66	Joint engagement (Cohen's *f*) = 0.32 Initiating joint attention = 0.32 Initiating behavior request = 0.33 Functional play = 0.31	Receptive language = NG Expressive language = NS
Goods et al. (2013)	Adequate	36–60	15	Play = 0.81 Time spent unengaged = 1.63 Initiating joint attention = NS Requests = 1.51	—
Kasari et al. (2006) Kasari et al. (2008)[a]	Strong	36–48	58	Initiating joint attention = 1.01 Joint engagement = 0.83	Expressive Language = 0.59
Kasari et al. (2010)	Adequate	21–36	42	Response to joint attention = 0.74 Functional play = 0.86 Joint engagement = 0.87	—
Kasari, Kaiser, et al. (2014)	Adequate	60–96	61	Total social-communicative utterances = 0.62 Total different word roots = 0.29 Total comments = 0.44	—
Kasari, Lawton, et al. (2014)	Strong	24–60	112	Joint engagement = 0.21 Initiating joint attention = 0.14 Play = 0.30	—
Kasari et al. (2015)	Strong	22–36	86	Joint engagement (Cohen's *f*) = 0.69	Initiating joint attention = NS Functional play (Cohen's *f*) = 0.06
Lawton & Kasari (2012)	Adequate	36–60	16	Class observation: joint attention = 1.85 Teacher–child interaction: supported joint engagement = 1.24 Object engagement = 1.41	NS
Shire et al. (2017)	Strong	24–36	113	Joint engagement = 0.68 Initiating joint attention = 0.24 Initiating behavior request = 0.41 Initiating joint attention language = 0.34–0.45 Functional play = 0.82	Initiating joint attention (standardized) = 0.39 Clinical global impression = 0.37–0.48

Key: JASPER, Joint Attention, Symbolic Play, Engagement, and Regulation; NG, not given; NS, nonsignificant.

[a]Kasari et al., 2008 is a follow-up study that reported on the long term expressive language outcomes of the Kasari et al., 2006 sample.

interventions, and the play intervention improved play to a greater extent than did the other interventions. In other words, when joint attention and play were specific targets of the intervention, these skills improved in children with ASD (Kasari et al., 2006). This was one of the first demonstrations of improvements in core deficits of children with ASD as a result of early intervention.

Given that all of the children received priming prior to working on the integration of the skill into play, researchers do not know if priming helped the children learn skills faster. They do know that each target that was selected for a child required, on average, only four or five sessions to master at the table and was similarly mastered on the floor in the same session (Wong et al., 2007). Thus, this finding speaks more to importance of the developmental selection of the target (the child was ready to learn this target) and the ways in which generalization was integrated naturally into the sessions so that generalization did not need to be programmed separately, as often reported in more traditional ABA programs, such as DTI.

One unexpected finding was that parents, who were not part of the treatment with their children, were observed to have more joint engagement with their children if their children received either the joint attention or the play intervention (Kasari et al., 2006). Researchers hypothesized that joint engagement was the common element between the two experimental interventions and perhaps why they performed similarly in the prediction to language outcomes. This finding of joint engagement as the mechanism for improving language has since been borne out in a subsequent study (Shih et al., accepted).

In a follow up study of this sample, researchers also found that children with the least amount of language (fewer than five words) actually improved more if they received the joint attention intervention as opposed to the play or treatment-as-usual conditions (Kasari et al, 2008). These data fit the hypothesis that joint attention skills are critical for developing language and that improvements in joint attention are associated with language above and beyond improvements in joint engagement.

These initial findings led researchers to 1) combine the play and joint attention modules and rename the intervention *JASPER*, 2) enhance the focus on joint engagement and regulation (both necessary to learning new skills), 3) teach different implementers of the intervention (parents, teachers), and 4) conduct a series of subsequent studies focused on particular subgroups of children (e.g., younger children, underresourced children, and minimally verbal school-age children).

Studies Teaching Parents to Implement JASPER

Three parent-mediated studies have been published, two with toddlers (Kasari et al., 2010; Kasari et al., 2015) and one with preschoolers (Kasari, Lawton et al., 2014), in which parents were taught to implement JASPER. In addition, parent training has been added to other studies that involve therapist-mediated JASPER, including one with school-age children who were minimally verbal (Kasari, Kaiser, et al., 2014). Three hundred children and their parents have been involved in these studies, and another few hundred are currently in trials just completed or in progress. In each of these studies, joint engagement between children and parents increased over the comparison condition. In addition, children's development in joint attention and play skills improved, as noted in sessions with the caregiver and/or from independent assessments of joint attention and play.

First tests of the new JASPER intervention (Kasari et al., 2010) involved teaching parents to implement the intervention with their toddlers (18–36 months of age). The rationale at the time was that these children would have the least amount of language (and therefore could benefit from a targeted social-communication intervention; Kasari et al., 2010). The first study was also conducted in the context of the Early Intervention (EI) program at the University of California–Los Angeles, which had just begun toddler services. Thus, all toddlers received 30 hours per week of ABA services. Their parents were not receiving any training as part of the program. Therefore, researchers randomized children and their parents to receive JASPER parent training or to receive training after a wait-list period. The intervention lasted 8 weeks with three sessions per week and a 1-year follow up.

Researchers designed the intervention with a series of modules that could be flexibly applied. They reasoned that parents were as heterogeneous as their children, with some dyads able to engage easily and others needing more support to do so. Contingent on the parent's level of skill in JASPER prior to the beginning of intervention, researchers thought modules might have different implementation orders depending on need. They found, however, that the modules had a logical order and were applied in similar fashion across dyads. This order is reflected in the current JASPER model. Although the order in which clinicians teach the modules is consistent, it is worth noting that dyads are heterogeneous, with some requiring more attention on some topics (e.g., strategies for regulation) than for others (e.g., communication). Therapists collected data on the parents' confidence, enthusiasm, ability to implement, and use of strategies across the intervention period, and parents reported on their own confidence and willingness to use the strategies at home. These data provided important information on feasibility and acceptability of the intervention.

Results indicated that parents found the intervention feasible and acceptable. In general, reports from parents were positive, the intervention was acceptable to them, and researchers found useful information about the feasibility of the intervention from interventionists' reports. According to therapist reports, parents varied in their confidence and comfort with strategies, and these data were associated with child outcomes (Kasari et al., 2010). Overall, parents implementing JASPER with their children could do so at high levels of fidelity, and their children were better able to be jointly engaged with them. On experimental assessments carried out by researchers unfamiliar to the children, children receiving JASPER had greater diversity in their functional play outcomes and more responding to joint attention bids than children in the EI wait-list control group. These gains were maintained over the 1-year follow up.

Several more studies with parents were carried out following this initial small study. In a second toddler study (Kasari et al., 2015), where toddlers were also receiving the 30-hour per week EI ABA program, clinicians asked whether they could give parents information that would help them engage their children and improve their communication or if parents needed to do hands-on, one-to-one JASPER training to improve child outcomes. This larger study of toddlers (86 dyads) randomized dyads to hands-on JASPER practice with a trained therapist/coach or to an evidence-based early intervention parent education program based on Brereton and Tonge's intervention manual (2005). The study involved 20 hours of intervention over 10 weeks (two half-hour sessions per week for JASPER dyads or 1-hour-long session once per week for parent education sessions; Kasari et al., 2015).

Results of the Kasari et al. study (2015) yielded findings similar to those of a previous study. Parents in the JASPER group improved their ability to keep their child engaged, and children were better able to initiate joint engagement with their parents. Children in the JASPER group demonstrated higher levels of play and more diversity in their play. Their skills also generalized to their classroom, as observed by blinded observers, and were maintained over a 6-month follow-up.

A third randomized, controlled parent-mediated intervention was conducted using a similar design, a psychoeducation model versus hands-on JASPER (Kasari, Lawton, et al., 2014). However, this study included preschoolers (ages 2–5 years) who were primarily from families with low income, and intervention was carried out in the child's home for 24 sessions over 12 weeks. The study was relatively large (112 participants) and included five sites across the United States. Researchers found that, similarly to the toddler study, the hands-on JASPER program resulted in better child outcomes. Children receiving JASPER had better child-initiated joint engagement with their parents, more initiation of joint attention, and more symbolic play. These skills were maintained over a 3-month follow up (Kasari, Lawton, et al., 2014).

The information learned from these studies reinforces a few points made earlier. One is to expect significant change in a brief period of time—3 months at most. Second, the outcomes of intervention need to be considered developmentally. Over a short-term intervention, the change that is expected will be consistent with a child's developmental status. It is more likely that toddlers will increase in functional play and preschoolers in symbolic play, given their age, although there will be variability. Similarly, one might expect changes in responding to joint attention in groups of toddlers and initiations of joint attention in preschoolers. Thus, developmental readiness and difficulty of skill is associated with children's developmental age, reinforcing the importance of targeting skills within a child's ZPD. Next, JASPER was applied to older children who were still learning language (classified as minimally verbal).

JASPER for Minimally Verbal Children With ASD

In a study of school-age children who were minimally verbal, researchers began with 3 months of therapist-mediated intervention and backed parents into intervention during the second 3 months. Parents observed the intervention during the first 3 months of the therapist-mediated intervention. Researchers found that parents picked up strategies with their children just by observing. However, in the first month of hands-on intervention, their ability to engage their child significantly increased (Shire et al., 2015). These data reinforce the importance of JASPER strategies for helping parents to better engage their children (Kasari, Kaiser, et al., 2014). Moreover, most parents obtained high levels of fidelity, and those parents with fidelity higher than 75% had children with better spoken language outcomes (Shire, Shih, & Kasari, 2018).

This study with older children who are minimally verbal with ASD involved a novel research design (sequential, multiple assignment, randomized trial—**SMART design**; Collins et al., 2007), blending it with another intervention, Enhanced Milieu Teaching (EMT), that had been used with preschoolers with developmental delays who are verbal. EMT focuses on direct instruction of vocabulary (Kasari, Kaiser et al., 2014). The question in this study was whether blending JASPER and EMT with or without the additional benefit of a tablet with speech-generating software enhanced spoken language in school-age children with ASD who were minimally verbal. The SMART design employs a systematic method to personalize intervention on the basis of a child's response to intervention. In this case, researchers increased sessions for children who were slow responders (not improving in spoken language at the 3-month mark) or gave them the tablet-based speech-generation program if they did not initially receive it. The study found that the tablet-based speech-generation program significantly and rapidly improved spoken language outcomes over the blended intervention alone (Kasari, Kaiser et al., 2014). Thus, one important point from this study is that tablet-based speech-generation programs within JASPER may help children who are minimally verbal learn language faster. Clinicians now use tablets with younger children who have limited language as well as with those over the age of 5 years.

Studies on Teacher-Implemented JASPER

Three studies from our laboratory have investigated teacher-delivered JASPER. One pilot study (Lawton & Kasari, 2012) focused on whether teachers could deliver an intervention that would improve joint attention skills in preschool-age children with autism. This study was small and served as a proof-of-concept study. Results indicated that teachers could indeed teach children with autism to improve joint attention skills, as assessed during classroom time and on independent assessments. Following this study, two studies examined the extent to which teachers and paraprofessionals could deliver JASPER in their classrooms and whether their implementation improved child outcomes (Chang et al., 2016; Shire, et al. 2017). The first studied implementation in preschool center rotations where teachers and their paraprofessionals implemented JASPER strategies in two of the 20-minute rotations. Children who were randomized to the JASPER classrooms improved in their play, joint attention, and language outcomes compared to children in classrooms waiting for the intervention (Chang et al., 2016).

In the second implementation study(Shire et al., 2017)., nonspecialist paraprofessionals working one-to-one with toddlers with autism implemented JASPER, and these toddlers were compared with toddlers who received a nonspecific, group socialization program. Results of this study involving 113 toddlers indicated improvements in joint engagement, joint attention, and play skills in the JASPER group, and these improvements were maintained over follow-up.

Independent Replications

Finally, an investigation outside our laboratory examined the replication of our initial investigation of applying a joint attention module in preschool classrooms (Kaale et al., 2012). This study found similar results to the original 2006 and 2008 studies with improvements in children's initiations of joint attention and time in joint engagement with their caregiver. Moreover, there was maintenance a year later, also consistent with our earlier work (Kaale et al., 2014).

In another partial replication using JASPER strategies (Wong, 2013, teachers were taught to sequentially teach play or joint attention to their students). Children gained time jointly engaged and increased joint attention and play skills.

Summary

This series of studies indicates JASPER has a strong evidence base. It is effective with a variety of children (toddlers, children who are minimally verbal, and children with high language use), across a variety of contexts (home, school, clinic), and when implemented by different people (parents, therapists, teachers, nonprofessionals).

Importantly, JASPER as a module confers benefit beyond those of other interventions the child may be regularly receiving, even when those other interventions are implemented at high dose (e.g., classroom-based interventions, home-based ABA interventions). Thus, JASPER is flexible and can be implemented in a variety of contexts and in conjunction with other interventions to improve social-communication, play, and engagement outcomes.

PRACTICAL REQUIREMENTS

The only materials required to implement JASPER are a small space on the floor, a table and chairs that fit the child, toys at the child's developmental level, and containers to keep the toys organized (bags, bins, or shelves within reach). If the child uses an augmentative and alternative communication (AAC) system, visual symbols, or other supports, these can be incorporated as well.

There are two primary demands on those who wish to carry out JASPER. The first is the time spent in therapy with children. JASPER strategies can be used throughout the day across many different contexts, such as in schools, the home, or a clinic. However, when therapists are seeing a child one to one or are teaching others to use JASPER strategies, sessions typically range from 30 to 60 minutes. Sessions occur 2–4 times per week with only about 15 minutes needed to prepare for and plan a session.

The second demand is the time spent being trained in JASPER. Anyone can be trained to implement JASPER, from therapists to parents to teachers, as long as they have sufficient child experience and motivation to implement the intervention as designed. Like most interventions for complex conditions such as ASD, JASPER relies on in-person, hands-on training to reach fidelity and deliver the intervention. There have been three basic training models applied to teach JASPER. In each of these models, the first component is always to provide the trainee with foundational knowledge of the targets, key components, and strategies of the intervention as well as a basic overview of ASD and JASPER's operationalization of its core deficits (i.e., engagement, joint attention, and play). The second component involves guided practice whereby the trainee receives feedback on his or her strategy implementation from an experienced JASPER coach. Finally, ongoing support and feedback is optionally provided to promote maintenance of skills and to troubleshoot individual cases. The way in which each of these three components—foundational knowledge, guided practice, and ongoing support—is delivered varies depending on the training population and available resources, with procedures being adapted to meet the unique needs of therapists, parents, and teachers.

The training model for one-to-one therapists to learn JASPER involves 5 days of lecture and guided practice with trainers followed by remote feedback and supervision as therapists practice strategies independently. The initial 5 days consists of daily lectures (to teach the foundational knowledge) and three to four sessions per day of guided practice (1-hour sessions). The week of training is followed by the trainee submitting videos weekly or biweekly for feedback and review until he or she reaches fidelity.

Overall, parents require less intense and more targeted training based on the profile of their child and the assumption that they will need to learn only JASPER strategies that are related to their own child. In our studies, the primary training model for parents involves brief sessions weekly (1–3) and over 3–6 months (20–48 sessions). Similar to therapist training, parent training entails foundational knowledge, tailored to their child, provided in brief moments during the session. Each parent is also provided written materials in a notebook that he or she can refer to before or after sessions. Sessions are active, with attention paid to the child as well as to the parent's comfort and needed supports. Information is layered in, with a structure that builds from previous sessions. Depending on how rapidly the parent is up-taking strategies, the therapist will vary the level of support he or she is providing with the goal of increased parent confidence, comfort, and acceptability of the intervention strategies, and together the coach and parent problem-solve and co-construct sessions. Ongoing booster sessions (periodic check-ins) are recommended to support maintenance of strategy use. Protocols are being tested to determine the feasibility of shifting the bulk of delivery of foundational knowledge and some of the initial live coaching to be delivered remotely. However, it is clear that live coaching, to some degree, is necessary to carry out the intervention with fidelity.

A model to train teachers and paraprofessionals in educational settings has been developed to address their specific needs, mainly their limited time available to devote to training. The initial delivery of foundational knowledge is often presented in a workshop, and guided feedback from a coach takes place in the classroom with children. The role of ongoing support is often shifted to a local supervisor who is a part of the educational team. This local supervisor takes on the role of providing feedback and coaching during sessions with children in the school and provides a more cost-efficient and feasible way to provide consistent feedback to trainees from someone who is familiar with the unique characteristics of the specific educational setting. Paraprofessionals and teachers have reached fidelity in JASPER with this model, and their children have seen subsequent gains in core social-communication challenges (Chang et al., 2016; Shire et al., 2017).

The manual for JASPER is currently under publication contract. The manual presents a thorough introduction to the domains, targets, and strategies of JASPER, thus providing the foundational knowledge component of the training procedure, but it does not provide sufficient training on its own. To reiterate, hands-on coaching and feedback are crucial to successful implementation of JASPER. Clinicians, parents, and teachers are assessed using the same criteria, which rates the quality and quantity of the strategies implemented across multiple aspects of the intervention (e.g., using environmental arrangement). A brief overview of the various components of the intervention is provided next.

KEY COMPONENTS

This section discusses the goals and strategies for JASPER sessions.

Goal of JASPER Sessions

The three social-communication domains that were discussed in detail previously (joint engagement, joint attention, and play) along with behavioral and emotional regulation, constitute the primary intervention goals within JASPER sessions. While systematic assessment, target setting, and monitoring are essential (see next), JASPER is a dynamic intervention. There are no linear guidelines for sessions: for example, there are no guidelines such as that session 1 targets addressing dysregulation, session 2 targets increasing engagement, and so on. All of the strategies are used consistently and in conjunction with each other to improve children's social-communication.

This flexible structure is essential, as each child has unique and nuanced goals that can and should change over the course of the intervention and even within a single session depending on the child's response. The goal in all sessions is to create a motivating context for the child to learn and engage with the adult in a productive way. This context is child led (to the extent possible) and seeks to create as many opportunities as possible to teach new skills. Within JASPER, the motivating context is referred to as a *play routine*, where both children and adults have equal roles in the social interaction.

Play Routines The overarching goal of play routines within JASPER sessions is to increase the amount of time that children are playing with toys and engaging productively with a social partner. Play routines are not seen as activities with a concrete beginning and end to be finished but rather as a natural, fluid process because play is for typically developing children. By emphasizing this natural interaction, longer periods of engagement are created, providing many opportunities to teach new play, social-communication, and regulation skills.

Equal and Active Roles JASPER is different from many other early intervention models for young children with ASD in that the therapist is deliberate and conscious of maintaining an equal and active role in the interaction. For the adult and child to have an equal and active role, they must be playing and communicating with each other in a similar way and taking a similar role in the routine. The communication the adult is using and the way the adult is playing should always be within the child's ZPD.

JASPER Strategies

Play is not easy for many children with ASD, and without support and structure, it might be difficult for them to stay in a high-quality play routine and to maintain flexibility and an equal and active role. Support and structure within JASPER comes in the form of the various intervention strategies that are each discussed in reference to play routines. Broadly, there are seven categories of strategies: 1) environmental arrangement; 2) imitating and modeling play; 3) establishing the base routine; 4) expanding routines; 5) imitating, modeling, and expanding communication; 6) programming; and 7) supporting engagement and regulation.

Environmental Arrangement In JASPER, environmental considerations are the most fundamental and important strategies to establish and maintain high-quality play routines. The strategy of **environmental arrangement** encompasses a wide range of decisions made before and during intervention sessions. Two main decisions regarding the environment are made prior to beginning a session. The first is selecting motivating and developmentally appropriate toys, that is, toys that are within the child's ZPD. The second decision relates to how the play area is set up. More (e.g., tabletop) or less (e.g., floor) structured environments should be selected on the basis of what can help the child engage most easily. In other words, the least restrictive setting that will allow the child to engage successfully with the play partner should be selected.

The environmental arrangement is used to maintain a distraction-free environment that has enough appropriate materials for the child to continue to play with the social partner. The goal of nearly all environmental arrangement strategies is to make it as easy as possible for the child to maintain engagement within play routines.

Imitating and Modeling Play   Imitation and modeling help to maintain longer play routines and to ensure that an equal and active role is maintained between the adult and child. *Imitation* refers to the adult's repetition of children's appropriate play acts (e.g., the child stacks a block and the adult also stacks a block), and *modeling* refers to the adult's demonstration of developmentally appropriate play acts. It is always preferable for the adult to imitate more than he or she models throughout the session. The adult imitating during a session indicates that the child is initiating more skills. If the child is not initiating and needs support, the adult can model to demonstrate an appropriate way to play at that moment in the play routine. Regardless of whether the adult is imitating or modeling, both the adult and child should take a relatively equal number of turns throughout the routine.

Establishing the Base Routine   A base routine is a series of play steps that the child can maintain. As an example, stacking blocks to make a tower and then putting a person on top are two separate play steps. These steps should be developmentally appropriate and motivating for the child; if the steps are too hard or too easy, the child is likely to disengage from the activity. The purpose of the base routine is to facilitate the child's comfort with the interaction and to build momentum within the play routine. During the base steps, as well as throughout the entire routine, the adult should be monitoring the child's engagement and regulation to support the child's play as needed.

Expanding Routines   Expanding routines involves adding new toys or steps to the base routine, as described previously. These new toys and steps accomplish a number of goals within the routine: 1) They provide opportunities for the child to learn new play skills (new types of play or higher levels of play). 2) Expansions help to keep the child interested and motivated by infusing novelty within the routine, which in turn can maintain engagement for longer periods of time. 3) Expansions teach flexibility and contribute to a fluid and natural play interaction.

Imitating, Modeling, and Expanding Communication   Communication strategies within JASPER are focused on facilitating child-initiated communication both to request and to share with the social partner. Adults place emphasis on being aware of the function and on timing of adult language during sessions. In particular, adults communicate primarily through commenting and gesture use. For example, if the adult places a baby onto a bed, he or she can comment, "Baby's sleeping." The adult would then wait and give time for the child to communicate, not speaking on the child's turn. This pause, simulating conversational turn-taking, gives the child a chance to communicate. Children with ASD often communicate to some capacity, even when they have not yet developed verbal language. The pause gives the child an opportunity to initiate the communication and also gives the adult a salient opportunity to respond to, expand on, and reinforce any communication attempts from the child. Just as with play, adults implementing JASPER are expected to imitate (either repeat or rephrase) any functional communication from the child and expand by adding one or two new words. This process of imitating and expanding is the most fundamental communication strategy within JASPER. Other communication strategies within JASPER include matching the child's mean length of utterance, limiting prompts, and avoiding directive language (e.g., "Put the block on").

Programming The basic communication strategies can build a child's communication; however, children with ASD benefit from clear and systematic opportunities to learn new ways to communicate. The process of modeling gestures during play routines (e.g., pairing commenting language with a joint attention gesture) and providing opportunities for the child to practice new skills is referred to as *programming* within JASPER. Programming involves setting up clear opportunities for the child to communicate within play routines. The therapist may give several puzzle pieces to the child while keeping several for him- or herself. The therapist may model a show of an animal puzzle piece before putting it in the puzzle board and say "dog" to label it. If the child does not imitate this action by showing the therapist his or her puzzle piece, the therapist may prompt the child to show ("Let me see"). Occasional modeling and prompting will occur as necessary to help the child communicate in as natural a manner as possible.

Supporting Engagement and Regulation Many of the strategies discussed previously, such as selecting the correct toys and establishing motivating base routines, are designed to support and maintain the child's engagement and regulation. These strategies are a proactive way to set the child up for success within the session. Examples of other strategies used during intervention sessions to support engagement include modulating affect (being excited or calm) to match the needs of the child and monitoring the pace of the routine (taking turns quickly to keep the child motivated or taking turns slowly to promote higher-quality joint engagement).

As is the case for other interventions based in behavioral principles, if the child becomes dysregulated (e.g., has tantrums, escapes), the adult works to identify the function of the behavior and respond appropriately based on the identified function. The appropriate response, for example, could be ignoring the behavior, redirecting, providing visual supports, or placing a clear demand that the child can follow through on.

Summary The difficulty in implementing these JASPER strategies lies not in understanding the strategies individually but in the coordination of the strategies together to facilitate a high-quality social interaction. Practice is essential to master how to appropriately balance all of the skills, such as deciding when to push for a new skill or to ease back to maintain engagement, whether to imitate or model, or when to expand from the base routine.

ASSESSMENT FOR TREATMENT PLANNING AND PROGRESS MONITORING

JASPER, in general, can be used with any child who is learning language and for whom play is appropriate. As a result, no specific assessments have been developed to determine the appropriateness of JASPER for a particular child. The child's age and the presence of any communication delay is all that is needed to decide whether JASPER is an appropriate intervention for him or her.

The two experimental measures, the ESCS (Mundy et al., 2003) and SPA (Ungerer & Sigman, 1981), described in the Empirical Basis section, have been used in all of the RCT studies to assess change in play and communication. Changes in engagement and regulation have been assessed using observational coding of adult–child play interactions with novel materials. These measures, while reliable and sensitive to change over short periods of time, are resource intensive both to administer and code and are difficult for clinicians to use. As a solution to these issues, Shire, Shih, Chang, and Kasari (2018) developed a shorter measure that combines the protocols of the ESCS and SPA, is easier to administer, and is better suited for treatment planning and progress monitoring.

This measure, called the **SPACE Assessment** (Short Play and Communication Evaluation; Shire, Shih, Chang, & Kasari, 2018), measures children's frequency of spontaneous initiations of joint attention, requesting skills, and play acts. It also allows the adult to generate an estimate of the children's amount of time jointly engaged and regulated during the assessment. The information gleaned from this assessment is crucial to a successful JASPER session. It gives information on the child's mastered play level and roughly aligns with the child's ZPD. This in turn allows the adult to select developmentally appropriate toys for the session. In addition, it gives information on the ways in which the child can communicate, specifically, what gestures the child can use spontaneously and whether he or she has functional language. For example, if the child consistently gave to share during the assessment but never showed or pointed to share, the latter skills would be the main joint attention target. Most programming opportunities for joint attention would then be centered around the selected target skill.

Multiple skills are targeted during every JASPER session, so traditional methods of teaching one particular skill to mastery before moving to the next or teaching a skill in isolation before mixing it with unlearned skills do not apply to JASPER. To inform toy choice and shifts in communication goals, the clinician should note the highest play level achieved in the session, the ways in which the child communicated, how much support the child needed to communicate, how long the child was engaged in play routines, and any new problem behaviors that may have occurred. The SPACE is typically repeated every 2–3 months as a systematic and consistent way to record progress. JASPER can be continued for as long as the two entry criteria—age and social-communication delays—are met.

IMPLICATIONS FOR INCLUSIVE PRACTICE

JASPER has been implemented in homes and schools. In homes, clinicians encourage parents to integrate JASPER strategies throughout their day and with other family members, including siblings. Collaboration with parents yields information on what parents need help with, such as engaging their child in play, mealtimes, bed and bath times, and going out into the community (Kasari, Lawton, et al., 2014). Parents do not need to work with their child for designated periods of time each day. Instead, they give information on what they are doing, how comfortable or easy they find the strategies to implement, and whether they are noticing change in their child (Kasari et al., 2010; Kasari, Lawton, et al., 2014, Kasari et al., 2015). The home situations for families are highly variable, and clinicians want to learn from them how best to adapt strategies to fit their particular situation.

At school, most studies have adopted a similar approach whereby collaboration has resulted in adaption of JASPER strategies to the particular educational context.

Most published JASPER studies have been carried out in special education preschool classrooms (Chang et al., 2016; Goods et al., 2013; Shire et al., 2017), although in one study, clinicians taught teachers JASPER strategies in inclusive preschools (Lawton & Kasari, 2012), and in another study, clinicians taught teachers in inclusive child care centers (Gulsrud et al., 2019). Because JASPER is modular in approach, it has worked across different classroom configurations.

For example, Chang and colleagues (2016) taught teachers to implement JASPER in two different existing classroom rotations that involved play, a block center, and a dress-up center. Teachers benefited from learning about play development and were able to assess and target the developmentally appropriate play level for each child. In this context, teachers also had to manage small groups of children, thus using play to facilitate peer interactions within the rotations.

Similarly, Shire and colleagues (2017) taught paraprofessionals to implement JASPER, but in this program, each toddler had a one-to-one assistant. One adaptation made in the program (and in collaboration with the school staff) was to pair two children and work on JASPER strategies within the peer dyad.

In inclusive preschools and child care centers, JASPER strategies have been distributed across the day in morning circle time, small-group time, and individual time (Gulsrud et al., 2019; Lawton & Kasari, 2012). Clinicians found it helpful to provide visual reminders to teachers, an idea developed by the teachers in the toddler program, who hung posters about play levels, programming for joint attention, and other JASPER-related concepts around their classrooms.

CONSIDERATIONS FOR CHILDREN FROM CULTURALLY AND LINGUISTICALLY DIVERSE BACKGROUNDS

JASPER studies have involved diverse populations of children with ASD. One study specifically recruited preschool-age children from low-income, culturally diverse backgrounds (Kasari, Lawton, et al., 2014). All of the children in the sample came from low-income backgrounds, but 66% of the children in the sample were also ethnically and culturally diverse, and 15% spoke a language other than English.

Other ongoing studies have included substantial proportions of culturally and linguistically diverse participants. In large part, this effort stemmed from community work in homes and schools and the fact that the student population served by the Los Angeles Unified School District is three-quarters Latino children. Of the more than 14,000 children with ASD in the school district, the overwhelming majority of children are Latino, with a high proportion also second-language English learners. Because JASPER is meant to be developmental, flexible, and collaborative between parents and/or teachers, the diversity in culture, ethnicity, and languages spoken has been viewed as a strength.

Cultural and linguistic diversity becomes a critical issue primarily for caregiver-mediated interventions. JASPER research has tried to limit the exclusion of individuals other than a parent in caregiver-mediated interventions (e.g., a grandparent, aunt) and of parents who speak languages other than English. The goal is for the intervention strategies to be generalizable and used with a representative population of families who have a child with ASD in the local context.

With such a diverse population of families, a diverse group of coaches and therapists is also necessary. Many of the coaches have been native Spanish or Korean language speakers. These two languages are the most common among participants; however, JASPER has been implemented both clinically and in research contexts using other languages as well, such as Vietnamese, Russian, Japanese, Farsi, and Mandarin. Some adaptions are needed as a result of this cultural and linguistic diversity. For example, there are, at times, cultural differences in how the caregivers interact with their children—they may be less likely to play with their child and instead would rather read or do other household activities with the child. The types of words or phrases used with the child may also vary.

These adaptions may be greater in countries other than the United States. Training parents and therapists in other countries (Japan, Macedonia, Kazakhstan, Vietnam, among others) also requires adaption to the context, the language, and the usual ways of caring for children. Overall, the adjustments have been relatively minor, probably because JASPER is rooted in development; most children around the world play, and children learn social-communication skills and language in social interactions with others.

Application to a Child

Parents requested help with their 3-year-old son, Jason, who was not talking. He had been diagnosed with ASD at age 2 and had immediately begun to receive 20 hours per week of ABA therapy, employing discrete trial instructions in the home. Although he had made progress in matching colors and discriminating shapes, he had not made progress in spoken language (he still had no words), nor could his parents engage him in play. He had no joint attention gestures, and he requested primarily by leading another's hand to what he wanted.

Clinicians assessed Jason using the ESCS and the SPA. He coordinated his looking between objects and the examiner twice but displayed no other gestures of joint attention. He reached to request a toy once. His mastered level of play was presentation combination. Along the developmental play hierarchy (Lifter et al., 1993), this level of play refers to the child being able to place an object into a clearly designated spot, such as placing a ring on a ring stacker. He was emerging in general combination play, the next level in the play hierarchy. General combinations involve putting together objects that do not necessarily go together (e.g., stacking blocks and cups together). In determining the types of toys to use given his mastered play level, clinicians chose a number of presentation combination toys as well as some general combination toys (a level above his mastered level). They also targeted a point to request and a point to share for social-communication targets. All skills were within Jason's ZPD.

In his first session of JASPER with a therapist, Jason was able to put small animals on pegs, taking turns with his therapist. When he had finished putting all of the animals on pegs, the therapist modeled a new action, taking an animal off and putting it on a tower. Jason began to cry. This is not what he had in mind. He had finished the task and was done. It was clear that Jason did not take much pleasure in playing. His idea about toys was more about completing a task then moving on. The therapist got a sense of what his parents were experiencing, as his mother talked about not being able to engage him in play and said that he preferred to be left alone. When he did play, he had to do things his way, on his own terms. In other words, he could not really play socially with another person.

Because the first session of JASPER was not very successful, adjustments needed to be made, particularly around toy choice. In the second session, Jason's therapist brought in a car ramp and cars—toys that were just below his mastered level of play and that did not have a clear visual cue to their completion (e.g., puzzles do). She also brought in a tablet with speech-generating software. She programmed eight pictures that said the corresponding words when pressed. The pictures represented nouns and verbs that related to the toys and activities she had prepared.

This session was much more successful. The therapist imitated Jason when he put the car on the ramp, putting her car on the ramp behind him. She also said "car," then pressed a picture of a car on the tablet, which also produced the word CAR. As they continued to take turns with the cars going down the ramp, the therapist continued to model spoken and augmented language, expanding both her play actions (the car drove into garage at end of ramp) and her language ("car goes down ramp"). In this session, the child imitated the therapist, pressing the button on the tablet and expanding his augmented talk to two words. He began to initiate on the tablet, and he was regulated and happy while playing. The change in toy choice and support of visual and auditory input from the tablet helped to regulate Jason so that he could learn from the interaction.

While Jason continued to develop his play and social-communication skills in the context of JASPER over the next many sessions, clinicians also continued to prompt his use of sounds and approximations for words. He began to pair vocalizations along with his use of the augmentative device. He also began to use more gestural communicative intent, pointing to request and to share events or activities during play.

Jason continued to use the tablet for communication, becoming fairly independent using it over the next 3 years. The tablet helped him to regulate his behaviors and to repair communication if the listener did not understand him. He was using a greater number of words but still using the tablet to communicate. He had many folders of icons and words on his device, and he could navigate through them quickly. At age 6, he lessened his dependence on the tablet, and now at age 7, he is always using spoken language to communicate.

Application to an Adult

JASPER is designed for young children (up to 9 years old) and thus is not appropriate for adolescents or adults.

To review an extended application and implementation of this intervention, see Case 6 about a child with ASD in the companion volume *Case Studies for the Treatment of Autism Spectrum Disorder*.

Future Directions

Several projects have recently been completed that test JASPER alone or in combination with other treatment models or strategies, and several more have been initiated. The goal of this work is to determine the best sequence or combination of intervention strategies that improve overall social communication and language abilities in children with autism and other neurodevelopmental disorders. Questions include the following: How long should clinicians wait to change something in the child's treatment plan? What characteristics of a child predict how he or she will do in the intervention and at what dose of intervention? Can clinicians disseminate JASPER into community settings with fidelity and have its implementation sustain past the life of a study? How does JASPER work? In what situations does it work and with which populations? Our current work focuses primarily on children with ASD who are minimally verbal or are very young children (12–21 months).

Because JASPER is modular with flexible implementation across a variety of settings and implementation by different individuals, we have many partnerships with other clinicians and researchers in various contexts. The goal of ongoing work is to improve the developmental trajectories of young children with ASD, and to this end, adaptive intervention designs allow us to tease apart various components of the intervention.

Suggested Readings

1. Gulsrud, A. C., Hellemann, G., Shire, S., & Kasari, C. (2016). Isolating active ingredients in a parent- mediated social communication intervention for toddlers with autism spectrum disorder. *Journal of Child Psychology & Psychiatry, 57*(5), 606–613. This article is one of the few studies of early intervention for children with ASD that focuses on the active ingredients of the intervention, that is, which particular components of the intervention are leading to change in children's outcomes. The results show that parents' appropriate and timely imitation and modeling within play routines (mirrored pacing) mediated the relationship between treatment and joint engagement.

2. Kasari, C., Gulsrud, A., Freeman, S., Paparella, T., & Hellemann, G. (2012). Longitudinal follow up of children with autism receiving targeted interventions on joint attention and play. *Journal of the American Academy of Child & Adolescent Psychiatry, 51*, 487–495. This study examines the cognitive and language outcomes of children with autism over a 5-year period after receiving targeted early interventions that focused on joint attention and play skills. This study confirms the importance of change in joint attention and play on later language and cognition, reiterating the importance of early interventions such as JASPER that target the core deficits of children with ASD.

3. Kasari, C., Lawton, K, Shih, W., Barker, T., Landa, R., Lord, C., Orlich, F., King, B., Wetherby, A., & Senturk, D. (2014). Caregiver mediated intervention for low resourced preschoolers with autism: An RCT. *Pediatrics, 134*, 72–79. This study was one of the early applications of JASPER that involved parent training. Particularly noteworthy is that this intervention took place in families' homes and that parents were able to uptake JASPER strategies at high fidelity. Not only did the parents' strategy use increase, but their children also saw subsequent gains in core deficits such as play and joint attention.

4. Shire, S. Y., Chang, Y. C., Shih, W., Bracaglia, S., Kodjoe, M., & Kasari, C. (2017). Hybrid implementation model of community- partnered early intervention for toddlers with autism: A randomized trial. *Journal of Child Psychology & Psychiatry, 58*(5), 612–622. In this study, clinicians taught paraprofessionals to use JASPER strategies within their classrooms. As was true for parents, the

paraprofessionals were able to uptake JASPER strategies at high fidelity, and children made gains across the targeted domains. This study also serves as a model for community-partnered research. The successful implementation of the intervention relied on support from within the educational agency, not just from research staff.

Learning Activities

1. Discuss the importance of early developing prelinguistic behaviors to later spoken language and the relation to children with ASD. Which prelinguistic behaviors are most connected to later cognitive and language skills, and how might these prelinguistic behaviors be scaffolded or modified to facilitate early language production?

2. Write a brief summary of each of the core component strategies of JASPER (e.g., environment arrangement, imitation, and modeling) in your own words. Which of these strategies do you believe would be the most difficult to implement, and why? Do any of the strategies align with your current intervention practices?

3. What modifications to early interventions and specifically to JASPER do you think would be relevant or helpful for the context in which you live or work? Think about both the physical setting and the materials as well as the cultural and resource-based adaptations that might be required.

Summary of Video Clip

*See the **About the Videos and Downloads** page at the front of the book for directions on how to access and stream the accompanying video to this chapter.*

The child in this video clip is a 20-month-old, at risk toddler whose primary presenting concerns include language, non-verbal communication delays, and difficulty with sustaining engagement. The primary goals in this session are to increase the time and quality of the child's joint engagement, build more diverse and flexible play, and increase the frequency of nonverbal and verbal communication bids.

We see in this clip strategies that are familiar to many early intervention providers, such as the therapist's high affect and immediate, high-quality responsiveness to all of the child's communicative bids. Throughout this clip there are other subtle yet important strategies used to support and maintain the high-quality interaction and simultaneously teach new skills. The therapist's consistent, engaged, and timely imitation of the child's play allows her to maintain an active and reciprocal role in the interaction and thus provides the child more time to practice and be exposed to high-quality and appropriate developmental communication. The therapist's use of the environment keeps the child from becoming unengaged or object focused; the therapist made developmentally appropriate toys available and has extra motivating materials easily accessible, placing the materials at eye level. The therapist's teaching of new nonverbal communication skills through consistent modeling and well-timed prompting episodes builds on the child's current communicative repertoire. In conjunction, these strategies, among others, work synergistically to provide a high-quality and natural learning environment for the child.

REFERENCES

Adamson, L. B., Bakeman, R., & Deckner, D. F. (2004). The development of symbol-infused joint engagement. *Child Development, 75*(4), 1171–1187.

Adamson, L. B., Deckner, D. F., & Bakeman, R. (2009). Early interests and joint engagement in typical development, autism, and Down syndrome. *Journal of Autism and Developmental Disorders, 40*(6), 665–676.

Brereton, A. V., & Tonge, B. J. (2005). *Pre-schoolers with autism: An education and skills training programme for parents: Manual for clinicians.* Jessica Kingsley Publishers.

Chang, Y., Shire, S. Y., Shih, W., Gelfand, C., & Kasari, C. (2016). Preschool deployment of evidence-based social communication intervention: JASPER in the classroom. *Journal of Autism and Developmental Disorders, 46*(6), 2211–2223.

Collins, L. M., Murphy, S. A., & Strecher, V. (2007). The multiphase optimization strategy (MOST) and the sequential multiple assignment randomized trial (SMART): New methods for more potent eHealth interventions. *American Journal of Preventive Medicine, 32*(5), S112–S118.

Cooper, J. O., Heron, T. E., & Heward, W. L. (2007). *Applied behavior analysis.* Macmillan.

De Giacomo, A., & Fombonne, E. (1998). Parental recognition of developmental abnormalities in autism. *European Child & Adolescent Psychiatry, 7*(3), 131–136.

Goods, K. S., Ishijima, E., Chang, Y. C., & Kasari, C. (2013). Preschool based JASPER intervention in minimally verbal children with autism: Pilot RCT. *Journal of Autism and Developmental Disorders, 43*(5), 1050–1056.

Gulsrud, A. C., Hellemann, G. S., Freeman, S. F., & Kasari, C. (2014). Two to ten years: Developmental trajectories of joint attention in children with ASD who received targeted social-communication interventions. *Autism Research, 7*(2), 207–215.

Gulsrud, A., Carr, T., Williams, J., Panganiban, J., Jones, F., Kimbrough, J., Shih, W., & Kasari, C. (2019). Developmental screening and early intervention in a childcare setting for young children at risk for autism and other developmental delays: A feasibility trial. *Autism Research, 12*, 1423–1433.

Kaale, A., Fagerland, M. W., Martinsen, E. W., & Smith, L. (2014). Preschool-based social-communication treatment for children with autism: 12-month follow-up of a randomized trial. *Journal of the American Academy of Child & Adolescent Psychiatry, 53*(2), 188–198.

Kaale, A., Smith, L., & Sponheim, E. (2012). A randomized controlled trial of preschool-based joint attention intervention for children with autism. *Journal of Child Psychology and Psychiatry, 53*(1), 97–105.

Kasari, C., Freeman, S., & Paparella, T. (2006). Joint attention and symbolic play in young children with autism: A randomized controlled intervention study. *Journal of Child Psychology and Psychiatry, 47*(6), 611–620.

Kasari, C., Gulsrud, A. C., Wong, C., Kwon, S., & Locke, J. (2010). Randomized controlled caregiver mediated joint engagement intervention for toddlers with autism. *Journal of Autism and Developmental Disorders, 40*(9), 1045–1056.

Kasari, C., Gulsrud, A., Freeman, S., Paparella, T., & Hellemann, G. (2012). Longitudinal follow-up of children with autism receiving targeted interventions on joint attention and play. *Journal of the American Academy of Child & Adolescent Psychiatry, 51*(5), 487–495.

Kasari, C., Gulsrud, A., Paparella, T., Hellemann, G., & Berry, K. (2015). Randomized comparative efficacy study of parent-mediated interventions for toddlers with autism. *Journal of Consulting and Clinical Psychology, 83*(3), 554–563.

Kasari, C., Kaiser, A., Goods, K., Nietfeld, J., Mathy, P., Landa, R., Murphy, S., & Almirall, D. (2014). Communication interventions for minimally verbal children with autism: A sequential multiple assignment randomized trial. *Journal of the American Academy of Child & Adolescent Psychiatry, 53*(6), 635–646.

Kasari, C., Lawton, K., Shih, W., Barker, T. V., Landa, R., Lord, C., Olrich, F., King, B., Wetherby A., & Senturk, D. (2014). Caregiver-mediated intervention for low-resourced preschoolers with autism: An RCT. *Pediatrics, 134*(1).

Kasari, C., Paparella, T., Freeman, S., & Jahromi, L. B. (2008). Language outcome in autism: Randomized comparison of joint attention and play interventions. *Journal of Consulting and Clinical Psychology, 76*(1), 125.

Kasari, C., & Smith, T. (2016). Forest for the trees: Evidence- based practices in ASD. *Clinical Psychology: Science and Practice, 23*(3), 260–264.

Kasari, C., Sturm, A., & Shih, W. (2018). SMARTer approach to personalizing intervention for children with autism spectrum disorder. *Journal of Speech, Language, and Hearing Research, 61*(11), 2629–2640.

Konstantareas, M. M., & Stewart, K. (2006). Affect regulation and temperament in children with autism spectrum disorder. *Journal of Autism and Developmental Disorders, 36*(2), 143–154.

Lawton, K., & Kasari, C. (2012). Teacher-implemented joint attention intervention: Pilot randomized controlled study for preschoolers with autism. *Journal of Consulting and Clinical Psychology, 80*(4), 687–693.

Lifter, K., Sulzer-Azaroff, B., Anderson, S. R., & Cowdery, G. E. (1993). Teaching play activities to preschool children with disabilities: The importance of developmental considerations. *Journal of Early Intervention, 17*(2), 139–159.

Lovaas, O. I. (1987). Behavioral treatment and normal educational and intellectual functioning in young autistic children. *Journal of Consulting and Clinical Psychology, 55*(1), 3–9.

Mundy, P., Delgado, C., Block, J., Venezia, M., Hogan, A., & Seibert, J. (2003). *Early Social-Communication Scales (ESCS).* University of Miami.

Mundy, P., Sigman, M., & Kasari, C. (1990). A longitudinal study of nonverbal joint attention and language development in young autistic children. *Journal of Autism and Developmental Disabilities, 20*, 115–128.

Mundy, P., Sigman, M., Ungerer, J., & Sherman, T. (1986). Defining the social deficits of autism: The contribution of non-verbal communication measures. *Journal of Child Psychology and Psychiatry and Allied Disciplines, 27*(5), 657–669.

Reichow, B., Volkmar, F. R., & Cicchetti, D. V. (2008). Development of the evaluative method for evaluating and determining evidence-based practices in autism. *Journal of Autism and Developmental Disorders, 38*, 1311–119.

Schreibman, L., Dawson, G., Stahmer, A. C., Landa, R., Rogers, S. J., McGee, G., Kasari, C., Ingersoll, B., Kaiser, A., Bruinsma, Y., McNerney, E., Wetherby, A., & Halladay, A. (2015). Naturalistic developmental behavioral interventions: Empirically validated treatments for autism spectrum disorder. *Journal of Autism and Developmental Disorders, 45*(8), 2411–2428.

Shih, W., Chang, Y. C., Shire, S., & Kasari, C. (2017). *Measuring small but meaningful change.* Symposium presented at the 2017 Gatlinburg Conference, Gatlinburg, TN, United States.

Shire, S. Y., Chang, Y. C., Shih, W., Bracaglia, S., Kodjoe, M., & Kasari, C. (2017). Hybrid implementation model of community-partnered early intervention for toddlers with autism: A randomized trial. *Journal of Child Psychology and Psychiatry, 58*(5), 612–622.

Shire, S. Y., Chang, Y. C., Shih, W., Bracaglia, S., Kodjoe, M., & Kasari, C. (2019). Sustained community implementation of JASPER intervention with toddlers with autism. *Journal of Autism and Developmental Disorders, 49*(5), 1863–1875.

Shire, S. Y., Goods, K., Shih, W., Distefano, C., Kaiser, A., Wright, C., Mathy, P., Landa, R., & Kasari, C. (2015). Parents' adoption of social-communication intervention strategies: Families including children with autism spectrum disorder who are minimally verbal. *Journal of Autism and Developmental Disorders, 45*(6), 1712–1724.

Shire, S. Y., Shih, W., Chang, Y. C., & Kasari, C. (2018). Short Play and Communication Evaluation: Teachers' assessment of core social-communication and play skills with young children with autism. *Autism, 22*(3), 299–310.

Shire, S. Y., Shih, W., & Kasari, C. (2018). Brief report: Caregiver strategy implementation—Advancing spoken communication in children who are minimally verbal. *Journal of Autism and Developmental Disorders, 48*(4), 1228–1234.

Sigman, M., Mundy, P., Sherman, T., & Ungerer, J. (1986). Social interactions of autistic, mentally retarded and normal children and their caregivers. *Journal of Child Psychology and Psychiatry, 27*(5), 647–656.

Sigman, M., Ruskin, E., Arbelle, S., Corona, R., Dissanayake, C., Espinosa, M., Kim, N., Lopez. & Zierhut, C. (1999). Continuity and change in the social competence of children with autism, Down syndrome, and developmental delays. *Monographs of the Society for Research in Child Development, 64*(1), i–139.

Skinner, B. F. (1957). *Verbal behavior.* Appleton-Century-Crofts.

Tager-Flusberg, H., & Kasari, C. (2013). Minimally verbal school-aged children with autism spectrum disorder: The neglected end of the spectrum. *Autism Research, 6*(6), 468–478.

Tomasello, M. (2000). First steps toward a usage-based theory of language acquisition. *Cognitive Linguistics, 11*(1/2), 61–82.

Tomasello, M., & Farrar, M. J. (1986). Joint attention and early language. *Child Development, 57*(6), 1454–1463.

Ungerer, J. A., & Sigman, M. (1981). Symbolic play and language comprehension in autistic children. *Journal of the American Academy of Child Psychiatry, 20*(2), 318–337.

Vygotsky, L. (1978). Interaction between learning and development. *Readings on the Development of Children, 23*(3), 34–41.

Wong, C. S. (2013). A play and joint attention intervention for teachers of young children with autism: A randomized controlled pilot study. *Autism, 17*(3), 340–357.

Wong, C. S., Kasari, C., Freeman, S., & Paparella, T. (2007). The acquisition and generalization of joint attention and symbolic play skills in young children with autism. *Research and Practice for Persons with Severe Disabilities, 32*(2), 101–109.

10

Enhanced Milieu Teaching

Ann P. Kaiser, Elizabeth A. Fuller, and Jodi K. Heidlage

INTRODUCTION

Enhanced Milieu Teaching (EMT) is an evidence-based language intervention that has been shown to be effective for a variety of developmental delays, including autism spectrum disorder (ASD; Hampton, Kaiser, & Fuller, 2020; Hampton et al., 2019; Kaiser & Roberts, 2013; Olive et al., 2007). EMT, founded in behavioral, developmental, and social interactionist theoretical perspectives, has been developed from milieu teaching and responsive interaction strategies. EMT appears to be highly effective with children who are in the early stages of language learning, particularly children who do not verbalize frequently and who are learning vocabulary or early word combinations.

EMT includes six components: 1) environmental arrangement, 2) responsive interaction, 3) language modeling, 4) language expansions, 5) time delays, and 6) milieu teaching prompts. When implementing EMT using these components, the adult sets up a context for communication by arranging the environment to set the stage for adult–child interactions and to increase the likelihood that the child will initiate to the adult (environmental arrangement). The adult uses responsive interaction strategies to respond contingently and reinforce a child's verbal and nonverbal communication (responsive interaction). During these responsive interactions, the adult models specific language targets appropriate to the child's skill level and connects to the child's play and focus of interest (language modeling). When the child communicates, the adult responds by adding content words, increasing the child's message complexity or vocabulary (**language expansions**). Lastly, the adult uses two strategies to elicit communication from the child. First, the adult uses time delay strategies, such as holding up alternative objects representing a choice or pausing in a routine, as a nonverbal cue to the child to communicate. The adult responds to the child's requests with prompts for elaborated language consistent with the child's targeted skills (milieu teaching) and functionally reinforces the child's production of prompted target forms in a variety of ways. Functional reinforcement can be provided by allowing access to requested objects (milieu teaching), continuing adult interaction (responsive interaction), offering feedback in the form of expansions (language expansions), or confirming the meaning and pragmatic functions of the child's utterances (responsive interaction).

TARGET POPULATIONS

There is empirical support for the effectiveness of EMT for children who have a diagnosis of ASD. Under the *Diagnostic and Statistical Manual of Mental Disorders, Fifth Edition* (DSM-5), a diagnosis of ASD requires that children have 1) persistent deficits in social communication and social interaction and 2) restricted, repetitive patterns of behavior, interests, or activities (American Psychiatric Association [APA], 2013). EMT is specifically designed to improve social-communication. Because EMT is a conversational, dyadic intervention, it is particularly well suited for children with deficits in social and verbal communication. EMT addresses the lack of back-and-forth conversation, limited sharing of interest or attention, and failure to initiate and respond to a social partner—all symptoms described in the DSM-5 as associated with both ASD and social-communication disorder. Although research examining the effectiveness of EMT has not yet been conducted with children diagnosed with social-communication disorder, research on EMT has shown it is effective for children with a wide range of developmental disorders, indicating EMT would likely be appropriate for this population.

Evidence indicates that EMT is effective for children with intellectual disability (Kaiser & Roberts, 2013), specific language impairment (Roberts & Kaiser, 2015), Down syndrome (Wright et al., 2013), or cleft lip and/or palate (Kaiser et al., 2017), and it is currently being studied with children with hearing loss and children who are dual language learners (Peredo et al., 2017). Research across children with a range of complex communication needs suggests EMT may be appropriate for a range of young children with ASD, including children with comorbid disorders. Although historically EMT has been used primarily with children who are verbally imitative, more recent research has shown EMT to be effective for children with ASD who are minimally verbal (Hampton, Kaiser, & Fuller, 2020; Hampton et al., 2019; Kasari et al., 2014). EMT is most appropriate for children who are at early stages of verbal or preverbal communication. When children's mean length of utterance (MLU) is greater than 3.0, they can often learn efficiently with responsive interaction strategies alone (Kaiser et al., 1997; Kaiser et al., 1998). Whether EMT is appropriate for a child with ASD can be easily ascertained using a brief (20-minute) observation of the child, either with a familiar adult or with a trained examiner, as described under the Assessment for Treatment Planning section.

THEORETICAL BASIS

EMT is derived from a blend of three developmental perspectives of early language and communication development: behavioral theory, developmental theory, and social interactionist theory. EMT has been identified as a Naturalistic Developmental Behavioral Intervention (NDBI; Schreibman et al., 2015) because it draws from multiple theoretical bases.

Behavioral Theory

The behavioral theory of language development was largely influenced by Skinner (1957), who argued that children learn language through a series of reinforcement contingencies in which correct utterances are reinforced and incorrect utterances are not reinforced, resulting in the overall development of more complex words and sentences. Lovaas's (1987) flagship study, which showed large gains for children who received a high dosage of trial-based learning delivered using the concepts of behavioral theory, or applied behavior analysis (ABA), set the stage for interventions based in behavioral theory to be widely implemented in the field of ASD, including for the use of teaching language and communication. In a behavioral approach to language instruction, methods such as modeling, imitation, and prompted practice of expressive language skills are key. Adults prompt children to use language by presenting antecedent stimuli (models, time delays) that signal when to talk and what to say. When children respond to these prompts, they are reinforced by the consequences adults provide that are contingent on their communication. Contingent adult responding plays an important role in this behavioral paradigm because it presumably functions as a reinforcer that increases the frequency with which children communicate. In addition, it provides differential feedback for children's more complex language. Imitation and production practice, with contingent adult feedback, are essential child behaviors for learning language in this framework. In EMT, prompting procedures (elicitive model, mand model, time delay, incidental teaching) are strategies for facilitating more frequent child initiations. First, children learn to imitate when given adult models. Next, they learn to respond to questions of increasing complexity (mand-model). Finally, children initiate requests and comments (time delay, incidental teaching), thus becoming more independent language users.

EMT uses a contemporary model of ABA intervention, which addresses some of the criticisms of traditional ABA therapies, including limited generalization of treatment outcomes and the lack of flexibility in children's communication skills often seen when they complete traditional ABA therapy. Studies of milieu teaching and EMT including children with and without ASD have demonstrated systematic generalization across 1) settings (Kaiser & Roberts 2013; Wright et al., 2013), 2) partners (Hancock & Kaiser, 2002), 3) specific classes of language structures (Warren et al., 1994), and 4) global indicators of language development (Hampton et al., 2017; Kaiser & Roberts, 2013; Roberts & Kaiser, 2015). Adult prompts are faded within EMT from most supportive (models) to least supportive (open questions) as new language forms are being acquired. Fading encourages children to use their newly learned language skills more flexibly and independently than may occur when children participate in more traditional ABA instruction. Children with ASD have particular difficulty in generalizing social-communication skills across settings and people (Goldstein, 2002). Thus, teaching in everyday communicative contexts, teaching partners to provide support for communication across contexts, and including practice across different people and settings may be especially important for these children.

Social Interactionist Theory

Social interactionist theory is largely influenced by Lev Vygotsky (1978) and Jerome Bruner (1978). This theory of language development holds that language is acquired through social interactions in the natural environment, and it places an emphasis on the communication partner. The partner is a more knowledge-able other who provides meaning for events in the child's environment and mod-els language and communication at a level slightly higher than where the child currently falls, thereby scaffolding learning. Several EMT strategies draw upon this theory. First, the communication partner, most often the parent, establishes a back-and-forth interaction using strategies of environmental engagement. This dyadic interaction is the basis onto which the adult maps language teaching. Sec-ond, the adult uses *target-level language* and *proximal target-level language.* This means that during the established interaction, the adult models language at the child's developmental level for about half of the utterances and uses lan-guage that is slightly more advanced (proximal target) for the rest of the modeled utterances. In this way, the adult is modeling language in the "zone of proximal development" (Vygotsky, 1978, p. 86) and scaffolding learning of more advanced language. Communication partners create an important social-interactional con-text, which may be a motivating force for children to learn language to communi-cate (Bruner, 1974).

The social interactionist theory may be especially important for children with ASD and their parents given early disruptions in the child's social behaviors. Both children and parents are influenced by the context in which they interact and the supports provided as part of this context. For typically developing chil-dren, parents' linguistic input matches children's needs for systematic examples of the language system. Parents adjust their input and feedback on the basis of their children's responses, and there is a smooth bidirectional or transactional flow between adult and child partners. This degree of fit between children and parents is reflected in the adequacy of ongoing communication as well as in the children's acquisition of new communicative forms and strategies. However, children with ASD generally speak less often, are less likely to seek out a communication partner, use fewer words, and have greater difficulty understanding the meaning of parent talk than do their peers who are typically developing (Landa, 2007). Parents can have difficulty matching their linguistic input to their child's existing knowledge. A mismatch can occur between the language input needed for learning and the input parents provide. This mismatch may decrease the frequency as well as the useful-ness of these interactions from a communication and language learning transac-tional perspective. From an intervention perspective, the social interactionist model serves as a means for tailoring parent responses to children's utterances by using the children's current language level to inform the appropriateness of new input provided to them (Camarata & Yoder, 2002; Haebig et al., 2013a). Parent responsiv-ity to child communication attempts must be increased to scaffold or directly rein-force the child's attempts to communicate. Following children's lead in interactions and conversations, modeling language that describes the children's actions, and expanding their utterances will increase input that more closely matches the chil-dren's focus and conceptual understanding. Parents are ideal communication part-ners because they often understand children's communicative intent more easily than do other adults and consequently have more opportunities to model functional language for children to convey their meaning. Responsive interaction strategies (following the child's lead, equal turn taking, language modeling, and expansions) are associated with better language development outcomes when children, includ-ing children with ASD have significantly delayed language (Haebig et al., 2013b; Yoder & Warren, 2004).

Developmental Theory

EMT also draws on developmental theory of typical language development. Developmental theory lays out a sequence of behaviors in typical language development, ranging from early vocalizations to advanced syntactic development (Brown, 1973). EMT uses developmental theory to select skills and adjusts intervention goals to sequentially address developmental milestones. In target-level modeling of language, communication partners provide input at and slightly above the child's current developmental level. Modeling may progress from modeling a small set of vocabulary words to modeling classes of vocabulary (e.g., action verbs); semantic relations (e.g., agent + action, action + location); and short, grammatically complete sentences. Goals are chosen on the basis of initial assessments and are adjusted to meet the next step in development as the child progresses.

Naturalistic Developmental Behavioral Interventions

Given these theoretical roots, EMT falls under the definition of an NDBI (Schreibman et al., 2015). NDBIs include many evidence-based practices for children with ASD and define many of the interventions described in this book. NDBIs have three core components. First, learning targets are not taught discretely but are embedded in ongoing interactions, thus promoting the integration of skills across domains rather than learning skills in isolation. Second, NDBIs most often occur in socially engaging contexts, emphasizing the interaction and the relationship between the child and the partner as a key piece of the learning environment. Third, the strategies of NDBIs "work together to support high levels of success inside ecologically valid contexts, routines and materials within them" (Schreibman et al., 2015, p. 2417). EMT and its theoretical basis fit well within this definition.

Functional Outcomes and Target Areas of Treatment   EMT specifically targets social communication, one of the two core deficits observed in ASD. EMT is delivered in the context of play and everyday activities and targets the functional use of language. EMT goes beyond many language interventions that specifically target vocabulary or syntax development by using principles of behavior analysis and a responsive interaction approach to model and directly teach the social use of language in a generalized setting. The primary goal of EMT is to increase the frequency of functional communication, especially used spontaneously, across everyday contexts and partners. The secondary goals are to increase the diversity of utterances and the complexity of communication, which are done through modeling and prompting communication in a developmental sequence. Both primary and secondary treatment goals can be addressed using the child's mode of communication, including spoken language and AAC use. These treatment goals directly target a functional limitation in social communication associated with ASD.

EMT, like most NDBIs, is designed to be implemented by indigenous communication partners. EMT is a dyadic intervention, occurring between the child and one or more communication partners. Training naturally occurring partners such as parents, caregivers, and teachers in EMT strategies allows the child to gain access to language-promoting strategies in the natural environment.

A meta-analysis of 26 randomized, controlled trials (RCTs) enrolling young children with ASD indicated the largest gains in spoken language occurred when parents collaborated with therapists to deliver intervention (Hampton & Kaiser,

2016). For this reason, an evidence-based coaching method has been paired with EMT to enhance delivery: Teach-Model-Coach-Review (TMCR). TMCR has been shown to be effective in training parents to use the strategies of EMT at high fidelity (Roberts et al., 2014). TMCR builds on theories of adult learning to provide systematic instruction and reflective feedback (Trivette et al., 2009).

TMCR has four steps. The therapist begins each session by reviewing two specific intervention strategies (e.g., modeling and expanding language) with the caregiver (teacher). The therapist then models these strategies with the child, generally for a minimum of 10 minutes, while the caregiver watches. This modeling provides the child with a baseline dosage of the intervention from a skilled intervention, which is especially important at the beginning of training when the caregiver is not yet fluent in his or her skills. While modeling with the child, the therapist verbally highlights the use of those strategies (e.g., "When he vocalized while playing with the car, I said 'car' and activated the SGD [speech-generating device]"). After the therapist models with the child, the caregiver practices the strategies with the child and is coached by the therapist. During the coaching, the therapist provides materials to support play and engagement, makes suggestions for using the EMT strategies, praises the caregiver's use of the specific strategies, and gives corrective feedback as needed. The therapist ends the session by reviewing with the caregiver, pointing out specific instances in which the caregiver used the intervention strategies, verbally linking the caregiver's use of specific EMT strategies to the child's play and communication behaviors, and allowing the caregiver to reflect on the experience. The therapist and caregiver then make a plan for other times the caregiver will use the EMT strategies between coaching sessions to ensure that the child is getting daily exposure to the strategies.

EMPIRICAL BASIS

Across the last three decades, milieu teaching strategies have been expanded to include environmental arrangement and responsive interaction strategies as well as elicitive modeling, mand modeling, time delay, and incidental teaching. Since 1990, this expanded model of milieu teaching has been referred to as *Enhanced Milieu Teaching* (Kaiser, 1993). Initial studies of milieu teaching extended and specified the incidental teaching model of Hart and Risley (1968, 1975). Since then, more than 50 studies incorporating variants of milieu teaching have been conducted (Kaiser & Trent, 2007).

EMT blends six main components: 1) environmental arrangement to set the physical and interactional stage for promoting children's engagement with activities and communication partners (Ostrosky & Kaiser, 1991); 2) responsive interaction strategies to build a social, conversational interaction (Weiss, 1981); 3) modeling new language forms to expose children to a variety of words; 4) expanding children's communication and language to provide models that are aligned with the child's interest and communicative intent; 5) using time delay strategies to elicit communication without verbal prompts and to bridge the gap to spontaneous use of language; and 6) targeted milieu teaching episodes in response to children's requests. See Kaiser and Hampton (2016) for more detailed information about the empirical basis of EMT with children with general language impairments.

As discussed previously, EMT has been developed from early work in incidental teaching to incorporate aspects of responsive interaction and milieu teaching, and as such, several variants of EMT are currently implemented with children with ASD in the empirical literature. This section discusses the bases on which EMT has been used and tested, specifically with children with ASD, although EMT has also been used with children with specific language impairment, Down syndrome, cleft palate, developmental delays, and cochlear implants. The research on EMT with children with ASD included in this section used the key components of EMT as conceptualized today, including 1) occurring in typical routines across a day (play, snack, reading books), 2) using environmental arrangement strategies to promote child engagement and communication with a partner, 3) an emphasis on modeling and nonverbal elicitation strategies, and 4) balanced milieu teaching prompting procedures with responsive interaction strategies.

The studies included in this section represent the range of EMT studies conducted over the last 25 years that have included children with ASD (e.g., Hancock & Kaiser, 2002; Hancock et al., 2008; Kaiser et al., 2000; Kaiser et al., 2008). This evidence is separated into three noteworthy categories: 1) EMT implemented primarily by therapists (Hancock & Kaiser, 2002; Hampton et al., 2019); 2) EMT delivered by coaching caregivers to implement the intervention strategies, either as the primary therapist or together with a therapist (Hancock et al., 2008; Kaiser et al., 2000; Kaiser et al., 2008; Kaiser & Roberts, 2013); and 3) EMT when used in conjunction with other evidence-based practices or tools (Hancock et al., 2008; Kaiser et al., 2008; Kasari et al., 2014; Hampton, Kaiser, Nietfeld, & Khachoyan, 2021; Olive et al., 2007). See Table 10.1 for a summary of the levels of evidence.

Therapist-Implemented Enhanced Milieu Teaching

Two single-case studies have demonstrated the effectiveness of EMT for increasing language and communication for children specifically with ASD when delivered by a therapist.

In the first study, four preschool children with autism and their mothers participated (Hancock & Kaiser, 2002). The children ranged in age from 35 to 54 months, and their measured IQ scores ranged from <50 to 95. Expressive and receptive skills were in the 20- to 28- month range as measured by the Sequenced Inventory

Table 10.1. Enhanced Milieu Teaching research with levels of evidence categorized by overall design strength (Levels Ia–IV; Phillips et al., 2001) as well as quality of evidence for group and single-participant experimental designs (Reichow et al., 2008)

EMT implementation approach	Design type	Article	Level of evidence
Therapist implemented	III: SCD	Hancock & Kaiser (2002) Hampton, Kaiser, Nietfeld, & Kachoyan (2020)	Strong
	Ib: RCT	Hampton et al. (2019)	Strong
Parent implemented	III: SCD	Kaiser et al. (2000)	Strong
	III: SCD	Kaiser & Hancock (2003)	Moderate
	Ib: RCT	Hampton, Kaiser, & Fuller (2020)	Strong
Additional adaptations	III: SCD	Olive et al. (2007)	Strong
	Ib: RCT	Kasari et al. (2014)	Strong

Key: EMT, Enhanced Milieu Teaching; RCT, randomized, controlled trial; SCD, single-case design.

of Communication Development (SICD; Hedrick et al., 1975), and average MLU at entry was 1.29 (range 1.03–2.00).

The study used a multiple baseline across participants single case experimental design (Ledford & Gast, 2018). Children in this study completed either 5 or 7 baseline sessions, 24 intervention sessions, and 6 follow-up sessions (one each month for the 6 months after the intervention ended), with each session lasting 15–20 minutes. Therapists did not use EMT strategies during baseline play sessions but did use EMT strategies with a high level of precision and well above established levels of fidelity during intervention and follow-up sessions. Generalization of the children's use of social communication with their untrained parents was assessed in the families' homes in nine sessions: three each at baseline, intervention, and the 6-month follow-up.

In addition, the children were assessed on a battery of standardized language tests: the SICD (Hedrick et al., 1975), the Peabody Picture Vocabulary Test–Revised (PPVT-R; Dunn & Dunn, 1981), and the Expressive One-Word Picture Vocabulary Test–Revised (EOWPVT-R; Gardner, 1990). Two 30-minute language samples were completed during baseline, at the end of intervention, and again at the end of the follow-up phase. Based on these standardized assessments and observations, early semantic language targets were selected for each child, including two-word forms (viz., agent-action, action-object, attribute-object, two-word request) or three-word forms (viz., agent-action-object, three-word request).

Observational time series data indicated that all four children showed positive increases for specific target language use (prompted and unprompted) across the 24 intervention sessions, and these results were maintained through the 6-month follow-up observations (Hancock & Kaiser, 2002). There was also evidence of positive changes in the children's complexity (MLU increases for three children) and diversity of language (all four children) used during the intervention sessions. Three of the four children generalized these positive language effects to interactions with their mothers at home, with the greatest change seen immediately after the intervention ended.

Therapist-delivered EMT (Hancock & Kaiser, 2002) resulted in positive changes for children's social communication assessed across settings and measures. In addition, these changes generalized to interactions with their parents, who had not been trained in the EMT intervention. The results of this study indicate that shorter amounts of a powerful, focused intervention positively impact the language skills of children with ASD. Younger children whose language development was less delayed relative to their age showed the greatest increases in the acquisition, maintenance, and generalization of language skills. The single child who did not show the same level of changes as the other three children may have needed more than 24 intervention sessions or more intense sessions, that is, sessions lasting longer than 15–20 minutes, to show positive language changes.

A recent single case experimental design study examined the effects of EMT implemented in the context of a South African school for children with ASD (Hampton et al., 2019). Three children between ages 5 and 8, in a school for children with ASD in Cape Town, South Africa, participated in the study. Students were evaluated using the Preschool Language Scales–Fourth Edition (PLS-4; Zimmerman et al., 2002), a 20-minute naturalistic language sample, and a play-based assessment. All of the participants rated low in verbal communicators, with fewer than 10 words during the language sample and expressive language age equivalents on the PLS-4 between 1 and 2 years.

Following baseline assessments, therapist-implemented EMT was delivered in a multiple baseline design across participants (Hampton et al., 2019). During each session, the child participated in 30-minute one-to-one sessions with the therapist twice weekly in a small clinic room in the school. During baseline sessions, the therapist joined the child in play with the toys but did not implement the specific EMT intervention procedures. When the first participant showed a low and stable trend in the number of different words (NDW) used spontaneously during a 10-minute coded segment of the session, EMT for that child commenced. During EMT sessions, the therapist used the same setting and materials but used EMT strategies, including environmental arrangement, responsive interaction, modeling of target-level language, language expansions, and elicitation (time delays and milieu prompting). When the first participant demonstrated a clear and stable shift in level or trend on NDW, the next participant commenced the EMT session, and frequency of sessions for the first participant was reduced but continued to maintain the child's language skills.

The results of this study (Hampton et al., 2019) indicated a moderately strong functional relation between EMT and NDW. All three participants demonstrated a clear shift in level, trend, or variability concurrent with the onset of intervention. Furthermore, they each demonstrated an increase in level and variability of the frequency of their spontaneous utterances immediately following the introduction of the intervention. All three participants showed marked increases in NDW and spontaneous utterances from pretest to posttest during the language sample (with the therapist) and during the play assessment (with an adult untrained in EMT strategies), indicating some evidence of generalization of communication gains to novel contexts. This study is important because it shows that EMT can be an effective intervention for children in low-resource environments.

Parent-Implemented Enhanced Milieu Teaching

Given that EMT is a naturalistic intervention, the majority of research has included indigenous communication partners, particularly primary caregivers, as an implementer of the intervention. As a result, combining EMT with systematic strategies for teaching caregivers has been central to the development of an effective and useful naturalistic intervention (Kaiser & Roberts, 2013). This has been demonstrated across single case design studies and RCTs.

In a single case design study, Kaiser, Hancock, and Nietfeld (2000) examined the effects of training parents to implement EMT with their preschoolers with ASD. A modified single case research design across six families was used to assess the parent's acquisition and generalized use of EMT strategies. The six male children in this study ranged in age from 32 to 54 months and included three children who had a diagnosis of autistic disorder, two who had a diagnosis of pervasive developmental disorder-not otherwise specified (PDD-NOS), and one child who had an Asperger syndrome diagnosis. At entry, the children on average scored 24 months on the expressive section of the SICD and 25 months on the receptive section of the SICD. The children's average MLU at the beginning of the intervention was 1.48 (range 1.00–2.37). Their IQ scores ranged from <50 to 85; however, low scores were associated with nonresponsiveness during the testing (>50 is the lowest score possible). The participating parents were mothers who ranged in age from 30 to 37 and averaged 3 years of college. All parent training sessions and parent–child play sessions (baseline, intervention, follow-up) were conducted in a clinic setting. Generalization sessions were conducted and videotaped in the families' homes (baseline, end of intervention, follow-up).

Before intervention began, children were pretested using a battery of standardized language assessments, including the SICD, the PPVT-R, and the EOWPVT-R, parent report measures of children's language on the MacArthur-Bates Communication Development Inventories–Second Edition (MCDI-2; Fenson et al., 2007), and two 30-minute language samples taken from play interactions between the children and a trained research assistant. Based on these standardized assessments, observations, and parent input, early semantic language targets were selected for all children. Individual targets ranged from single nouns and action verbs to three-word requests or three-word forms, such as agent-action-object. The assessments were repeated at the end of intervention and again at the end of the follow-up phase.

Following the completion of the baseline phase, 24 intervention sessions were conducted with each parent and child. Intervention sessions lasted approximately 45 minutes and included providing the parent with information about EMT strategies, allowing the parent to practice EMT strategies in a play session with the child while the EMT therapist provided live coaching, and offering the parent suggestions for using the procedures at home. After the end of intervention, follow-up sessions were completed once a month for 6 months to assess parents' maintenance of EMT strategies and children's use of communication skills. No coaching or feedback was provided during these follow-up sessions.

Five of the six parents learned all of the EMT procedures to criterion levels within the 24 intervention sessions (see Roberts et al., 2014; Kaiser & Roberts, 2013 for specific criterion levels) and maintained their use of these EMT strategies during the follow-up, sometimes at higher levels than had been observed at the end of intervention but always well above baseline levels. Five of the six parents showed consistent generalization across most EMT procedures at the postintervention observation and sustained their performance during the follow-up observations.

All six children showed increases in their spontaneous use of language targets, which were maintained during the clinic follow-up sessions. Four of the six children showed increases in MLU or diversity of words used at the end of intervention, and all six children showed changes in these measures during the follow-up period. Children showed similar increases in targets, MLU, and diversity of words in the home generalization sessions with their parents. Evidence of developmental changes was indicated on standardized assessments for all six children on the SICD (average increase of 10 months on receptive communication from baseline to follow-up; average increase of 9 months on expressive communication from baseline to follow-up) and for all six children on the EOWPVT-R (average increase of 18 months from baseline to follow-up). In this first study of parent-implemented EMT with children with ASD, results indicated that parents could implement these strategies effectively and efficiently and that their children showed positive effects in their observed and assessed social-communication skills as a result of their parents' use of EMT.

In a second study, researchers investigated the effects of a parent- and therapist-implemented EMT intervention on the communication skills of three children with autism (Hancock et al., 2008; Kaiser et al., 2008S). These children and their parents were part of a larger study (Kaiser & Roberts, 2013) investigating the effects of two models of EMT on the language performance of children with cognitive deficits and significant language delays. The larger study of EMT randomly assigned children to two different delivery conditions: 1) when delivered by two skilled therapists in the clinic and at home and 2) when implemented by the children's trained parent and a skilled therapist (parent + therapist) in clinic and home. The children who participated in the single subject design study were the first three children with autism who were randomly assigned to the parent + therapist condition in the larger study.

The three children all had an autism diagnosis and included two boys and one girl ranging in age from 36 to 48 months. The children's average receptive language standard score was 50, and their average expressive language standard score was 58, as assessed by the PLS-4 (Zimmerman et al., 2002). The children's average MLU before beginning the intervention was 1.13 (range 1.04–1.22), and their nonverbal IQ scores ranged from 62 to 76 on the Leiter International Performance Scale–Revised (Leiter-R; Roid & Miller, 1997).

A multiple baseline design across participants was used to evaluate the effects of the parent + therapist EMT intervention on the children's language. Following the procedures for multiple baseline designs, baseline observations occurred for five to seven sessions or until stable levels and trends were observed in child and adult data. The intervention was introduced sequentially across three parent–child dyads. When the effects of the intervention were observed for the first child (6–10 sessions), the intervention was introduced for the next child. The same procedure was followed for the third child. The intervention continued until 36 sessions were completed. Follow-up intervention observations in the clinic occurred at 6 and 12 months after the intervention ended.

All three children had the same two-word target forms (agent-action, action-object, modifier-noun, two-word request) that were selected on the basis of their pretest assessments. Intervention sessions were conducted in the clinic (24 sessions) and in the children's homes (12 sessions interspersed with clinic sessions). Each clinic-based intervention session lasted approximately 1 hour and included four parts: 1) training on a specific EMT strategy, 2) the therapist-implemented EMT session, 3) the parent-implemented EMT session, and 4) a review of the day's session and a plan for the next session. During home intervention sessions, the parent coach supported the parent's use of the targeted strategy during four activities in the home: playing with the child's toys, snack, book reading, and a cleanup task.

By the end of intervention, parents implemented EMT at levels consistent with those of the skilled therapists who worked with their children. Two of the three children showed increases in their use of targets, MLU, and diversity of vocabulary during the intervention and at both the 6- and 12-month follow-up assessments. On average, the children showed an increase of 23 points on their PPVT-R standard scores from baseline to the 12-month follow-up and an increase of 28 points on their Expressive Vocabulary Test-2 (EVT-2) standard scores from baseline to the 12-month follow-up.

The results of this study (Kaiser et al., 2008) suggest that the parent + therapist–implemented EMT intervention may be an efficient and effective protocol for teaching new language skills to young children with ASD. Immediately upon entry into the intervention condition, children received systematic intervention to learn their targeted forms and more elaborated language with skilled therapists while their parents were learning each component of EMT to criterion. Children's increased communication initiations and responses primed by skilled therapists potentially provided parents with more opportunities to practice their newly learned EMT skills. As parents became proficient in their use of EMT strategies, they facilitated their children's use of new language skills on a daily basis at home and continued the intervention when the clinic intervention with the skilled therapist was completed.

In a recent RCT (Hampton, Kaiser, Nietfeld, & Khachoyan, 2021), 68 preverbal children ages 36–60 months with ASD and fewer than 20 words and their caregivers were randomly assigned to receive an EMT-based intervention with parent training or the business-as-usual control group. The study examined the effects of a multicomponent intervention that included training parents to implement EMT strategies during play and everyday activities. Children were assessed at baseline, postintervention (4 months), and follow-up (4 months) on a battery of language and developmental assessments, including language samples, the Early Social Communication Scales (ESCS; Mundy et al., 2003), the Mullen Scales of Early Learning (Mullen, 1984), the PLS-4 (Zimmerman et al., 2002), and the MCDI-2 (Fenson et al., 2007). On average, at pretest, children used 12 words during the language sample and had PLS-4 raw scores of 22 on both the receptive and expressive subscales, indicating a language age equivalent of about 18 months.

All parents and their children received an iPad programmed with Proloquo2go (AssistiveWare, 2012) to use throughout the study. The treatment group participated in 36 intervention sessions (two clinic and one home) each week for 4 months. During each 1-hour session, the therapist provided up to 15 minutes of discrete trial training (DTT; Smith, 2001) for four pivotal communication skills, modeled EMT with the child, and coached the caregiver to use EMT in play routines and in-home routines (e.g., snack, art, books, self-care).

At posttest, children in the intervention group, when compared to children in the treatment-as-usual control group, had significantly more instances of joint attention measured by ESCS; at follow-up, they had significantly more socially communicative utterances during the caregiver–child interaction. Caregivers trained in EMT demonstrated significantly higher use of matched turns, target language, language expansions, and time delay strategies, and these gains generally remained significant at follow-up. Maintenance of parents' use of EMT paired with children's continued growth in socially communicative utterances suggests caregivers' use of EMT may have promoted continued growth even after the primary implementation of multicomponent intervention ended.

Adaptations of Enhanced Milieu Teaching

Research on communication interventions for children with autism has expanded in the last decade, and new strategies for improving the foundations of social communication have emerged (Fuller & Kaiser, 2020). Traditional EMT strategies have been expanded to include new strategies (e.g., modeling nonverbal joint attention behaviors [point, show, give], modeling and expanding play) and modes of communication (e.g., augmentative and alternative communication [AAC]) to improve outcomes for children with ASD.

EMT has been adapted to include use of AAC, specifically SGDs that provide digitized or recorded voice output based on programmable software controlling touch-based screen. Increased access to iPads and similar tablets, and flexible software (e.g., Proloquo2go and GOTalk) has made these systems convenient, portable, and socially acceptable (Sennott & Bowker, 2009). Numerous studies have demonstrated SGD use can be taught to children with ASD, resulting in a functional communication system. For example, van der Meer and Rispoli (2010) reviewed

29 interventions that taught 51 children with ASD to use SGDs. They reported increases in communication or SGD-related skills for 86% of the children enrolled in the studies.

In a multiple probe across participants design, Olive and colleagues (2007) tested the effects of EMT using an SGD for three children with ASD. Three children between 45 and 66 months old and their teacher participated in the study. None of the three children communicated with functional words, and each received scores above 42 on the Childhood Autism Rating Scale (CARS, Schopler et al., 1986), indicating severe autism. Baseline and intervention occurred in 5-minute play-based sessions in the children's classroom. In the baseline sessions, the teacher played and talked as she normally did but did not use EMT strategies, and although the SGD was present, she did not model its use. During intervention sessions, the teacher used EMT strategies, with the one adaptation that when a child initiated a nonverbal request (e.g., reach, grab), the teacher followed the milieu prompting procedure but prompted the child to respond using the SGD. Phase changes were based on consistent changes affecting the dependent variable (i.e., correct and independent requesting using the SGD), in level, trend, or variability co-occurring with the onset of intervention.

All three children showed an increase in SGD use to request following intervention. In addition, all three children showed an increase in total communication following the intervention, including gesture, vocalization, and SGD use. These findings suggest that EMT used with an SGD can increase children's rate of communication.

A second adaptation of EMT, building on the use of EMT with an SGD, was the addition of Joint Attention, Symbolic Play, Emotional Regulation (JASPER; Kasari et al., 2006). JASPER uses toy play as a context for increasing joint attention and engagement behaviors that are considered to be foundational in ultimately improving social communication (see Chapter 9 for a complete description). JASPER specifically teaches symbolic play skills and the use of communicative gestures (point, show, give) for commenting and requesting. EMT and JASPER interventions, when blended into a single intervention (J-EMT), teach both basic social communication and expressive language. J-EMT uses the language support strategies of EMT (e.g., modeling, expansions, milieu teaching episodes) combined with JASPER strategies to teach symbolic play and joint engagement (e.g., modeling progressively higher levels of play, scaffolding joint engagement). In a sequential RCT, J-EMT with spoken language only was compared to J-EMT using an SGD plus spoken language. Sixty-one minimally verbal children with ASD ages 5–8 years were initially randomly assigned to the J-EMT with spoken language only or the J-EMT with spoken language plus an SGD (Kasari et al., 2014). After 12 weeks of treatment (Phase 1), children were assessed to determine response to treatment. Children who were identified as nonresponders were rerandomized to receive the addition of the SGD in their J-EMT with spoken language only intervention or to receive a more intensive dosage of J-EMT with spoken language only (Phase 2). During Phase 2, parents in both groups were trained to implement J-EMT. After 6 months of intervention, children who received the J-EMT with SGD intervention in Phase 1 and Phase 2 showed significantly greater gains in spoken language compared to the children who received J-EMT with spoken language only. In addition, children who received the SGD only in Phase 2 demonstrated more spoken language than children who received a higher dosage of J-EMT but no SGD in Phase 2. Two aspects of these results are important to note. First, children in both groups showed progress in spoken language across the 6 months of intervention combining therapist- plus parent-implemented J-EMT, with an average increase of 20 socially communicative utterances in a 20-minute language sample over the 24-week intervention. Second, children who received the therapist- plus parent-implemented J-EMT intervention that incorporated an SGD had better immediate and long-term outcomes at the 6-month follow-up, showing an average of 21.6 more socially communicative utterances during the 20-minute language sample than children in the J-EMT group without an SGD at the end of the 24-week intervention. For children with ASD who have minimal verbal social communication, a blended intervention (J-EMT with use of SGD) implemented by therapists and parents may be an effective strategy for teaching spoken language.

Hampton, Kaiser, and Fuller (2020) extended the therapist plus parent-implemented J-EMT with SGD intervention to include therapist-implemented DTT to teach foundational communication skills (e.g., joint attention, imitation, receptive language, basic SGD operations) to preverbal preschoolers with ASD. The intervention included brief (10–15 minutes), structured, direct teaching with a relatively high number of teaching trials (approximately 15–30, depending on child attention to the task) and systematic reinforcement of child responses with social and tangible consequences. The goal was to provide direct instruction for foundational skills in a structured context to improve children's response to the naturalistic, caregiver-implemented EMT intervention. The findings indicated that this multicomponent intervention was effective in increasing joint attention and social communication with a caregiver after about 100 hours of intervention (3 hours per week for 36 weeks), including time spent teaching parents the intervention across clinic and home.

The findings of these studies suggest that EMT can be blended with additional evidence-based strategies to improve early communication for children with autism who have limited spoken language. The blended interventions have potential for tailoring components to fit specific profiles of children with ASD. For example, more intensive DTT or a more naturalistic teaching of joint attention skills might be implemented with children who have low social communication and few skills for learning language in naturalistic EMT interactions. Within the Kasari and colleagues (2014), Hampton, Kaiser and Fuller (2020), Hampton, Kaiser, Nietfeld, and Khachoyan (2021) studies, adaptations were implemented to address children's entry communication skills; however, additional research is needed to replicate and extend these adaptations. Ongoing studies are furthering the examinations of beneficial adaptations by including a blended DTT, JAPSER, and EMT intervention for school-age children and EMT for children with ASD under age 3.

Summary of the Evidence to Date

The seven studies previously described (Hampton et al., 2019; Hampton, Kaiser, Nietfeld, & Khachoyan, 2021; Hancock & Kaiser, 2002; Kaiser et al., 2000; Kaiser et al., 2008; Kasari et al., 2014; Olive et al., 2007) provide empirical evidence of the effectiveness of EMT when implemented by parents or therapists with children with ASD. Together, they represent systematic replication of EMT, progressive development of this model, and consistent evidence of generalization by children and parents trained in EMT. Further, they demonstrate the ability to adapt the intervention to meet the needs of the full spectrum of children with ASD, including those who are minimally verbal. Ongoing and future studies of EMT with children who have ASD will address key limitations of these studies: 1) the majority of these studies were completed by the same research team, 2) variability in child outcomes suggests that further tailoring of intervention may be needed for children who are initially unresponsive to treatment, and 3) longitudinal evaluations of sequential intervention to move from simple functional communication to social language use are needed.

PRACTICAL REQUIREMENTS

Implementing EMT at high levels of fidelity requires a significant time commitment, and most parents who participated in EMT training reported that the positive outcomes for their children far outweighed the time devoted to training and practice. Many parents in our research program brought their children to a university clinic twice each week for EMT sessions. About one third of participating parents drove more than 50 miles to participate in the training. Over time, we modified aspects of the protocol to reduce parents' time commitments and to promote better generalization to the home setting. One third (12) of the intervention sessions in our last study were conducted at home (Hampton, Kaiser, Nietfeld, & Khachoyan, 2021). When needed, a second staff member accompanied the parent coach and provided care for siblings so that the parent and the parent coach could focus on practicing the intervention with the target child. Home intervention sessions were conducted using routine activities (e.g., snack, cleanup, reading a book, and play) and materials and settings within the home that had been identified by the family.

Although interventionists do not need to meet any specific professional requirements to receive training in EMT, most have an educational background in speech and language sciences, psychology, or special education and have previous experience with young children who have special needs, including children with ASD. Interventionists receive training in EMT through observing and coding the discrete behaviors of EMT, attending an intensive interactive workshop on the principles and components of EMT, and implementing EMT strategies with practice children while receiving systematic coaching and feedback from experienced staff. After successful completion of the EMT training program, interventionists are paired with experienced staff who provide ongoing feedback on their implementation of EMT strategies with children. Interventionists also receive systematic feedback through coded and summarized session data and support through weekly research meetings.

For those interventionists who want to become a parent coach, additional training is provided (Kaiser & Hancock, 2003; Kaiser et al., 2007; Kaiser & Roberts, 2013). Even when an interventionist is skilled in implementing EMT with several children, giving feedback to another adult about the intervention requires an entirely different skill set. Information about effective parent training and coaching strategies are provided in readings, handouts, and video examples. Interventionists then learn to apply this information in an apprentice model with an experienced parent coach who provides ongoing feedback and support (see Kaiser & Hancock, 2003; Kaiser et al., 1998, for more detailed information about training parent coaches). The entire training process for an EMT interventionist who also trains parents in the intervention from learning to code to functioning as a primary parent coach takes 6 months to 1 year to complete. This apprentice approach ensures that children and parents receive the most effective intervention while trainees are fully supported in becoming skilled and independent.

KEY COMPONENTS

Refer to Table 10.2 for specific examples of the first four of the six components of EMT: 1) environmental arrangement, 2) responsive interaction, 3) specific language modeling, 4) language expansions, 5) time delay, and 6) milieu teaching prompts. Children with ASD frequently exhibit behaviors that make implementation of EMT procedures more difficult. These behaviors include restricted interests in activities and toys, limited joint attention skills, limited social engagement with adults during activities, perseverative behavior, verbal echolalia, and other challenging behaviors (e.g., throwing materials, physical aggression). Specific adaptations of EMT strategies to accommodate children with ASD and make the intervention more effective and functional for them have been developed. These adaptations are included in the following discussion of the six components of EMT.

Environmental Arrangement

The purpose of environmental arrangement is to create a context for teaching and learning language. Selecting and arranging materials and activities of interest supports child engagement and increases interactions with adults. Generally, when children are interested in activities, they are motivated to engage with adults in communication interactions for longer periods of time. Selecting interesting materials and activities for children with ASD, however, can be challenging because these children often have restricted interests. In addition, sometimes children with ASD find a particular toy or material so interesting that they exclude the adult from the interaction either by focusing exclusively on the toy or by refusing to allow the adult to enter into the play. Inviting the child to choose a toy from a set of moderately preferred toys (and not offering toys that set the occasion for exclusionary play) provides an immediate assessment of child interest. For children with limited attention or few play skills, toy choices may be offered at the beginning of a play session and at several intervals during the session when the child loses interest. Selecting sets of materials that are presented sequentially can extend the time spent in shared play (e.g., introducing a toy garage and cars followed by people who fit into the cars, sponges and buckets for washing cars, brushes and pretend paint for painting cars). This serves two purposes. First, including a variety of toys, activities, and play schemes allows adults to model a range of vocabulary and syntax forms. Novel materials and actions introduced into an established play routine can be used to draw attention to the verbal model of the label and the action. Routines provide repeated opportunities to model sequences of utterances that describe cohesive action schemes ("The boy feeds the cows, then they go into the barn, and then they go to sleep"). Second, having a variety of choices allows children to maintain engagement with the adult either by extending the routine, or by transitioning to a new routine with limited time spent in transition.

Children with ASD often have restricted interests in toys and play routines, which can limit opportunities for modeling and prompting diverse language forms. There is often a delicate balance between providing a toy with which the child will play for an extended time and exposing the child to different toys so the adult can model a variety of vocabulary. Some balance can be achieved by allowing the child to play with a favorite toy while the adult slowly introduces novel, attractive materials to the toy. Then the adult may require the child to play with these newly introduced materials for increasingly long periods of time before accessing the favorite

Table 10.2. Rationales and examples of the Enhanced Milieu Teaching components

EMT Strategies	Rationale	Examples
Environmental Arrangement	Promote child engagement	Select and arrange materials and activities that are of interest to the child
		Provide a number of choices to allow for changing preferences
	Maintain and extend the child's play and interaction with the adult	Provide additional materials like water when playing with the farm so child can give animals a bath or a drink
	Prevent and manage child behavior problems by arranging physical surroundings	Designate a play space with a physical cue like a carpet square; limit number of toys/materials that are within the child's reach
Responsive interaction	Engage children in positive interactions	Follow the child's play or conversational lead so there is no pressure for the child to perform.
	Prime child for responding	Mirror child's actions and verbally map corresponding language, which supports the child in orienting to adult communication.
	Maintain space for the child to engage in conversations	Pace the interaction so there is plenty of time (at least 5 seconds) for the child to participate as an equal conversation partner.
	Reinforce child for any and all communication attempts	Respond contingently to any verbal, vocal, or nonverbal child turn.
Modeling child target and target level language	Provide child with salient, specific models of target language	Model all of the child's selected language targets in the context of child interest.
	Prime child to imitate targets spontaneously	Map language onto mirrored actions that are close to the child's attentional focus.
Language expansions	Scaffold language for more complex vocabulary, grammar, and syntax	Expand child language by adding one to three words to model more complex language at a time when the child is motivated to communicate.
Time delay	Provide nonverbal and context cues to reduce dependence on verbal prompts	Respond to child reach for toy by naming and giving the toy.
	Language models contingent on child requests are most likely to be imitated	Give a choice by presenting two objects; when the child chooses, model the label and give object the child chooses.
	Access to preferred items reinforces communication attempts	
Milieu Teaching prompts	Children are highly motivated to respond when prompting follows a request	When a child requests using a gesture, prompt use of a spoken word ("<u>Tell me</u> what you want.")
	Prompts support practice of target level language in functional context	Following child use of a single word ("open"), prompt a two-word utterance by modeling (Say: "open box")
	A least-to-most sequence of prompts provides the level of support the child needs for target language	If child does not respond to an open question (e.g., "What do you want?") follow up with a choice prompt (e.g., "Puzzle or truck?").

toy. For example, if a child perseverates on trains, the adult may begin the play session with a train and add other materials or expand play to build an extended play scheme. The adult might have the train go down the track to the train-washing station where the child can spray soap and water to wash the train. The train may transport animals or people. Each train car may carry a piece of Mr. Potato Head that is assembled when the train reaches the station. Expanding play by modeling and prompting new actions helps children with ASD extend their time playing and increases the diversity of play actions.

Children with ASD, like most children, may have varying attention spans or fleeting interest in toys and activities. For this reason, it is important to have a variety of materials available. However, it is also important to maintain control of the environment. This means that some toys may be kept on a shelf or out of view and brought out when needed. Toys should be cleared away when not in use to maintain an orderly environment but should remain out should the child want to return to the routine.

Although in ideal situations toys should be arranged on the floor or at a small table and the child should be able to roam freely so that the adult can follow the child's lead, in some cases, more structure or a restricted space may be required. If the child spends most of his or her time roaming the room without choosing a toy or an activity, this is an indication that more structure is needed. Consider arranging the environment so there is less space to roam or with the child seated at a table. The adult should always be seated across from or next to the child to promote eye contact and shared attention.

Responsive Interaction

Following the child's lead in play and conversation, verbal and nonverbal turn taking, and mirroring actions while providing verbal descriptions or mapping child actions are core strategies included in the **responsive interaction** component of EMT. The purpose of these strategies is to engage the child in nonverbal and verbal interactions that provide the opportunities for modeling new language forms and increase the likelihood that the child will interact with the adult as a conversational partner. Play with toys and nonverbal engagement between the child and adult set the context for language modeling; however, implementing these responsive interaction strategies is challenging when children with ASD have limited functional play skills, engage in repetitive or inappropriate actions with toys, or have low rates of engagement with adults.

Following the child's lead and nonverbal mirroring are intended to promote connection between the child and adult and extend nonverbal engagement; however, these strategies also reinforce existing behavior when the adult responds contingently. To use these strategies effectively, the adult must wait until the child performs an appropriate action or play behavior. In addition, following the child's lead or mirroring the child's actions is often sufficient to promote a nonverbal connection between the child and the responsive adult. However, these strategies also must be balanced with moving the child to a more complex play schema or routine by expanding the child's play actions with new materials or by modeling new actions.

Language Modeling

Language modeling provides children with salient, specific models of targeted language forms in ongoing interactions with adults. Each child has an identified language level, determined by initial assessments or observations during intervention.

About half of the adult's utterances should be at the child's target level. By modeling target language, the adult primes the child to imitate language that is in the child's developmental range. The other half of the adult's utterances should model language slightly above the child's target, exposing the child to more complex language.

Modeling targets at the child's selected language level, however, can be problematic for some children with ASD. Adults may need to pay particular attention to modeling diverse vocabulary, which can be difficult when children have restricted interests. Supplementing children's restricted toy interest with additional materials may provide adults with opportunities to model more diverse vocabulary. Adults may need to pay particular attention to modeling when interacting with children who are imitative and initiate language with a pronoun reversal, saying *you* when they mean *I*. Prompting the child to use *I* is one way for the child to practice using pronouns correctly, especially when the child is requesting, but it does not necessarily support the child's ability to comment appropriately. Having the adult model *I* when he or she is mirroring a child's actions and mapping language that corresponds to the actions can be an important strategy for supporting children who are learning to comment about their own actions. For instance, when the adult and child are scooping and pouring beans, the adult can map the action by saying, "I scoop the beans." When the child imitates this statement in the ongoing play activity, he or she is commenting about his play, using *I* correctly. This practice may make it easier for the child to spontaneously comment about what he or she is doing in future activities.

Language Expansions

When a child is communicating verbally, this is an indication that the child is motivated by the particular situation. Language expansions capitalize on this motivation. When a child says an utterance, the adult responds with an expansion, or an utterance that is one or two words longer than the child's utterance. This strategy allows the adult to slowly model longer and more complex utterances. Sometimes language expansions may require an additional action. For example, if the child says "ice cream" while playing with pretend food, the adult might respond by saying, "Eat the ice cream," while modeling a new part of the routine—eating. In this way, the adult is expanding the language and the routine concurrently.

It is important to note that not every utterance should be expanded. Sometimes children who are frequent imitators can get into unnatural feedback loops that become rote. In this case, the adult should respond with diverse and flexible language.

Time Delay

EMT includes two strategies for the purpose of eliciting communication. The first is **time delay**. A time delay provides a nonverbal cue for communication and is sometimes considered a special class of environmental arrangement. Typically, the adult sets up a nonverbal cue for the child to request. A time delay includes the adult pausing and focusing his or her attention on the child plus holding up a choice, stopping during familiar routine, setting up a situation in which the child needs assistance, or giving the child a small amount of a preferred item. For example, an adult might provide the material of interest to the child in a container that only the adult can open so the child will have to engage the adult by requesting assistance in opening it, or the adult might pause in the middle of a tickling routine and wait for the child to ask for more. The purpose of time delays is to get the child to communicate at a higher rate without creating a reliance on overt prompts (e.g., verbal question, "say" prompts). It is important that time delays are used sparingly so as not to interrupt the flow of the interaction. Time delays that upset the child or cause the child to disengage should be avoided. Presenting a time delay only when the child is requesting (explicitly by reaching, giving an object, or asking or implicitly by looking or vocalizing) and the adult is willing to provide the requested object or continued action as a consequence for communication ensures that the interaction is positive and likely reinforcing for the child.

Milieu Teaching

The prompting procedures of milieu teaching are designed to facilitate children's productive use of new communication forms. Milieu teaching prompts are used only in response to a child initiation, which ensures that the child is motivated to respond. A child initiation could include a reach, grab, or verbal response that is lower than the child's prescribed target. In milieu teaching, the sequence of prompts follows a least-to-most support strategy. The adult starts with an open question (e.g., "What do you want?"), followed by a choice question ("Do you want the dog or the lion?"), and finally a controlling prompt ("Say 'dog'"). Three characteristics of the verbal behavior of children with ASD may interfere with effective use of the milieu teaching prompts: 1) indiscriminate imitation or verbal echolalia, 2) fleeting attention, and 3) resistance to verbal prompting. Based on individual children's specific verbal response, milieu teaching prompting procedures may require modifications to be effective for children with ASD. When children imitate the controlling prompt in modeling episodes, the controlling prompt can be eliminated or given minimal emphasis. The modeling procedure begins with the controlling prompt "say," signaling the child to imitate the adult model. When children with ASD repeat the complete adult utterance, including the prompt "say," the adult may drop the cue "say" and state emphatically what he or she wants the child to say so it is clear that the intent is for the child to imitate. For example, when the adult prompts the child, "Say, 'want juice'" as the child reaches for juice and the child says, "Say want juice," the adult may prompt saying only, "Want juice." Children with verbal echolalia may repeat a choice mand rather than making the choice. For example, if the adult says, "Play with bubbles or the ball?" and the child responds by imitating the question "Bubbles or ball?" the adult may provide more support by offering a visual referent concurrent with the verbal choice. The adult shows the child bubbles and the ball, while saying "Play with bubbles or the ball?" With the concurrent visual and verbal prompts, the child may be able to process the choices visually while having the labels embedded in the question. Even if the child imitates the adult's prompt again, he or she will usually signal a choice by reaching for the preferred object or looking at it. At that point, the adult can provide a model so that the child is fully supported in responding with an accurate request.

Children with ASD often have limited persistence and lose interest or shift interest during a long prompting sequence. In a least-to-most prompting sequence, a child may become frustrated in having to wait for the controlling prompt if he or she needs that level of support. In this case, the adult should go directly to the level of prompt the child requires, with a goal of reducing the level of prompt over time. When implementing any milieu teaching prompting procedure, the adult needs to balance providing sufficient time for the child to respond with holding the child's interest.

Finally, some children with ASD who have participated in therapies that involve repeated prompts for verbal behavior in a drill-and-practice format may refuse to respond to prompts embedded in the EMT procedures. Alternatively, these children may respond *only* when prompted and may not independently initiate language. In these situations, it may be useful to initially limit prompting. Increasing child verbal and nonverbal engagement using responsive interaction and time delay strategies should be the first phase of intervention. Even without prompting, modeling in context and expanding child nonverbal and verbal communication by modeling new forms of language can be a powerful intervention. To increase responding to EMT prompts with prompt-resistant children, adults should choose very-high-probability occasions to prompt (i.e., the child has requested a preferred object and is highly motivated to respond). Reducing the frequency of prompting when intervening with children who are prompt dependent may initially decrease the frequency of child verbalizations; however, responding, expanding, and commenting contingent on child spontaneous communication attempts should increase child frequency over the course of two to six sessions. Because the goal of EMT is productive, spontaneous, and meaningful communication using new language forms, it is important to address, early in the intervention process, the challenges posed by children who are either prompt resistant or prompt dependent.

ASSESSMENT FOR TREATMENT PLANNING

Children with ASD who have been included in our intervention research are screened for eligibility using a global language measure such as the Preschool Language Scale-5 (PLS-5; Zimmerman et al., 2011), and an observational assessment, such as a naturalistic language sample or a caregiver questionnaire. Having both a standardized assessment that measures children's ability to communicate (using prompting and/or elicitation) and a naturalistic assessment to understand children's functional use of language is important with children who have ASD. Although vocabulary knowledge and MLU are important indicators of language potential, these measures are not always the best indicators of children's functional communication skills. Also, children with ASD may appear to have an inflated MLU if they frequently use rote phrases that are longer than their functional, spontaneous speech. Therefore, we ask parents to list their children's rote phrases, and we exclude these phrases when estimating the number of different words produced and MLU on the basis of transcripts of interactions analyzed with Systematic Analysis of Language Transcripts (SALT; Miller & Iglesias, 2012). This approach provides a more accurate estimate of the complexity and variety of children's functional language as a basis for selecting targets for teaching. Children with ASD who are reliant on prompting may do well on standardized tests that present items by asking questions, but they often display very low rates of language, particularly spontaneous language in observational. Therefore, it is important to use both standardized and observational assessments to fully understand a child's verbal communication abilities.

In addition to a standardized and naturalistic assessment, other assessments should be used to understand the child's range of communication across contexts. These additional assessments may include a receptive vocabulary assessment such as the PPVT-4 (Dunn & Dunn, 2007), a productive vocabulary assessment such as the EVT-2 (Williams, 2007), or a parent-reported vocabulary measure such as the MCDI-2 (Fenson et al., 2007) to provide broader information about children's vocabulary knowledge. For many children with ASD, verbal communication is not the primary mode. It may be important to adapt the MCDI-2 to allow caregivers to indicate how the child uses vocabulary: spoken, sign, Picture Exchange Communication System (PECS; Bondy & Frost, 2001), SGD, or other AAC. It is helpful to have multiple natural observations of children's language obtained with one or two unfamiliar therapists and the parent across different settings (clinic and home) and across various activities (play, snack, book reading, and clean up). Children's utterances are transcribed and analyzed using SALT (Miller & Iglesias, 2012). A speech production measure, such as the Arizona Articulation Proficiency Scale-third revision (Fudala, 2000) can be used to capture a child's ability to produce speech sounds; this information is helpful in choosing target vocabulary. Lastly, it is important to gain information from the parent on the child's communication in everyday routines. This can be done using a formal assessment such as a Routines-Based Interview (RBI; McWilliam et al., 2009). By understanding when the child is currently communicating, we can select routines and activities that the child prefers or that the child engages in frequently as a starting point.

This multidimensional assessment approach provides a more accurate estimate of the complexity and variety of children's functional language as a basis for selecting targets and contexts for teaching.

ASSESSMENT FOR PROGRESS MONITORING

Effective intervention requires ongoing monitoring of both adults' use of the EMT strategies and children's communication progress. When conducting research on applications of EMT, we employ a comprehensive data-collection process that includes videotaping adult–child interactions, transcribing adult and child utterances, coding adult and child behavior, and summarizing and graphing the data. A SALT analysis is completed on each transcribed session to provide data on child and adult MLU, diversity, and number of utterances. This level of data collection allows us to monitor whether the adult is implementing the EMT strategies with high levels of fidelity and whether the child is progressing in the use of targeted language forms. Because this level of data collection is time and cost intensive, we have developed other data-collection strategies for professionals in the field who are implementing EMT.

To track a child's progress across EMT sessions, an adult can complete a data-sheet based on audio or video recording of the session or can have another adult observe the session and record the child's behaviors as they occur. Data can be collected on whether a child's target was spontaneously produced, imitated, or prompted or elicited by the adult. Each of the child's targets can be listed, and the adult can record examples of each target or tally the occurrence of each form. When determining how to code a child's utterance, a spontaneous production is a child utterance that is different from the preceding adult utterance. Determining whether a child utterance is spontaneous can sometimes be difficult when a child with ASD has delayed echolalia and imitations do not occur directly after the imitated adult utterance. In general, we code an imitation when a child utterance is stated within 5 seconds of the adult utterance and repeats all or part of that preceding utterance. A prompted utterance is recorded when the child uses the target form response within 5 seconds of a milieu teaching prompt, such as a model ("Say 'dog'") or choice question ("Want the dog or cat?"). A child response to an open question or a time delay is recorded as elicited; although these utterances are generated by the child, they still require some scaffolding from the adult. The adult can also record specific models or expansions if this information is important to implementation of the overall EMT package. Tracking whether children use targeted language forms spontaneously or through prompting provides the adult with information about whether the child has mastered those forms or needs more adult support to learn them.

Depending on the child's social-communication targets, it may also be important to track the child's communication functions during a session. For many children with ASD, increasing child commenting can be key to the child becoming a conversational partner. Therapists or parents can also track language behaviors that are specific and important to monitor for each child. For example, if a child uses mostly scripted talk when interacting with an adult, it might be important to track the number or percentage of utterances that include scripted talk to determine if the child is beginning to communicate in more spontaneous and flexible ways. Summarizing each session and graphically displaying the child's use of targets and the adult's implementation of EMT is essential for the data-based evaluation of progress. Such data can be used to report progress to parents and track progress toward individualized education program goals (see Figure 10.1 for a sample datasheet).

Date Activity	Activity-specific examples	Prompt: SP, TD, MT-O, MT-M, MT-EI	Child responses	Child functions
Target 1				
Target 2				
Target 3				
Total		Spontaneous Prompted	Total target 1 Total target 2 Total target 3 Total all	Comments Requests Others

Figure 10.1. Sample child target-tracking sheet. *Key:* SP, spontaneous, no prompt; TD, time delay; MT-O, milieu teaching prompt–open question; MT-M, milieu teaching prompt–mand; MT-EI, milieu teaching prompt–elicited imitation.

IMPLICATIONS FOR INCLUSIVE PRACTICE

As discussed previously, EMT strategies are designed to be used in typical routines across a day (play, snack, reading books) in interactions when a child is engaged and communicating with a partner. EMT places an emphasis on modeling language and using responsive interaction strategies; these strategies can be used in response to child communicative initiations throughout the day. For example, in a classroom snack time routine, a child might reach across the table toward the milk to indicate that he or she wants more to drink. The teacher can *notice* this communication and *respond* contingently by pouring the child milk and modeling "milk" or "more milk." Similarly, if the child reaches and verbally says "more," the teacher could give the child more milk and *expand* on the child's language by saying "more milk." These strategies should be used during incidental teaching opportunities throughout the day in situations in which adults often ask children questions ("Oh, do you want some more milk?"). In the previous example, by responding to the function of the child's communication (requesting more milk), the teacher has reinforced the child for initiating communication. Providing a verbal model ("milk") provides the child with a language model that he or she can imitate and practice using. Expanding on the child's language ("more milk") links the child's language to new and diverse forms of language, increasing the complexity of the child's communication. When these teaching opportunities are used throughout the day, the child can access a naturally occurring reinforcement in response to his or her communication. Providing these opportunities across classroom routines increases the likelihood that the child will generalize to novel partners, contexts, and materials and that he or she will initiate more frequently in the future.

In addition to using a responsive interaction style throughout the day, a therapist can work closely with a teacher to identify one or two classroom routines that occur consistently and are enjoyable for the child (maximizing the likelihood that the child will be engaged and motivated to communicate). The therapist and the teacher can develop a lesson plan to identify environmental arrangement strategies to promote and increase child engagement and communication with a partner as well as a plan for how and when to balance milieu teaching prompting procedures with responsive interaction strategies.

These routines could be classroom activities such as hand washing, snack, meals, transitions, small-group activities (e.g., circle, academic), or free play. It is important to consider the classroom culture when identifying these routines. Routines identified for focused language teaching should be routines during which either the teacher or another staff member (paraprofessional, speech-language pathologist) can work directly with the child. The teacher should identify who is managing the classroom and/or activity and who is working directly with the target child. If behavior management strategies are needed to help the child stay engaged, these should be identified ahead of time. Clear steps should be identified for each routine (e.g., get lunchbox out of cubby, take lunchbox to table, open lunchbox, take food out, open food, eat, clean up lunchbox, return to cubby). Once steps are identified, use assessments (language sample, standardized assessments) to identify the child's target-level language based on how the child is communicating. Identify target language according to the steps of your routine. For example, with a child who is using one-word targets, you might use the following vocabulary words during a snack routine: *juice, sandwich, crackers, bag, open, close, eat,* and *drink.* Finally, plan three to four time delays and/or milieu teaching episodes for each 10- to 15-minute routine based on the materials that are available for each routine (e.g., pause in routine to open lunchbox, choice between juice and crackers, pause in routine to open sandwich container). As the child learns the expectations and steps of the routine and the teacher becomes more familiar with the strategies, you may consider incorporating a peer in the interaction by teaching the peer how to model language for the target child. It is important to remember that peer buddies will need prompting and reinforcement for using key strategies.

CONSIDERATIONS FOR CHILDREN FROM CULTURALLY AND LINGUISTICALLY DIVERSE BACKGROUNDS

EMT has been shown to be effective both for children with ASD who are primarily English-speaking (Kasari et al., 2014; Roberts & Kaiser, 2012) and for children from culturally and linguistically diverse backgrounds (Hampton, Kaiser, Nietfeld, & Khachoyan, 2021; Hampton et al., 2019; Olive et al., 2010; Wang, 2008). EMT has also been shown to be effective for children with identified language delays who are dual language learners (Peredo et al., 2017). Several factors should be considered when making systematic adaptions to the EMT intervention informed both by the cultural values and linguistic environment of each family. One main consideration when setting up the intervention is the fit of the materials chosen for intervention and the context where intervention will take place. Coaches should work with the family to choose toys and materials for intervention to ensure that the activities are appropriate for the family's culture and values; these activities should be embedded in routines in which parents and children typically interact. Traditionally, EMT is implemented in both play and everyday routines. If the family does not typically engage in play routines with their child, it would be important to begin intervention in home routines that are enjoyable for both the child and adult. After these routines are successful, the therapist could use materials in the home to help the parent engage in joint play routines with their child to supplement existing home routines.

For children with ASD who are dual language learners, it is important to make evidence-based decisions about language targets based on research in bilingual language development. The adult who is working with the child should be relatively competent in the language in which he or she is teaching. Language competence is important for selecting target-level language, for understanding the grammatical structure of the language both for expanding child language, and for systematically adapting target language as the child learns and changes targets. Caregivers should be encouraged to speak to children in the languages they speak with fluency so that they can model rich and more complex language. In addition, language targets should mirror typical language development in the languages spoken by the child and caregiver. It is important to support language development in both languages. Children should be encouraged to use their home language to maintain family culture and connections as well as to support healthy social-emotional development (Kohnert & Derr, 2012). For parents who are not fluent in English, a parent plus therapist model should be considered where the therapist prioritizes teaching in English and the parent uses EMT strategies in the home language.

Although children with ASD are variable in their presentation of speech, language, and communication skills, breakdowns in early communication skills (e.g., eye contact, joint attention) affect the child's ability to learn and use language socially with a partner. Therefore, targets for each child should be selected on the basis of the child's unique characteristics and needs. When considering target language for dual language learners who have ASD, it is important to identify and prioritize language targets for both languages according to the child's linguistic abilities. For example, for a child using one-word targets with a relatively limited vocabulary in both languages, a list of 5 to 10 target words could be identified and prioritized in each language on the basis of the play and/or home routines that were identified by the parent and therapist and the child's specific linguistic needs within each language.

One final cultural consideration is in the implementation of specific EMT strategies. It is important to understand how EMT strategies intersect with the cultural and linguistic values of each family. For example, in the English language, the major emphasis of target-level language and proximal target-level language is to increase the child's linguistic complexity mainly by increasing the child's MLU. In the Spanish language, many complex verb forms are frequently used. Therefore, for Spanish-speaking families, a linguistic adaption for target-level language would be to use more verbs and to model specific verb conjugations, such as first-person plural and third-person singular inflection of verbs (Jackson-Maldonado, 2012). See Peredo and Kaiser (2015) for more information on cultural and linguistic considerations for adapting EMT.

Application to a Child

The following is a brief description of a child who participated in our intervention and for whom the EMT strategies were both appropriate and effective. For a more comprehensive description of this case, please refer to Chapter 7 in the companion volume *Case Studies for the Treatment of Autism Spectrum Disorder.*

Sierra was 34 months old and recently diagnosed with ASD when she participated in our intervention. Sierra's mother, Becky, reported that Sierra had approximately 10 consistent word approximations that she used mostly for requesting. She rarely made eye contact when she was requesting and had limited gesture use. Our evaluations confirmed Becky's report. Sierra's MLU during the language sample was 1.15, and she produced seven different words. Her score for the standardized tests were more than 1.5 standard deviations below the mean, although her score for the auditory comprehension subscale of the Preschool Language Scales was higher than her score for the expressive subscale score.

As a participant in a study, Sierra and her mother participated in 36 sessions of parent-implemented EMT in which the therapist coached the parent to implement the EMT strategies both in the clinic setting and at home. In addition, Becky participated in three workshops where the therapist explained each strategy and gave specific examples, including video examples from Sierra's sessions. During each session, either at home or at the clinic, the therapist and Becky chose toys and activities that they felt Sierra enjoyed and that would be appropriate for engaging her in a dyadic interaction. The therapist then chose one or two strategies for Becky to focus on with Sierra during that session. Over the course of the 36 sessions, the therapist covered all six EMT strategies with Becky. During each 1-hour session, the therapist reviewed the rationale of the strategy. In Sierra's case, consistent with most children, the therapist began with responsive interactions. She explained to Becky all the ways Sierra might be communicating, both verbally and nonverbally (e.g., "She just pointed to the doll to request, so I responded by saying 'doll' and gave it to her"). She then modeled EMT with Sierra for approximately 10 minutes while highlighting all the times she was using responsive interaction strategies. The therapist then invited Becky to practice. While Becky was playing with Sierra, the therapist helped maintain the interaction by handing Becky toys, cleaning up the environment, and giving suggestions of when to use key strategies. The therapist also provided frequent positive feedback to Becky and tied her behavior into Sierra's behavior (e.g., "That was a great way to notice and respond to her point. When you said 'ball,' she imitated you"). At the end of the session, the therapist talked with Becky about how the strategy felt and addressed any questions Becky had. They then made a plan for Becky to use the strategies during everyday interactions. They discussed how Becky could try the same strategies during snack time and bath time, two of Sierra's favorite routines.

Over the course of the 36 sessions, the therapist continued to introduce the remaining EMT strategies and was able to fade her support over time as Becky became more fluent with the EMT strategies. At the end of 36 sessions, Sierra was reassessed using the battery first used during the screening/baseline period. Sierra made consistent changes in her communication in play sessions with her mother in the clinic and at home, showing increases in the number of total and spontaneous targets she used, her MLU, and the diversity of her vocabulary. Furthermore, Becky said she felt confident as a language teacher for Sierra, and she and the therapist made a plan for how she could continue to use the strategies as Sierra's language continues to grow.

**To review an extended application and implementation
of this intervention, see Case 7 in the companion volume
Case Studies for the Treatment of Autism Spectrum Disorder.**

Future Directions

EMT has been implemented effectively with children who have ASD and are between 2.5 and 5 years of age (Hancock & Kaiser, 2002; Hancock et al., 2008; Kaiser et al., 2000; Kaiser et al., 2008). J-EMT has been implemented effectively with minimally verbal children with ASD who are 5–8 years of age and who are minimally verbal despite being involved in at least 2 years of intervention (Kasari et al., 2014). In this study examining a combined JASPER and EMT approach, children in both intervention groups (with and without the addition of an SGD) made gains in their language. J-EMT with the addition of SGD plus DTT has also been implemented effectively for children with ASD (ages 3–5) who are in preverbal stages of linguistic development. We are currently finishing a research project looking at the effects of parent-implemented J-EMT for young children 24–36 months old who were recently identified with ASD (Kaiser & Roberts, 2016–2020).

Results from previous studies indicate that EMT is effective for young children with ASD in early stages of linguistic development (ages 2.5–8) with ASD. Although EMT was effective for both groups (SGD, no SGD) in the study examining school-age minimally verbal children with ASD (Kasari et al., 2014), the group receiving the SGD had significantly more spoken words than the group without the SGD. Currently, we do not understand how the SGD functions and for whom. Although J-EMT with an SGD and the addition of DTT was shown to be effective with young, preverbal children with ASD (Hampton et al., 2020), we still do not understand the optimal dosage for rapidly accelerating language growth both for the DTT intervention and the J-EMT intervention. Finally, we do not know the effects of EMT on dual language learners with ASD. The next steps for EMT appear to be determining how to make decisions around incorporating an SGD into intervention, identifying the optimal intervention dosage for rapidly accelerating language learning, and determining the effects of EMT on dual language learners with ASD.

Suggested Readings

1. Kaiser, A. P., & Hampton, L. H. (2016). Enhanced milieu teaching. In R. McCauley, M. Fey, & R. Gilliam (Eds.) *Treatment of language disorders in children* (2nd ed., pp. 87–120). Paul H. Brookes Publishing Co. This chapter provides an overview of EMT procedures and their theoretical and empirical bases with a specific emphasis on parent-implemented applications. It includes detailed information about the six components of EMT and illustrates the application of EMT through case histories of two children.

2. Hancock, T. B., & Kaiser, A. P. (2002). The effects of trainer-implemented enhanced milieu teaching on the social communication of children who have autism. *Topics in Early Childhood Special Education, 22*(1), 39–54. This study examines the effects of EMT on the social-communication skills of preschool children with ASD when delivered by trained interventionists. Observational data indicated that all of the children showed positive increases for specific target-language use at the end of 24 intervention sessions, and these results were maintained through the 6-month follow-up.

3. Kaiser, A. P., & Roberts, M. Y. (2013). Parents as communication partners: An evidence-based strategy for improving parent support for language and communication in everyday settings. *Perspectives on Language Learning and Education, 20*(3), 96–111. This work provides recommendations for teaching parent-implemented EMT to families of toddlers and preschoolers with significant language delays based on single-case and group design studies.

Learning Activities

1. List the ways EMT can be adapted when implementing it with children who have ASD.

2. This chapter listed several common behavior challenges (restricted interests, issues in joint attention, limited engagement with others in activities, perseveration, echolalia) to address when implementing EMT with a child who has ASD. Choose another behavior challenge you have encountered when working with children who have ASD, and list how you would adapt the components of EMT (environmental arrangement, responsive interaction, language modeling, language expansions, milieu teaching) so that EMT can be used most effectively with that child.

3. Write a script of what you would say when talking with parents about why EMT may be an effective language intervention for their child with ASD.

Summary of Video Clip _____

*See the **About the Videos and Downloads** page at the front of the book for directions on how to access and stream the accompanying video to this chapter.*

This video shows an EMT session with a therapist and a preschool-age boy whose language targets are one-word nouns, verbs, and requests. During this session, the therapist sits directly across from the child to facilitate social-communication, centers her language on his focus of interest, and paces her talk at a rate that allows him time to process her language and then imitate it. The therapist sets up opportunities for the child to functionally communicate and request in ways that are both fun and meaningful. The therapist also verbally responds to all of the boy's communicative attempts and expands any verbal utterance made by the boy, thus reinforcing his use of language. The EMT approach looks deceptively simple, but the power and effectiveness of this intervention lies in the adult's connecting with the child in a way that makes it possible for the adult to map the child's meaning into specific models of what the child would say and then providing the child with the time and space to practice this functional language.

REFERENCES

American Psychiatric Association. (2013). *Diagnostic and statistical manual of mental disorders, fifth edition (DSM-5).* Author.

AssistiveWare. (2012). AssistiveWare-Proloquo2Go™. http://www.assistiveware.com/product /proloquo2go

Bondy, A., & Frost, L. (2001). The picture exchange communication system. *Behavior Modification, 25*(5), 725–744.

Brown, R. (1973). *A first language: The early stages.* George Allen & Unwin.

Bruner, J. S. (1974). From communication to language—A psychological perspective. *Cognition 3*(3): 255–287.

Bruner, J. S. (1978). The role of dialogue in language acquisition. In A. Sinclair, R., J. Jarvelle, and W. J. M. Levelt (Eds.), *The child's concept of language.* Springer-Verlag.

Camarata, S., & Yoder, P. (2002). Language transactions during development and intervention: Theoretical implications for developmental neuroscience. *International Journal of Developmental Neuroscience, 20*, 459–467.

Dunn, L. M., & Dunn, D. M. (2007). *Peabody Picture Vocabulary Test–Fourth Edition.* NCS Pearson.

Dunn, L. M., & Dunn, L. M. (1981). *Peabody Picture Vocabulary Test–Revised.* American Guidance Service.

Fenson, L., Marchman, V. A., Thal, D., Dale, P. S., Reznick, J. S., & Bates, E. (2007). *The MacArthur-Bates Communicative Development Inventories: User's guide and technical manual* (2nd ed.). Paul H. Brookes Publishing Co.

Fudala, J. B. (2000). *Arizona 3: Arizona Articulation Proficiency Scale, third revision.* Western Psychological Services.

Fuller, E. A., & Kaiser, A. P. (2020). The effects of early intervention on social-communication outcomes for children with autism spectrum disorder: A meta-analysis. *Journal of Autism and Developmental Disabilities, 50*(5), 1683–1700.

Gardner, M. F. (1990). *Expressive One-Word Picture Vocabulary Test–Revised.* Academic Therapy Publications.

Goldstein, H. (2002). Communication intervention for children with autism: A review of treatment efficacy. *Journal of Autism and Developmental Disorders, 32*(5), 373–396.

Haebig, E., McDuffie, A., & Weismer, S. E. (2013a). Brief report: Parent verbal responsiveness and language development in toddlers on the autism spectrum. *Journal of Autism and Developmental Disorders, 43*(9), 2218–2227.

Haebig, E., McDuffie, A., & Weismer, S. E. (2013b). The contribution of two categories of parent verbal responsiveness to later language for toddlers and preschoolers on the autism spectrum. *American Journal of Speech-Language Pathology, 22*(1), 57–70.

Hampton, L., Harty, M., Fuller, E., & Kaiser, A. (2019). Enhanced milieu teaching for children with autism spectrum disorder in South Africa. *International Journal of Speech-Language Pathology, 21*(6), 635–645.

Hampton, L. H., & Kaiser, A. P. (2016). Intervention effects on spoken-language outcomes for children with autism: A systematic review and meta-analysis. *Journal of Intellectual Disability Research, 60*(5), 444–463.

Hampton, L. H., Kaiser, A. P., & Fuller, E. A. (2020). Multi-component communication intervention for children with autism: A randomized controlled trial. *Autism: International Journal of Research and Practice, 24*(8), 2104–2116.

Hampton, L. H., Kaiser, A. P., Nietfeld, J. P., & Khachoyan, A. (2021). Generalized effects of naturalistic social-communication intervention for minimally verbal children with autism. *Journal of Autism and Developmental Disorders, 50*(1), 75–87.

Hampton, L. H., Kaiser, A. P., & Roberts, M. R. (2017). One-year language outcomes in toddlers with language delays: An RCT follow-up. *Pediatrics, 140*(5), e20163646.

Hancock, T. B., & Kaiser, A. P. (2002). The effects of trainer-implemented enhanced milieu teaching on the social-communication of children who have autism. *Topics in Early Childhood Special Education, 22*(1), 39–54.

Hancock, T. B., Ton, J., & Crowe, C. (2008). *The effects of parent and therapist implemented enhanced milieu teaching on the language production of children with autism.* Poster presented at the 6th Biennial Conference on Research Innovations in Early Intervention, San Diego, CA, United States.

Hart, B. M., & Risley, T. R. (1968). Establishing the use of descriptive adjectives in the spontaneous speech of disadvantaged preschool children. *Journal of Applied Behavior Analysis, 1,* 109–120.

Hart, B. M., & Risley, T. R. (1975). Incidental teaching of language in the preschool. *Journal of Applied Behavior Analysis, 8,* 411–420.

Hedrick, D. L., Prather, E. M., & Tobin, A. R. (1975). *Sequenced Inventory of Communication Development.* University of Washington Press.

Jackson-Maldonado, D. (2012). Verb morphology and vocabulary in monolinguals, emerging bilinguals, and monolingual children with primary language impairment. In B. Goldstein (Ed.), *Bilingual language development and disorders in Spanish-English speakers* (2nd ed., pp. 153–174). Paul H. Brooks Publishing Co.

Kaiser, A. P. (1993). Functional language. In M. E. Snell (Ed.), *Enhancing children's communication: Research foundations for intervention* (pp. 347–379). Paul H. Brookes Publishing Co.

Kaiser, A. P., & Hampton, L. H. (2016). Enhanced Milieu Teaching. In R. McCauley, M. Fey, & R. Gilliam (Eds.), *Treatment of language disorders in children* (2nd ed., pp. 87–120). Paul H. Brookes Publishing Co.

Kaiser, A. P., & Hancock, T. B. (2003). Teaching parents new skills to support their young children's development. *Infants and Young Children, 16,* 9–21.

Kaiser, A. P., Hancock, T. B., & Lambert, W. (1997). *The effects of teaching parents two naturalistic language-teaching strategies.* Paper presented at the 30th Annual Gatlinburg Conference on Research and Theory in Mental Retardation and Developmental Disabilities, Riverside, CA, United States.

Kaiser, A. P., Hancock, T. B., & Nietfeld, J. P. (2000). The effects of parent-implemented enhanced milieu teaching on the social-communication of children who have autism. *Journal of Early Education and Development, 11*(4), 423–446.

Kaiser, A. P., Hancock, T. B., & Trent, J. A. (2007). Teaching parents communication strategies. *Early Childhood Services: An Interdisciplinary Journal of Effectiveness, 1*(2), 107–136.

Kaiser, A. P., Lambert, W., Hancock, T. B., & Hester, P. P. (1998). *Differential outcomes of naturalistic intervention on vocabulary growth.* Paper presented at the 32nd Annual Gatlinburg Conference on Research and Theory in Mental Retardation and Developmental Disabilities, Charleston, SC, United States.

Kaiser, A. P., McFarland, T., & Hancock, T. B. (2008). *Individual differences in parent-implemented enhanced milieu teaching: Effects on children with ASD.* Paper presented at the 41st Annual Gatlinburg Conference on Research and Theory in Intellectual and Developmental Disabilities, San Diego, CA, United States.

Kaiser, A. P., & Roberts, M. Y. (2016–2020). An efficacy trial of J-EMT: Enhanced milieu teaching language intervention plus joint attention, engagement and regulation intervention for toddlers with autism. Institute for Educational Sciences, US Department of Education (R324A150094), in progress.

Kaiser, A. P., & Roberts, M. Y. (2013). Parents as communication partners: An evidence based strategy for improving parent support for language and communication in everyday settings. *Perspectives on Language Learning and Education, 20*(3), 96–111.

Kaiser, A. P., Scherer, N., Frey, J., & Roberts, M. (2017). The effects of Enhanced Milieu Teaching with phonological emphasis on the speech and language skills of young children with cleft palate: A pilot study. *American Journal of Speech-Language Pathology, 26*(3), 806–818.

Kaiser, A. P., & Trent, J. A. (2007). Communication intervention for young children with disabilities: Naturalistic approaches to promoting development. In S. L. Odom, R. H. Horner, M. E. Snell, & J. Blacher (Eds.), *Handbook of developmental disabilities* (pp. 224–245). Guilford Press.

Kasari, C., Freeman, S., & Paparella, T. (2006). Joint attention and symbolic play in young children with autism: A randomized controlled intervention study. *Journal of Child Psychology and Psychiatry, 47*, 611–620.

Kasari, C., Kaiser, A. P., Goods, K., Nietfeld, J., Mathy, J., Landa, R., Murphy, S., & Almirall, D. (2014). Communication interventions for minimally verbal children with autism: Sequential multiple assignment randomized trial. *Journal of the American Academy of Child & Adolescent Psychiatry, 56*(6), 635–646.

Kohnert, K., & Derr, A. (2012). Language intervention with bilingual children. In B. Goldstein (Ed.), *Bilingual language development and disorders in Spanish-English speakers* (2nd ed., pp. 337–356). Paul H. Brooks Publishing Co.

Landa, R. (2007). Early communication development and intervention for children with autism. *Mental Retardation and Developmental Disabilities Research Reviews, 13*, 16–25.

Ledford, J. R., & Gast, D. L. (Eds.). (2018). *Single case research: Applications in special education and behavioral sciences* (3rd ed.). Routledge.

Lovaas, O. I. (1987). Behavioral treatment and normal educational and intellectual functioning in young autistic children. *Journal of Consulting and Clinical Psychology, 55*(1), 3.

McWilliam, R. A., Casey, A. M., & Sims, J. (2009). The routines-based interview: A method for gathering information and assessing needs. *Infants & Young Children, 22*(3), 224–233.

Miller, J., & Iglesias, A. (2012). Systematic Analysis of Language Transcripts (SALT), Research (Version 2012) [Computer software]. SALT Software, LLC.

Mullen, E. M. (1984). *Mullen Scales of Early Learning (MSEL).* American Guidance Service.

Mundy, P., Delgado, C., Block, J., Venezia, M., Hogan, A., & Seibert, J. (2003). *A manual for the Abridged Early Social-Communication Scales (ESCS).* University of Miami Psychology Department.

Olive, M. L., de la Cruz, B., Davis, T. N., Chan, J. M., Lang, R. B., O'Reilly, M. F., & Dickson, S. M. (2007). The effects of enhanced milieu teaching and a voice output communication aid on the requesting of three children with autism. *Journal of Autism and Developmental Disorders, 37*(8), 1505–1513.

Olive, M. L., Kim, H. M., Kong, N., Kang, S., Choi, H., & O'Reilly, M. F. (2010). *Examining the use of enhanced milieu teaching with Korean families* [Unpublished manuscript]. University of Texas–Austin.

Ostrosky, M. M., & Kaiser, A. P. (1991). Preschool classroom environments that promote communication. *Teaching Exceptional Children, 23*(4), 6–10.

Oxford Centre for Evidence-based Medicine: Levels of Evidence (March 2009). https://www.cebm.ox.ac.uk/resources/levels-of-evidence/oxford-centre-for-evidence-based-medicine-levels-of-evidence-march-2009

Peredo, T. N., & Kaiser, A. P. (2015). *EMT en Español: A cultural and linguistic adaptation of caregiver-implemented language intervention.* Presentation at the annual meeting of the American Speech and Hearing Association, Denver, CO, United States.

Peredo, T. N., Zelaya, M. I., & Kaiser, A. P. (2017). Teaching low-income Spanish-speaking caregivers to implement *EMT en Español* with their young children with language impairments: A pilot study. *American Journal of Speech and Language Pathology, 27*(1), 136–153.

Phillips, B., Ball, C., Sackett, D., Badenoch, D., Straus, S., Haynes, B., & Dawes, M. (2001). Oxford Centre for Evidence-based Medicine levels of evidence. Centre for Evidence-based Medicine, Oxford, United Kingdom.

Reichow, B., Volkmar, F. R., & Cicchetti, D. V. (2008). Development of the evaluative method for evaluating and determining evidence-based practices in autism. *Journal of Autism and Developmental Disorders, 38*(7), 1311–1319.

Roberts, M., & Kaiser, A. (2012). Assessing the effects of a parent-implemented language intervention for children with language impairments using empirical benchmarks: A pilot study. *Journal of Speech, Language, and Hearing Research, 55*(6), 1655–1670.

Roberts, M. Y., & Kaiser, A. P. (2015). Early intervention for toddlers with language delays: A randomized controlled trial. *Pediatrics, 134*(4), 686–693.

Roberts, M. Y., Kaiser, A. P., Wolfe, C., Bryant, J., & Spidalieri, A. (2014). The effects of the Teach-Model-Coach-Review instructional approach on caregiver use of language support strategies and children's expressive language skills. *Journal of Speech, Language, and Hearing Research, 57*(5), 1851–1869.

Roid, G., & Miller, L. (1997). *Leiter-R: Leiter International Performance Scale–Revised.* Stoelting.

Schopler, E., Reichler, R. J., & Renner, B. R. (1986). *The Childhood Autism Rating Scale (CARS): For diagnostic screening and classification of autism.* Irvington.

Schreibman, L., Dawson, G., Stahmer, A. C., Landa, R., Rogers, S. J., McGee, G. G., & Halladay, A. (2015). Naturalistic developmental behavioral interventions: Empirically validated treatments for autism spectrum disorder. *Journal of Autism and Developmental Disorders, 45*, 2411–2428.

Sennott, S., & Bowker, A. (2009). Autism, AAC, and Proloquo2Go. *Perspectives on Augmentative and Alternative Communication, 18*, 137–145.

Skinner, B. E. (1957). *Verbal behavior.* Appleton-Century-Crofts.

Smith, T. (2001). Discrete trial training in the treatment of autism. *Focus on Autism and Other Developmental Disabilities, 16*, 86–92.

Trivette, C. M., Dunst, C. J., Hamby, D. W., & O'Herin, C. E. (2009). Characteristics and consequences of adult learning methods and strategies. *Practical Evaluation Reports, 2*(1), 1–32.

van der Meer, L., & Rispoli, M. (2010). Communication interventions involving speech-generating devices for children with autism: A review of the literature. *Developmental Neurorehabilitation, 13*, 294–306.

Vygotsky, L. S. (1978). *Mind in society: The development of higher psychological processes.* Harvard University Press.

Wang, P. (2008). Effects of a parent training program on the interactive skills of parents of children with autism in China. *Journal of Policy and Practice in Intellectual Disabilities, 5*(2), 96–104.

Warren, S. F., Gazdag, G. E., Bambara, L. M., & Jones, H. A. (1994). Changes in the generativity and use of semantic relationships concurrent with milieu language intervention. *Journal of Speech and Hearing Research, 51*, 924–934.

Weiss, R. S. (1981). INREAL intervention for language handicapped and bilingual children. *Journal of the Division for Early Childhood, 4*, 40–52.

Williams, K. T. (2007). *EVT-2: Expressive Vocabulary Test* (2nd ed.). Pearson Assessments.

Wright, C. A., Kaiser, A. P., Reikowsky, D. I., & Roberts, M. Y. (2013). Effects of naturalistic sign intervention on expressive language of toddlers with Down Syndrome. *Journal of Speech, Language, and Hearing Research, 56*, 994–1008.

Yoder, P. J., & Warren, S. F. (2004). Early predictors of language in children with and without Down syndrome. *American Journal on Mental Retardation, 109*, 285–300.

Zimmerman, I. L., Steiner, V. G., & Pond, R. E. (2002). *PLS-4: Preschool Language Scales–Fourth Edition.* Psychological Corporation.

Zimmerman, I. L., Steiner, V. G., & Pond, R. E. (2011). *PLS-5: Preschool Language Scales–Fifth Edition.* Pearson.

11

Early Social Interaction

Juliann J. Woods, Amy Wetherby, Abigail Delehanty,
Shubha Kashinath, and Renee Daly Holland

INTRODUCTION

Early Social Interaction (ESI) is an intervention model for toddlers who are at risk for or have a diagnosis of autism spectrum disorder (ASD) and their families. It was originally developed as a model demonstration project funded by the Office of Special Education Programs of the U.S. Department of Education (2002–2006) and has been extended through multiple research projects with funding from Autism Speaks, the Institute of Education Sciences, and the National Institute of Mental Health An efficacy trial of ESI with toddlers with ASD who were 18 months old at the beginning of treatment was the first parent-implemented treatment with significant differential effects on children's outcomes (Wetherby et al., 2014). This chapter describes the essential features of ESI and the rationale for its implementation with young children and their caregivers.

ESI was first designed to incorporate the National Research Council (NRC; Lord & McGee, 2001) recommendations within the context of a family-guided, natural-environments approach, consistent with the delivery of Individuals with Disabilities Education Improvement Act (IDEA) of 2004 Part C services and supports (American Speech-Language-Hearing Association, n.d.-a, n.d.-b; Goode, S., Lazara, A., & Danaher, J., 2008; IDEA, 2004; Sandall et al., 2005). Although the NRC recommendations were based primarily on research reviews of preschool programs, situating their recommendations within the Part C guidelines for delivery of early intervention services facilitated the development of a model that would promote the use of evidence-based practices and allow replication within statewide service delivery systems by early intervention teams. ESI was initially developed and continues to be refined to promote community-based access for all children and families, including those typically underrepresented in early intervention services and supports.

As additional models were developed and evidence accumulated on interventions that were effective, efficient, and specific to children younger than those in the NRC recommendations, commonalities among these approaches were discerned. The Autism Speaks Toddler Treatment Network (ASTTN) reviewed parent-mediated interventions for young children and brought together a working group of autism experts to identify the evidence-based practices and to operationalize the active ingredients of these models. This step was critical to further the application of research to community-based practice. The term *Naturalistic Developmental Behavioral Interventions* (NDBIs) was developed to describe these common features. Broadly, two core components are central to all NDBIs: 1) the use of the principles and science of applied behavior analysis (ABA) and 2) the integration of developmentally based intervention strategies and sequences to guide functional goals and outcomes individualized for each child (Schreibman et al., 2015). Additional features vary across NDBI models and include common instructional strategies such as natural reinforcement, balanced turns in routines, environmental arrangements, modeling, prompting, and fading procedures (Schreibman et al., 2020).

ESI is an NDBI; it is implemented in natural settings utilizing natural contingencies and encourages child-initiated interactions and deliberate teaching to extend child interest and motivation. ESI includes more than specific intervention strategies for social-communication delays associated with ASD. It is a comprehensive developmental model that incorporates processes and procedures for initial and ongoing assessment for program planning, individualized family service plan (IFSP) development and monitoring, intervention, transition, teaming, and parent coaching and support that is congruent with Part C legislation and adaptable to meet various state standards and guidelines. The specific components of the approach are described in the chapter.

TARGET POPULATIONS

ESI is designed for infants and toddlers and their families when an infant or toddler is identified as at risk for social-communication deficits or demonstrates early red flags for ASD (e.g., lack of response to name; limited sharing of warm, joyful expressions). More than 88% of children from birth to age 3 in the United States receive Part C services in home-based settings most appropriate for a parent-implemented model (U.S. Department of Education, 2016). In the ESI model, families meaningfully participate with their children throughout the evaluation, assessment, and intervention process. They describe their priorities and concerns, identify their preferred activities and routines as well as those that are challenging for them, and actively participate in the development of an individualized plan for the child and caregivers. Observations of the child and parent within typical play and caregiving routines are combined with standardized and curriculum-based measures described later to identify functional and meaningful outcomes. In addition to parent-implemented interventions at home, caregivers in community programs can use ESI to support young children in early care and education, play and recreation groups, and other family-identified activities.

Early identification and intervention specific to ASD significantly improve children's outcomes (Dawson et al., 2010; Lord & McGee, 2001; Wetherby et al., 2014) and together are the greatest tools available to reduce the societal cost of treating ASD. Early intervention is particularly critical for children with ASD because without intervention, early social attention deficits associated with ASD often lead to secondary delays in learning and developmental outcomes (Dawson et al., 2012; Wetherby et al., 2007). Parents benefit by learning social-communication interventions that promote their self-efficacy and increase interactions with their children (Dunst et al., 2019). The ESI model can be implemented with children as soon as parents identify concerns because, as evidence clearly establishes with ASD, the earlier intervention begins, the better.

THEORETICAL BASIS

As mentioned previously, ESI is a comprehensive early intervention approach for toddlers with ASD and their families, incorporating evidence-based active ingredients and designed to be consistent with requirements of the IDEA Part C early intervention program. The ESI model incorporates the following features: 1) family-centered capacity-building approach; 2) learning in natural environments; 3) collaborative coaching to support parent learning and generalization; 4) developmental framework to prioritize child outcomes; 5) systematic instruction using evidence-based strategies; 6) intensity needed for children with ASD; and 7) technology to support family informational, emotional, and intervention needs.

Family-Centered Capacity-Building Approach

A family-centered capacity-building approach addresses the family's needs, concerns, and priorities throughout the assessment and intervention process. Respecting family members' perceptions, priorities, and preferences; developing active participatory and relational partnerships; and building capacity and unity are key components of an effective family-centered program. Families are more involved in the achievement of goals when they have been stakeholders in their development (Bransford et al., 2000; Dunst et al., 2019).

Learning in Natural Environments

Natural environments are defined in IDEA Part C as the everyday activities, routines, and settings typical for any family, including home, child care, and community locations such as the park or grocery store. Everyday activities such as mealtime, play, caregiving, and family chores provide authentic opportunities to embed teaching of objectives that are functional to the activity and therefore naturally support acquisition and generalization of skills. Working in the natural environment builds on the strengths of the family by supporting their interactions with their children rather than delivering instruction directly to the child with the parent observing in a passive role (Schertz et al., 2011).

Collaborative Coaching to Support Parent Learning and Generalization

Within ESI, a systematic coaching plan is developed for the parent congruent with the child's intervention plan. Goals for the child and the parent are identified, discussed, and implemented to build the capacity of the parent within an adult learning framework. This means that each parent is recognized as a unique learner with varying preferences and motivations for learning. Specific teaching or coaching practices are identified and matched to the caregiver to improve existing abilities, develop new skills, and gain a deeper understanding of his or her practices for use in current and future situations.

Research syntheses on adult learning provide evidence for the implementation of effective consulting and coaching strategies that are applicable to parent-implemented interventions (Bransford et al., 2000; Donovan et al., 1999; Dunst & Trivette, 2009; Fixsen et al., 2005). Findings that are essential to the implementation of ESI include, first, the importance of establishing what the learner—the parent—knows and believes when entering a learning environment. Adult learning espouses that, initially, each learner has preconceived ideas about a subject matter. For example, parents may be expecting the intervention to be conducted by the interventionist and believe that the interventionist as expert can offer intervention of a quality that is superior to what they as parents can provide. They may also be expecting therapy in the sense of that offered in a medical or educational model and be suspicious of the use of everyday activities, play, and their own objects rather than specialized toys and therapy materials.

Second, to develop a deep level of understanding in a particular area, the learner must 1) have a solid base of factual knowledge, 2) understand these facts within the context of a conceptual framework, and 3) organize the information to facilitate generalization (Bransford et al., 2000; Merriam & Baumgartner, 2020; National Academies of Sciences, Engineering, and Medicine, 2018). Because families are often new to ideas and terminology associated with early intervention systems, child development, a diagnosis of ASD, and the constructs of teaching and learning, there is much to learn. Expecting parents to grasp all of the facts and details of this information immediately is unrealistic. It requires a consistent continuum of supports with frequent review and rechecks to ensure knowledge and skills are developing.

Third, learners must acquire a metacognitive approach in which they assess their own level of understanding, establish learning goals, and measure progress (Bransford et al., 2000; Merriam & Baumgartner, 2020; NAS, 2018; Snyder et al., 2015). In order for learners to gain deep knowledge of a particular content area, they must develop an understanding of how that knowledge not only may be used in a specific context but also may be generalized to other situations (Dunst & Trivette, 2009). The application of these adult learning principles is currently being adapted and evaluated in coaching practices to promote adoption and use of embedded intervention practices by parents in their everyday activities (Friedman et al., 2012; Kemp & Turnbull, 2014).

Developmental Framework to Prioritize Child Outcomes

As an NDBI, ESI utilizes a developmental framework for goal setting and intervention planning. Working within a developmental model, however, should not imply teaching to a developmental checklist. Rather than merely offering a guideline for sequencing objectives, a developmental framework provides a reference for understanding a child's behavioral competencies and for individualizing appropriate and developmentally sensible goals and objectives. Developmental approaches, including ESI, focus on addressing the core deficits of ASD, because improvement or lack thereof predict later cognitive, social, and language outcomes in children with ASD. Skills emphasized in these core deficit areas include expanding the use of gestures, initiating verbal and nonverbal communication, understanding and using words with referential meaning, initiating and responding to joint attention, and demonstrating reciprocity in interaction. Because of the importance of skill building in the core deficit areas, ESI interventionists advocate for the use of nonspeech communication systems (e.g., gesture, sign language, or picture communication) to jump-start the speech system and boost cognitive and social underpinnings. Nonspeech communication systems can provide an important bridge between parents and their children to reduce challenges that frequently occur because of the child's communication deficits. Therefore, developmental interventions focus not only on targeting goals directly on the ASD core deficits of the child but also on targeting strategies for the parent to use that support social-communication development.

ESI uses The SCERTS® Model, a manualized curricular-based assessment and intervention, as a framework to identify goals and objectives and monitor progress (Prizant et al., 2006). SCERTS refers to Social Communication (SC), Emotional Regulation (ER), and Transactional Support (TS), which are the primary dimensions targeted to support learning and development for children with ASD and their families. The SCERTS curricular-based assessment includes parent report and observation forms administered in the child's home with the family to identify priority goals and objectives. The SC and ER domains delineate specific, measurable goals and objectives for the child and are organized by communication stage, beginning with the Social Partner Stage, before the development of any words. The TS domain delineates goals and objectives for the parent or other communication partners and includes teaching strategies and learning supports that are selected to help the child meet individualized goals and objectives. SC targets for toddlers with ASD include expanding the use of gestures, sounds, and words; initiating spontaneous verbal and nonverbal communication; understanding the meaning of words; initiating and responding to joint attention; increasing functional object use and pretend play; and extending reciprocity in interaction. ER targets for toddlers with ASD include being available for learning and expressing emotion, expanding self-regulatory strategies to calm self when dysregulated, using communication to help regulate emotion when frustrated or when help is needed, and using regulatory strategies to stay engaged in activities and handle new and changing situations. SC and ER targets are integrated to prevent the development of problem behavior, consistent with tenets of positive behavior support.

Systematic Instruction Using Evidence-Based Strategies

Children with ASD can learn from everyday activities and experiences when learning opportunities are structured and systematic techniques are used to foster active engagement. ESI incorporates systematic instruction using evidence-based naturalistic-behavioral strategies that are developmentally sensible for toddlers. Ongoing monitoring with corresponding adjustments in programming is based on observational data. Parents learn to use intervention strategies matched to priority objectives within daily activities to increase opportunities for teaching and learning when the activity occurs.

Intensity Needed for Children With ASD

The intensity needed for children with ASD is achieved through the integration of the core features of ESI. Parents partner with professionals to plan an individualized intervention program to address the impact of autism symptoms on learning. Professionals coach parents on how to competently and systematically use intervention strategies throughout the day in typical activities. A minimum of 25 hours per week of active engagement in learning activities has been recommended as soon as children are suspected of having ASD. Embedding strategies within everyday activities the family is already participating in supports parent implementation of 25 hours per week of active child engagement. While the intensity of intervention necessary to provide optimal outcomes is not yet determined for infants and toddlers at risk for ASD, research suggests that more time spent in active, positive engagement results in better outcomes for preschoolers. ESI provides a way to maximize intensity of intervention and reduce professional time.

Technology to Support Family Informational, Emotional, and Intervention Needs

Technology is clearly used by families for many reasons and is an integral component of the ESI model. Research on technology-supported intervention for families of children with ASD includes both asynchronous online learning (e.g., information, resources, training modules) and individualized interventions using a coaching approach. The Baby Navigator and Autism Navigator tools and courses offer families and interventionists a range of resources for use when implementing ESI (https://babynavigator.com; https://autismnavigator.com). Addressing a major limitation in previous technology-supported studies, the technology supports in ESI are interactive, individualized, focused on application, and alternated with face-to-face coaching opportunities by professionals to ensure knowledge is applied and sustained (Meadan & Daczewitz, 2015; Wainer & Ingersoll, 2013).

EMPIRICAL BASIS

Parent-Implemented Intervention With Young Children With ASD

While it is broadly accepted that parent-implemented interventions can have positive effects on child communication, there is less high-quality research on parents implementing intervention in their typical daily routines and activities and even less that supports generalization of implementation across multiple contexts. Details of studies on ESI are provided in Table 11.1.

In an early study of ESI, Kashinath and colleagues (2006) examined the effects of facilitating generalized use of naturalistic teaching strategies designed to help the parents of five preschool students with ASD synchronize with their child's attentional focus and increase communication. Results of this multiple baseline design study were that all parents demonstrated proficient use of teaching strategies, including environmental arrangement, natural reinforcement, time delay, contingent imitation, modeling, and gestural and/or visual cue. Parents were also observed to generalize their use of strategies across different routines both in the same class and across classes of routines such as play, outdoor or recreation, caregiving routines (e.g., diapering, bath and mealtime, household chores), community activities, and other health or comfort routines. The intervention had positive effects on communication outcomes for four of the five children. All five parents perceived the intervention to be useful in facilitating their child's communication.

Wetherby and Woods (2006) reported on a pretest–posttest quasi-experimental study as a preliminary effort to evaluate the effects of ESI on social-communication outcomes in a group of 17 children with ASD who entered ESI in the second year of

Table 11.1. Level of evidence and overall strength of the design. All studies supported the intervention and provided strong evidence.

Design strength	Description of design level	Studies with strong evidence	Studies with adequate evidence	Studies with weak evidence
Ia	Meta-analysis of >1 randomized controlled trial (RCT)			
Ib	RCT	Wetherby et al. (2014)		
IIa	Controlled study without randomization			
IIb	Quasi-experimental study	Wetherby & Woods (2006)		
III	Single-participant experimental designs	Brown & Woods (2015) Kashinath, Woods, & Goldstein (2006)		

Note: Levels Ia–IV (Philips et al., 2001) as well as quality of evidence for group and single-participant experimental designs (Reichow et al., 2008).

life. Parents were taught naturalistic teaching strategies in two weekly sessions in natural environments over the course of a year. Intervention goals were individualized and selected from a developmental framework targeting social interaction, joint attention, communication, imitation, play, and emotional regulation (Prizant et al., 2000). Results indicated significant improvement with large effect sizes on 11 of 13 social-communication outcomes measured with the Communication and Symbolic Behavior Scales Developmental Profile™ (CSBS DP™; Wetherby & Prizant, 2002). It is particularly noteworthy that significant changes were demonstrated in initiating and responding to joint attention, because few studies have demonstrated significant changes on these measures.

In an effort to strengthen this design, the ESI group of 17 children was compared with a no-treatment contrast group of 18 children with ASD who entered early intervention during the third year of life. Social-communication measures were collected from the contrast group at the same age as the ESI group at post-test and compared to the ESI group. The contrast group was comparable to the ESI postintervention group on communicative means and play but had significantly poorer performance, with moderate to large effect sizes on all other measures of social communication. At a mean age of 31 months, 77% of the ESI group was using words compared to 56% of the contrast group. A weakness of the study was that it was not possible to determine that the groups were comparable in the second year of life because children in the contrast group had not been identified and tested at a younger age.

Most recently, multisite randomized controlled trial (RCT) of ESI with 82 toddlers with ASD and their families compared two parent-implemented intervention conditions for 9 months each: 1) individual ESI offered in two to three weekly sessions at home to teach parents how to embed strategies to support social-communication skills for 25 hours a week within everyday routines, activities, and places; and 2) group ESI offered once a week to offer information, education, and group (Wetherby et al., 2014). Toddlers with ASD were recruited at 18 months of age and randomly assigned to the individual or group condition, and then, using a crossover design, received the other condition. After 9 months of intervention, children in both conditions showed significant improvement on all three composites of the CSBS, expressive and receptive language as measured by the Mullen Scales of Early Learning (Mullen, 1995), and communication as measured by the Vineland Adaptive Behavior Scales (Sparrow et al., 2005). Children receiving individual ESI made significantly greater gains on the social composite of the CSBS and receptive language on the Mullen scales and significantly greater gains on the Vineland scales. On the Autism Diagnostic Observation Schedule (ADOS; Lord et al., 1999), children in both conditions showed a significant decrease in symptom severity on social affect scores and no significant change in restrictive and repetitive behavior.

The NRC (Lord & McGee, 2001) recommended monitoring children with ASD for progress at least every 3 months to make programming decisions and guide refinements to intervention in the case of minimal measurable progress. Wetherby and colleagues (2018) recently examined child active engagement using a Measure of Active Engagement (MAE) and found that the MAE offered strong psychometric features that were sensitive to change after 3 months of treatment for toddlers with ASD who participated in the RCT of ESI. In addition, MAE scores were found to predict outcomes on measures of social communication (CSBS), developmental level (Mullen), adaptive behavior (Vineland), and autism symptoms (ADOS). The results from the measure of AE opens a window into making informed decisions for the child and family. The lens of AE is a guidepost for parent support within everyday activities. Treatment responders may be identified by the end of the first 3 months, informing the team of the effect of ESI for the child and family. Researchers continue to examine the psychometric properties of the Measure of Active Engagement and Transactional Supports (MAETS: Wetherby et al., 2013); however, preliminary studies have indicated good interobserver reliability. Taken together, these findings support the effectiveness of ESI as a cost-effective, community-viable intervention. They are particularly important in light of the lack of main effects on standardized assessments of child outcomes in other parent-implemented interventions for toddlers with ASD.

In summary, coaching parents to embed intervention strategies during everyday activities is an innovative method to achieve the intensity of active engagement needed for very young children with ASD. The effectiveness of parent-implemented interventions for children with developmental disabilities has been well established; however, fewer studies have included or focused on children with ASD and established positive outcomes for both caregiver and child learning (e.g., Brown & Woods, 2015; Kashinath et al., 2006; Landa et al., 2011; Rogers et al., 2014; Wetherby et al., 2014; Wetherby et al., 2018). Empirical evidence supports that parents can learn specific techniques, such as modeling, contingent imitation, and prompting, to prevent the full unfolding of symptoms of ASD and minimize associated secondary impact on brain development and cognitive skills (Brown & Woods, 2016).

PRACTICAL REQUIREMENTS

Providing coordinated and comprehensive intervention of adequate intensity for very young children with ASD is challenging for the health care and education systems (Adams & Tapia, 2013). Services delivered by professionals within Part C of IDEA (IDEA, 2004) average 2 to 3 hours per week, or less in many regions of the

United States. In only a few states that have developed guidelines for intensive services for children with ASD will services be as high as 20 or more hours per week. Again, although the intensity of intervention for optimal outcomes is not yet determined for infants and toddlers with ASD, it has been shown that amount of time spent in active and productive engagement affects outcomes for preschoolers, with a critical minimum threshold of at least 5 hours per day, 5 days per week (Lord & McGee, 2001). See Figure 11.1 for an example of how intervention delivered in the natural environment by parents offers more opportunities for intervention than that delivered only through direct services. Children with ASD participating in activities with other children would not be expected to learn simply by being there. Inclusive opportunities must have adequate support for the child with ASD to learn from engagement with the materials, activities, and other children. Providing intervention in the natural environment is a way to maximize learning throughout the day and thus achieve the intensity of active engagement that is critical for children with ASD. However, it presents some additional programmatic considerations.

The ESI approach, although congruent with Part C recommended practice, goes beyond the generalized knowledge and skills necessary to serve most children with other types of delays and disabilities and their families; it requires personnel to receive specialized training for working with children with ASD and their families. As a result, there are several areas of specialized training that have been identified in this chapter. ESI providers first must be knowledgeable of the core deficits of ASD

Play routines		Caregiving routines	
Play with objects/constructive play	Pretend play	Comfort	Dressing-related routines
Playing ball Bowling games Hammer/ball toy Cars and planes	Feeding Batman Cooking dinner with Mom or Dad	Rocking with Dad Beanbag/music in living room	Getting dressed/undressed Putting on shoes
Physical play	Social games (roles)	Hygiene-related routines	Food-related routines
Backyard run Basketball Walking in neighborhood Run and catch, kickball Slide/swing at park	Hide and seek Rough and tumble play with Dad	Hand washing Diaper/potty Bath time	Snack Breakfast Lunch Dinner Juice/getting a drink
Learning and literacy routines		Family routines and transitions	
Reading books	Songs and rhymes	Family errands	Family chores
Ladybug *Finding Nemo* *Old MacDonald*	Listening to music on the computer with sister	Grocery shopping Siblings activities	Folding laundry Cooking, setting table
Computer, video	Fluid play	Transitions	Recreation
Any Disney movie Music on computer	Coloring with crayons and markers Playdough	Clean up before bed Packing backpack for car trip Countdown to outside play	Library hour Church park and playground Eating out Visiting family in different towns

Figure 11.1. Intervention in a natural environment: Jay's family routine categories.

as well as the typical and atypical behaviors toddlers with ASD are likely to exhibit. When personnel use ESI with very young children, they also need knowledge of early red flags for ASD; changes that may occur during the second and third years as the child's social-communication behaviors improve, plateau, or regress; and the possible sequence or point in time when behaviors become red flags (e.g., less interest in people than in objects, repetitive movements with objects). ESI interventionists must also be prepared to implement positive behavior interventions and supports (PBIS) to teach communication as replacements for challenging behaviors if they develop. ESI providers must be fluent in child assessment and intervention planning using The SCERTS Model®. Learning to use SCERTS requires time in both training and feedback for proper implementation. However, it provides a comprehensive approach for team members and a coordinated plan for implementation in early intervention, preschool and elementary programs.

Finally, learning to coach families using a systematic process of interventionist–caregiver supports to promote caregiver competence and independence may also be a new knowledge and skill set for the interventionist. ESI providers must be both skilled interventionists working with children and competent coaches supporting adult learners to implement interventions within their daily routines and activities. The ability to apply coaching strategies that facilitate the caregiver's capacity to promote child learning with diverse caregivers also takes experience and performance feedback from other skilled interventionists or team members.

KEY COMPONENTS

The key components of the approach—everyday activities and routines, individualized child and family curriculum, parent-implemented embedded intervention, collaborative coaching, positive behavior interventions and supports, and caregiver–team coordination—are described in the following sections.

Everyday Activities and Routines

Intervention practices in Part C emphasize the delivery of supports and services within the context of the child and family's everyday routines, activities, and places (NECTAC, 2008). Embedding the intervention into the family's daily routines and activities supports the caregiver's role as the child's communication partner, playmate, and parent. ESI may be implemented in the home, in a community-based parent–child playgroup, and within community early care and education programs. While the routines, activities, and opportunities afforded parents and children are different in the settings, the goals are similar. In all settings, the role of the interventionist is to coach parents and caregivers how to interact positively with the child, to support the child's engagement in the interactions, to increase frequency of interactions between caregiver and child, and to guide the caregiver's use of evidence-based intervention strategies to practice social communication and emotional regulation goals that are functional, predictable, and meaningful for the child and likely to occur throughout the day.

Intervention sessions are scheduled to accommodate the child's attention, family's preferences, work and/or school schedules, and the specific routines (e.g., interactive play, dressing, snack and meals, bath time, play with siblings) that are identified for intervention. We recommend two home visits per week to facilitate parent implementation and to monitor child progress initially. The number of home visits that actually take place each week varies, primarily due to family circumstance (e.g., work schedules, birth of new siblings, vacations, family illness) and the capacity of the family to embed intervention within their daily routines successfully. It takes time for most families to learn how to embed interventions with their child throughout the day at a level sufficient to provide adequate intensity for learning. The interventionists offer make-up sessions to maintain intensity when possible, and they maintain contact via text, email, and web conferencing to ensure that families are supported.

Although **everyday routines** appropriate for intervention may seem obvious, they are individual to the family based on their interests, beliefs, and unique characteristics. To ensure an individualized contextual match is provided for each child and family (Bernheimer & Weismer, 2007), families are encouraged to go beyond describing the schedule of their day, evenings, and weekends in order to also consider their interests, hobbies, favorite times with their child, challenging routines or activities, community participation, regular appointments, and so on. The conversation seeks to identify the child's current interests and motivators as well as his or her level of engagement, independence, and participation within the activities and routines (Woods & Lindeman, 2008; Woods et al., 2011). Observing the parent and the child in routines promotes an understanding of the strategies the caregiver is already using that are supporting or preempting the child's participation and communication.

ESI advances the practice of routines-based intervention for young children with ASD through the careful selection of routines and activities that support the teaching and learning priorities for both the child and parent. The family and interventionist choose routines and play activities from the list that was generated in the interview that 1) either do, or could, occur at high frequency; 2) are motivating to the child and parent; and 3) include multiple opportunities for joint interaction, communication, and other core intervention targets (Kashinath et al., 2006). After an initial set of routines is implemented, additional routines are added to the plan to expand practice opportunities (e.g., hand washing expands to toothbrushing and combing hair), include additional play or communication partners (e.g., grandpa after school, trips to the playground), increase types of routines and activities to support generalization (e.g., snacks at a friend's house, a trip to a restaurant), and promote development of new skills (e.g., initiating play with peers at the park, taking care of the family pet). The total number of routines and play activities as well as the rate of implementation are individualized for each family and child. Although the numbers will vary, a variety of routines and play activities for each family is always used to encourage dispersing learning opportunities throughout the day, participation within functional and meaningful events in the family life, and promoting the child's growth and development.

Another feature of ESI that is compatible with the Part C practices is the use of objects, toys, and materials that belong to the family and are used within their routines and settings. For example, indoor play routines include the child's favorite toys, music, or constructive materials, whereas outdoor play materials consist of the child's ball, swing set, or scooter. No special equipment or materials are brought into the home setting. It is also important to point out that within each routine, the interventionist supports the parent's use of controlled variations to decrease the likelihood the routine will become a ritual and to increase opportunities for additional practice through the introduction of moderate novelty

Individualized Child and Family Curriculum

SCERTS is used as a curriculum for home visitation, within playgroups, and in community settings as a mechanism that links assessment with individualized goals and objectives and as a tool to monitor progress. The SC and ER are the primary developmental dimensions targeted to support the development of children with ASD, and the TS are the targets for their families. In SCERTS, it is recognized that most learning in childhood occurs in the social context of daily activities and experiences (Prizant et al., 2003; Prizant et al, 2006). Interventionists teach families how to target SC and ER goals and objectives by implementing transactional supports within daily activities. These are taught across home and community settings and in both individual and group sessions in order to help communication partners who will be interacting with the child with ASD in everyday learning contexts.

Parent-Implemented Embedded Intervention

ESI is a parent-implemented intervention approach. Following the identification of the child's priority goals and initial routines and play, the interventionist and parent begin the process of embedding goals within routines using a variety of general and specific intervention strategies and parent supports. Within the SCERTS curriculum, multiple evidence-based strategies are identified for each child active engagement target and parent transactional support. The interventionist systematically consults with each parent on the strategies or cluster of strategies that are appropriate for the child's identified priority goals and are the best fit for the child and parent's current knowledge and skills. Building on the developmental model for children and adult learning for parents, the ESI interventionist select the supports that are most immediately relevant to improve the parent's ability to encourage the child to initiate social communication and follow the child's attentional focus.

Collaborative Coaching

ESI interventionists individualize the methods for coaching parents to embed interventions within their routines just as they individualize for the children's phase of learning. Parents can choose from easy-to-read handouts, videos, or demonstrations of specific strategies and examples of their use in family-identified routines. Interventionists follow the continuum of teaching, demonstrate and explain the strategies within the routines, guide the parents' practice as needed, and provide feedback as the parent engages with the child (see Figure 11.2). They also encourage the parents to reflect on what works or what does not work, and they problem-solve other options together.

   Parents and interventionists discuss strategy use and possible barriers to implementation and identify additional instances of potential strategy use across routines. Parent input is solicited regarding types of teaching methods used to increase their satisfaction and ownership of the intervention. Parents are also encouraged to evaluate "what works best for me?" during the summary and planning time with the interventionist. Each week, the interventionist observes the parent's implementing the intervention within the routines selected. If the parent does not embed the goal or use the intervention strategy as coached, the interventionist demonstrates and reviews the training to facilitate problem solving about what is working and what is challenging for the parent. They practice together to increase caregiver's

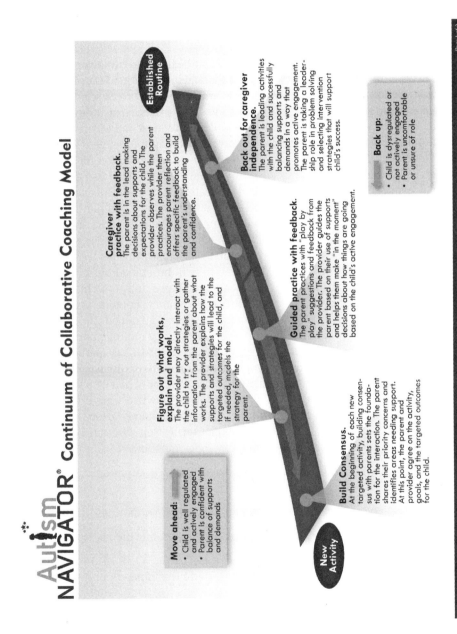

Figure 11.2. Collaborative coaching model. From Autism Navigator, LLC. Copyright © 2020, Florida State University. All rights reserved.

competence and develop another plan. If the caregiver is implementing as planned, then they discuss what the next steps are for the child to further enhance the quality of the interaction or expand the level of the child's independence or sophistication in communication. Parents who feel good about their ability to engage their child actually will engage more frequently in intervention. Therefore, time spent on increasing the parent's feelings of self-efficacy influences child outcomes. In ESI, we focus not only on what parents should learn to do but also on how they feel about what they are doing.

ESI is implemented systematically to achieve both child and caregiver outcomes. For example, the interventionist introduces a specific intervention strategy, such as contingent imitation for the caregivers to use with the child to expand turn taking and increase initiations during bath and play with cars. Each strategy is chosen specifically with the caregiver to address the child's outcomes and is relevant to the identified routines on each visit. This is in contrast to other approaches that teach a general principle or strategy, such as imitation, without consideration for the child's current targets or the context to practice it functionally. Attention is also given to the caregiver's learning curve. In this example, the strategy is new for the caregiver and is embedded in two familiar and preferred child routines, bath and play. The interventionist supports the caregiver by demonstrating contingent imitation and guiding practice in the routines, observing the caregiver and child and offering feedback. As the caregiver's confidence increases, the interventionist provides less hands-on support and more indirect feedback. The strategy will be embedded in additional appropriate routines to continue to expand the child's use and to facilitate generalization. Problem solving is used throughout by the interventionist as a learning check for caregiver understanding, to increase caregiver confidence through verbal rehearsal, and to use the problem-solving power provided by multiple perspectives.

Caregivers have opportunities to determine the easiest-to-use methods of collecting data on the child's goals and the implementation of the strategies within routines. For example, one parent may identify the use of a daily diary or log sheet is easiest for noting the child's participation, and another may use wipe-off boards in the bathroom and on the refrigerator to take notes immediately after the routine. Treatment fidelity is monitored through the completion of a self-assessment checklist to ensure that each home visit includes the following components:

- Initial review of child and family outcomes and intervention intensity since the previous visit

- Observation of and participation by the parent in multiple routines

- Guided practice in implementing the intervention for specific goals within the routines

- Discussion about what, when, how often, and where the intervention would occur between visits

- Development of a plan for the next visit

Positive Behavioral Interventions and Supports

ESI interventionists are trained in functional assessment and implementation of PBIS, methods designed to limit the occurrence of problem behaviors. Children enrolled in ESI may or may not need PBIS within their intervention plan. Initial energies are focused on development of early communication and social interaction skills, and if successful, the need for PBIS can be prevented; however, if children are not identified early enough or do not develop early communication that is easily understood, the likelihood of challenging behaviors developing increases (Fox et al., 2003). PBIS is incorporated in the ESI approach on a child-by-child basis. However, features of PBIS, such as environmental arrangements to prevent challenging behavior, the use of visual supports, and the importance of responding to the child's communication, are also common features of ESI and therefore provide common foundations for learning appropriate communication and social interaction.

Caregiver and Team Participation

ESI has the most impact on younger children and may not be suitable for all families and settings. Although few families have discontinued the project to date, some have questioned the time commitment of the family members, and others preferred an interventionist-directed approach. For those questioning how they could possibly engage their child for 25 hours a week with only 2–4 hours of support from the early intervention team, the ESI handout *Do the Math for Jeremy and Jamaal* was helpful to illustrate what they were doing and the amount of time spent without setting aside special times for therapy when they embedded intervention strategies in routines (see Figure 11.3).

A primary caregiver is essential to provide the majority of the embedded intervention with the child. However, support to any additional partners becomes a part of the child's program to ensure consistency of implementation. Although intensity is crucial, it is not essential that only one parent deliver the intervention, and over time, additional partners can support generalization. Examples include Grandpa bringing Larry's big brother home after school to provide a consistent outdoor play partner for 60–90 minutes most days. Jose's mom and dad divided routine types and different times of day to maximize opportunities, increase controlled variations, and enhance generalization. The use of multiple caregivers can enhance outcomes for children and their families but does create an important consideration for the interventionist, who must ensure that all partners are competent and coordinated in their efforts.

The importance of interprofessional education and ongoing collaboration must be emphasized and recognized as an important role for all members of the team (Coufal & Woods, 2018). It also necessitates time, attention, and ongoing communication. As with any team, multiple providers must coordinate child outcomes, intervention plans, strategies, and caregiver supports to ensure consistency. When multiple providers are not coordinated and family centered, we have seen ownership transferred to professionals so that, for example, snack time belongs to the occupational therapist to work on sensory concerns and feeding, whereas stories and play are the domain of the speech-language pathologist (SLP) to increase communication. In ESI, routines or activities do not belong to different disciplines but rather to the child and family. Our view is that families should not be asked to become three or four different types of interventionists and divide their day between specialized procedures; they are parents. The use of MAETS that emphasizes the child's active engagement and the caregiver's transactional supports to intentionally embed intervention increases the individualization of the plan for each child and family and the identification of the most appropriate targets for identified activities rather than specific skills from a developmental domain or discipline.

Autism NAVIGATOR

Do the Math: Who receives more intervention? James

Day	MON	TUES	WED	THURS	FRI	Total Time
Activity	Occupational Therapy • Moves with music and swings	Speech Therapy • Names picture cards and takes turns activating toys		Occupational Therapy • Moves with music and swings	Speech Therapy • Names picture cards and takes turns activating toys	
Professional Time	45 Minutes	45 Minutes		45 Minutes	45 Minutes	3 Hours
Child Time	45 Minutes	45 Minutes		45 Minutes	45 Minutes	3 Hours

Jamaal

MON	TUES	WED	THURS	FRI	Total Time

MON

Morning – 45 minutes:
- Requests food and drink items at breakfast
- Plays social games (peek, twinkle) during diaper change
- Fills turn in songs during dressing

Playtime – 30 minutes:
- Takes turns in simple action games (rolls ball, stacks block, activates toy)
- Chooses book and points to pictures
- Requests more (bubbles, swing, music)

Chores – 15 minutes:
- Gives toys to mom during pick up
- Reaches up to mom to request pick up or comfort when chores are done
- Puts laundry in baskets and puts stuffed toys on bed during room pick up

Lunch – 45 minutes:
- Requests food and drink items at breakfast
- Plays social games (peek, twinkle) during diaper change
- Fills turn in songs during hand washing

TUES / WED / THURS

Getting Ready for Nap – 15 minutes:
- Reaches up to mom to request pick up
- Plays a social game with music while rocking to sleep

Playtime – 30 minutes:
- Takes turns in simple action games (rolls ball, stacks block, activates toy)
- Chooses book and points to pictures
- Requests more (bubbles, swing, music)

Car Travel – 15 minutes:
- Sing songs with mom on school pick up

Outside Play – 30 minutes:
- Swings and plays ball with his big brother

Dinner – 45 minutes:
- Requests food and drink items at dinner
- Carries cups and plates to dad for clean up, takes turn labeling

Bath/Bedtime – 30 minutes:
- Requests toys for tub
- Takes turns with dad in dump and fill play
- "Finds" body parts in songs

FRI

Morning – 30 minutes:
- Requests food and drink items at breakfast
- Plays social games (peek, twinkle) during diaper change
- Fills turn in songs during dressing

Playgroup – 90 minutes:
- Plays with parent and peers

Lunch – 45 minutes:
- Requests food and drink items at lunch
- Plays social games (peek, twinkle) during diaper change
- Fills turn in songs during hand washing

Getting Ready for Nap – 15 minutes:
- Reaches up to mom to request pick up
- Plays a social game with music while rocking to sleep

Mother's Play Date – 1 Hour:
- Games, songs, play, snack with friends

Dinner – 30 minutes:
- Requests food and drink items at dinner
- Carries cups and plates to dad for clean up, takes turn labeling

Bath/Bedtime – 30 minutes:
- Requests toys for tub
- Takes turns with dad in dump and fill play
- "Finds" body parts in songs

	Professional Time	Child Time
	Two 1 Hour Home Visits Per Week	5 Hours Daily
FRI	90 Minutes	5 Hours
Total Time	3:30 Hours	25 Hours

Figure 11.3. Opportunities for parent-implemented intervention in natural environments. From Autism Navigator, LLC. Copyright © 2020, Florida State University. All rights reserved.

The ESI interventionist may be identified by the team to serve as the family service coordinator. Service coordination includes multiple roles around quality assurance, family satisfaction, and accomplishment of program goals and services. The interventionist also assists the family to access resources, complete referrals for other services and supports, and provide information. All team members, and especially the ESI interventionist, share information with caregivers. Along with the how-to coaching that caregivers are anxious to learn, the interventionist provides information to explain the what and why of ASD and to address family concerns, such as family acceptance of the diagnosis of autism, feeding problems, or the prevention of the development of challenging behaviors. Addressing the information and resource needs of families enhances their capacity to use the information for problem solving, decision making, and generalization to other settings and routines.

Bringing families together within parent–child playgroups can facilitate the sharing of information and resources between parents and fosters support and socialization for the parents. As children increase their social-communication skills, opportunities to join peers in community activities are facilitated. Combination home, early care, and education programs are a natural progression in ESI. Family preferences and access to group settings are highly variable depending on resources, family values, and geographic availability. ESI providers offer initial training to child care providers and preschool teachers; help to arrange the environment to support communication, interaction, and positive behavior; develop visual supports as needed; and practice with the child to facilitate transition to the setting. Just as with the parent, the continuum of consultation supports is provided for the teacher. As the child is successful and the teacher gains confidence, the ESI interventionist decreases time with the child in the program and establishes regular consultation visits to review the program, add new or revise existing outcome targets, and problem-solve with the teacher, thereby increasing his or her capacity to generate additional social-communication and play opportunities between peers.

DATA COLLECTION TO SUPPORT DECISION MAKING

Based on the belief that the earlier the intervention, the better the outcomes for the child, ESI collects data at multiple levels. First, it is important to know that the intervention is being implemented. Data on time spent in intervention are collected by the interventionist and include the time provided by early intervention, other team members, and the parents. During each session, families share information with the interventionist on the routines they completed between visits, time spent in community activities, and new routines or activities initiated. When intensity drops or is consistently low, problem solving between the parent and interventionist is initiated. Solutions may include identification of other potential partners (e.g., grandpa, older sibling, high school volunteer) or activities (e.g., mother's morning out, Early Head Start) to promote the child's practice or a reorganization of the current routines and activities to provide more time for parents at the end of the day when their other children return home from school.

Child data are collected throughout sessions on the specific intervention targets observed and are updated using the MAETS, as discussed shortly. Child targets need to be monitored closely to ensure progress is occurring, and if not, then revisions in the plan need to occur immediately. Again, time is of the essence. Finally, on a less formal basis, parents' use of supports and strategies is monitored and shared with them during home visits as feedback.

To be efficient and useable within early intervention programs, data collection must be manageable. ESI interventionists use a home visit note to record samples of child outcomes, routines and activities implemented, and caregiver utilization. Planning for what is to occur between visits by the parent is an important component of the home visit that sets the stage for the next round of data collection on what actually occurred. Families report data on specific targets and routines throughout the week using a variety of methods, including refrigerator logs or tally sheets, wipe-off boards, e-mails, or video clips. Increased access to technology by families makes data collection a very dynamic process. Videos shared via cellphones are becoming more frequent.

ASSESSMENT FOR TREATMENT PLANNING AND PROGRESS MONITORING

We use standard sampling procedures (Wetherby & Prizant, 2002) to derive measures of the child's use of social communication from the CSBS DP sample. A parent joins the evaluator and is present during a warm-up caregiving routine and play interaction and a complete communication evaluation. Parents are instructed to respond naturally but not to direct the child's behavior, instead encouraging spontaneous communication and play. The communication evaluation begins after the 10-minute warm-up and lasts approximately 30 minutes. The evaluator first presents the child with a series of communicative temptations (e.g., a wind-up toy, a balloon, bubbles, a jar containing food, a bag with toys, and books designed for young children from the test kit) to entice spontaneous communication. Next, the evaluator offers the child a feeding toy set and stuffed animal for symbolic play and blocks for constructive play to assess knowledge of play behaviors. The sample consists of six activities during which the child's skills are rated. Also included are probes of gaze/point follow and comprehension of object names, person names, and body parts that are interspersed between activities. Information about the reliability and validity of the CSBS DP is included in several publications (see Wetherby et al., 2002; Wetherby et al., 2003; Wetherby & Prizant, 2002). For a child being considered for ESI, the CSBS DP may be administered in a clinical setting or the child's home in cooperation with the local early intervention program or upon referral from the early intervention program, family, physician, or other community agencies.

Child Measure of Language Stage

During the collection of each behavior sample, we describe the child's language stage using criteria based on expressive language use that were established by Tager-Flusberg and colleagues (2009). Those criteria include *Preverbal*—0 or 1 word; *Early one-word stage*—2–5 different words; *Late one-word stage*—6–9 different words; *Multiword stage*—10 or more different words and 2 or more different word combinations.

Child Measure of Autism Symptoms

Early red flags of ASD (https://autismnavigator.com) that the child is showing are coded from a video recording of the behavior sample of the CSBS, which lasts approximately 20 minutes. Red flags from each domain of the *Diagnostic and*

Statistical Manual of Mental Disorders, Fifth Edition (DSM-V; American Psychiatric Association, 2013), diagnostic criteria for ASD—Impairment in Social Communication and Social Interaction (SC) and Restricted Repetitive Behaviors, Interests, and Activities (RRB) are coded. Some behaviors measured are a lack of typical behaviors (SC). Other behaviors are unusual or not expected in typical development (RRB). Coding may also be completed during an ongoing interaction of the child and one or more adults, such as a semistructured home observation during which the parent tries for 1 hour to engage the child in interaction during six different activities (e.g., play with objects, play with people, caregiving, snacks and meals, book sharing, and family chores). Whatever interactional context is chosen, it is important to include structured and unstructured activities so that a lack of typical milestones of social-communication development as well as the presence of unusual behaviors may be observed. Video recordings may also provide additional clinical utility, as they can be used as a reference to build consensus with families on observed red flags.

Curriculum-Based Assessment and Progress Monitoring: Measure of Active Engagement and Transactional Supports

MAETS quantifies the proportion of time the child is actively engaged (AE) and the caregiver's use of transactional supports (TS) during a home observation of everyday activities and routines. The MAETS operationalizes AE and TS into components (see AE definitions in Wetherby et al., 2018) that correspond to the ESI framework for child outcomes targeted by parents. The MAETS is rated from videos of home observations lasting approximately 1 hour, collected throughout treatment; however, live in vivo scoring is also possible. Ongoing home observations used to monitor progress can be done in 10–15 minutes before and after a home visit and used to score MAETS. Selected intervals of each observation are coded using a three-point rating scale for each component.

MAETS includes measures of eight components of child active engagement: 1) emotional regulation; 2) productivity; 3) social connectedness; 4) gaze to face; 5) response to bids for interaction; 6) initiated, directed communication; 7) flexibility; and 8) generative language. It also includes eight caregiver TS dimensions: 1) promoting participation and a productive role, 2) providing structure to make activities predictable, 3) using language that follows the child's focus of attention, 4) promoting child initiations, 5) providing a balance of communicative turns, 6) supporting the development of child comprehension, 7) providing verbal and nonverbal models, and 8) caregiver creates appropriate expectations and demands.

IMPLICATIONS FOR INCLUSIVE PRACTICE

Inclusivity and meaningful family participation are integral to the ESI process from the beginning. Family priorities, concerns, challenges, meaningful activities and routines, and preferences are identified, and families actively participate in the development of their intervention plan. Intervention sessions are scheduled to accommodate family circumstances and to include extended family members to facilitate generalization. In addition to the home-based sessions, children can participate in a parent–child playgroup guided by ESI interventionists either face to face or online. Each playgroup is flexibly structured with predictable opening and closing songs, book times, and new play centers each week, encouraging individualization for the parent and child dyads and opportunities to expand participation in novel activities. Through playgroups such as these, families may have opportunities to focus on interacting with their child, to support peer interaction with other participants, and to receive feedback on their strategy use. The interventionists provide information to families through discussion and handouts, responses to questions, modeling, and individual coaching by setting up opportunities and making suggestions. Further, the playgroups offer the families opportunities to observe their child in a group with same-age peers and to network with other parents of children with and without ASD, which may be helpful to parents in adjusting to the realization that their child has ASD.

As children increase their social-communication skills, opportunities to join peers in community activities are facilitated. Combination home, early care, and education programs are a natural progression in ESI. Family preferences and access to group settings is highly variable depending on resources, family values, and geographic availability. Some ESI families have identified child care or mother's morning out options for a morning or two a week initially, whereas others have sought a more formal nursery or preschool program. Still others have developed community cooperative programs and play dates to support social interaction as a less formal or inexpensive option. Whatever the family choice, ESI providers offer initial training to child care or preschool teachers; help to arrange the environment to support communication, interaction, and positive behavior; develop visual supports as needed; and practice with the child to facilitate transition to the setting. Just as with the parent, the continuum of collaborative coaching supports are provided for the teacher. As the child is successful and the teacher gains confidence, the ESI interventionist decreases time with the child in the program and establishes regular consultation visits to review the program, add new or revise existing outcome targets, and to problem-solve with the teacher, thereby increasing his or her capacity to generate additional social-communication and play opportunities between peers.

CONSIDERATIONS FOR CHILDREN FROM CULTURALLY AND LINGUISTICALLY DIVERSE BACKGROUNDS

Family-centered capacity-building services and supports are, by definition, culturally responsive and respectful (Woods & Wetherby, 2003). ESI builds on this principle by joining in the families' daily routines and activities rather than assigning specific lessons or therapeutic activities. The provider works with the family as a partner through the intervention process, establishing a relationship that honors the family's beliefs as well as their priorities and concerns for their child's social-communication needs. The individualized curriculum for the child and the family allows the ESI provider to build upon the child's and family's strengths and interests and choose from the menu of evidence-based instructional strategies that are most comfortable and compatible with the family's culture and learning style. For some children and families, this may mean starting with play or familiar social interaction games and songs that promote joint attention and turn taking before evolving into more typical caregiving routines or household chores. Other families want to make the most of what they do and find that embedding outcomes during bath time or while folding laundry increases opportunities for interaction between caregiver and child, promotes active engagement, and supports activities important to the family's well being. ESI is often the entry point to early intervention for the child and family.

We believe the family education component of the individualized curriculum is key to successful child and family outcomes. Families are not just new to ESI and early intervention but are new to a diagnosis and the recognition that their child is at risk for or has autism. At this time, families are often concerned about the impact of the diagnosis and are in a particularly vulnerable place. They may be experiencing a range and intensity of emotions from remorse to blame, anger, frustration, and denial, and they may be questioning the diagnosis. Education of the family in the ESI approach is an integral part of each home visit and is integrated throughout the session using conversations, information sharing, and problem-solving strategies to answer questions, clarify family understanding, apply content to the family's contexts, and address immediate family concerns. The specific coaching strategies used are individualized for the family and the relationship established with the provider. Strategies are jointly identified to be compatible with the family's preferences, culture, and learning style.

Content that is core to child progress but may be affected by culture is addressed with families to increase their understanding and implementation. For example, sometimes families are comfortable with a quiet child who only responds and does not initiate or a child who entertains him- or herself. Through ongoing parent education as well as coaching during the session, the provider demonstrates the value of joint attention and engagement to enhance communication and interaction. Whether it is family culture, history, education, or expediency, some families preempt opportunities for their child to gain independence and would prefer to complete the routine *for* their child to show their love for their child and their competence as a parent. Again, the ESI provider supports family members along the continuum of coaching to gain understanding of the importance of child opportunities for practice and independence.

To date, the ESI model has been studied across multiple geographic regions, which has informed the intervention procedures and process. The cumulative sample reported in this chapter has included families representing the demographic distribution of urban and suburban areas in New York, Georgia, Florida, and Michigan and has included white, African American, Hispanic, Haitian, and Asian families. We are continuing to explore diverse samples globally, including in South Africa (Chambers et al, 2018), Brazil, and Canada, and anxiously await learning more about the ESI components and their adaptability to diverse cultural, linguistic, and socio-educational populations.

Application to a Child

Jay was referred at 18 months and began intervention. He was at the SCERTS Social Partner Stage because he did not yet have recognizable words or symbols. The profile summary from his home observation in a variety of everyday activities indicated relative strengths and challenges in SC and ER. Jay was just beginning to use intentional communication. He directed his gaze to others occasionally but was not yet coordinating his gaze, gestures, and vocalizations. He smiled and laughed occasionally but did not share positive affect with others or respond with laughter differentially. His rate of communication was low, and he used communication primarily to request comfort or continuation of a social game. If not redirected, Jay spent much of his time rolling objects, which seemed to be a self regulation strategy. Jay's family identified favorite play routines as listening to music in the family room and in the car, swinging, and collecting and rolling small objects. Although Jay did not participate in many family or caregiving routines without considerable adult support, he did request favorite foods and drinks with vocalizations and was comforted by rocking in his rocking chair.

Using the MAETS, the initial goals for Jay were to shift his gaze between people and objects, to request comfort when distressed, to combine a vocalization and gesture to gain attention, to imitate familiar actions in a turn-taking sequence, to use familiar objects functionally, and to make choices with gestures. The ESI interventionist and the family members discussed how Jay's specific goals would be practiced within routines as they occurred throughout the day. Goals for his parents included increasing their consistency in responding immediately to any communication initiation by Jay by imitating him, using environmental arrangements such as limiting access to preferred materials until he communicated a request or choice, and marking clear beginnings and endings to the routines so Jay knew what was expected of him. Within the first few weeks, he began to imitate actions with his dad in favorite games. His parents reported an increase in distress when objects were removed or when they required him to transition to another activity without advance warning.

Jay's parents learned how to use positioning to support Jay's participation; make activities predictable with balanced turns; respond to his gestural, vocal, and facial signals to request and to stop interaction; and wait for Jay to take a turn or communicate a choice. Intervention strategies were embedded in cereal and drink routines, in which he was given a choice of juice or water or of a type of cereal at breakfast but was given smaller portions so that he could vocalize to request more. Jay's father is usually responsible for breakfast while his mother drives older siblings to school. The father pulled up his chair to face Jay in his highchair, watched for him to make his initial drink request, and offered him the choices and then modeled the label of the choice that he made (i.e., apple juice). He took a turn drinking his coffee after Jay took a drink, then he watched for Jay again and responded. The process of embedding the goals would occur within each routine as appropriate and would be jointly planned by the family members and service providers. Routines would be added over time, as illustrated in Figure 11.3, to help his family learn how to embed intervention strategies in routines 25 hours per week to promote Jay's active engagement.

Application to an Adult

The ESI is designed for toddlers and thus is not appropriate for adolescents or adults with ASD.

> **To review an extended application and implementation of this intervention, see Case 8 about a child with ASD in the companion volume *Case Studies for the Treatment of Autism Spectrum Disorder.***

Future Directions

Early identification of red flags for ASD provides a unique opportunity for prevention of significant social and communication delays and an interruption of the progression of the disorder. Families served by ESI voiced concerns about their child's development and identified multiple red flags by age 12–18 months. With increased public and physician awareness, earlier identification of red flags is occurring. Consequently, our research will continue to explore avenues for ESI to be used with families earlier. We have developed a streamlined family education program to help families get ahead of ASD when red flags are identified. Educating parents through individual sessions or parent–child playgroups may serve as a prevention tool. Appropriate education goals in such contexts would support responsive interaction, increased engagement in family-identified meaningful activities, and focus with the parents on the development of joint attention skills. An emerging body of literature has identified telepractice as an effective intervention tool for providing services in a cost- and time-effective manner to children with autism and their parents (National Autism Center, 2015; Vismara et al., 2013; Wainer & Ingersoll, 2015).

The next step in our research is to determine ways to make the ESI model more portable and to incorporate innovative technology to support scalability and sustained practice change in community early intervention systems. We have developed a Seamless Path for Families by maximizing technology supports—beginning with online tools that teach parents early social-communication milestones (learn more at https://autismnavigator.com/family-resources). For families with a positive screen for autism, our Seamless Path offers an online introductory course, Autism Navigator About Autism in Toddlers, to learn the early signs of autism with video clips of more than a dozen toddlers with ASD. For families who suspect their child has ASD, the Autism Navigator How-To Guide for Families is an interactive online self-paced course that has 10 hours of interactive slides and 5 hours of video libraries. It puts in the hands of families hundreds of video illustrations of evidence-based intervention techniques they can implement in everyday activities to support their child's learning as soon as they suspect autism. This course teaches families how to embed strategies and supports into their everyday activities. These online tools and courses provide technology-supported resources that are interactive, individualized, and focused on application to ensure knowledge is applied and sustained, which was a major limitation in previous technology-supported studies (Meadan et al., 2016; Wainer & Ingersoll, 2013). This How-To Guide for Families is instrumental for early intervention providers coaching with the ESI model to help families they serve learn more efficiently so that coaching sessions can focus on changing developmental trajectories of toddlers with ASD and supporting their families. A further advantage of the Autism Navigator web platform is that it is available for use by multidisciplinary teams of early intervention providers to increase coordination and implementation fidelity of ESI strategies. It also is integrated with an online screening and monitoring system, and the family tools and resources grow with the child and can help improve early detection (learn more at https://babynavigator.com).

For ESI to be effective in the local early intervention arena, it is essential to identify competencies for personnel training and for developing user friendly and easily accessible continuing education and mentoring opportunities. Efforts are underway to develop training materials and manuals that can be available on the Internet with video illustrations (https://babynavigator.com; https://autismnavigator.com). However, without support to learn the consultation or coaching strategies described as essential for families to become skilled at engaging their children in embedded intervention, it is unlikely that providers will gain the confidence and competence to implement the procedures with a high degree of fidelity. Consultation and coaching intervention approaches are believed to be effective but still not used widely in the field in meaningful ways to build caregiver capacity (Dunst et al., 2019). Fixsen and colleagues (2005) identify complexity, distance from familiar and comfortable practice, and the need for additional training as reasons why providers are unlikely or unwilling to utilize procedures. Although ESI was designed for and implemented collaboratively within an IDEA Part C early intervention program, the ESI providers in the published studies were highly qualified providers with ongoing training and mentoring. Each of the components of the approach (i.e., family-guided routines, individualized child and family curriculum, parent-implemented embedded intervention, collaborative coaching, team-based community coordination, positive behavior supports) necessitates competence by interventionists in a bundle of practices that, although recommended, are not currently implemented with fidelity (Lord & McGee, 2001; Schreibman et al., 2020). Therefore, an important future direction for ESI is to disseminate training and mentoring opportunities more widely; technology supports are a low-cost and highly accessible option under development and evaluation.

Suggested Readings

1. Early Social Intervention Project, http://esi.fsu.edu. The ESI website is a repository for materials developed for the original model-demonstration project as well as for its ongoing research. New materials or links are posted as developed. This site also has links to Baby Navigator (https://babynavigator.com), First Words Project (https://firstwords.fsu.edu), and Autism Navigator (https://autismnavigator.com), which provide information and resources on early social-communication development, identification, and intervention.

2. Autism Navigator About Autism in Toddlers, https://autismnavigator.com/courses/#everyone. This free online course for families, professionals, or anyone interested in learning more about ASD includes video clips of more than a dozen toddlers with ASD at 18–24 months of age. Simply register and log in to learn about core diagnostic features of autism, critical importance of early detection and early intervention, and current information on prevalence and causes of autism.

3. Wetherby, A., Guthrie, W., Woods, J., Schatschneider, C., Holland, R., & Morgan, L. (2014). Parent-implemented social intervention for toddlers with autism: An RCT. *Pediatrics, 134*(6), 1084–1093. Results of the large-scale RCT are shared with physicians to demonstrate the importance of early intervention and offer implication for early detection.

4. Wetherby, A. M., Woods, J., Guthrie, W., Delehanty, A., Brown, J. A., Morgan, L., Holland, R. D., Schatschneider, C., & Lord, C. (2018). Changing developmental trajectories of toddlers with autism spectrum disorder: Strategies for bridging research to community practice. *Journal of Speech, Language, and Hearing Research, 61*(11), 2615–2628. This paper extends the research on ESI, explores clinical implications, and suggests future research.

5. National Center for Pyramid Model Innovations, https://challengingbehavior.cbcs.usf.edu. The NCPMI, sponsored by the Office of Special Education Programs, offers extensive information for families, team members, and administrators on evidence-based practice and tool kits to support implementation.

Learning Activities _____

1. Identify how the processes and procedures of ESI reflect an NDBI.

2. Identifying and building intervention activities and routines that are meaningful to the family and provide multiple opportunities for the child's communication and engagement can appear to be challenging initially. ESI does not provide a list of best options but rather encourages joint identification by the family and the team, as no children and families are alike. Develop a checklist of important considerations to ensure you are jointly identifying the most authentic and functional contexts with the family that also ensure sufficient intervention intensity and dosage.

3. Cara's mom and dad agree that she has social-communication delays and would benefit from early intervention, but they cannot see why *you* just don't do it. They are sure you have more expertise than they do, and they fear they will just be in your way. What would you tell them?

4. Jamal says several single words and sometimes uses them to label favorite foods and toys. His dad is convinced he is verbal and wants you to work on two- and three-word combinations so he sounds more like the other kids at his child care. You are concerned about his limited joint attention, turn taking, response to communicative bids, and participation in productive roles. How would you proceed to work closely with Jamal's dad to increase his understanding of Jamal's essential targets and choose appropriate early communication and social interaction outcomes?

5. The team, including the family members, has been pleased with Tyler's progress. He is initiating social interactions; coordinating gaze, gestures, and a few words in familiar routines; playing with his toys functionally; and beginning to combine actions more flexibly. In addition, he has decreased his repetitive spinning behaviors. Everyone agrees the next step is to integrate him into a small group or classroom setting. The teacher at the community program the family chose is not sure she has time to collaborate and be coached. How can the team use the continuum of caregiver supports in an early care and education program to support Tyler and his teacher?

Summary of Video Clip _____

See the **About the Videos and Downloads** page at the front of the book for directions on how to access and stream the accompanying video to this chapter.

This video clip depicts a little boy with autism interacting with his mom and dad. He first began early intervention at age 18 months in the Early Social Interaction Project. His intervention focuses on joint attention and building early language. The video depicts his interactions in four routines. In the first routine, Julius and his dad are engaged in a turn-taking game. You will notice Julius's vocalizations, movements, and gaze shifts. The father supports imitation and shared attention. The second activity is a dressing routine in which Julius has opportunities to follow directions and learn new words. During this activity, Julius initiates a social game, and the father follows his son's lead. In the next routine, the SLP coaches the parent to extend pretend play. The final routine is book reading. The mother pauses during book reading, which allows Julius to imitate and add words.

REFERENCES

Adams, R. C., & Tapia, C. (2013). Early intervention, IDEA part C services, and the medical home: Collaboration for best practice and best outcomes. *Pediatrics, 132*(4), e1073–e1088.

American Psychiatric Association. (2013). *Diagnostic and statistical manual of mental disorders, fifth edition* (DSM-5). Author.

American Speech-Language-Hearing Association. (n.d.-a). *Autism* (Practice Portal). Retrieved January 15, 2021, from https://www.asha.org/Practice-Portal/Clinical-Topics/Autism

American Speech-Language-Hearing Association. (n.d.-b). *Core knowledge and skills in early intervention speech-language pathology practice* [Knowledge and Skills]. Retrieved January 15, 2021, from https://www.asha.org/policy/KS2008-00292

Bernheimer, L., & Weismer, T. (2007). "Let me tell you what I do all day . . .": The family story at the center of intervention research and practice. *Infants and Young Children, 20*(3), 192–201.

Bransford, J. D., Brown, A., & Cocking, R. (2000). *How people learn: Mind, brain, experience, and school.* National Academy Press.

Brown, J. A., & Woods, J. J. (2015). Effects of a triadic parent-implemented home-based communication intervention for toddlers. *Journal of Early Intervention, 37*(1), 44–68.

Brown, J. A., & Woods, J. J. (2016). Parent-implemented communication intervention: Sequential analysis of triadic relationships. *Topics in Early Childhood Special Education, 36*(2), 115–124.

Chambers, N. J., de Vries, P. J., Delehanty, A. D., & Wetherby, A. M. (2018). Feasibility of utilizing Autism Navigator® for primary care in South Africa. *Autism Research, 11*(11), 1511–1521.

Coufal, K. L., & Woods, J. J. (2018). Interprofessional collaborative practice in early intervention. *Pediatric Clinics, 65*(1), 143–155.

Dawson, G., Bernier, R., & Ring, R. H. (2012). Social attention: A possible early indicator of efficacy in autism clinical trials. *Journal of Neurodevelopmental Disorders, 4*(1), 11.

Dawson, G., Rogers, S., Munson, J., Smith, M., Winter, J., Greenson, J., Donaldson, A., & Varley, J. (2010). Randomized, controlled trial of an intervention for toddlers with autism: The Early Start Denver Model. *Pediatrics, 125*(1), e17–e23.

Donovan, M. S., Bransford, J. D. & Pellegrino, J. W. (Eds., 1999). How people learn: Bridging research and practice. The National Academies Press.

Dunst, C. J., Hamby, D. W., & Raab, M. (2019). Modeling the relationships between practitioner capacity-building practices and the behavior and development of young children with disabilities and delays. *Educational Research and Reviews, 14*(9), 309–319.

Dunst, C. J., & Trivette, C. M. (2009). Using research evidence to inform and evaluate early childhood intervention practices. *Topics in Early Childhood Special Education, 29*, 40–52.

Fixsen, D. L., Naoom, S. F., Blase, K. A., Friedman, R. M., & Wallace, F. (2005). *Implementation research: A synthesis of the literature.* University of South Florida.

Fox, L., Dunlap, G., Hemmeter, M. L., Joseph, G. E., & Strain, P. S. (2003). The Teaching Pyramid: A model for supporting social competence and preventing challenging behavior in young children. *YC Young Children, 58*(4), 48–52.

Friedman, M., Woods, J., & Salisbury, C. (2012). Caregiver coaching strategies for early intervention providers: Moving toward operational definitions. *Infants & Young Children, 25*(1), 62–82.

Goode, S., Lazara, A., & Danaher, J. (2008). Part C updates. National Early Childhood Technical Assistance Center (NECTAC). University of North Carolina-Chapel Hill.

Individuals with Disabilities Education Improvement Act (IDEA) of 2004, PL 108-446, 20 U.S.C. § 1400 *et seq.* (2004; 2012).

Kashinath, S., Woods, J., & Goldstein, H. (2006). Enhancing generalized teaching strategy use in daily routines by parents of children with autism. *Journal of Speech, Language, and Hearing Research, 49*(3), 466–485.

Kemp, P., & Turnbull, A. P. (2014). Coaching with parents in early intervention: An interdisciplinary research synthesis. *Infants & Young Children, 27*(4), 305–324.

Landa, R. J., Holman, K. C., O'Neill, A. H., & Stuart, E. Z. (2011). Intervention targeting development of socially synchronous engagement in toddlers with autism spectrum disorder: A randomized controlled trial. *Journal of Child Psychology and Psychiatry, 52*(1), 13–21.

Lord, C., & McGee, J. P. (Eds.). (2001). *Educating children with autism*. Committee on Educational Interventions for Children with Autism, Commission on Behavioral and Social Sciences and Education, National Research Council. National Academy Press.

Lord, C., Rutter, M. L., DiLavore, P. S., & Risi, S. (1999). *Autism Diagnostic Observation Schedule—Generic*. Western Psychological Services.

Meadan, H., & Daczewitz, M. E. (2015). Internet-based intervention training for parents of young children with disabilities: A promising service-delivery model. *Early Child Development and Care, 185*(1), 155–169.

Meadan, H., Snodgrass, M. R., Meyer, L. E., Fisher, K. W., Chung, M. Y., & Halle, J. W. (2016). Internet-based parent-implemented intervention for young children with autism: A pilot study. *Journal of Early Intervention, 38*(1), 3–23.

Merriam, S. B., & Baumgartner, L. M. (2020). *Learning in adulthood: A comprehensive guide* (4th ed.) Jossey-Bass.

Mullen, E. M. (1995). *Mullen Scales of Early Learning* (pp. 58–64). American Guidance Service.

National Academies of Sciences, Engineering, and Medicine. (2018). How people learn II: Learners, contexts, and cultures. National Academies Press.

National Autism Center. (2015). *National Standards Project, Phase 2: Addressing the need for evidence-based practice guidelines for ASD*. https://www.nationalautismcenter.org

Oxford Centre for Evidence-based Medicine: Levels of Evidence (March 2009). https://www.cebm.ox.ac.uk/resources/levels-of-evidence/oxford-centre-for-evidence-based-medicine-levels-of-evidence-march-2009

Prizant, B. M., Wetherby, A. M., Rubin, E., & Laurent, A. C. (2003). The SCERTS® Model: A transactional, family-centered approach to enhancing communication and socioemotional abilities of children with autism spectrum disorder. *Infants and Young Children, 16*(4), 296–316.

Prizant, B. M., Wetherby, A., Rubin, E., Laurent, A., & Rydell, P. (2006). *The SCERTS® Model: A comprehensive educational approach for children with autism spectrum disorders*. Paul H. Brookes Publishing Co.

Prizant, B. M., Wetherby, A. M., & Rydell, P. J. (2000). Communication intervention issues for children with autism spectrum disorders. In A. M. Wetherby & B. M. Prizant (Eds.), *Autism spectrum disorders: A transactional developmental perspective* (pp. 193–224). Paul H. Brookes Publishing Co.

Reichow, B., Volkmar, F. R., & Cicchetti, D. V. (2008). Development of the evaluative method for evaluating and determining evidence-based practices in autism. *Journal of Autism and Developmental Disorders, 38*(7), 1311–1319.

Rogers, S. J., Vismara, L., Wagner, A. L., McCormick, C., Young, G., & Ozonoff, S. (2014). Autism treatment in the first year of life: A pilot study of infant start, a parent-implemented intervention for symptomatic infants. *Journal of Autism and Developmental Disorders, 44*(12), 2981–2995.

Sandall, S., Hemmeter, M. L., Smith, B. J., & McLean, M. E. (2005). *DEC recommended practices: A comprehensive guide for practical application in early intervention/early childhood special education*. Sopris West Educational Services.

Schertz, H. H., Baker, C., Hurwitz, S., & Benner, L. (2011). Principles of early intervention reflected in toddler research in autism spectrum disorders. *Topics in Early Childhood Special Education, 31*(1), 4–21.

Schreibman, L., Dawson, G., Stahmer, A. C., Landa, R., Rogers, S. J., McGee, G. G., Kasari, C., Ingersoll, B., Kaiser, A. P., Bruinsma, Y., McNerney, E., & Wetherby, A. (2015). Naturalistic Developmental Behavioral Interventions: Empirically validated treatments for autism spectrum disorder. *Journal of Autism and Developmental Disorders, 45*(8), 2411–2428.

Schreibman, L., Jobin, A. B., & Dawson, G. (2020). Understanding NDBI. In Y. Bruinsma, M. Minjarez, L. Schreibman, & A. Stahmer (Eds.), *Naturalistic Developmental Behavioral Interventions for autism spectrum disorder* (pp. 3–20). Paul H. Brookes Publishing Co.

Snyder P., Hemmeter, M. L., & Fox L. (2015). Supporting implementation of evidence-based practices through practice-based coaching. *Topics in Early Childhood Special Education, 35*, 133–143.

Sparrow, S., Cicchetti, D. V., & Balla, D. A. (2005). *Vineland Adaptive Behavior Scales* (2nd ed). American Guidance Service.

Tager-Flusberg, H., Rogers, S., Cooper, J., Landa, R., Lord, C., Paul, R., Rice, M., Stoel-Gammon, C., Wetherby, A., & Yoder, P. (2009). Defining spoken language benchmarks and selecting measures of expressive language development for young children with autism spectrum disorders. *Journal of Speech, Language, and Hearing Research, 52*(3): 643–652.

U.S. Department of Education. (2016). *Thirty-eighth annual report to congress on the implementation of the Individuals with Disabilities Education Act.* Office of Special Education and Rehabilitative Services. https://www2.ed.gov/about/reports/annual/osep/2016/parts-b-c/index.html

Vismara, L. A., McCormick, C., Young, G. S., Nadham, A., & Monlux, K. (2013). Preliminary findings of a telehealth approach to parent training in autism. *Journal of Autism and Developmental Disorders, 43*(12), 2953-2969.

Vismara, L. A., Young, G. S., & Rogers, S. J. (2012). Telehealth for expanding the reach of early autism training to parents. *Autism Research and Treatment, 2012,* 1–12.

Wainer, A. L., & Ingersoll, B. R. (2013). Disseminating ASD interventions: A pilot study of a distance learning program for parents and professionals. *Journal of Autism and Developmental Disorders, 43*(1), 11–24.

Wainer, A. L., & Ingersoll, B. R. (2015). Increasing access to an ASD imitation intervention via a telehealth parent training program. *Journal of Autism and Developmental Disorders, 45*(12), 3877–3890.

Wetherby, A. M., Allen, L. Cleary, J., Kublin, K., & Goldstein, H. (2002). Validity and reliability of the communication and symbolic behavior scales developmental profile with very young children. *Journal of Speech, Language, and Hearing Research, 45*(6), 1202–1218.

Wetherby, A. M., Goldstein, H., Cleary, J., Allen, L., & Kublin, K. (2003). Early identification of children with communication disorders: Concurrent and predictive validity of the CSBS Developmental Profile. *Infants and Young Children, 16*(2), 161–174.

Wetherby, A. M., Guthrie, W., Woods, J., Schatschneider, C., Holland, R. D., Morgan, L., & Lord, C. (2014). Parent-implemented social intervention for toddlers with autism: An RCT. *Pediatrics, 134*(6), 1084–1093.

Wetherby, A. M., Morgan, L., & Holland, R. (2013). *Measure of Active Engagement and Transactional Supports* [Unpublished manual]. Florida State University.

Wetherby, A., & Prizant, B. (2002). *Communication and Symbolic Behavior Scales Developmental Profile™–First Normed Edition.* Paul H. Brookes Publishing Co.

Wetherby, A. M., Watt, N., Morgan, L., & Shumway, S. (2007). Social-communication profiles of children with autism spectrum disorders late in the second year of life. *Journal of Autism and Developmental Disorders, 37*(5), 960–975.

Wetherby, A., & Woods, J. (2006). Effectiveness of early intervention for children with autism spectrum disorders beginning in the second year of life. *Topics in Early Childhood Special Education, 26,* 67–82.

Wetherby, A., Woods, J., Guthrie, W., Delehanty, A., Brown, J. A., Morgan, L., Holland, R. D., Schatschneider, C., & Lord, C. (2018). Changing developmental trajectories of toddlers with autism spectrum disorder: Strategies for bridging research to community practice. *Journal of Speech, Language, Hearing Research, 61*(11), 2615–2628.

Woods, J., & Lindeman, D. (2008). Gathering and giving assessment information with families. *Infants and Young Children 21*(4), 272–284.

Woods, J., & Wetherby, A. (2003). Early identification and intervention for infants and toddlers at-risk for autism spectrum disorders. *Language, Speech, and Hearing Services in Schools, 34,* 180–193.

Woods, J. J., Wilcox, M. J., Friedman, M., & Murch, T. (2011). Collaborative consultation in natural environments: Strategies to enhance family-centered supports and services. *Language, Speech, and Hearing Services in Schools, 42*(3), 379–392.

12

Peer-Mediated Support Interventions for Students With ASD

Erik W. Carter

INTRODUCTION

Schools are rich contexts for peer interaction, friendship formation, and shared learning among diverse students. Opportunities for establishing social connections usually abound within the classrooms, cafeterias, clubs, playgrounds, and other settings in which students spend their days. Yet many students with autism spectrum disorder (ASD) remain on the peripheries of the interactions and collaborative experiences that can make school enjoyable and engaging (Carter et al., 2008; Lipscomb et al., 2017).

Enhancing the social and communication outcomes of students with ASD has long been considered a critical focus of high-quality schooling and effective special education. Through interactions with their peers, children and youth with ASD can develop important social-communication and language skills, learn academic and functional life skills, access emotional and instrumental supports, establish friendships, and participate more actively in the life of their school (Huber & Carter, 2019). The relationships students experience can also contribute to their sense of belonging, encourage independence, increase school engagement, and promote overall well-being and quality of life (Carter, 2018; Ryan & Ladd, 2012). Recognizing these multiple benefits, researchers and practitioners have emphasized the importance of adopting strategies that improve social outcomes within inclusive schools.

Although educators, related services providers, parents, and other adults can be instrumental in enhancing student outcomes, peers can also play a powerful role in promoting social, communication, and other educational outcomes for children and youth with ASD. Peer-mediated support interventions focus on equipping one or more peers to provide ongoing social or academic support, or both, to similar-age students with ASD under the guidance of educators, paraprofessionals, or other school staff (Carter & Kennedy, 2006). These interventions typically involve identifying students with ASD and their peers who would benefit from involvement in these interventions, orienting peers to their new roles, providing regular opportunities for the students to interact within instructional or noninstructional school settings, and offering needed guidance and support to ensure all participating students are benefiting as anticipated. As students gain experience working together, adults incrementally fade their proximity and their direct support to promote independence.

A broad array of peer-mediated instruction and intervention strategies have been described and evaluated in the professional literature (see reviews by Carter et al., 2010; Watkins et al., 2015). This chapter focuses on two approaches with strong empirical support: peer support arrangements and peer network interventions. **Peer support arrangements** are individually tailored interventions that involve equipping two or more peers without disabilities to provide academic and social support to a classmate with ASD throughout the semester in a general education classroom. **Peer network interventions** involve establishing a cohesive social group of three to six students that meets formally and informally across an entire semester or school year and emphasizes social connections for students with ASD beyond the classroom. Both approaches 1) involve peers in providing ongoing and direct support (vs. occasional or incidental support) to their classmates with ASD; 2) have been implemented in inclusive elementary, middle, or high school settings (i.e., Grades 1–12); and 3) work to enhance social interactions among similar-age students with ASD and their peers without disabilities. The focus on peer social interaction contrasts with other interventions that focus instead on acquisition of social skills, interactions with adults, or interactions with other classmates with disabilities.

TARGET POPULATIONS

Peer-mediated support interventions were developed primarily for school-age individuals with moderate to severe disabilities who require extensive or pervasive supports to participate fully within inclusive classes, extracurricular activities, and other school-sponsored activities (Carter, 2017). Because these interventions are delivered in schools, researchers often describe participating students using special education categories rather than the *Diagnostic and Statistical Manual of Mental Disorders, Fifth Edition* (DSM-V; American Psychiatric Association, 2013) diagnostic criteria. In addition to being served under the special education category of autism, these students have also been served under the categories of intellectual disability and/or multiple disabilities. Most students involved in studies of peer support arrangements have been eligible for their state's **alternate assessments** for individuals with significant cognitive impairments. However, a substantial number of peer network intervention studies have also focused on students with ASD who do not have coexisting intellectual disability (e.g., Carter et al., 2017; Kamps et al., 2015; Kasari et al., 2016; R. L. Koegel et al., 2012). Autism symptomology—typically reported using the Childhood Autism Rating Scale (Schopler et al., 1988)—has varied widely across studies. Nonetheless, the persistence of social-communication deficits and a paucity of social interactions across school contexts characterizes these students. Most of these students also have substantial language impairments.

As with all special education programming, decisions about intervention appropriateness, design, and delivery for an individual should be determined within collaborative teaming models (Biggs et al., 2017; Hunt et al., 2003). Typically, peer-mediated support interventions are considered appropriate for students with ASD who exhibit one or more of the following characteristics: 1) have **individualized education program (IEP)** goals addressing the quality and/or quantity of their interactions or relationships with peers; 2) experience limited interactions with same-age peers, despite being in close proximity (e.g., enrollment in the same class, club, or school activity); 3) evidence substantial impairments in social and/or communication skills; and, 4) require additional support to participate in classroom or school activities. Students' interest in working with and receiving support from their peers should also be a primary consideration.

Direct observation is the primary approach used to determine the appropriateness and focus of peer-mediated support interventions for school-age children with ASD. For example, observations can be conducted by educators, paraprofessionals, or other school staff to identify those settings (e.g., specific classrooms, extracurricular activities, cafeteria, hallways, playground) and instructional contexts (e.g., large-group lecture or discussion, small-group activities, independent seat work) during which peer-mediated supports may be particularly beneficial (Huber & Carter, 2016). These observations should focus on existing interaction opportunities within particular school settings, the extent to which and ways in which students with ASD are accessing those opportunities, and potential factors that may influence social participation. At the same time, because peer support interventions also involve peer-delivered academic supports, consideration should be given to the nature of students' educational goals within the general education curriculum.

As they enter adolescence and approach adulthood, students with ASD should become more actively involved in determining their own supports within and beyond the classroom. This includes having a voice in whether and how peer-mediated supports are utilized (Carter, Biggs, et al., 2016; Huber et al., 2018). Although the perspectives of students are infrequently sought, person-centered planning and preference assessments offer avenues for giving students a voice in determining how they receive support and from whom. For students with complex communication challenges or who lack speech, alternative avenues for determining these preferences should be explored. For example, a student might use pictures of his or her classmates to indicate with whom he or she would like to work. Similarly, peers should have say regarding their involvement in these interventions. Although educators can use a wide variety of recruitment approaches (e.g., class or school announcements, personal invitations, staff recommendations), the experience is always voluntary.

THEORETICAL BASIS

A variety of factors can converge to limit the peer interactions, friendships, and sense of belonging students with ASD experience within their schools. Figure 12.1 identifies four especially salient factors: opportunity barriers, support-related barriers, peer-related barriers, and student-related barriers (Carter et al., 2014). Multiple components of peer support arrangements and peer networks can serve to overcome or obviate these barriers. Both types of peer-mediated support interventions have been associated with substantial improvements in social interaction outcomes (e.g., peer interactions, initiations, responses, social engagement) for school-age children and youth with ASD (Brock & Huber, 2017; Huber & Carter, 2019).

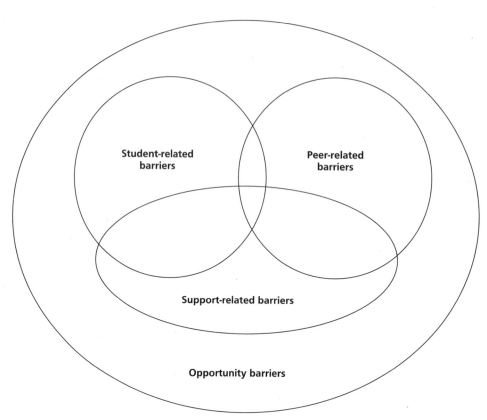

Figure 12.1. Barriers that can impact social opportunities for students with autism spectrum disorder. *Source:* Carter, Bottema-Beutel, & Brock (2014).

Opportunity Barriers

Despite legislative initiatives and school reform efforts challenging schools to promote greater access to the general education curriculum for students with disabilities, most children and youth with ASD spend much of their school day outside the general education classroom and apart from their peers without similar disabilities (Morningstar et al., 2016). Specifically, only 39% of students with autism spend most (i.e., more than 80%) of their school day in general education classes alongside a wide range of schoolmates. Among the remaining students, 18% spend a mix of time in general and special education classes (i.e., between 40% and 80% of their school day), 33% spend most of their day in special education classes (i.e., more than 60%), and 9% are served in other settings altogether (U.S. Department of Education [DOE], 2016). Peer interactions and relationships remain limited when students with and without ASD do not participate in shared activities throughout the school day. In other words, encounters must precede interactions. Peer-mediated support interventions ensure such encounters occur regularly throughout the school year.

Even within inclusive classrooms, students with ASD may be on the periphery of ongoing activities or may be pulled to other locations for individualized instruction (Feldman et al., 2016). For example, an observational study of inclusive high school classrooms found that students with severe disabilities—half of whom had

ASD—were not sitting in proximity to any other classmate during 58% of the class period (Feldman et al., 2016). Instead, students were sitting next to a paraprofessional, working separately with other students with disabilities, or were absent from the classroom (e.g., arriving late, leaving early). Moreover, many teachers draw heavily on instructional arrangements such as lectures or independent seatwork during which interactions among students are discouraged or diminished. **Peer-mediated interventions** establish regular, teacher-sanctioned opportunities for students with and without autism to interact with one another within the context of ongoing, shared activities (Kennedy, 2001).

Support-Related Barriers

One widespread approach for supporting inclusion in classrooms and other school activities is through the **individually assigned paraprofessionals.** Across the country, the number of paraprofessionals now exceeds the number of special education teachers (DOE, 2016). This heavy reliance on adult-delivered supports can negatively impact peer interactions and relationships in multiple ways (Carter et al., 2008; Carter, Asmus, et al., 2016). First, paraprofessionals can inadvertently become substitute social partners or mediators of interactions among students. For example, peer initiations may become directed to staff rather than students, students may ask questions of staff rather than classmates, or the constant presence of an adult inadvertently narrows or closes off a student's social circle. Second, the regular presence of an adult can be stigmatizing. Peers may perceive that their interactions must always be relayed through an adult or assume that their classmates with ASD are not capable of communicating on their own or working with others. Third, paraprofessionals often receive limited training on facilitating social interactions or supporting shared activities within inclusive settings (Carter et al., 2009). As a result, they may directly address the academic and social needs while unintentionally crowding out peers. Peer-mediated support arrangements communicate expectations that students with and without ASD should learn from and interact with one another. Moreover, they provide a supportive context for students to spend time together. Such approaches also more closely reflect the typical avenues through which students participate in classroom activities—alongside their peers and with their support. Finally, these interventions can diminish stigma by reducing the heavy reliance on specialized and adult-delivered supports (Carter, Biggs, & Blustein, 2016; Giangreco et al., 2012).

For students without intellectual impairments who perform at or near grade level academically, the absence of any supplemental support can also be problematic (Huber & Carter, 2019). Such students may still struggle socially yet lack ongoing and planned opportunities to spend time with or learn alongside other students. Peer-mediated support interventions formally connect students with ASD to a consistent cadre of peers within (peer support arrangements) or beyond (peer network interventions) the classroom (Carter et al., 2017).

Peer-Related Barriers

The influence of peers on the social opportunities and outcomes of students with ASD is also critical to consider. The attitudes, beliefs, priorities, and experiences of peers can directly impact the occurrence of interactions and the development of relationships with their schoolmates with ASD (Schaefer et al., 2016). For example, some peers initially might be hesitant to initiate conversations with a student who has extensive support needs, engages in stereotypical or atypical behaviors, or demonstrates aggressive or self-injurious behavior. Other students might be unsure of how to interact with someone who has limited speech, uses an AAC device, or has no reliable form of communication. This reluctance may be amplified if peers have had limited experiences with individuals with disabilities in the past. Although attitudes toward and knowledge about ASD continue to improve over time, peers may still hold inaccurate information or perceptions of people with ASD that diminish their desire to seek out or develop relationships with their classmates (Griffin, 2019; Tonnsen & Hahn, 2015). For example, they may assume that all students with ASD are disinterested in relationships, do not experience or express emotions, or have cognitive impairments.

Peer-mediated support interventions ensure peers are confident and comfortable working and interacting with their classmates and schoolmates with ASD. The information and training peers receive as part of their initial orientation—along with the ongoing support and facilitation provided to them by educators and paraprofessionals—can enable them to feel confident and able to interact with and support their classmates with ASD. For example, recruited peers often receive general information about ASD, individualized information about the students with whom they will be spending time (e.g., interests, backgrounds, strengths, communication preferences, and school activities), guidance on the types of support they should and should not provide, and accurate answers to the questions they consider most pressing. Peers also participate alongside one or more other peers, giving them confidence that they are not alone in their roles or commitments. As peers spend time with their schoolmate with ASD, they serve as models to other students in their class or school. Seeing their peers developing new relationships and providing support to classmates with ASD may entice other students in the class to do the same.

Student-Related Barriers

The difficulties related to verbal and nonverbal communication, social skills, social-emotional reciprocity, and developing and maintaining relationships experienced by children with ASD can affect the quality and quantity of their interactions with peers (Lyons et al., 2016). A small proportion of students have complex communication needs or limited symbolic language that require **augmentative and alternative communication (AAC)** systems (Kearns et al., 2011). Peer-mediated support interventions equip multiple peers without disabilities to prompt, model, and reinforce the social, academic, and other individualized behaviors of their partners with ASD. During initial orientation sessions led by special educators, paraprofessionals, or other school staff, peers are shown how to elicit and encourage specific social and communicative behaviors by their classmates with ASD, deliver verbal or other reinforcement when those behaviors are appropriately demonstrated, and model their effective use when they are not. Arranging for students with and without disabilities to interact with one another within shared activities in and beyond the classroom expands the opportunities students with ASD have to practice critical social behaviors, receive **natural support,** obtain feedback from peers, and connect with new communities of reinforcement. Moreover, the close and continuous proximity of peers expands the number of conversational initiations directed to students with ASD and simultaneously increases the likelihood that students' communication attempts will be reinforced. In other words, these interventions create structured contexts within which the social and communication efforts of students with ASD are encouraged, facilitated, and supported by peers. In addition, the involvement of multiple peers within most of these intervention approaches may promote generalized social outcomes by embedding multiple exemplars of prosocial behavior (Stokes & Baer, 1977). Rather than addressing skill-related difficulties as a prerequisite to peer interaction, social and communication skills are instead taught within the context of ongoing peer interaction.

Increases in interactions among students with ASD and their peers without disabilities may also be attributed to observational learning. Social learning theory (Bandura, 1977) posits that people learn through the process of observing behaviors exhibited by others in their environment and witnessing the outcomes—both positive and negative—of those behaviors. Within peer-mediated support interventions, participating peers serve as both explicit and incidental models of age-appropriate social, communication, academic, and other related skills for their partners with ASD. Through participation in shared activities, students with ASD encounter increased opportunities to observe their peers interacting effectively with other classmates and to observe the positive consequences of those behaviors within the context of social interactions. When students with ASD are enrolled in inclusive classrooms and other school activities, these peer models may already be present. However, peer support arrangements and peer networks increase the proximity and number of peer models accessible to students with ASD as well as the appropriateness and salience of those models. For example, educators often identify **peer partners** who are competent communicators, possess age- and context-appropriate interpersonal skills, and have high social status (e.g., Garrison-Harrell et al., 1997; Jackson & Campbell, 2009).

EMPIRICAL BASIS

A total of 27 studies have included students with ASD in their evaluations of school-based peer support arrangements and peer network interventions. A study by Asmus and colleagues (2016) evaluated both. Most of these studies have been published in the last decade, reflecting the field's growing interest in enhancing social outcomes within inclusive school settings. This section first reviews the two intervention approaches separately before providing a summary of key methodological features across all of the studies.

Peer Support Arrangements

Broadly defined, these semester-long interventions involve arranging for students without disabilities to provide ongoing social and academic support to their same-age classmates with disabilities while receiving initial training and ongoing guidance from paraprofessionals or special educators in general education classrooms (Carter et al., 2009; Carter et al., 2015). These approaches are highly individualized according to the needs of participating students and the inclusive classrooms in which they are enrolled. Ten experimental studies involving 39 students with ASD have been published to date. Most participating students were reported to have a moderate to severe intellectual disability and required additional support to meaningfully access the general education curriculum. Moreover, most received individually assigned paraprofessional support within these classrooms. As a result, the study samples all include a mix of students with and without ASD. It is important to note that this literature addresses only older students enrolled in middle and high school. Table 12.1 summarizes selected features of these studies, and Table 12.2 summarizes the evidence in support of these studies.

Table 12.1. Summary of 10 studies examining peer support arrangements

Study	Students with ASD / Sex, race/ethnicity	School level(s) / School setting(s)	Primary questions / Design	Primary social-related outcomes for students with ASD
Asmus et al. (2016)	2 of 3 students / 1F, 1M / 2W	High school / Art, ceramics, social studies	What are the effects of the IV relative to adult support models? How socially valid is the IV? / Pilot randomized controlled trial	Increases in peer interaction (particularly responses) across both peer partners and other classmates (2/2), as well as increases in both social contacts and reported friendships (2/2)
Brock et al. (2016)	3 of 4 students / 1F, 2M / 1B, 2W	Middle school / Art, computer science	Can a teacher-delivered training package improve paraprofessional implementation of the IV? What are the effects of the IV relative to adult support models? How socially valid is the IV? / Multiple-baseline across participants	Increases in peer interactions during the IV (3/3)
Brock & Carter (2016)	1 of 4 students / 1F / 1B	Middle school / Math, science	Can a teacher-delivered training package improve paraprofessional implementation of the intervention? What are the effects of the IV relative to adult support models? How socially valid is the IV? / Multiple-baseline across participants	Increases in peer interactions during the IV (1/1)
Carter et al. (2005)	2 of 3 students / 1F, 1M / 2W	Middle/high school / English, science	How does the number of peer partners (one vs. two) impact student outcomes? / ABAB, BABA	More frequent social interactions with peer partners when working with two peers (2/2); no differences in overall quality of interaction or interaction frequency with other classmates (2/2)
Carter, Asmus, et al. (2016)	22 of 51 students / 22NR / 22NR	High school / Art, band, computer technology, culinary arts, dance, digital arts, language arts, math, music, science, social studies, theater, wellness	What are the effects of the IV relative to adult support models? What supports do peer partners provide? How socially valid is the IV? / Randomized controlled trial	IV associated with significantly more peer interactions ($d = 0.42$), more contributions to interactions ($d = 0.34$), greater number of peers contacted ($d = 0.50$), greater social goal attainment ($d = 0.79$), and greater friendship gains ($d = 1.02$); no differences in social skill ratings ($d = 0.17$)

Study	Participants	Setting/Subjects	Research question & design	Findings
Carter et al. (2017)	4 of 4 students 4M 1B, 3W	High school *Business, math, physical education, science*	What are the effects of the IV without adult facilitation? How socially valid is the IV? *Nonconcurrent multiple-baseline across participants*	Increases in peer interactions during the IV (4/4), primarily with peer partners; modest increases in social initiations (2/4)
Huber et al. (2018)	2 of 3 students 2M 2W	High school *Art, nutrition, world history*	What are the effects of the IV relative to adult support models? Can structural analyses be used to refine and improve the IV? How socially valid is the IV? *Multiple-baseline across participants*	Increases in social initiations and responses that more closely approximated normative rates (3/3); further improvements in social responses after refining the IV (1/1)
Schaefer et al. (2018)	1 of 3 students 1M 1W	Middle school *Science, social studies*	What are the effects of the IV relative to adult support models? How is instructional format associated with outcomes? To what extent do interactions generalize to other settings? *Multiple-baseline across participants*	More frequent social interactions with trained and untrained peers (1/1) during both independent work and group activities
Shukla et al. 1998	1 of 3 students 1F 1W	Middle school *English, math, piano*	How does adult involvement influence the peer partner outcomes? How are students impacted by involvement in the IV? *ABACABAC, ACABACAB*	More frequent social interactions with peer partners during the IV (1/1); more social interactions with untrained peers in (C) (1/1)
Shukla et al. (1999)	1 of 3 students 1F 1W	Middle school *Art, social studies, math, industrial arts*	What are the effects of the IV relative to adult support models? *ABAB, ABABAB, BABAB*	More frequent and increased duration of social interactions with peer partners and untrained peers as well as more frequent social support behaviors (1/1) during IV

Key: X of X students refers to number of all study intervention recipients who had autism spectrum disorder (ASD). F, female; M, male; NR, not reported; B, black/African American; W, white; IV, peer support intervention.

Table 12.2. Studies supportive of peer support arrangements and peer network interventions

Design strength	Description of design level	Peer support arrangements			Peer network interventions		
		Studies with strong evidence	Studies with adequate evidence	Studies with weak evidence	Studies with strong evidence	Studies with adequate evidence	Studies with weak evidence
Ib	Randomized controlled trial	Carter et al. (2016)	—	Asmus et al. (2016)	—	Asmus et al. (2017); Kamps et al. (2015)	Asmus et al. (2016); Kasari et al. (2016)
IIa	Controlled study without randomization	—	—	—	—	—	—
IIb	Quasi-experimental study	—	—	—	—	—	—
III	Single-participant experimental designs	Brock et al. (2016); Brock & Carter (2016); Huber et al. (2018); Schaefer et al. (2018)	Carter et al. (2005); Carter et al. (2017); Shukla et al. (1998); Shukla et al. (1999)	—	Bambara et al. (2016); Bambara et al. (2018); Biggs et al. (2018); Hochman et al. (2015); Kamps et al. (2014); Mason et al. (2014); Sreckovic et al. (2017)	Gardner et al. (2014); Garrison-Harrell et al. (1997); Haring et al. (1992); Kamps et al. (1997); R. L. Koegel et al. (2012); L. K. Koegel et al. (2012); R. L. Koegel et al. (2013)	—

Note: Interventions categorized by overall strength of the design (Levels Ia–IV; Philips et al., 2001) as well as quality of evidence for group and single-participant experimental designs (Reichow et al., 2008).

In most of these studies, a primary focus has been on comparing peer support arrangements to a baseline condition in which students receive support primarily from an individually assigned adult. Shukla and colleagues (1998, 1999) used single-case withdrawal designs to compare the effects of individually assigned adult support versus adult support that was augmented by peer support on the social interactions of students with severe disabilities who were enrolled in a variety of inclusive middle school classes. During baseline conditions, paraprofessionals or special educators provided one-to-one support (e.g., systematic instruction, adapting activities, implementing behavior supports) while seated directly next to the focus students. Peer support arrangements were systematically introduced and withdrawn for participating students throughout the semester. The social interactions of students with ASD in these classrooms were both longer and more frequent when they received support from peers rather than exclusively from adults. Moreover, students received a greater variety of social support behaviors (i.e., greetings, information, access to others, material aid, emotional support, companionship) when working with their classmates.

Similarly, Schaefer and colleagues (2018) used a multiple-baseline across participants design to examine the effects of peer support arrangements for middle school students with severe disabilities enrolled in core academic classes. Students rarely interacted with peers when supported exclusively by adults during the baseline condition. The shift in support approaches produced immediate and substantial increases in social interactions with peers during the class. These social outcomes were accompanied by increases in academic engagement. However, most interactions took place with participating peer partners rather than with other classmates. Moreover, interactions in the classroom did not generalize to lunch or recess. In contrast, Carter and colleagues (2017) implemented peer support arrangements with high school students with ASD who did not have a significant intellectual disability. Using a nonconcurrent multiple-baseline across participants design, the researchers established peer support arrangements comprising one to six peer partners for each of the students. Clear increases in interactions with peers were evident in the class without negatively impacting the academic engagement of participating students.

Only two studies have adopted group designs to evaluate this intervention approach. Carter, Asmus, and colleagues (2016) examined the efficacy of peer support arrangements for 51 high school students with severe disabilities (20 of whom had ASD) in a variety of academic and elective general education classrooms. Paraprofessionals or special educators selected, trained, and supported 106 peers to provide individualized academic and social assistance to the 51 students with severe disabilities throughout one semester. Effect sizes (ES), Cohen's d using unstandardized regression coefficients, were calculated. Relative to a comparison group of 48 students (22 of whom had ASD) who received support only from adults, students receiving support from peers experienced increased social interactions (ES = 0.42), increased academic engagement (ES = 0.50), more progress on individualized social goals (ES = 0.79), greater social participation in the classroom (ES = 0.42), and an increase in the number of new friendships reported by teachers (ES = 1.02). Moreover, a modest proportion of peer relationships lasted one (43%) and two (40%) semesters later after the intervention had concluded. Asmus and colleagues (2016) conducted a pilot study as a prelude to this larger study. Although there were similar findings, the study was not adequately powered.

Two of the studies examined the extent to which teachers (rather than researchers) could equip paraprofessionals to implement peer support arrangements in inclusive classrooms. Brock and Carter (2016) used a multiple-baseline across participants design to examine whether teacher-delivered professional development could enable paraprofessionals to implement peer support arrangements with adequate fidelity and whether their implementation of peer support arrangements would improve outcomes for middle school students with severe disabilities. Paraprofessionals successfully implemented the intervention with fidelity, and three of the four students substantially increased their peer interactions while maintaining their levels of academic engagement. Likewise, Brock and colleagues (2016) used a multiple-baseline design to investigate a model in which the teacher delivered training to paraprofessionals on intervention fidelity and target student outcomes. All four paraprofessionals were able to implement peer support arrangements in ways that substantially increased the extent to which students with disabilities received support from and had interactions with their peers. Moreover, three of four students with disabilities experienced growth on their individualized goals within the classroom. Findings from both studies are important in their demonstration that these interventions can be implemented by local educators in public schools without extensive external support.

Finally, some research suggests that varied intervention configurations may differentially affect the outcomes experienced by participating students. Shukla and colleagues (1998) examined the impact of the adult supervision component of the intervention on the active engagement of peer partners. Specifically, they compared the academic engagement of peers when they 1) received adult assistance while being a peer partner, 2) received adult assistance while working independently, and 3) received no adult assistance while working independently. Carter and colleagues (2005) used a single-case withdrawal design to examine the effects of varying the number of peers involved in these intervention approaches. Substantially higher levels of social interaction among students with and without disabilities were evident when two versus one peer supported middle and high school students with disabilities within inclusive core academic classrooms (e.g., English, science). Across the two- versus one-peer conditions, differences were not evident in the quality of students' interactions nor in the percentage of intervals during which students interacted with other classmates not directly involved in the intervention. Huber and colleagues (2018) explored the addition of structural analysis as a data-based approach for further refining peer support arrangements in order to enhance their impact within high school classrooms. Specifically, they systematically examined how different contextual factors (e.g., whole- versus small-group activities, instructional versus noninstructional tasks) influenced student outcomes before incorporating those factors into the intervention. The initial introduction of the intervention produced substantial increases in social initiations and responses for all three students with severe disabilities, and subjective ratings of interaction quality tended to be higher. At the same time, academic engagement maintained or improved modestly for all participants. Structural analyses were used to refine aspects of each intervention (e.g., number of peer partners, choice of tasks) and led to increased social initiations for one student.

Peer Network Interventions

Peer network interventions involve establishing a cohesive social group (e.g., two to six peers) that meets regularly with a student with a disability around shared activities during noninstructional times of day (e.g., lunch, recess, free periods, before or after school) and with facilitation by school staff (Carter et al., 2013). These semester-long interventions also are highly individualized with regard to the selection of peers, activities, locations, and adult roles. To date, 18 experimental studies involving 208 students with ASD have been published. All but four of these studies used single-case methodology. Unlike peer support arrangements, this literature includes a more heterogenous group of participants with ASD, including those with a wide range of intellectual abilities. Moreover, these studies span elementary, middle, and high school levels. Table 12.3 summarizes selected study features, and Table 12.2 summarizes the support for these studies.

Seven of these studies were implemented in elementary schools. A series of experimental studies by Kamps and colleagues (1997) highlights the impact peer network interventions can have on social interactions outcomes for younger students. The researchers used a multiple-probe across activities design to evaluate the efficacy of peer network interventions across up to six settings. In addition to training peers without disabilities and scheduling regular interactive activities, adults provided verbal feedback and visual reinforcement to peers at the end of each activity. Students with ASD demonstrated substantial increases in their duration of peer interaction across all settings, with some generalization to untreated settings noted for two students. Garrison-Harrell and colleagues (1997) examined the effects of peer networks embedded within a multicomponent intervention package for three elementary students with ASD who had severe disabilities. Participating peers received training in the use of AAC systems and relevant social skills (e.g., initiating, responding, turn taking, sharing), and students with ASD received training on the use of the communication system. Interaction opportunities among students with disabilities and their network members were arranged across at least three different school activities (e.g., reading, language arts, lunch, computers, recess, library). Introduction of the peer network intervention within a multiple-baseline design was associated with substantial increases in the frequency and duration of social interactions, functional verbal behavior, and augmentative communication system use. Kamps and colleagues (2014) used a multiple-baseline across participants design to evaluate peer network interventions implemented three times per week. All of the students had ASD, and none had an intellectual disability. The intervention incorporated direct instruction of social skills (e.g., sharing, requesting, commenting, play organizers), scripted practice involving the student and peers, visual cues, and free play—all within the context of a fun game and preferred items (e.g., games, puzzles, books). This was followed by a short time of feedback. Although up to six peers comprised each network, only two participated with the student on any given day. The intervention package produced substantial increases in total communication acts for all four students and increased initiations for three students. Mason and colleagues (2014) used a multiple-baseline across participants design to evaluate the impact of a peer network intervention—each involving two peers—delivered during recess to students with ASD who did not have an intellectual disability. The intervention began with brief instruction on a targeted social skill, followed by a period of group play during which a teacher provided occasional prompting and behavior

Table 12.3. Summary of 18 studies examining peer network interventions

Study	Students with ASD Sex Race/ethnicity	School level(s) School setting(s)	Primary questions Design	Primary social-related outcomes for students with ASD
Asmus et al. (2016)	2 of 3 students 2M 1B, 1W	High school NR	What are the effects of the IV? How socially valid is the IV? Pilot randomized trial	Increases in both social contacts and reported friendships with peers without disabilities (2/2)
Asmus et al. (2017)	24 of 47 students 24NR 24NR	High school Cafeteria, conference room, staff office, gym, school coffee shop, other	What are the effects of the IV? Do the effects generalize across locations and time? How socially valid is the IV? Randomized controlled trial	IV associated with significant increases in teacher-reported social contact gains ($d = 1.39$) and friendship gains ($d = 1.39$); gains maintained one semester later; no differences in social skill ratings ($d = -0.13$)
Bambara et al. (2016)	3 of 3 students 1F, 2M 3H	High school Cafeteria	What are the effects of introducing facilitative strategies into a peer network? Is there a collateral effect on commenting? How socially valid is the IV? Multiple-baseline across participants	Increases in conversational acts (3/3); initiations and follow-up questions increased when related strategies were introduced (3/3)
Bambara et al. (2018)	4 of 4 students 1F, 3M 1B, 2H, 1W	High school Cafeteria	What are the effects of introducing facilitative strategies into a peer network? Is there a collateral effect on assertive acts? Do the effects generalize to other peers? How socially valid is the IV? Nonconcurrent multiple-baseline across participants	Increases in conversational initiations (4/4); follow-up questions increased when related strategies were introduced (4/4); some indication of generalization of initiations
Biggs et al. (2018)	3 of 4 students 2F, 1M 2H, 1W	Elementary school Classroom, school lobby near cafeteria	What is the effect of the IV for students who use AAC? What is the added effect of embedding peer-implemented AAC modeling? How socially valid is the IV? Multiple-probe across participants with two IV phases	Peer networks produced increases in peer interaction (4/4) but not symbolic communication (1/4); the addition of peer modeling increased symbolic communication (3/4)

	Participants	Setting	Research question/design	Outcomes
Gardner et al. (2014)	2 of 2 students 2M 1H, 1W	High school *Advisory periods*	What are the effects of the IV? Which IV components were most challenging for facilitators to implement? How socially valid is the IV? *ABAB and ABA within multiple-baseline*	Increases in social engagement (2/2) as well as interactions to and from peers (2/2)
Garrison-Harrell et al. (1997)	3 of 3 students 1F, 2M 3NR	Elementary school *Classrooms, cafeteria, library, recess*	What are the effects of an IV incorporating AAC? Do the effects generalize across settings, activities, and peers? *Multiple-probe across settings, nested within multiple-baseline across participants*	Increased frequency and duration of peer interactions (3/3); increased total duration of using AAC during interactions (2/3)
Haring & Breen (1992)	1 of 2 students 1M 1NR	Middle school *Cafeteria, hallways, school field, special education classroom*	What are the effects of the IV? How socially valid is the IV? *Multiple-baseline across participants*	Increased number of social interactions with network peers (1/1); increased appropriate responding (1/1)
Hochman et al. (2015)	4 of 4 students 4M 2B, 1H, 1W	High school *Cafeteria*	What are the effects of the IV? Do the effects generalize across times? How socially valid is the IV? *Multiple-baseline across participants*	Increases in social interactions and social engagement with peers (4/4), with limited generalization (1/4); improvements on social-related goals (4/4)
Kamps et al. (1997)	3 of 3 students 3M 3NR	Elementary school *Cafeteria, classrooms, recess*	What are the effects of the IV? Do the effects generalize across settings? *Multiple-probe across activities*	Increased total duration of social interactions with peers (3/3)
Kamps et al. (2014)	4 of 4 students 4M 4W	Elementary school *Resource room, speech therapy room*	What are the effects of the IV that incorporates scripted lessons and visual cues? How socially valid is the IV? *Multiple-baseline across participants*	Increases in total communication acts (4/4) and social initiations (3/4)
Kamps et al. (2015)	56 of 56 students 7F, 49M 4A, 4B, 2H, 46W	Elementary school *Empty classrooms, hallways, speech therapy room*	What are the effects of the IV? Do the effects generalize across settings? Are there differences based on length of intervention? How socially valid is the IV? *Randomized controlled trial*	IV associated with significantly greater growth differences in initiations to peer (including in generalization probes) but not responses or total communication

(continued)

Table 12.3. *(continued)*

Study	Students with ASD Sex Race/ethnicity	School level(s) School setting(s)	Primary questions Design	Primary social-related outcomes for students with ASD
Kasari et al. (2016)	80 of 80 students 19F, 61M 14A, 4B, 12H, 39W, 5O, 6NR	Elementary school *Recess*	How do the effects of the IV compare to those of a social skills intervention? *Randomized controlled trial*	No significant differences in social network salience by groups, though a moderated effect of teacher–child relationship was found. Playground engagement was significantly lower for IV group.
R. L. Koegel et al. (2012)	3 of 3 students 3M 3NR	Middle/high school *Classroom or courtyard*	What are the effects of the IV designed around the perseverative interests of students? *Multiple-baseline across participants with reversals for one student*	Increases in social engagement with peers (3/3) and initiations (3/3)
L. K. Koegel et al. (2012)	3 of 3 students 1F, 2M 3NR	Elementary school *Libraries, cafeteria, sports fields, summer day camp program*	What are the effects of the IV designed around the perseverative interests of students? *Nonconcurrent multiple-baseline across participants with reversal for one student*	Increases in social engagement with peers (3/3) and unprompted verbal initiations to peers (3/3)
R. L. Koegel et al. (2013)	7 of 7 students 1F, 6M 4H, 2M, 1W	High school *Classrooms during lunch, school lawn, basketball court*	What are the effects of the IV? Do the effects generalize across time and contexts? How socially valid is the IV? *Multiple-baseline across participants*	Increases in social engagement with peers (7/7) and rate of initiations (7/7); generalization was mixed
Mason et al. (2014)	3 of 3 students 3M 3NR	Elementary school *Playground*	What are the effects of the IV? *Multiple-baseline across participants*	Increases in total communication acts (3/3)
Sreckovic et al. (2017)	3 of 3 students 3M 1M, 2W	High school *Cafeteria or outside, conference room, empty classroom*	What are the effects of the IV? Do students perceive changes in bullying victimization? Do the effects generalize across time and contexts? How socially valid is the IV? *Multiple-baseline across participants*	Increases in total social interactions (3/3), as well as initiations and responses (3/3); generalization was mixed

Key: X of X students refers to number of all study intervention recipients who had autism spectrum disorder (ASD); F, female; M, male; NR, not reported; A, Asian; B, black/African American; H, Hispanic; M, multiracial; O, other; W, white; AAC, augmentative and alternative communication; IV, peer network intervention.

specific praise. All students immediately and substantially increased the number of verbal communicative acts they directed to their peers on the playground. Finally, Kamps and colleagues (2015) conducted a randomized, controlled trial to evaluate a comprehensive peer network intervention that combined both peer training, direct instruction in social skills (e.g., requests and shares, comments, niceties, play organizers), and reinforcement and feedback from teacher facilitators. The intervention took place three times per week over 6 months. Early elementary students with ASD (without severe intellectual disability) who received the intervention showed significantly more growth in initiations to peers in natural settings than did a closely balanced comparison group of students for whom peer networks were not established. No differences in responses or total communication frequency were found.

Two other elementary studies compared peer networks with a second intervention approaches. Biggs and colleagues (2018) used a multiple-probe across participants design to evaluate a paraprofessional-facilitated peer network intervention with elementary students who were learning to use aided AAC (i.e., speech-generating device, communication book) and had severe disabilities. The network involved an initial orientation for students and peers, followed by twice-weekly meetings around a variety of shared activities with occasional adult facilitation. Although the intervention substantially increased students' overall interactions with peers, no changes in symbolic communication were observed. A second intervention phase was introduced in which peers received instruction and coaching to implement aided AAC modeling within the peer network. This additional component increased most students' use of symbolic communication within interactions with peers. Kasari and colleagues (2016) compared a didactic social skill instruction intervention (i.e., SKILLS) with a peer network intervention (i.e., ENGAGE) for elementary students with ASD who did not have an intellectual disability. Eighty students received the ENGAGE intervention, and 57 received the SKILLS intervention. Two to three peers joined each network and, with support from an adult facilitator, the shared interests of the group were used to identify activities. Although modest improvements in social network salience (i.e., social prominence within one's classrooms) were found for both interventions, no differences were found between groups. The social skill instruction intervention produced greater gains in joint engagement on the playground than did the peer network intervention.

Eleven of these 18 studies were implemented in secondary schools. In the earliest of these studies, Haring and Breen (1992) used a multiple-baseline design to examine the efficacy of peer networks for two students with severe disabilities, one of whom had both ASD and repetitive and noncompliant behaviors. The network consisted of four to five peers without disabilities, weekly 30-minute planning meetings with adult facilitation and feedback, intentional scheduling of interactions during noninstructional times (e.g., hallways, cafeteria, before and after school), teacher-delivered social skills training, and peer-delivered reinforcement of the students' social behavior. The introduction of the peer network intervention was associated with substantial increases in the frequency of social interactions, appropriate responding, and contact with peers.

Sreckovic and colleagues (2017) focused their intervention evaluation on three high school students with ASD who did not have an intellectual disability. The peer networks involved three to six peers, met twice weekly in quiet rooms on campus over 5 weeks, and focused on games selected on the basis of student preferences. Immediate increases in social interactions—both initiations and responses—were observed after the initial orientation. Evidence of both maintenance and generalization to other settings was apparent. Moreover, some decreases in bullying victimization were reported for two students. A pair of studies by Bambara and colleagues (2016, 2018) also focused on peer networks implemented during lunchtime. In this intervention variation, peers were taught by researchers to implement three strategies during regular network meetings: 1) support conversational interactions, 2) promote initiations, and 3) encourage follow-up questions made by high school students with ASD, most of whom did not have an intellectual disability. Students with ASD were also taught to use written text cue cards to initiate conversation and to ask follow-up questions. Bambara and colleagues (2018) used nonconcurrent multiple-baseline participants, whereas Bambara's earlier group of colleagues (2016) used a multiple-baseline design across participants. Both studies documented increases in conversational acts and specific interactive behaviors related to the training. Assertive acts also increased for most students, and some generalization was noted in the later study.

A series of studies by Carter and colleagues did not incorporate an explicit social skills instruction component in the peer network intervention. Gardner and colleagues (2014) used withdrawal designs embedded within a multiple-baseline design to evaluate peer networks for two high school students with severe disabilities. The incorporation of the withdrawal component enhanced the ability to draw causal interpretations. The networks each involved three peers, took place during an advisory period (i.e., a period in which teachers meet with students for the purpose of advising them about academics or future planning), and involved joint activities or conversations (e.g., card games, trivia, discussing current or school events). The intervention produced increased levels of peer interaction and social-related goal attainment. Hochman and colleagues (2015) used a multiple-baseline across participants design to evaluate the impact of lunchtime peer network interventions on four high school students with both ASD and an intellectual disability. During baseline, interactions remained rare in the midst of a cafeteria filled with peers. Upon introduction of the networks—which met weekly and involved shared activities—substantial and sustained increases in peer interactions and social engagement occurred. However, interactions did not generalize to peers not involved in the network. Asmus and colleagues (2017) used a randomized, controlled trial to examine the efficacy of peer network interventions for 47 high school students with severe disabilities. The groups—each comprising three to six peers—met weekly or biweekly throughout the semester and received ongoing facilitation from a school staff member (e.g., coach, paraprofessional, special educator). Compared to a business-as-usual control group ($n = 48$ students), students receiving peer networks gained significantly more new social contacts and friendships. Although many peer relationships were maintained one and two semesters later, limited spillover was found beyond the school day. Asmus and colleagues (2016) conducted a small-scale pilot study that preceded this study. As noted in the previous section, although similar findings were obtained, the study was not powered to support causal claims.

Finally, a trio of studies (R. L. Koegel et al., 2012; L. K. Koegel et al., 2012; R. L. Koegel et al., 2013) incorporated the perseverative or preferred interests of middle and high school students with ASD into the design of the peer network. Each of the participating students—none of whom had an intellectual disability—was interviewed to determine their preferred interests in an effort to integrate those interests into new or existing club activities during lunchtime. The clubs included a wide range of other peers and were facilitated by an adult. As with the prior set of studies, formal social skills instruction was not part of the intervention. Using multiple-baseline across participant designs, all three studies demonstrated substantial increases in social engagement and initiations with peers. Generalization to other activities was demonstrated in R. L. Koegel and colleagues (2013).

Limitations on the Existing Literature

The existing literature has several limitations related to the types of experimental designs, the narrow range of social outcomes, consideration of implementation fidelity, and limited attention to generalization and maintenance.

Experimental Designs   Given the low incidence of autism and intellectual disability, as well as the heterogeneity among students served under these special education categories, it is not surprising that the majority of studies (81%) utilized single-case research designs to examine efficacy. Among these, 19 studies employed variants of the multiple-baseline design and four employed variants of withdrawal and/or reversal designs (one study incorporated both designs). Because many studies included heterogeneous samples comprised of both students with and without ASD, nine of the single-case studies included fewer than three replications of intervention effects for participants with ASD, and one group design study (Carter, Asmus, et al., 2016) did not disaggregate results for students with and without ASD. The literature also includes relatively few comparative studies examining which of these intervention approaches is most effective and few parametric and/or component analyses examining how intervention variations influence outcomes. As a result, limited guidance is available to inform which intervention approach is likely to prove most effective for particular outcomes and students.

Social-Related Intervention Outcomes   Discrete measures of peer interaction (e.g., overall interactions, initiations, responses) represented the primary intervention outcomes in these studies. Qualitative aspects of conversational exchange—such as affect, conversational topics, appropriateness, interaction quality, and social support behaviors—were explored less frequently and often only descriptively (e.g., Carter et al., 2005; Gardner et al., 2014; Huber et al., 2018; Shukla et al., 1999). Likewise, only a few studies addressed the extent to which new friendships developed (Asmus et al., 2016, 2017; Carter, Asmus, et al., 2016). Future studies need to examine the collateral effects of these interventions on students' language and communication skill acquisition, social status, or stereotypical and challenging behaviors.

Intervention Fidelity   Most studies (74%) indicated that intervention fidelity data were collected. Exceptions were older studies conducted before reporting of procedural fidelity was emphasized (Garrison-Harrell et al., 1997; Haring & Breen, 1992; Shukla et al., 1998, 1999) or were part of a series of more recent peer network studies (R. L. Koegel et al., 2012; L. K. Koegel et al., 2012; R. L. Koegel et al., 2013). When fidelity data were reported, high levels of treatment integrity were documented. This is noteworthy, as many of the more recent interventions were implemented by school staff. However, it is important to emphasize that most of these interventions were individually tailored in some way to address the unique needs of participating students with ASD and the settings in which they were delivered. In other words, most interventions appear to have both essential and flexible components, though the distinctions between the two were rarely addressed in the studies (e.g., Carter, Asmus, et al., 2016).

Generalization and Maintenance   The extent to which intervention effects were maintained over time was assessed in only seven studies (26%). Within these studies, intervention effects generally were maintained at or above intervention levels for up to 2 months postintervention, supporting the short-term impact of these interventions. Among those looking at longer-term impact were studies by Asmus and colleagues (2017) and Carter, Asmus, and colleagues (2016) that tracked social connections up to 1 year later. The degree to which improvements in social outcomes generalized to additional settings or peers other than those represented in the intervention condition was assessed in only 11 studies (41%). Additional efforts to promote generalization (e.g., using multiple exemplars, programming common stimuli across settings and peers) may be essential to ensuring more widespread outcomes.

Social Validity

Considerable attention has focused on assessing the social validity of these interventions. Nineteen studies (70%) incorporated some measure of acceptability or feasibility from the vantage point of implementers, teachers, or participating students and peers. When some indicator of social validity was offered, the goals of these interventions were considered important and the social outcomes considered desirable. When asked, most facilitators affirmed the feasibility of the intervention procedures. These findings echo descriptive studies indicating that general educators, special educators, paraprofessionals, and other school staff consider peer-mediated support interventions to be effective at increasing interaction among students with and without disabilities and fairly feasible to implement given resources available to educators (Carter, Dykstra Steinbrenner, & Hall, 2019; Carter & Pesko, 2008). Similarly, children and youth without disabilities who serve as peer partners affirm their willingness to participate and attribute considerable benefits to their involvement (e.g., Copeland et al., 2004; Schaefer et al., 2016).

PRACTICAL REQUIREMENTS

Researchers studying the adoption of educational interventions have cautioned that even effective practices are unlikely to be adopted and implemented with fidelity if they do not align with everyday instructional practices or are simply too difficult to implement (Boardman et al., 2005; Carter, Dykstra Steinbrenner, & Hall, 2019). Fortunately, research addressing the implementation of peer-mediated support interventions with students with ASD suggests that educators value peer-mediated strategies and consider them feasible. Several practical requirements typically are associated with implementing peer support arrangements and peer network interventions (Biggs & Carter, 2017).

Special Educators

Although peers without disabilities play a direct role in providing support to their schoolmates with ASD, special education staff remains actively involved in selecting, initiating, monitoring, and supervising peer-mediated support interventions.

Special educators have primarily assumed responsibility for planning and implementing these interventions, particularly for students with more extensive support needs. In part, this is because many students with severe disabilities have traditionally received one-to-one support from individually assigned adults within inclusive classrooms, extracurricular activities, and other school activities. Moreover, these are the school staff typically most familiar with students' individualized educational goals, support needs, and instructional history. Special educators typically lead orientation and training activities (see the Key Components section) for peers without disabilities involved in these interventions, particularly when this training requires meeting with students outside of class. For example, a teacher might hold orientation sessions with students without disabilities involved in a peer network or peer support arrangement during a couple of lunch periods, before or after school, during recess, or during a free period. The time required to carry out this initial training depends on the nature of the support peers will be asked to provide, the number of peers involved, the characteristics of the students who will be receiving support, and the school settings in which they will require support. For both kinds of interventions described in this chapter, only one or two initial meetings (about 20–45 minutes long) with peers are likely to be required. In addition, some peers will benefit from one or more follow-up meetings during which they can discuss their experiences, share any concerns, and address any challenges.

Paraprofessionals

Paraprofessionals also have a role in implementing these interventions for some students. Many schools rely extensively on individually assigned paraprofessionals to support the general education participation and extracurricular involvement of students with ASD and other disabilities (Giangreco et al., 2012). As a result, they may be involved in facilitating peer support arrangements in inclusive classrooms. As peers begin working alongside their classmates with ASD, one-to-one paraprofessionals gradually fade their direct support and assume a more flexible role in which they provide ongoing feedback and assistance to all of the students involved in these interventions. For example, paraprofessionals may model the use of appropriate support strategies as students work together, facilitate peer interactions and collaborative work, collect data on student outcomes, and/or troubleshoot any challenges that arise. Given their regular presence in the classroom, it can be helpful to involve paraprofessionals in the initial orientation and training of peers. Paraprofessionals also must maintain regular communication with general educators, special educators, club sponsors, or providers of related services. Paraprofessionals report that they appreciate the clarity these interventions bring to their roles, the guidance they receive from fellow school staff, and the opportunity to work with additional students.

General Educators

Within inclusive classrooms, general educators often assume an active—albeit typically less direct—role in establishing and supporting peer-mediated support interventions. General educators usually assume primary responsibility for determining the curricular content and instructional approaches that characterize a classroom; they often are most familiar with the academic standards and learning objectives that students must meet. Thus, it is essential that they discuss their expectations and recommendations for peer support arrangements with the special educators and paraprofessionals who support students with ASD in their classroom. General educators also assist with identifying students without disabilities who might serve effectively in providing support to their classmates with disabilities. Beyond the classroom, general educators may be invited to facilitate peer networks that take place during noninstructional times. Their connections to a wide range of peers can help them identify network members who share interests and experiences with participating students with ASD.

Related Services Providers

Related services providers can also support the design and implementation of peer-mediated support interventions. For example, speech-language pathologists can help identify specific social and communication skills needed within peer interactions and suggest strategies for encouraging their development. Behavior analysts can suggest strategies for addressing challenging and stereotypical behaviors that can hinder interactions with peers or participation in inclusive activities. Occupational therapists can suggest technologies, adaptations, and other approaches that enable students with and without ASD to participate in shared activities within and beyond the classroom. Such an interdisciplinary focus expands the expertise and creativity that can be drawn upon in the design and delivery of peer-mediated support interventions.

Team-Based Planning

Collaborative teaming is critical to the success of **inclusive education.** Supporting meaningful participation for students with ASD typically requires special educators, general educators, paraprofessionals, and related service providers to work collaboratively to identify and address a student's social and educational goals. Peer-mediated support interventions are certainly no exception, particularly when intervention approaches span multiple contexts within a school (i.e., peer network interventions) or take place beyond the special education classroom (i.e., peer support arrangements). Several individualized planning models can be used by educational teams to outline the specific peer-mediated and adult-delivered supports students with ASD will need to participate in various school contexts, including the Instructional Activities Assessment (Cushing et al., 2005), Unified Plans of Support (Hunt et al., 2003), Peer Support and Communication Opportunity Plans (Biggs et al., 2017), Student Support Plans (Kuntz, 2019), and the Beyond Access Model (Sonnenmeier et al., 2005).

Training

Early evaluations of peer-mediated support interventions occur within the context of close collaborations among researchers and educators. The involvement of non–school staff in the design and delivery of these intervention is more intensive and leaves open the question of whether similar outcomes could be obtained in the absence of research involvement. For example, university staff may have developed the intervention plan, trained the peers, and facilitated student interactions. More recent studies, however, have examined implementation and outcomes when peer network interventions and peer support arrangements are carried out by local school staff with limited external support. Such studies have shown that educators and paraprofessionals can learn to implement the interventions with fidelity in ways that lead to improved outcomes for students. To enable widespread implementation, staff from within the school community must be equipped to design and deliver these interventions. Studies suggest they can learn to do so with just 2.5 to 4.5 hours of professional development (e.g., Asmus et al., 2016; Brock et al., 2016; Brock & Carter, 2016).

KEY COMPONENTS

As suggested in the previous sections, peer-mediated support strategies are individually tailored to address the particular needs of students in specific settings. Moreover, the implementation of the interventions—especially peer networks—has varied somewhat across research groups. However, the core components of these interventions typically involve 1) identifying students with ASD and their peers who would benefit from involvement in these interventions, 2) equipping peers to provide support, 3) arranging ongoing opportunities for students to interact with and support one another, and 4) monitoring students and their peers and offering needed guidance to students involved in the intervention. The following sections elaborate on each of these steps and highlight variations that may be associated with peer support arrangements and peer networks. Example fidelity checklists are included in Figure 12.2.

Recruiting and Selecting Peers

The specific procedures and criteria employed when recruiting peers without disabilities for these interventions has garnered relatively little attention in the professional literature (Schaefer et al., 2016). The recruitment process typically involves determining 1) the number of participating peers, 2) the attributes peers should possess, and 3) the approaches used to extend invitations. The number of peers typically involved in these interventions depends on the specific approach being implemented. For example, peer support arrangements typically involve students working within dyads (one peer) or triads (two peers), primarily because of the academic focus of peer-delivered supports. Research suggests that triadic arrangements may be associated with higher rates of social interaction, but comparable rates of academic engagement (Carter et al., 2005). Peer network interventions involve recruiting a somewhat larger number of peers (i.e., three to six) determined primarily by the activities students will do together and settings in which they will spend time (e.g., transitions, lunch, recess, before or after school).

Although the literature includes no established criteria for determining which students without disabilities will participate most effectively within peer-mediated support interventions, several qualities and characteristics of peers have been identified as potential considerations during recruitment (Carter, 2017; Brock & Huber, 2017). For example, peers who already know the focus student with ASD, have regular school attendance, exhibit age-appropriate social skills, and share some interests with the student with ASD often are asked to participate. When a desired intervention outcome involves the development of friendships, gender, social status, and where peers live may be relevant considerations. Relationships may be more likely to develop when peers themselves have an established network of friends, when students are the same gender, and when students live close enough to see one

Peer Support Fidelity

☐ **Facilitator recruits at least one to three peers for the intervention.**

☐ **Facilitator addresses all relevant topics at the initial peer orientation meeting.**

☐ **Facilitator supports peer partners and students as they work collaboratively.**

☐ Facilitator facilitates interactions during class when appropriate.

☐ Facilitator provides reminders and feedback to peer partners before, during, or after class.

☐ Facilitator provides praise and feedback to students with ASD during or outside of class.

☐ **Peer partners are in close proximity to focus student throughout class.**

☐ Students sit next to each other as appropriate.

☐ Students remain in close proximity during out-of-seat activities.

☐ During small-group and lab activities, students join the same group.

☐ **Peer partners interact with the student throughout the class.**

☐ Peer partners greet the student (e.g., "Hi," "See you later").

☐ Peer partners involve the student in interactions with other classmates.

☐ **Peer partners assist the student academically throughout the class.**

☐ Peer partners help the student participate in class activities.

☐ Peer partners repeat or rephrase instructions for student.

☐ Peer partners appropriately prompt the student.

☐ Peer partners provide appropriate feedback to the student.

☐ Students work together on classroom activities.

☐ Students share class materials.

Peer Network Fidelity

☐ **The facilitator recruits a minimum of two peers for the intervention.**

☐ **The facilitator addresses all topics at the initial peer orientation meeting.**

☐ **A minimum of two peers attend network meetings.**

☐ **The facilitator provides support for peer partners and the student during network meetings.**

☐ The facilitator provides structure and facilitates network meetings, as needed.

☐ The facilitator checks with peer partners weekly about interactions with the student.

☐ The facilitator monitors interactions during the meeting, as appropriate.

☐ The facilitator provides praise and feedback to all students (in or outside of the meeting).

☐ **Peer partners and the student interact during the meeting.**

☐ The students greet each other.

☐ The student initiates interactions with peer partners.

☐ Peer partners initiate interactions with the student.

☐ The students engage in a game or shared activity together.

☐ The students engage in conversation together.

☐ **Peer partners and the student report interactions occurring outside of the meeting.**

Figure 12.2. Example fidelity checklists for peer support arrangements and peer network interventions. *Note:* Core intervention components are bold. Flexible components are listed below. (Adapted from Asmus, J. M., Carter, E. W., Moss, C. K., Born, T. L., Vincent, L. B., Lloyd, B. P., & Chung, Y. C. [2016]. Social outcomes and acceptability of two peer-mediated interventions for high school students with severe disabilities: A pilot study. *Inclusion, 4,* 195–214; and Carter, E. W., Asmus, J., Moss, C. K., Amirault, K. A., Biggs, E. E., Bolt, D., Born, T. L., Brock. M. E., Cattey, G. N., Chen, R., Cooney, M., Fesperman, E., Hochman, J. M., Huber, H. B., Lequia, J. L., Lyons, G., Moyseenko, K. A., Riesch, L. M., Shalev, R. A., Vincent, L. B., & Wier, K. [2016]. Randomized evaluation of peer supports arrangements to support the inclusion of high school students with severe disabilities. *Exceptional Children, 82,* 209–233.)

another outside of school (Carter et al., 2009). When the primary purpose is supporting access within inclusive classrooms, peers should evidence a willingness and capacity to learn basic instructional and support strategies. Although academically successful peers are often identified for academic-focused interventions, research suggests that peers who are struggling academically may also benefit from assuming these support roles (Shukla et al., 1998). Selection and identification of these factors in potential peer recruits have been based primarily on the perceptions of school staff. Prior research has not focused on how these considerations are weighed or their impact on fidelity or student outcomes.

Similarly, a variety of methods have been used to recruit peers. To the greatest extent possible, the preferences of students with ASD should be sought when determining which peers to involve in these interventions. However, some students with complex communication challenges or limited existing friendships within a classroom may have difficulty expressing their perspectives. Likewise, peers should always express an interest in and willingness to assume these support roles. It is important to ensure that these interventions are mutually beneficial for all participating students. Often-used approaches for recruiting peers include soliciting recommendations from teachers or club sponsors, general class or school announcements, Circle of Friends procedures (Miller et al., 2003), and teacher-determined pairings. Permission to participate is sought from the parents of both the students with disabilities and their peers.

Equipping Peers and Students

After agreeing to participate, peers receive initial training from school staff on their roles and responsibilities within peer-mediated support interventions. The information and strategies addressed during these orientation sessions—as well as the avenues through which training is delivered—varies somewhat depending on the intervention approach being implemented. Moreover, the content addressed is tailored to reflect the individualized social and educational support needs of participating students with ASD within specific school settings. In more recent studies (e.g., Carter et al., 2017; Sreckovic et al., 2017), students with ASD have also attended these orientation sessions in order to share information about themselves or to learn about what it will look like to work together as a group.

Regardless of whether the students with ASD are included in orientation sessions, several common topics are typically addressed during initial meetings with peer recruits. When students do not already know one another well, peers may be provided general information about their partner's interests, strengths, hobbies, school activities, and broad educational goals (e.g., to meet more of her classmates, to participate more actively in small-group work, to use his communication device more frequently). Such information provides a launching point for initial conversations among students. The importance of using respectful language and maintaining confidentiality also are emphasized. Because some peers may have had limited knowledge about and experience with disability, training for peers has historically emphasized disability awareness elements.

The primary focus of training typically involves teaching peers targeted strategies for supporting the communication, social participation, and/or academic engagement of their partner with ASD. When social and communication outcomes are the primary intervention focus, conversation-enhancing skills often receive particular emphasis. For example, peers may be shown specific strategies for eliciting initiations, prompting use of an AAC device, extending conversational turns, interacting with someone who uses a communication device, redirecting inappropriate conversations, reinforcing conversation attempts, and modeling relevant social skills (e.g., Biggs et al., 2018; Bambara et al., 2016, 2018).

Within peer support arrangements that also emphasize academic participation, peers may learn systematic instruction techniques, such as prompting, modeling, reinforcement, and corrective feedback. Peers also are shown strategies for promoting academic engagement through working together on assignments, providing feedback effectively, reviewing course content, highlighting key concepts, sharing class materials, or modeling self-management strategies. Other relevant student-specific information might also be shared with peers, such as explanations of the communicative intent of any stereotypical or challenging behaviors their partner might exhibit or guidance on how to respond appropriately to these behaviors. Providing students with relevant information and equipping them with targeted skills is expected to increase their confidence and effectiveness as they undertake their new support roles. In addition, peers must know when they should turn to adults (e.g., paraprofessionals, special educators, related services providers) for needed assistance and which support roles they should not assume (e.g., feeding, toileting, responding to behavioral challenges, such as physical aggression).

Special educators and/or paraprofessionals (see Practical Requirements section) typically lead the initial training sessions, although other school staff could also assume this responsibility. Within most research studies, training has been delivered to peers by pulling them aside from ongoing class activities or meeting with them separately in a different location within the school (e.g., another classroom, during recess or lunch). As with other elements of these intervention approaches, the number of initial training sessions will vary widely depending on the approach being used, the individualized support needs of participating students with ASD, and the abilities of participating peers. Overall, most intervention evaluations have required relatively few training sessions (e.g., one to three) of approximately 45–60 minutes in length to produce substantial improvements in social interaction outcomes.

Arranging Interaction Opportunities

After completing recruitment efforts and initial training, educators next establish regular opportunities for students with and without disabilities to interact with one another during the school day. Establishing shared activities during which interaction is both allowed and encouraged is an essential component of peer-mediated support interventions. In the general education classroom, increasing environmental support for interaction typically involves either relocating students with and without ASD so they are sitting next to one another or designing interactive activities during which all students can readily converse with one another (e.g., small-group projects, play-based activities). Within peer support arrangements, students with ASD sit next to participating peers throughout the duration of the class or during specified instructional times. As students work together within these interdependent instructional arrangements, the social interactions they have with one another are both encouraged and reinforced by the classroom teacher, creating interaction opportunities that might not otherwise have existed.

When interventions are implemented outside the classroom, designated times are established for students to spend time together during lunch, at recess, between classes, or within extracurricular activities. Although these represent noninstructional times during which social opportunities naturally exist, many students with ASD rarely access these opportunities. Coordinating students' schedules and arranging intentional social supports increases the social and communication opportunities that students with ASD encounter as well as the likelihood that their conversational initiations will be reciprocated.

Prior research suggests that the types of activities arranged for students with and without disabilities can influence the nature and extent of their interactions with one another (Hughes et al., 2002; McMahon et al., 1996). Specifically, recreational and leisure activities appear to promote social conversations more typical of interactions occurring among friends, whereas academic and instructional activities tend to promote more task-related interactions. These findings suggest that educators should consider carefully the contexts in which they implement peer-mediated interventions, particularly in light of the specific social and communication outcomes they hope to promote.

Feedback and Guidance

As students with and without ASD participate in shared activities, adults thoughtfully monitor their interactions to ensure that peers are delivering supports effectively and interacting meaningfully. In addition, adults ensure that all students are benefiting from their involvement in the intervention. When students begin working together, the supervision that adults provide is more intensive. For example, a special educator might watch students to determine whether peers are using support strategies correctly and consistently and might check in to make sure they have the information and direction they need. In addition, the teacher might observe whether the student with ASD has effective avenues for communicating with his or her peers, appears to enjoy spending time with them, and continues to make adequate progress toward his or her individualized goals. As needed, adults might provide additional assistance by sharing ideas for including focus students in ongoing activities, suggesting alternative support strategies, modeling new instructional approaches, redirecting students when they are off-task, brainstorming solutions to unexpected challenges, or introducing adaptations and modifications to promote greater participation of students with disabilities. Moreover, adults initially provide rich schedules of verbal and/or written reinforcement for students and their peers. Often, this feedback can be provided within the flow of ongoing class activities as students work together.

As students with and without disabilities gain experience working together, adults fade their direct involvement and assume more facilitative roles in which they provide feedback and guidance to students only as needed. Within peer support arrangements, peers may soon need to check in with educators or paraprofessionals only at the beginning or end of the class period or as specific needs arise. Within peer network interventions, adult facilitators gradually turn leadership responsibilities for network meetings over to peers as they gain more experience and confidence, remaining available as needed to address unanticipated challenges or to redirect the group. Adults should find the appropriate balance between encouraging student independence and providing just enough support to promote meaningful interaction. Because the curriculum and instructional strategies typically change as the school year progresses, adults should periodically check with peers and students with disabilities to discuss their experiences, address their concerns, and solicit ideas for refining the intervention.

ASSESSMENT FOR TREATMENT
PLANNING AND PROGRESS MONITORING

Peer-mediated support interventions are appropriate for students with ASD who have goals related to increasing peer interactions, improving social-related skills, and developing social relationships. Moreover, they are helpful for promoting the active participation of students in class and school activities. Figure 12.3 displays a set of steps and considerations when planning these interventions. This decision-making chart can be used to determine whether to pursue peer support arrangement or peer network interventions—or both—for particular students with ASD.

Implementation steps	Peer support arrangement	Peer network intervention
1. Establish a collaborative planning team	Typically includes general educators, special educators, and paraprofessionals	Typically includes special educator, related service providers, and paraprofessionals
2. Identify which social, communication, and other goals should be addressed	Social, communication, behavioral, academic, and class participation goals	Social, communication, and school participation goals
3. Select the appropriate peer-mediated support intervention approach(es)	Supporting learning and social connections within inclusive classrooms	Supporting social skills and relationships across noninstructional times
4. Identify and prepare a facilitator to implement the intervention(s)	Paraprofessionals, special educators, general educators	Club leaders, coaches, school counselors, special educators, paraprofessionals
5. Recruit and select peer partners	One to two peers from within the same classroom	Two to six peers from within the school with shared interests and availability
6. Orient peers to their roles	One to two orientation sessions for peers outside of the classroom	One initial orientation session for peers and students during the first network meeting
7. Support students as they spend time together	Prompting, reinforcing, and providing information for social *and* academic interactions, checking in	Prompting, reinforcing, and providing information for social interactions, checking in
8. Evaluate student outcomes through direct observations and interviews	Examples include academic engagement, task- and social-related interactions, targeted social-related skills	Examples include social interactions, reciprocity, appropriate play, targeted social-related skills
9. Refine intervention(s) as needed	Examples include retraining peers, selecting new peer, further adapting class activities	Examples include additional peer training, incorporating skill instruction, selecting new peers or activities
10. Maintain the intervention(s)	Intervention typically lasts one semester	Intervention typically lasts one to two semesters

Figure 12.3.   Decision-making chart for planning peer-mediated support interventions.

Direct observations represent the primary approach used to determine whether peer-mediated support interventions are working as intended and promoting desired outcomes, as well as whether additional refinements or alternative approaches may be necessary. Observing students as they spend time together enables school staff to ascertain the extent to which peers are delivering social and instructional supports with sufficient fidelity and whether students with ASD are benefiting through communication and social interactions outcomes. For example, observations might focus on characteristics of students' social interactions (e.g., reciprocity, appropriateness, conversational topics, overall quality), the social and communication skills used by students (e.g., initiations, responses, extensions, affect, communication mode), the contexts within which these interactions occur (e.g., small groups, large groups, transitions, free time), and the individuals involved in these interactions (e.g., peer supports, other classmates, adults). Recognizing the complexity of peer relationships and the numerous dimensions along which peer interaction might be assessed, teachers should prioritize and operationally define desired social outcomes. Paraprofessionals, special educators, or related services providers can conduct formal classroom or other school-based observations before and after initiating peer-mediated interventions. Observational approaches and measures used in the studies described in this chapter (see Tables 12.1 and 12.2) can be readily adapted and implemented by school staff.

At the same time, direct observations should be supplemented with student and teacher interviews. Educators can ask students with ASD about 1) their experiences receiving support from their peers, 2) whether they enjoy spending time with their classmates, 3) other classmates they would like to work with or get to know better, and 4) whether they would like to continue receiving social and/or academic support from their peers. Educators should ask participating peers their perspectives regarding 1) their emerging relationships with their partner with disabilities; 2) their perceptions of how they and their partner are benefiting from their ongoing interactions; 3) support strategies that are and are not working well; and 4) additional information, assistance, or supports that they think would enhance their interactions with their partner. As noted elsewhere, peers have a unique perspective into the social culture of the school and often can share insightful ideas and recommendations for enhancing the social participation of their classmates with disabilities. Finally, conversations with other teachers and school staff can reveal whether an intervention is producing noticeable improvements in social and communication outcomes, aligns well with other instructional and intervention approaches being used, is practical to initiate and maintain, and produces broad improvements in students' social participation across multiple school contexts. Finally, educators can ask families about the impact they see at home, including whether interactions are extending outside of school.

CONSIDERATIONS FOR CHILDREN FROM CULTURALLY AND LINGUISTICALLY DIVERSE BACKGROUNDS

Schools across the country are serving an increasingly diverse population of students with ASD (DOE, 2016). The effectiveness of peer-mediated support interventions has been demonstrated with a wide range of students in varied geographic locales (e.g., California, Kansas, North Carolina, Texas, Washington, Wisconsin) and district types (e.g., rural, suburban, urban). Moreover, students with ASD from diverse racial/ethnic backgrounds have participated in these studies, including 46% who were white, 11% who were Hispanic, 7% who were Asian American, 6% who were African American, 3% who were multiracial or from other backgrounds, and 27% from whom race/ethnicity was not reported. Unfortunately, relatively little information about the linguistic backgrounds of participating students has been reported, nor has socioeconomic status frequently been addressed.

Culture can shape when, where, and how students spend time together at their school. It can influence views about disability and inclusion. Finally, it can impact students' views on various intervention approaches and support models (Biggs & Carter, 2017). Supporting student and family involvement in the intervention planning process offers one primary avenue for ensuring that the goals and intervention procedures associated with these strategies reflect the priorities and values of these culturally and linguistically diverse individuals. During educational planning meetings, the team should ask parents for their input into the design and delivery of peer-mediated supports. Moreover, parents can provide information about whether and how their child talks about his or her relationships with peers at school. Parent involvement becomes especially critical if intervention efforts are intended to facilitate peer interactions and relationships that extend beyond the school day.

Application to a Child

Keagan (age 9) was a third-grade student served under the special education category of autism. She was included in general education classes throughout the school day but received speech and language therapy in a separate room several times per week. Keagan had IEP goals focused on increasing the frequency and appropriateness of her conversational initiations, using her voice output communication aid with greater fluency, and improving the quality of her social interactions with her classmates. However, observations within the classroom indicated that Keagan rarely used her communication device, never interacted with her classmates, and received most of her instruction and support from an individually assigned paraprofessional. Informal conversations with several classmates indicated that they felt unsure of how to interact with someone who used a communication device and did not understand why Keagan engaged in certain stereotypical behaviors (e.g., rocking, hand waving). The general education teacher met with a special educator to consider how a peer support arrangement could be established for Keagan. They also sought input from Keagan's parents and Keagan herself. Together, they identified two girls from the class who had expressed an interest in getting to know Keagan and who worked well together. After securing parent permission, the special educator and paraprofessional met with the girls during two lunch periods to orient them to their roles. They discussed the importance of friendships and provided general information about Keagan's interests, strengths, and abilities; shared ideas for conversational topics; discussed strategies for gaining Keagan's attention and encouraging her to use her AAC device; and brainstormed ways the students could help Keagan participate during different aspects of the class (e.g., whole-group, small-group, centers). As the students began working together, the paraprofessional modeled ways of communicating with Keagan and involving her in class activities. As the students got to know one another and felt more comfortable working together, the paraprofessional gradually faded her direct involvement and began working with a wider range of students within the classroom. However, she continued to monitor Keagan's interactions with her class-mates and collected data on her progress toward her social-related IEP goals. Throughout the semester, Keagan was observed interacting more frequently with her peer partners as well as with other students in the class with whom she was not formally paired. She also began initiating more conversations with her communication device and participating more actively in class activities.

Application to an Adolescent

Ms. Hatty, a special educator at Northbrook High School, noticed that several of her students with ASD seemed disconnected from the larger student body and rarely par-ticipated in schoolwide events. She approached her principal to discuss the idea of establishing peer networks to help her students meet other schoolmates. Ms. Hatty reached out to several other educators at her school who seemed to be kid magnets and asked if they would be interested in helping foster greater inclusion at the school. For John, a freshman who had autism and a significant intellectual disability, the peer network seemed especially appropriate. Mr. Smith, a sociology teacher and the boys' track coach, volunteered to facilitate John's peer network. He and Ms. Hatty spoke with John and his mom to ask their thoughts about whom to involve and what informa-tion would be appropriate to share with others. A girl from John's art class, her friend, and two boys from the track team—all of whom were involved in the school's drama program—agreed to get involved. The idea of hanging out with John during first-hour lunch each week sounded fun. Initially, Mr. Smith suggested some games the students could play while eating lunch in his classroom. Ms. Hatty also gave the students some guidance on social skills they could help John practice. The peers came to appreci-ate John's unique sense of humor. Before long, John could be seen roaming the halls between classes with his new friends—giving high-fives and sharing his charming smile. Mr. Smith checked in with students outside of the lunch meeting to make sure things were going well and to answer any questions. Ms. Hatty also asked John how his peer network was going whenever he was in her classroom. As the students got to know each other throughout the school year, they began connecting with one another out-side of school. For example, they went to the opening night of the school play together and periodically went to see movies together. Of course, this took coordination with John's mom, who was eager to see her son's social relationships grow throughout his first year of high school.

> **To review an extended application and implementation**
> **of this intervention, see Case 9 about a child with ASD**
> **and intellectual disability in the companion volume**
> *Case Studies for the Treatment of Autism Spectrum Disorder.*

Future Directions

Although nearly thirty studies have examined these peer-mediated support inter-ventions for school-age children with ASD, additional research is needed to fur-ther refine these interventions and increase our understanding of their impact on participating students. First, the steps taken to select and train peers to provide support are salient factors that likely influence the outcomes associated with these intervention approaches. Few studies have examined how the characteristics of peers or the content and delivery of initial training to peers affect subsequent social interactions or skill acquisition. Such considerations warrant closer examination. Second, although the proximal impact of peer-mediated support interventions is well documented, only a few studies have examined the extent to which the social interactions and relationships established within these arrangements 1) extend to other peers not directly involved, 2) spill over to other contexts during or beyond the school day, or 3) are maintained over multiple semesters or school years. Future research should explore how best to promote the generalized and longitudinal impact of these interventions. Third, although peer-mediated support interventions promote increases in social interaction, less is known about their impact on the communication and language skill acquisition of students with ASD. A few studies have examined the acquisition of individualized, targeted skills (e.g., Bambara et al., 2016, 2018; Kamps et al., 2014) as part of peer networks. This focus has been more limited within peer support arrangements (e.g., Brock et al., 2016). Therefore, use of measures designed to examine these outcomes should be undertaken more routinely in research on peer-mediated interventions.

Fourth, the increasing involvement of youth and young adults with ASD in postsecondary education raises questions regarding the implementation and efficacy of peer-mediated support strategies within inclusive college programs (Carter, Gustafson, et al., 2019) and integrated workplaces (Hughes & Carter, 2019). Although the focus of this chapter was on school-age children with ASD, research examining the extension of these strategies to other contexts and ages is needed.

Suggested Readings

1. Carter, E. W. (2017). The promise and practice of peer support arrangements for students with intellectual and developmental disabilities. *International Review of Research in Developmental Disabilities, 52,* 141–174. This review article addresses key issues related to designing, delivering, and evaluating peer support arrangements in ways that enhance efficacy and its feasibility.

2. Carter, E. W., Asmus, J., Moss, C. K., Cooney, M., Weir, K., Vincent, L., Born, T., Hochman, J., Bottema-Beutel, K., & Fesperman, E. (2013). Peer network strategies to foster social connections among adolescents with and without severe disabilities. *TEACHING Exceptional Children, 46*(2), 51–59. This article outlines 10 steps for launching and maintaining peer networks and providing checklists for holding orientation meetings using case examples.

3. Carter, E. W., Cushing, L. S., & Kennedy, C. H. (2009). *Peer support strategies for improving all students' social lives and learning.* Paul H. Brookes Publishing Co. This step-by-step planning guide provides information to educators and administrators on how to implement peer support arrangements in elementary, middle, and high schools.

Learning Activities

1. Students with and without ASD have unique insight into the barriers to peer interaction existing in their school as well as the factors that could enhance relationships. Talk with students to learn their perspectives regarding the information, supports, and opportunities that would enable them to work together

and encourage them to get to know one another. In addition, ask how they see their roles in promoting relationships and social connections within their school.

2. Most peers are quite willing to play a role in supporting their classmates with ASD when invited by educators. Often, the challenge is determining which and how many peers to invite. When deciding which peers to involve in these interventions, what qualities and characteristics would you consider to be most important? How might your answer change depending on the primary focus of the peer-mediated support intervention and the specific social and communication outcomes you hope to obtain? What steps could you take to make sure students with ASD have a meaningful voice in determining which peers will be involved in providing support?

3. Research findings describing the effectiveness and feasibility of peer-mediated support strategies are very promising. As with all educational interventions, however, questions may arise about the implementation of these strategies. What concerns might teachers, paraprofessionals, administrators, parents, or others raise about implementing peer-mediated support interventions for students with ASD? Consider how you could address or reduce each of these concerns when establishing and maintaining these interventions.

REFERENCES

Asterisk (*) indicates research studies discussed in the Empirical Basis section of this chapter.

American Psychiatric Association. (2013). *Diagnostic and statistical manual of mental disorders, fifth edition* (DSM-V). Author.

*Asmus, J. M., Carter, E. W., Moss, C. K., Biggs, E. E., Bolt, D. M., Born, T. L., Bottema-Beutel, K., Brock, M. E., Cattey, G. N., Cooney, M., Fesperman, E. S., Hochman, J. M., Huber, H. B., Lequia, J. L., Lyons, G. L., Vincent, L. B., & Weir, K. (2017). Efficacy and social validity of peer network interventions for high school students with severe disabilities. *American Journal on Intellectual and Developmental Disabilities, 122*, 118–137.

*Asmus, J. M., Carter, E. W., Moss, C. K., Born, T. L., Vincent, L. B., Lloyd, B. P., & Chung, Y. C. (2016). Social outcomes and acceptability of two peer-mediated interventions for high school students with severe disabilities: A pilot study. *Inclusion, 4*, 195–214.

*Bambara, L. M., Cole, C. L., Chovanes, J., Telesford, A., Thomas, A., Tsai, S. C., Ayad, E., & Bilgili, I. (2018). Improving the assertive conversational skills of adolescents with autism spectrum disorder in a natural context. *Research in Autism Spectrum Disorders, 48*, 1–16.

*Bambara, L. M., Cole, C. L., Kunsch, C., Tsai, S. C., & Ayad, E. (2016). A peer-mediated intervention to improve the conversational skills of high school students with autism spectrum disorder. *Research in Autism Spectrum Disorders, 27*, 29–43.

Bandura, A. (1977). *Social learning theory.* General Learning Press.

Biggs, E. E., & Carter, E. W. (2017). Supporting the social lives of students with intellectual disability. In M. L. Wehmeyer and K. A. Shogren (Eds.), *Handbook of research-based practices for educating students with intellectual disability* (pp. 235–254). Routledge.

*Biggs, E. E., Carter, E. W., Bumble, J. L., Barnes, K., & Mazur, E. L. (2018). Enhancing peer network interventions for students with complex communication needs. *Exceptional Children, 85*, 66–85.

Biggs, E. E., Carter, E. W., & Gustafson, J. R. (2017). Efficacy of collaborative planning and peer support arrangements to increase peer interaction and AAC use in inclusive classrooms. *American Journal on Intellectual and Developmental Disabilities, 122*, 25–48.

Boardman, A. G., Argüelles, M. E., Vaughn, S., Hughes, M. T., & Klingner, J. (2005). Special education teachers' views of research-based practices. *Journal of Special Education, 39*, 168–180.

*Brock, M. E., Biggs, E. E., Carter, E. W., Cattey, G., & Raley, K. (2016). Implementation and generalization of peer support arrangements for students with significant disabilities in inclusive classrooms. *Journal of Special Education, 49*, 221–232.

*Brock, M. E., & Carter, E. W. (2016). Efficacy of teachers training paraprofessionals to implement peer support arrangements. *Exceptional Children, 82*, 354–371.

Brock, M. E., & Huber, H. B. (2017). Are peer support arrangements an evidence-based practice? A systematic review. *Journal of Special Education, 51*, 150–163.

Carter, E. W. (2017). The promise and practice of peer support arrangements for students with intellectual and developmental disabilities. *International Review of Research in Developmental Disabilities, 52*, 141–174.

Carter, E. W. (2018). Supporting the social lives of secondary students with severe disabilities: Critical elements for effective intervention. *Journal of Emotional and Behavioral Disorders, 26*, 52–61.

*Carter, E. W., Asmus, J., Moss, C. K., Amirault, K. A., Biggs, E. E., Bolt, D., Born, T. L., Brock. M. E., Cattey, G. N., Chen, R., Cooney, M., Fesperman, E., Hochman, J. M., Huber, H. B., Lequia, J. L., Lyons, G., Moyseenko, K. A., Riesch, L. M., Shalev, R. A., Vincent, L. B., & Wier, K. (2016). Randomized evaluation of peer supports arrangements to support the inclusion of high school students with severe disabilities. *Exceptional Children, 82*, 209–233.

Carter, E. W., Asmus, J., Moss, C. K., Cooney, M., Weir, K., Born, T. L., Hochman, J. M., Bottema-Beutel, K., & Fesperman, E. (2013). Peer network strategies to foster social connections among adolescents with and without severe disabilities. *Teaching Exceptional Children, 46*(2), 51–59.

Carter, E. W., Biggs, E. E., & Blustein, C. L. (2016). Relationships matter: Addressing stigma among students with intellectual disability and their peers. In K. Scior & S. Werner (Eds.), *Intellectual disability and stigma: Stepping out from the margins* (pp. 149–164). Palgrave McMillan.

Carter, E. W., Bottema-Beutel, K., & Brock, M. E. (2014). Social interactions and friendships. In M. Agran, F. Brown, C. Hughes, C. Quirk, & D. Ryndak (Eds.), *Equity and full participation for individuals with severe disabilities: A vision for the future* (pp. 197–216). Paul H. Brookes Publishing Co.

Carter, E. W., Cushing, L. S., Clark, N. M., & Kennedy, C. H. (2005). Effects of peer support interventions on students' access to the general curriculum and social interactions. *Research and Practice for Persons with Severe Disabilities, 30*, 15–25.

Carter, E. W., Cushing, L. S., & Kennedy, C. H. (2009). *Peer support strategies for improving all students' social lives and learning.* Paul H. Brookes Publishing Co.

Carter, E. W., Dykstra Steinbrenner, J. R., & Hall, L. J. (2019). Exploring feasibility and fit: Peer-mediated interventions for high school students with autism spectrum disorder. *School Psychology Review, 48*, 157–169.

Carter, E. W., Gustafson, J. R., Mackay, M. M., Martin, K., Parlsey, M., Graves, J., Day, T. L., McCabe, L. E., Lazarz, H., McMillan, E. D., Schiro-Geist, C., Williams, M., Beeson, T., & Cayton, J. (2019). Motivations and expectations of peer mentors within inclusive higher education programs for students with intellectual disability. *Career Development and Transition for Exceptional Individuals, 42*, 168–178.

*Carter, E. W., Gustafson, J. R., Sreckovic, M. A., Steinbrenner, J. R. D., Pierce, N. P., Bord, A., Stabel, A., Rogers, S., Czerw, A., & Mullins, T. (2017). Efficacy of peer support interventions in general education classrooms for high school students with autism spectrum disorder. *Remedial and Special Education, 38*, 207–221.

Carter, E. W., & Kennedy, C. H. (2006). Promoting access to the general curriculum using peer support strategies. *Research and Practice for Persons with Severe Disabilities, 31*, 284–292.

Carter, E. W., Moss, C. K., Asmus, J., Fesperman, E., Cooney, M., Brock, M. E., Lyons, G., Huber, H. B., & Vincent, L. (2015). Promoting inclusion, social connections, and learning through peer support arrangements. *Teaching Exceptional Children, 48*(1), 9–18.

Carter, E. W., O'Rourke, L., Sisco, L. G., & Pelsue, D. (2009). Knowledge, responsibilities, and training needs of paraprofessionals in elementary and secondary schools. *Remedial and Special Education, 30*, 344–349.

Carter, E. W., & Pesko, M. J. (2008). Social validity of peer interaction intervention strategies in high school classrooms: Effectiveness, feasibility, and actual use. *Exceptionality, 16*, 156–173.

Carter, E. W., Sisco, L. G., Brown, L., Brickham, D., & Al-Khabbaz, Z. A. (2008). Peer interactions and academic engagement of youth with developmental disabilities in inclusive middle and high school classrooms. *American Journal on Mental Retardation, 113,* 479–494.

Carter, E. W., Sisco, L. G., Chung, Y., & Stanton-Chapman, T. (2010). Peer interactions of students with intellectual disabilities and/or autism: A map of the intervention literature. *Research and Practice for Persons with Severe Disabilities, 35,* 63–79.

Copeland, S. R., Hughes, C., Carter, E. W., Guth, C., Presley, J., Williams, C. R., & Fowler, S. E. (2004). Increasing access to general education: Perspectives of participants in a high school peer support program. *Remedial and Special Education, 26,* 342–352.

Cushing, L. S., Clark, N. M., Carter, E. W., & Kennedy, C. H. (2005). Access to the general education curriculum for students with severe disabilities: What it means and how to accomplish it. *Teaching Exceptional Children, 38,* 6–13.

Feldman, R., Carter, E. W., Asmus, J., & Brock, M. E. (2016). Presence, proximity, and peer interactions of adolescents with severe disabilities in general education classrooms. *Exceptional Children, 82,* 192–208.

*Gardner, K. F., Carter, E. W., Gustafson, J. R., Hochman, J. M., Harvey, M. N., Mullins, T. S., & Fan, H. (2014). Effects of peer networks on the social interactions of high school students with autism spectrum disorders. *Research and Practice for Persons with Severe Disabilities, 39,* 100–118.

Garrison-Harrell, L., Kamps, D., & Kravits, T. (1997). The effects of peer networks on social-communicative behaviors for students with autism. *Focus on Autism and Other Developmental Disabilities, 12,* 241–254.

Giangreco, M. F., Doyle, M. B., & Suter, J. C. (2012). Constructively responding to requests for paraprofessionals: We keep asking the wrong questions. *Remedial and Special Education, 33,* 362–373.

Griffin, W. B. (2019). Peer perceptions of students with autism spectrum disorders. *Focus on Autism and Other Developmental Disabilities, 34*(3), 183–192.

*Haring, T. G., & Breen, C. G. (1992). A peer-mediated social network intervention to enhance the social integration of persons with moderate and severe disabilities. *Journal of Applied Behavior Analysis, 25,* 319–333.

*Hochman, J. M., Carter, E. W., Bottema-Beutel, K., Harvey, M. N., & Gustafson, J. R. (2015). Efficacy of peer networks to increase social connections among high school students with and without autism spectrum disorder. *Exceptional Children, 82,* 96–116.

*Huber, H. B., Carter, E. W., Lopano, S. E., & Stankiewicz, K. C. (2018). Using structural analysis to inform peer support arrangements for high school students with severe disabilities. *American Journal on Intellectual and Developmental Disabilities, 123,* 119–139.

Huber, H. B., & Carter, E. W. (2016). Data-driven individualization in peer-mediated interventions for students with ASD: A literature review. *Review Journal of Autism and Developmental Disorders, 3,* 239–253.

Huber, H. B., & Carter, E. W. (2019). Fostering peer relationships and shared learning for students with autism spectrum disorders. In R. Jordan, J. Roberts, & K. Hume (Eds.), *The SAGE handbook of autism and education* (pp. 265–278). Sage.

Hughes, C., Carter, E. W., Hughes, T., Bradford, E., & Copeland, S. R. (2002). Effects of instructional versus non-instructional roles on the social interactions of high school students. *Education and Training in Mental Retardation and Developmental Disabilities, 37,* 146–162.

Hunt, P., Soto, G., Maier, J., & Doering, K. (2003). Collaborative teaming to support students at risk and students with severe disabilities in general education classrooms. *Exceptional Children, 69,* 315–332.

Jackson, J. N., & Campbell, J. M. (2009). Teachers' peer buddy selections for children with autism: Social characteristics and relationships with peer nominations. *Journal of Autism and Developmental Disorders, 39,* 269–277.

*Kamps, D., Mason, R., Thiemann-Bourque, K., Feldmiller, S., Turcotte, A., & Miller, T. (2014). The use of peer networks to increase communicative acts of students with autism spectrum disorders. *Focus on Autism and other Developmental Disabilities, 29,* 230–245.

*Kamps, D. M., Potucek, J., Lopez, A. G., Kravits, T., & Kemmerer, K. (1997). The use of peer networks across multiple settings to improve social interaction for students with autism. *Journal of Behavioral Education, 7,* 335–357.

*Kamps, D., Thiemann-Bourque, K., Heitzman-Powell, L., Schwartz, I., Rosenberg, N., Mason, R., & Cox, S. (2015). A comprehensive peer network intervention to improve social communication of children with autism spectrum disorders: A randomized trial in kindergarten and first grade. *Journal of Autism and Developmental Disorders, 45*, 1809–1824.

*Kasari, C., Dean, M., Kretzmann, M., Shih, W., Orlich, F., Whitney, R., Landa, R., Lord, C., & King, B. (2016). Children with autism spectrum disorder and social skills groups at school: A randomized trial comparing intervention approach and peer composition. *Journal of Child Psychology and Psychiatry, 57*, 171–179.

Kearns, J. F., Towles-Reeves, E., Kleinert, H. L., Kleinert, J. O., & Thomas, M. K. (2011). Characteristics of and implications for students participating in alternate assessments based on alternate academic achievement standards. *Journal of Special Education, 45*, 3–14.

Kennedy, C. H. (2001). Social interaction interventions for youth with severe disabilities should emphasize interdependence. *Mental Retardation and Developmental Disabilities Research Reviews, 7*, 122–127.

*Koegel, L. K., Vernon, T. W., Koegel, R. L., Koegel, B. L., & Paullin, A. W. (2012). Improving social engagement and initiations between children with autism spectrum disorder and their peers in inclusive settings. *Journal of Positive Behavior Interventions, 14*, 220–227.

*Koegel, R. L., Fredeen, R., Kim, S., Danial, J., Rubinstein, D., & Koegel, L. (2012). Using perseverative interests to improve interactions between adolescents with autism and their typical peers in school settings. *Journal of Positive Behavior Interventions 14*, 133–141.

*Koegel, R. L., Kim, S., Koegel, L., & Schwartzmann, B. (2013). Improving socializations for high school students with ASD by using their perseverative interests. *Journal of Autism and Developmental Disorders, 43*, 2121–2134.

Kuntz, E. M. (2019). *Evaluation of a collaborative planning framework for general educators teaching students with severe disabilities* [Unpublished doctoral dissertation]. Vanderbilt University.

Lipscomb, S., Haimson, J., Liu, A. Y., Burghardt, J., Johnson, D. R., & Thurlow, M. L. (2017). *Preparing for life after high school: The characteristics and experiences of youth in special education.* U.S. Department of Education.

Lyons, G. L., Huber, H. B., Carter, E. W., Chen, R., & Asmus, J. A. (2016). Assessing the social skills and problem behaviors of adolescents with severe disabilities enrolled in general education classes. *American Journal on Intellectual and Developmental Disabilities, 121*, 327–345.

*Mason, R., Kamps, D., Turcotte, A., Cox, S., Feldmiller, S., & Miller, T. (2014). Peer mediation to increase communication and interaction at recess for students with autism spectrum disorders. *Research in Autism Spectrum Disorders, 8*, 334–344.

McMahon, C. M., Wacker, D. P., Sasso, G. M., Berg, W. K., & Newton, S. M. (1996). Analysis of frequency and type of interaction in peer-mediated social skills intervention: Instructional vs. social interactions. *Education and Training in Mental Retardation and Developmental Disabilities, 31*, 339–352.

Miller, M. C., Cooke, N. L., Test, D. W., & White, R. (2003). Effects of Circle of Friends on the social interactions of elementary age students with mild disabilities. *Journal of Behavioral Education, 12*, 167–184.

Morningstar, M. E., Kurth, J. A., & Johnson, P. E. (2016). Examining national trends in educational placements for students with significant disabilities. *Remedial and Special Education, 38*, 3–12.

Ryan, A. M., & Ladd, G. W. (Eds.). (2012). *Peer relationships and adjustment at school.* Information Age Publishing.

*Schaefer, J. M., Cannella-Malone, H., & Brock, M. E. (2018). Effects of peer support arrangements across instructional formats and environments for students with severe disabilities. *Remedial and Special Education, 39*, 3–14.

Schaefer, J. M., Canella-Malone, H. I., & Carter, E. W. (2016). The place of peers in peer-mediated interventions for students with intellectual disabilities. *Remedial and Special Education, 37*, 345–356.

Schopler, E., Reichler, J., & Renner, B. (1988). *The Childhood Autism Rating Scale.* Western Psychological Services.

*Shukla, S., Kennedy, C. H., & Cushing, L. S. (1998). Adult influence on the participation of peers without disabilities in peer support programs. *Journal of Behavioral Education, 8*, 397–413.

*Shukla, S., Kennedy, C. H., & Cushing, L. S. (1999). Intermediate school students with severe disabilities: Supporting their social participation in general education classrooms. *Journal of Positive Behavior Interventions, 1*, 130–140.

Sonnenmeier, R., McSheehan, M., & Jorgensen, C. (2005). A case study of team supports for a student with autism's communication and engagement within the general education curriculum: Preliminary report of the Beyond Access model. *Augmentative and Alternative Communication, 21*, 101–115.

*Sreckovic, M. A., Hume, K., & Able, H. (2017). Examining the efficacy of peer network interventions on the social interactions of high school students with autism spectrum disorder. *Journal of Autism and Developmental Disorders, 47*, 2556–2574.

Stokes, T. F., & Baer, D. M. (1977). An implicit technology of generalization. *Journal of Applied Behavior Analysis, 10*, 349–367.

Tonnsen, B. L., & Hahn, E. R. (2015). Middle school students' attitudes toward a peer with autism spectrum disorder: Effects of social acceptance and physical inclusion. *Focus on Autism and Other Developmental Disabilities, 31*, 262–274.

U.S. Department of Education. (2016). *State level data files*. Retrieved from https://www.ideadata.org

Watkins, L., O'Reilly, M., Kuhn, M., Gevarter, C., Lancioni, G. E., Sigafoos, J., & Lang, R. (2015). A review of peer-mediated social interaction interventions for students with autism in inclusive settings. *Journal of Autism and Developmental Disorders, 45*, 1070–1083.

13

Pivotal Response Treatment

Lynn Kern Koegel, Kristen Strong, and Elizabeth Ponder

INTRODUCTION

Pivotal Response Treatment® (PRT) is a naturalistic intervention model derived from applied behavioral analysis (ABA) approaches (Koegel & Koegel, 2019). Rather than targeting each individual behavior one at a time, PRT targets core, **pivotal areas**, such as motivation, self-regulation, and initiations (R. L. Koegel & Egel, 1979; L. K. Koegel, Koegel, et al., 2010; L. K. Koegel et al., 1992). Research has shown that focusing on these pivotal areas results in widespread, collateral improvements in other untreated social, communicative, and behavioral areas (L. K. Koegel, Koegel, Harrower, & Carter, 1999). PRT can be implemented across the lifespan, with studies showing that procedures are effective with infants through adults with autism spectrum disorder (ASD) and related disabilities (Ashbaugh et al., 2017; Vernon et al., 2012). Furthermore, PRT can be used during all stages of language development, from teaching first words to full sentences and improving advanced social conversation such as empathy and reciprocal interactions (Bradshaw et al., 2017; L. K. Koegel et al., 2016).

PRT is a package intervention that includes specific motivational procedures: child choice, interspersing maintenance and acquisition tasks, **contingent reinforcement, natural rewards,** and **rewarding attempts** (R. L. Koegel, Dyer, & Bell, 1987; R. L. Koegel et al., 1988; R. L. Koegel & Williams, 1980; Williams et al., 1981). The individual with ASD plays a large role in guiding the activities that will be used during intervention (e.g., if the child likes puzzles, then treatment can be implemented in the context of doing a puzzle). The PRT provider is responsible for mixing in easy and hard tasks, rewarding the good attempts, and providing immediate reinforcement that is directly related to the individual's response (e.g., if the child says "ba" as an attempt at the word *ball*, the adult gives the child a ball rather than giving a piece of candy as a reward). These procedures are described in more detail throughout the chapter.

PRT is considered an established evidence-based treatment for ASD (e.g., National Autism Center, 2015; Verschuur et al., 2014; Wong, et. al., 2015). Research has shown that PRT is effective in improving a range of communication skills, including the number and length of utterances, speech intelligibility, syntax, initiations, question-asking, a diversity of responses to questions, and conversation skills (L. K. Koegel et al., 2016; R. L. Koegel, Bradshaw, et al., 2014; Koegel et al., 1998; L. K. Koegel, Koegel, et al., 2010; Weiss & Harris, 2001). In addition, PRT can be used to teach academics, cooperative play, motor skills, daily living activities, and advanced social skills (L. K. Koegel, Singh, & Koegel, 2010; R. L. Koegel et al., 2005). Research has shown that children's disruptive and stereotypic behaviors decrease during and following PRT intervention and that child and parent affect improve when program-specific motivational components are incorporated (R. L. Koegel et al., 1996; R. L. Koegel et al., 1992). Studies have also used functional magnetic resonance imaging (fMRI) to show that neural systems supporting social perception are malleable through implementation of PRT (Voos et al., 2013).

PRT can be implemented through many different service delivery models. Treatment can be provided individually by clinicians in the home, school, community, or clinic settings. In addition, PRT therapists can teach parents to work collaboratively with them so that intervention can be implemented throughout the individual's waking hours and beyond the official PRT sessions (Coolican et al., 2010; Nefdt et al., 2010). Several programs have demonstrated that parents can be educated individually or in a group format to successfully implement PRT with their children (Gillett & LeBlanc, 2007; Hardan et al., 2015). Further, teachers, paraprofessionals, peers, and siblings can effectively deliver PRT to children with autism (Harper et al., 2008; Smith & Camarata, 1999). Thus, PRT is unique in that a variety of individuals can assist with delivery of the intervention in any type of setting, which leads to greater treatment intensity and more rapid acquisition and generalization of goals than previous adult-driven interventions (Koegel & Koegel, 2019).

TARGET POPULATIONS

The bulk of studies demonstrating the effectiveness of PRT have focused on preschool and elementary-school-age children with ASD (L. K. Koegel, Koegel, Shoshan, & McNerney, 1999; Mohammadzaheri et al., 2014). However, PRT procedures can also be used with infants (L. K. Koegel, Singh, et al., 2014; Steiner et al., 2013), adolescents (R. L. Koegel et al., 2012; R. L. Koegel et al., 2013), and adults (L. K. Koegel et al., 2013). In short, PRT can be used with individuals with ASD across the lifespan.

PRT was developed collaboratively by speech-language pathologists (SLPs) and psychologists, and treatment focuses on improving the core deficits and diagnostic features of ASD according to the *Diagnostic and Statistical Manual of Mental Disorders, Fifth Edition* (DSM-5; American Psychiatric Association [APA], 2013). PRT emphasizes improving social communication skills, such as language, social-emotional reciprocity, and social skills that aid in developing relationships. Children with ASD and language delays, difficulties with expressive communication, and challenges with reciprocal social interactions are very good candidates for PRT. It can also be used with individuals diagnosed with social communication disorder (APA, 2013), Asperger syndrome (APA, 2000), a variety of developmental disorders, cognitive delays, and individuals without a clinical diagnosis who are experiencing social and communication difficulties. Although PRT is designed to help individuals with ASD or social-communication impairments, it is important to note that intervention involves more than just the individual. Parents are heavily involved in PRT programs, and siblings, peers, and other professionals who are a part of the life of the individual with ASD are also incorporated as much as possible.

THEORETICAL BASIS

PRT is a naturalistic behavioral treatment that is based on the principle that learning is improved when individuals' motivation is high. PRT is a form of ABA that uses a developmental approach and incorporates specific strategies to increase motivation (Koegel & Koegel, 2019). This section describes the theoretical explanation and basis of the PRT approach discusses areas that are frequently targeted in treatment.

Theoretical Explanation

PRT was developed as a form of therapy based on the theory of learned helplessness. Research suggests that behavioral and communication challenges for individuals with ASD may be due to a lack of motivation associated with **learned helplessness,** not a lack of ability (Barnhill & Myles, 2001; R. L. Koegel & Egel, 1979; R. L. Koegel & Mentis, 1985; R. L. Koegel et al., 1988). Learned helplessness occurs when, because of noncontingent consequences, individuals behave as if they are helpless and do not respond as if their behavior has an impact on outcome. This theory has been a topic in psychological research since the 1960s when studies showed that when noncontingent punishment is administered, study participants begin demonstrating lethargy and a lack of responding (Maier & Seligman, 1976; Miller & Seligman, 1975; Seligman & Maier, 1967). In a simple example, imagine that are you are traveling and attempt to order food in a foreign language. If the waiter does not understand you or responds unfavorably, it is probable that you will stop trying to speak the foreign language and will either point to the item or get frustrated and give up. Consequently, the next time you are at a restaurant, it is likely that you will just point to the item and not try to speak the foreign language. You have theoretically learned that your attempts to verbally communicate are ineffective. In contrast, if the waiter rewards your attempts to converse and brings you the desired food, it is probable you will continue trying the foreign language in the future.

Since the 1960s, the concept of learned helplessness has subsequently been applied to a variety of human behaviors and disorders, including ASD. Children and adolescents with ASD often appear to lack the desire to engage or attempt tasks (R. L. Koegel & Mentis, 1985), which suggests that they may be more capable than some of their behavior suggests. It is possible that if children with ASD experience little or low levels of success and positive outcomes from their attempts to communicate, then they may reduce their attempts to use language and interact with others. For example, if a child with autism is learning first words and is not understood or takes a while to respond, a well-meaning adult may attempt to communicate for the child. Similarly, children with ASD may try to socially interact with peers, but communication and socialization impairments may cause their peers to respond in an unfavorable manner. That is, the child may make an attempt at social communication that is not rewarding. After a while, the child may stop trying to use language and socialize. In fact, other behaviors, such as grabbing or crying, that can lead to more efficient reinforcement may occur. Moreover, the child will often get reinforced without using words or word attempts (e.g., an adult gives the child a cookie without appropriate communication). Thus, over time, the child may begin to learn that language does not result in any reinforcement. When such patterns occur, children may begin developing symptoms of learned helplessness that reduce their likelihood to communicate in future situations (R. L. Koegel & Mentis, 1985). Therefore, the motivational principles of PRT aim to help individuals with ASD overcome symptoms of learned helplessness by teaching them that their behavior (e.g., communication) can have a positive impact on the outcome.

It is also important to point out that PRT is a naturalistic intervention designed to be implemented throughout everyday routines. **Naturalistic interventions** embed procedures in the context of naturally occurring, typical activities, and these strategies have been shown to improve generalization across settings and increase maintenance following intervention. Table 13.1 describes naturalistic versus structured (analog) treatment procedures. As opposed to analog procedures that are directed by a clinician, involve drilling of the target behavior until acquisition is reached, and incorporate arbitrary reinforcers, PRT strategies are interspersed into everyday activities across multiple settings by many individuals who work with the child (Koegel & Koegel, 2006; R. L. Koegel, O'Dell, & Koegel, 1987). During PRT sessions, stimulus items are functional and chosen by the child, communicative attempts are rewarded, and natural reinforcers are provided that directly relate to the task (R. L. Koegel, O'Dell, & Koegel, 1987; R. L. Koegel & Williams, 1980; Mirenda-Linne & Melin, 1992). Procedures are implemented in the environment where the skills will be needed (i.e., home, school, community), so individuals with ASD can rapidly produce gains and generalize and maintain them after intervention (Brown & Odom, 1995; Koegel & Koegel, 2006; McGee et al., 1984).

PRT supports the principle that parents are a necessary, integral, and essential part of the intervention program (R. L. Koegel et al., 1998; Koegel & Koegel,

Table 13.1.　Analog versus Pivotal Response Treatment procedures

	Analog condition	Pivotal Response Treatment condition
Stimulus items	Clinician chooses the item.	Child chooses the item.
	Clinician repeats the stimulus until criterion is met.	Clinician varies items every few trials.
		Clinician places age-appropriate items in the child's natural environment.
Prompts	Prompts are manual (e.g., touch tip of tongue or hold lips together).	Clinician models the name of the item.
Interaction	Clinician holds up stimulus item; stimulus item is not functional within the interaction.	Clinician and child play with the stimulus item; stimulus item is functional within the interaction.
Response	Clinician reinforces only correct responses or successive approximations.	This is a looser shaping contingency; clinician reinforces attempts and good tries at verbal responses.
Consequence	Clinician pairs edible reinforcers with social reinforcers (e.g., "Good job!").	Clinician pairs natural reinforcer (e.g., opportunity to play with the requested item) with social reinforcers.

1996; R. L. Koegel, O'Dell, & Koegel, 1987; R. L. Koegel & Williams, 1980; McGee et al., 1984; Mirenda-Linne & Melin, 1992). Research has shown that parents of children with autism can effectively implement behavioral, social, and communication procedures and that including parents results in greater gains and generalization of skills (Alpert & Kaiser, 1992; R. L. Koegel et al., 1978; Koegel & Koegel, 2006; Minjarez et al., 2011). PRT highly emphasizes parent education by providing hands-on practice with feedback so that parents can directly work with their child on target goals.

Underlying Assumptions

An important belief underlying PRT is that children with ASD have the potential to and are capable of learning to communicate and socially interact. Historically, researchers were uncertain whether individuals with ASD were unable to learn or whether variables could be adjusted to increase their learning ability (R. L. Koegel & Egel, 1979; R. L. Koegel & Mentis, 1985). Research revealed that many children with ASD do in fact have the ability to perform targeted behaviors and learn new skills, but teaching procedures often have to be modified. PRT modifies traditional teaching by allowing the child to direct activities in teaching and by providing natural reinforcement for responses and attempts. Through these procedures, responses are meaningful and produce positive outcomes, and therefore, individuals are more motivated to engage in the teaching interactions. PRT approaches social-communication challenges as both a skill and performance difficulty, and the intervention strives to reduce the gap in what individuals with ASD are capable of performing and what they actually perform in their day-to-day life.

Functional Outcomes

PRT first targets an individual's motivation to participate in intervention, which has then been shown to produce rapid and broad gains. By increasing a child's motivation to engage during the habilitation process, acquisition of goals is more rapid. By using naturalistic behavioral strategies, children learn the meaning and function of communication skills. The goal is that children learn socially significant skills that will have a meaningful impact on their long-term outcome and quality of life.

Since PRT focuses on pivotal areas and motivating the child, teaching each distinct behavior is not necessary. To demonstrate the power of motivation and targeting pivotal areas, consider a common application of PRT. The procedures are often implemented to help increase a child's motivation to ask questions (e.g., what, where, who questions). By targeting question-asking, the child will also experience collateral improvements in vocabulary, pronouns, prepositions, and social interaction. As well, improved long-term outcomes have been noted when children are taught to initiate, such as learning how to ask questions to show interest and engage in reciprocal interactions (L. K. Koegel, Koegel, Shoshan, & McNerney, 1999). Furthermore, increasing children's motivation to use verbal language to communicate their wants and needs and socially interact collaterally decreases their use of escape-, attention-seeking-, and avoidance-motivated disruptive behaviors (R. L. Koegel et al., 1992; Mohammadzaheri et al., 2014) and results in improved affect during their interactions (Dunlap, 1984). To summarize, PRT focuses on core, pivotal areas in order to produce broad gains and many positive and functional outcomes.

Target Area of Treatment

PRT is an intervention that can be used with individuals during all stages of language development. As previously mentioned, PRT is effective with infants (L. K. Koegel, Singh, et. al., 2014), school-age children (Mohammadzaheri et al., 2014), and adolescents (R. L. Koegel et al., 2013), and adults (L. K. Koegel et. al., 2013), and the therapy can be applied from basic to advanced language and communication skills. Extensive studies have shown that PRT is effective in increasing language and communication skills for individuals with ASD (see Table 13.2). The same core

Table 13.2. Levels of evidence for selected studies of treatment efficacy for Pivotal Response Treatment

Level	Description	References supporting the intervention
Ia	Meta-analysis of >1 randomized, controlled trial (RCT)	Bozkus-Genc & Verun (2013) Bozkus-Genc & Yucesoy-Ozkan (2016) Cadogan & McCrimmon (2015) Lei & Ventola (2017) Verschuur et al. (2014)
Ib	RCT	Gengoux et al. (2015) Hardan et al. (2015) Mohammadzaheri et al. (2014) Mohammadzaheri et al. (2015) Nefdt et al. (2010)
IIa	Controlled study without randomization	**Core Components** of Pivotal Response Treatment (PRT) ***Motivation*** R. L. Koegel & Egel (1979) ***Child Choice*** R. L. Koegel, Dyer, & Bell (1987) ***Reinforcing Attempts*** R. L. Koegel et al. (1988) ***Task Variation*** Dunlap & Koegel (1980) ***Natural Reinforcers*** R. L. Koegel & Williams (1980) Williams et al. (1981) ***Initiations as a Pivotal Area*** L. K. Koegel, Koegel, et al. (2010) L. K. Koegel et al. (2003) L. K. Koegel et al. (1998) ***PRT With Infants*** L. K. Koegel, Singh, et al. (2014) Steiner et al. (2013) ***PRT With Adolescents and Adults*** Ashbaugh et al. (2017) R. L. Koegel et al. (2013) ***PRT for Academics*** L. K. Koegel et al. (1997) L. K. Koegel, Singh, & Koegel (2010)

Table 13.2. *(continued)*

Level	Description	References supporting the intervention
		PRT for Disruptive Behavior L. K. Koegel et al., Koegel, Hurley, & Frea (1992) Koegel, Koegel, & Surratt (1992)
		PRT for Speech and Language Koegel, O'Dell, & Koegel (1987) Koegel, Camarata, Koegel, Ben-Tall, & Smith, (1998) Smith & Camarata (1999)
		PRT for Social Skills Harper, Symon, & Frea (2008) Koegel, Kuriakose, Singh, & Koegel (2012) Pierce & Schreibman (1995) Stahmer (1995)
		PRT Parent Education Coolican, Smith, & Bryson (2010) Gillett, & LeBlanc (2007) Laski, Charlop, & Schreibman (1988)
		Neurology and PRT Venkataraman, Yang, Dvornek, Staib, Duncan, Pelphrey, & Ventola (2016) Ventola, Yang, Friedman, Oosting, Wolf, Sukhodolsky, & Pelphrey (2015) Voos, Pelphrey, Tirrell, Bolling, Vander Wyk, Kaiser, McPartland, Volkmar, & Ventola (2013)
IIb	Quasi-experimental study	Duifhuis, den Boer, Doornbos, A., Buitelaar, Oosterling, & Klip (2017)
III	Nonexperimental studies (i.e., correlational and case studies)	Buckley, Ente, & Ruef (2014)
IV	Expert committee report, consensus conference, clinical experience of respected authorities	National Autism Center (2015) National Research Council (2001) Wilczynski (2010) Wong, Odom, Hume, Cox, Fettig, Kucharczyk, Brock, Plavnick, Fleury, & Schultz (2015)

Note: A sample of studies were selected from the many that have been conducted for the sake of brevity. No studies were found that did not support the intervention.

components of PRT can be used to target a variety of different language and social-communication skills, including the following:

- Communicative intent

- Speech intelligibility

- First words

- Two-word combinations

- Responsiveness to multiple cues rather than focusing on a single, often irrelevant, cue

- Verb diversity and verb tenses

- Full sentences

- Syntax

- Question-asking ("What's that?" "Where is it?")

- Initiations and social bids

- Social conversation (greeting, expressing interest, commenting, responding, empathy)

In addition to expressive language skills, PRT can be used to target the following areas:

- Social interaction during play dates

- Academics (e.g., math, writing, reading)

- Motor skills (e.g., writing)

- Socialization

- Daily living skills

- Executive functioning

- Employment skills

EMPIRICAL BASIS

The effectiveness of incorporating PRT motivational procedures has been documented in hundreds of single-subject design studies (Koegel & Koegel, 2019) as well as randomized clinical trials (Gengoux et al., 2015; Hardan et al., 2015; Mohammadzaheri et al., 2015). PRT has been determined to have strong empirical support by the National Standards Project (Wilczynski, 2010), by the National Research Council (2001), and in peer-reviewed publications (Wong et al., 2015). Table 13.2 summarizes some of the strongest studies conducted on PRT. The table is not exhaustive given the very large number of studies that have been undertaken.

Substantial research supports each of the motivational components of PRT in addition to the packaged intervention (Dunlap & Koegel, 1980; R. L. Koegel, Dyer, & Bell, 1987; R. L. Koegel et al., 1992; R. L. Koegel et al., 1988; Williams et al., 1981). First, research has shown that if an individual has a choice over the activities during teaching sessions, he or she will perform better, sustain engagement, and display less disruptive behavior (R. L. Koegel, Dyer, & Bell, 1987). Studies also support task variation, and research shows that interspersing previously mastered (maintenance) tasks with the more difficult target (acquisition) tasks results in faster learning, decreased disruptive behavior, and improved affect (Dunlap, 1984). Furthermore, there is evidence that tying the reward directly to the child's response results in greater learning (Williams et al., 1981). Lastly, research supports the strategy of rewarding attempts. Reinforcing a child's clear attempt, even if it is not perfect, will increase acquisition of verbal communication (R. L. Koegel et al., 1988).

PRT combines the motivational components described previously with substantial research to show that the packaged intervention can have a significant impact in the areas of language, communication, social skills, and academics (Koegel & Koegel,

2019). Initially, the empirical evidence showed that these components could be combined as a package to increase verbal communication in children with significant communication delays (R. L. Koegel, O'Dell, & Koegel, 1987). In this early study, children who were nonverbal increased their verbal responding when the traditional ABA approach was manipulated to include motivational components now regularly used in PRT. The approach, then referred to as the **Natural Language Paradigm** (NLP), led to the development of PRT.

Since this initial study in 1987, the primary motivational variables and components of PRT have remained largely the same. Research has shown that parents could easily learn to implement the NLP/PRT procedures (Laski et al., 1988). Further, children with ASD exhibited lower levels of untreated disruptive behavior when these motivational variables were incorporated into the intervention sessions (R. L. Koegel et al., 1992). This improvement was notable, as many children with ASD demonstrated disruptive behaviors when the traditional ABA intervention (without the motivational components incorporated) was implemented. Decreases in avoidance- and escape-motivated disruptive behavior fortuitously reduced the need for punishment. Further research also showed that parents demonstrate lower levels of stress when motivational components were incorporated (R. L. Koegel et al., 1996). This is important because clinicians recruit parents to be active participants in PRT, so they must assure them that the demands of implementing intervention are decreasing their stress. Subsequent to this initial research showing that the PRT motivational procedures were effective for teaching first words and language while also reducing disruptive behavior, additional studies showed that the PRT motivational procedures resulted in improvements in other behaviors, including symbolic play (Stahmer, 1995), socio-dramatic play (Thorp et al., 1995), social behavior (Pierce & Schreibman, 1997), speech intelligibility (R. L. Koegel et al., 1998), and academics such as math and writing (L. K. Koegel, Singh, & Koegel, 2010).

Randomized control trials have compared PRT with a more structured ABA approach in a school setting (Mohammadzaheri et al., 2014; Mohammadzaheri et al., 2015). In the first study by Mohammadzaheri and colleagues (2014), data indicated that the PRT approach was significantly more effective than ABA in improving targeted and untargeted areas after 3 months of intervention. Specifically, the mean length of utterance (MLU) of children in the structured ABA group improved slightly but nonsignificantly following intervention, whereas children in the PRT group showed significantly greater gains in MLU [$F(1, 27) = 6.97, p = .01$]. Another randomized control trial by Mohammadzaheri and colleagues (2015) used the same dataset to evaluate disruptive behavior during language intervention in public schools. Results showed that while the adult-directed ABA group showed a statistically significant change in disruptive behavior over time ($t = 4.5, p < .001$), the magnitude of those changes was small (1.2 minutes). The PRT group showed statistically significant ($t = 30, p < .0001$) and large decreases in levels of disruptive behavior over time (9.9 minutes). These results are consistent with the single case experimental designs that show when motivational components are included in the intervention, then disruptive behaviors are lower and targeted gains are greater (R. L. Koegel et al., 1992).

Other research showed that implementing the motivational procedures during standardized test taking could produce highly different test outcomes in regard to vocabulary, language, and intelligence scores (L. K. Koegel et al., 1997). That is, a study by L. K. Koegel and colleagues (1997) implemented 44 testing sessions across six children who demonstrated high levels of disruptive behavior. When motivation was included during the testing (which was administered according to the standard protocol), the children always scored higher on the tests. In fact, some of the children were scored as having severe intellectual and linguistic disabilities when the motivational variables were not incorporated and within average range when they were. This is important, as many children with ASD have difficulty responding on standardized tests, which can have implications for placement and goals. In addition to improvements in targeted areas, research has shown collateral gains in untreated areas when using the motivational procedures, including decreases in disruptive behavior (mentioned previously), improvements in joint attention (Vismara & Lyons, 2007), decreases in restricted and repetitive behaviors (Koegel, Koegel, & Surratt, 1992), and improved child affect (Dunlap, 1984).

Various methods of PRT dissemination have been evaluated. Since parents often experience lengthy wait lists before securing early intervention services, researchers have assessed whether PRT can be effectively implemented and beneficial with different short-term parent education models. Hardan and colleagues (2015) conducted a randomized controlled trial to evaluate a PRT parent training group for targeting language impairments in young children with ASD. In this study, 84% of parents in the PRT parent training group met **fidelity of implementation** (FoI) after 12 weekly training sessions. Furthermore, compared to children in the parent psychoeducation group, children in the PRT parent training group demonstrated greater frequency of utterances [$F(2, 43) = 3.53$, $p = .038$, $d = 0.42$]. A follow-up study by Gengoux and colleagues (2015) assessed maintenance of treatment effects 3 months after completion of the PRT parent training group. Results of this study indicated a significant improvement in frequency of functional utterances, with maintenance at 3-month follow-up [$F(2, 21) = 5.9$, $p = .009$]. Data also showed that children made significant gains on the Vineland Communication domain standard score [$F(2, 12) = 11.74$, $p = .001$] and the Mullen Scales of Early Learning composite score [$F(1, 20) = 5.43$, $p = .03$]. These studies indicate that parents can learn how to effectively implement PRT and that children produce more frequent utterances, with gains maintained posttreatment (Gengoux et al., 2015; Hardan et al., 2015). Such research shows the flexibility of PRT and that it can be effectively implemented in a time- and cost-efficient manner through a parent education model and a group educational format.

PRACTICAL REQUIREMENTS

Children receiving PRT services are typically provided with 10–30 hours per week of intervention services provided by a trained professional, with parent education being an important component. There are three levels of professionals working within the treatment team, although the exact implementation may vary depending on the needs of the child. The team typically includes one to three clinicians who work individually with the child and conduct the majority of the direct intervention hours with the child, a program supervisor/parent educator, a master's- or doctoral-level clinical supervisor, and the parent(s).

The main role of the clinician is to conduct direct intervention and record ongoing data on the child's goals. Clinicians must have a strong knowledge of the history and methodology of PRT, as well as hands-on training and supervised experience delivering it. Whenever possible, clinicians implement the intervention sessions across all environments in which the child regularly participates, including home, school, extra-curricular activities (e.g., sports, clubs, child care), and other community settings. Clinicians are also trained in data-collection procedures and are adept at recording representative probe data throughout the intervention sessions.

The role of the program supervisor/parent educator is to help determine appropriate goals for the child in coordination with the parents/caregivers and the supervisor, conduct parent education sessions, collect and analyze data, supervise the clinician, and assist with progress report writing. The program supervisor/parent educator typically conducts parent education sessions a minimum of 2–3 hours per week with a family. During parent education sessions, the parent is provided with hands-on training on how to implement the intervention strategies through practice with feedback. The parent educator first models the intervention for a particular target behavior, then steps back and, while providing guidance and feedback, has the parents practice working directly with their child. To ensure that the parent knows exactly what techniques he or she is implementing correctly or incorrectly, the parent educator regularly assesses the parent's FoI. Procedures for assessing PRT FoI are described later in the chapter. When reviewing for FoI, it is important that the parent educator provides both praise in procedures that the parent is implementing well and constructive feedback and ideas for improvement in procedures that are not being implemented or are being implemented incorrectly. It is sometimes helpful to videotape the parent working with the child to review one-to-one with the parent, but most frequently feedback is provided in vivo.

A clinical supervisor leads the child's treatment program and must have at least a master's-level education and extensive experience with PRT. Clinical supervisors often have a PhD and are licensed (generally in psychology, speech-language pathology, or a related area) or are certified with the Behavior Analyst Certification Board. Their role within the team is to help determine appropriate goals for the child, conduct assessments, write progress reports, and supervise the program supervisor or parent educator and clinicians.

If individuals want to become trained PRT therapists, there is a PRT certification program. The goal of the PRT certification program is to provide professionals with an effective and efficient mechanism for receiving training in PRT in order to achieve FoI in each core procedural area. There are five levels of certification; more information on these levels can be found at http://www.autismprthelp.com.

KEY COMPONENTS

The key components of PRT include motivating the child, improving the child's verbal expressive communication, encouraging initiations and self-management, and fostering participation of peers and siblings. Dosage and fidelity of implementation are also important aspects of intervention.

Motivational Components

The PRT intervention model comprises a package of six motivational components: offering child choice, varying the nature of the task, interspersing maintenance and acquisition tasks, using natural rewards, and reinforcing attempts. Two other

Table 13.3. Motivational components of Pivotal Response Treatment

Pivotal Response Treatment procedure	Description	Example
Clear prompts	Get the child's attention and provide a clear and concise prompt for language (model, verbal, or time delay prompt).	Put a desired item in sight but out of reach, get child's attention, and prompt "help?"
Child choice	Child directs activities used for teaching; adult has control over the activity.	Use child's favorite toys or activities (e.g., book, tickle), and prompt child to say the word to request the toy or activity.
Task variation	Intersperse many easy tasks with a few acquisition tasks in teaching.	Prompt child for mostly single words (e.g., *car*) and occasionally a two-word utterance (e.g., *want car*).
Contingent reinforcement	Immediately reward child for appropriate response; do not reward child for no response or inappropriate response.	Child says "bubbles," and adult immediately blows bubbles; child whines and grabs bubbles, and adult does not blow bubbles.
Direct and natural reinforcement	Reward directly relates to the language spoken by child.	Child says "ball" and then gets to play with a ball.
Reinforce attempts	Reasonable attempts that are clear and goal oriented are reinforced.	Child says "cook" for cookie or "wawa" for water, and child is immediately given a cookie or water.

components include providing clear prompts and contingent reinforcement (see Table 13.3). The following section provides a description of each key component of PRT.

Offering Child Choice **Child choice** refers to a variety of techniques used to incorporate a child's interests into the intervention. When child choice is incorporated into the intervention, there is an increase in responsiveness and engagement and a reduction in avoidance behaviors (R. L. Koegel, Dyer, & Bell, 1987). Child choice can include using stimulus items and activities that are highly preferred by the specific child, allowing the child (as opposed to the adult) to direct the flow of learning or providing choices during otherwise nonpreferred or neutral activities. For example, if a child enjoys turning lights on and off, using a variety of light-up toys and prompting language related to turning the toys on and off can be incorporated during intervention. Opportunities for choice can also be provided throughout all of the child's natural routines, such as breakfast (e.g., cereal or fruit), getting dressed (e.g., blue pants or green pants), homework (e.g., table or desk, pen or pencil), and bath time (e.g., different toys to play with in the bath, bubbles).

Varying the Nature of the Task **Task variation** refers to a change made to the more traditional ABA approach of providing opportunities and tasks in a drill-type format. Rather than providing the same opportunity or demand repeatedly, opportunities are interspersed into play and natural routines. For example, rather than drilling the child on the color blue 10 trials in a row, an interventionist may be playing Legos with the child and prompt "blue" for a blue Lego. Then, the next opportunity might be the prompt "put it on" to put a Lego block on top of another, then "red" for a red Lego, and so forth. This task variation helps to ensure that the child remains engaged and interested in the learning opportunities, leading to higher levels of successful responding (Dunlap & Koegel, 1980).

Interspersing Maintenance and Acquisition Tasks   Interspersing maintenance and acquisition tasks refers to the importance of not only introducing new acquisition tasks during intervention sessions but also incorporating previously acquired maintenance tasks that the child can successfully complete with relative ease. When only acquisition tasks are presented, children can become frustrated and motivated to leave the session. However, when children are presented with a string of easier maintenance tasks for which they can be reinforced, they are motivated to engage in the session and are more likely to respond when an acquisition task is presented, most likely because of behavioral momentum. With the interspersal of maintenance and acquisition, again, we see improved affect and faster treatment gains (Dunlap, 1984).

Using Natural Rewards   Using natural rewards that are directly related to the behavior being taught is another motivational component that leads to faster acquisition of targets and increased generalization (R. L. Koegel & Williams, 1980). In the more traditional ABA approaches, reinforcement was often social praise paired with an edible reinforcer. For example, if a child correctly labeled a picture of a train, the interventionist would say, "Good job," or "That's right," and hand the child a candy. When using natural rewards, the reinforcement is either an item or action directly related to the behavior. So, if the goal were to teach a child the word *train*, the interventionist would give the child a toy train to play with as the reinforcer for making a good verbal attempt at the word.

Reinforcing Attempts   Reinforcing attempts refers to rewarding a child's efforts, rather than only correct responses or closer approximations. Within the PRT framework, any reasonable response that is clear, unambiguous, and goal oriented should be rewarded. When a child is rewarded for trying, rather than only for successive approximations, he or she will be more responsive and engaged during teaching sessions, leading to faster gains (R. L. Koegel et al., 1988). For example, if a child is learning two-word combinations and says "boo bah" while reaching for a blue ball, the pronunciation may not be perfect, but it is very clear what the child is requesting, and so he or she should be immediately reinforced by being handed the blue ball to play with even if the response was not as good as or better than the previous attempt.

Using Clear Prompts and Contingent Reinforcement   In addition to the core motivational components described previously, providing clear prompts and contingent reinforcement also play important roles within the PRT framework. Gaining the child's attention prior to providing a prompt is essential to setting up a successful opportunity. Once you have the child's attention, use straightforward language to make the expectation very clear. Appropriate prompts for language include full verbal model prompts (i.e., say the exact word or phrase you want the child to repeat), open-ended questions (e.g., "What do you want?"), and time delays (i.e., holding up an item or pausing in a sequence of actions and waiting expectantly for the child to make a verbal request). Then, as soon as the child makes a good attempt at the target utterance, immediately provide the naturally reinforcing item or action. If the child does not respond appropriately or engages in disruptive or inappropriate behavior (e.g., grabbing, hitting, crying), do not provide reinforcement. Instead, either present the prompt again or put that item or activity away and move on to something else. Providing contingent reinforcement means that the child's access to the motivating item or action is dependent on his or her appropriate verbalization.

The motivational components described previously are consistently used in treatment, whether the target goal is communication, academics, play, socialization, or self-help areas. More detailed information about each PRT component and how to implement procedures can be found in *Pivotal Response Treatment®: Using motivation as a Pivotal Response* (L. K. Koegel, 2011). This manual is available at www.autismprthelp.com or on Amazon.

Teaching Verbal Expressive Communication

One of the main focuses of PRT is improving the child's verbal expressive communication, so this is often the first area addressed, with the bulk of the intervention hours often focusing on social communication. For example, when teaching a child his or her first words, a clinician will start by finding items or activities that are highly preferred for the specific child in order to motivate the child to make expressive verbal communicative attempts. The clinician models the word as a communicative prompt (e.g., "ball?" "tickle?" "cookie?" "swing?"), and when the child makes a verbal attempt or produces the correct word, he or she is immediately reinforced by being provided with that corresponding natural reinforcer (e.g., the chance to play with a ball, be tickled, get a cookie, be pushed on the swing). There should be a direct and functional connection between the prompt for language, the child's behavior (i.e., verbal attempt), and the delivery of the reinforcer. (See Figure 13.1 for an illustration of this sequence.) Often, this requires replacing the previous communicative behavior (e.g., crying, grabbing, whining) with the appropriate word or word attempt. Thus, these earlier communicative behaviors need to be ignored so they become nonfunctional for the child. Despite this, clinicians remain

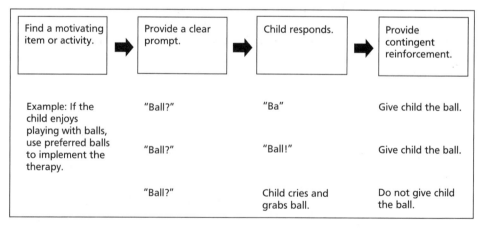

Figure 13.1. Teaching verbal communication through clear prompts and contingent reinforcement.

playful during sessions. The goal is not to punish the child but to teach the child that appropriate communication can have a positive outcome and is more useful than disruptive or inappropriate communicative behaviors. Opportunities for verbal communication are created as often as possible and can be requests for items (e.g., milk), social interaction (e.g., up), or activities (e.g., swing). Once the child is using a large number of single words to communicate, clinicians can target more complex language. The goal is to provide frequent and ongoing teaching opportunities, as research indicates that the greatest outcomes are correlated with parents who provide very frequent PRT opportunities for their child with high FoI (Koegel & Koegel, 2019).

Other Pivotal Areas

In addition to motivation, initiations and self-management are considered pivotal areas and are therefore important elements of PRT methodology. Teaching children to initiate is an important goal in PRT. Research has shown that when motivational components, such as child choice and natural rewards, are incorporated into teaching initiations, the children not only learned to ask spontaneous *wh-* questions (e.g., "What's that?" "Where is it?" "Whose is it?" "What happened?") and generalized these initiated questions outside of sessions but also made improvements in their vocabulary and use of prepositions, appropriate verb endings, and pronouns (L. K. Koegel, Koegel, Shoshan, & McNerney, 1999). For example, to teach the question, "What's that?" clinicians place child preferred items in an opaque bag and then prompt the child to ask, "What's that?" As soon as the child makes a good verbal attempt, clinicians take a preferred item out of the bag, label it for the child, and hand it to the child as the natural reward. Eventually, clinicians add novel items to the bag and prompt the question within natural routines (e.g., if a child shows interest in a new item that he or she does not know the label for). Other types of initiations, such as asking for help, seeking attention from others, and initiating social conversation can also be taught and allow the individual to become a more active participant in his or her environment and to engage in increased and improved social interactions.

Self-management involves teaching an individual to discriminate, monitor, and modify his or her own behavior. Essentially, the individual is taught the target behavior, then he or she records each occurrence of the behavior and receives a reward once the goal has been reached. For example, a child may be given the goal of asking five questions during a social conversation. During the conversation, the child marks down each time he or she asks a question, and once he or she has reached five, the child gets to play a favorite game. Through the use of self-management procedures such as these, behavioral control is transferred from the interventionist to the individual with ASD, thereby promoting independence and reducing the need for supervision and prompting from another person. Self-management procedures can be effectively utilized across a wide variety of target behaviors, including social conversation skills, appropriate replacement behaviors for disruptive or repetitive behavior, and daily living skills (L. K. Koegel et al., 1992; L. K. Koegel, Park, & Koegel, 2014). More information about how to teach initiations and self-management can be found in training manuals available at http://www.autismprthelp.com/books-and -manuals.php or on Amazon.

Participation of Peers and Siblings

In addition to parents and caregivers, siblings and peers are included in the intervention whenever possible. Siblings and peers are especially important when working on social skills and can and should be included when targeting other areas as well. Siblings and peers can be included as play partners and can also learn how to prompt and reinforce the child with ASD. In addition to learning to interact with adults, it is important for the child with autism to learn to respond to and initiate communications with similar-age individuals.

Dosage

Typically, formal intervention sessions are conducted once per day, five times per week. Depending on the number of intervention hours authorized (typically by the family's insurance provider, school, or another third-party payer) and individual need, such sessions usually range from 1 to 3 hours. Nonetheless, as mentioned throughout this chapter, parents, caregivers, teachers, and others are trained in how to incorporate PRT techniques into their natural daily routine so that children can receive consistent PRT intervention throughout the day, outside of designated therapy sessions. Therefore, although a child may be spending 10 hours per week engaged in intervention sessions conducted by or in coordination with a PRT professional, in theory, the child should receive a consistent PRT intervention program throughout all of his or her waking hours.

Fidelity of Implementation

Scoring clinicians and team members for FoI is a key element of PRT, designed to ensure that the child is receiving effective treatment. If a child is getting 30 or more hours a week of intervention, but the person implementing that intervention is not doing it correctly, it is unlikely that the child will make significant progress. These FoI checks can be assessed in either vivo during live sessions or through video review, depending on individual availability and preference.

FoI checks are typically 10-minute probes, broken down into 1-minute intervals. The implementer is asked to interact with the child and use PRT to target verbal language. For each interval, the participant is scored on his or her implementation of each core component of PRT: clear opportunities, child choice (shared control), interspersal of maintenance and acquisition tasks/task variation, contingent reinforcement, natural reinforcement, and reward attempts. To receive a passing score for one interval in one component, the participant must have correctly implemented that component across the majority of his or her language opportunities provided during that interval. For example, consider a clinician who gives three language opportunities in minute 5. During two of those opportunities, she has the child's attention, but during one of the opportunities, the child is distracted by another toy. Because she had the child's attention during the majority of opportunities given in that minute, she would still receive a passing score for clear opportunities for minute 5. However, if she had the child's attention for only one of the three opportunities, she would not receive a passing score for that minute interval. If no language opportunities are given in a minute interval, each component is scored as not passing for that interval. To receive a passing score for the entire 10-minute FoI probe, the participant must receive at least 80% (8 of 10 intervals) passing scores across all six components, and at least two trials per minute must be implemented. See Figure 13.2 for a sample FoI datasheet.

One-minute intervals	Clear prompts	Child choice (shared control)	Task variation	Contingent (immediate) reinforcement	Natural reinforcers	Reward attempts
1						
2						
3						
4						
5						
6						
7						
8						
9						
10						
Percentage (%)						

TOTAL:_____

Directions

Score each category as + or −.

Score entire 1-minute interval as − if no opportunities for language are provided.

Operational definitions

1. *Clear prompts.* Parent provides concise commands, clear opportunities for verbal responses, or clear instructions to the child (e.g., showing a toy, asking a clear question, labeling an object) and is able to maintain the child's attention either to the task or to the adult while presenting the instructions during the entire 1-minute interval.

2. *Child choice.* Parent does any of the following: 1) provides two or more alternatives from which the child may choose, 2) allows the child to accept or reject an activity, 3) prompts the child to select an activity from an open-ended question, 4) follows the child's lead in selecting activities by responding to the child's verbal or nonverbal initiations of choosing an activity.

3. *Task variation.* Parent provides many maintenance tasks (tasks that are easy and familiar and that the child has already mastered) in addition to acquisition tasks (more difficult tasks that the child is still learning). *Do not score unless you know the child.*

4. *Contingent (immediate) reinforcement.* Parent provides a reward immediately following the child's correct verbal response or attempt. Parent does not provide a reward if the child does not respond or responds inappropriately (i.e., disruptive). *If the parent is not contingent, he or she automatically receives a − for natural reinforcers and reward attempts.*

5. *Natural reinforcers.* Parent provides a contingent reward that is directly related to the child's expressive verbalizations rather than providing a reward that is unrelated to the child's expressive verbalization.

6. *Reward attempts.* Parent provides contingent rewards that are delivered following both the child's functional expressive verbal attempts and the child's fully correct verbal responses.

Figure 13.2. Fidelity of implementation scoring sheet.

ASSESSMENT FOR TREATMENT PLANNING AND PROGRESS MONITORING

Standardized measures often are inaccurate for individuals with ASD. These measures may underestimate their abilities (L. K. Koegel et al., 1997), so direct observation across multiple environments is an important tool for identifying appropriate goals and should be included in each child's individualized intervention program. Direct observation generally includes the collection of language samples (usually with a parent and with peers) as well as behavioral observations in various settings. In addition, parent/caregiver interviews, such as the Vineland Adaptive Behavior Scales–Second Edition (Vineland-2; Sparrow et al., 2005), can also be used to assess behaviors that may not occur during the observations (e.g., self-help skills). Because PRT focuses on pivotal areas and motivating the child, teaching each individual behavior is not necessary. Rather, the focus is on determining socially significant goals that will have a meaningful impact on that individual's quality of life.

For the majority of treatment goals, probe data are collected. It is important to keep in mind that while data collection is necessary in order to track progress and monitor the effectiveness of the intervention, it should not be so cumbersome that it interferes with the actual intervention. Because PRT requires the interspersal of different targets rather than repeated trials, and it is done within the context of play and natural routines, an all-in-one datasheet that includes all of the goals on one page is the most effective way to collect data. Research suggests that when the clinician can take one sheet of paper with him or her and have quick access to record on all goals, the clinician can collect data more frequently (Renshaw & Kuriakose, 2011).

IMPLICATIONS FOR INCLUSIVE PRACTICE

PRT aims to provide opportunities for learning within the context of the individual's natural environments. As well, PRT encourages the child with ASD to participate in inclusive settings, such as general education classrooms, inclusive after-school activities, and other activities in which the child would participate if he or she did not have a disability (Harrower & Dunlap, 2001). PRT teaching can take place across many inclusive settings and should be implemented consistently by a variety of individuals as an effective means of increasing skill acquisition, generalization, and maintenance of gains (Brown & Odom, 1995; Koegel & Koegel, 2006; McGee et al., 1984).

Table 13.4 shows common natural and inclusive environments that are used in PRT. In such settings, natural and desired items and activities individualized for each child help them learn functional communication and promote the transfer of skills to everyday life (Kaiser & Trent, 2007; L. K. Koegel et al., 1998). As mentioned previously, a core component of PRT is child choice and direct and natural reinforcers. Thus, if the child is interested in trucks, trucks are used during teaching trials. If the child enjoys reading books, language opportunities can be created within the context of books. The same core components of PRT can be implemented in any environment and within any activity. Intervention should not be considered or designated as work time. Instead, trials are woven into enjoyable activities throughout the day.

Importantly, PRT has been researched and used in classroom settings (Stahmer et al., 2011). For example, teachers and paraprofessionals can be effectively taught

Table 13.4.   Implementing Pivotal Response Treatment in inclusive settings

Inclusive environments for Pivotal Response Treatment	Natural treatment providers
Inclusive classrooms	Parents
Summer camps	Siblings
Extracurricular activities	Peers
Parks	Teachers
Restaurants	Child care providers
Outside games	Extended family
Play dates	
Home	

to incorporate a child's interests into lessons, make sure the student is paying attention before providing a cue, provide a clear and appropriate cue, mix easy and difficult tasks, establish shared control, provide reinforcement that is naturally and directly related to the activity, present immediate and contingent reinforcement, and reinforce the student's attempts (Stahmer et al., 2011).

CONSIDERATIONS FOR CHILDREN FROM CULTURALLY AND LINGUISTICALLY DIVERSE BACKGROUNDS

Ecocultural theory states that it is critical to take into account the family's perspective when developing goals and treatment plans for individuals with ASD (Bernheimer et al., 1990). Before implementing intervention, it is important to understand the child's autism as it is perceived by the family; strive to understand the family's unique goals, values, and needs; and collaborate on how to incorporate the family's cultural beliefs and daily routines into treatment (Ennis-Cole et al., 2013; Koegel & Koegel, 2019; Ravindran & Myers, 2012). Although the components of PRT are specific, they are easily adaptable to each unique child and family.

Children diagnosed with ASD represent great diversity in regard to symptomology (Harrower & Dunlap, 2001). As well, learning curves vary depending on child characteristics, family support, access to services, family competency, and other environmental variables (Wilder et al., 2004). Treatment plans must consider cultural and linguistic diversity. Prior to beginning PRT intervention, providers should consider the family's culture, goals, values, and needs during assessment and intervention planning (Ennis-Cole et al., 2013; Harry et al., 1995; Wilder et al., 2004). It is also important to understand the child's and family's routines and priorities in order to create a treatment plan that is feasible for the family and mutually acceptable (Ennis-Cole et al., 2013; Ravindran & Myers, 2012). So much of the intervention is dependent on the child's interests, daily routines, and parent involvement that it is critical to understand the child and family before procedures are employed. In addition, the child's outcomes should be meaningful in relation to the family's beliefs and values. Although the provider may have his or her own idea about priorities to target with the child, it is important to collaborate and understand what skills and behaviors are important for the family. Discussing the short- and long-term goals for the child, family roles, expectations of treatment, potential barriers to treatment, and strengths of the family is critical if the family is expected to consistently implement the intervention (Ennis-Cole et al., 2013; Harry et al., 1995; Ravindran & Myers, 2012).

When implementing PRT to improve social skills and social interactions, it is especially important to take into account the cultural context. Different cultures and diverse backgrounds have varying social norms, expectations, and behaviors, and the first step in using PRT to teach social skills is understanding the appropriate social behaviors for the family (Ennis-Cole et al., 2013; Harry et al., 1995). It is critical to learn what the appropriate verbal and nonverbal behaviors are for the child and other family members in order to tailor treatment techniques. Areas such as greetings, commenting, question-asking, sharing, leading, empathy, nonverbal pragmatics, and affect may vary depending on the culture and background of the family (Wilder et al., 2004).

Clinicians should take the time to consciously explore the unique background, diversity factors, life experiences, and strengths of each child with autism. It is essential to cultivate understanding of the child as a whole individual rather than as a presenting problem (Harry et al., 1995). Clinicians and treatment providers should constantly strive to practice cultural awareness and consider multicultural and diversity issues as key components to case conceptualization and treatment planning (Koegel & Koegel, 2019).

Application to a Child

Videoclips of Anthony at his 1-year birthday party showed that he was nonverbal, did not respond to his name, and did not interact with other children or with adults. However, he did hum the first line of "Happy Birthday" repeatedly. At 1 year, his parents did not recognize the differences in his development. In fact, the video shows them attempting to explain his behavior; his dad called his name while filming, and when he failed to respond, his mother replied with, "He's busy eating his cupcake," to which his father responded, "He's just so stubborn. I want him to look." By his second birthday, Anthony was still nonverbal and began to demonstrate regular and frequent meltdowns. At that point, his parents realized that he was not stubborn; something was not right with his development. Within about 6 months, Anthony was diagnosed with ASD. When he came to the clinic, he was almost 3 and continued to be nonverbal.

Anthony had several items that he enjoyed, including bubbles, candy, chips, and a few musical toys. Clinicians used these items as motivators to encourage his first words. When he said a word or made a word attempt, clinicians immediately gave him the item he attempted to request. For example, when clinicians held up the bubbles and he said "bubu," they immediately blew bubbles, after which he joyfully ran around the room popping them. They also taught his parents how to use his favorite items to prompt communication. His parents were able to prompt words all day long by creating ongoing opportunities throughout his waking hours. It took a lot of effort, but consequently, words came in steadily, and within 6 months he had a huge vocabulary and readily and spontaneously requested items and activities using single words. At that point, clinicians began requiring him to combine words, which he used as requests, such as "blow bubbles" or "open chips." Soon thereafter, Anthony began creating slightly longer phrases, sometimes unprompted.

By then, he was quite verbal, but since all of his utterances functioned as requests, clinicians started working on question-asking, beginning with "What's that?" then "Where is it" and then "Whose is it?" After Anthony began using those early questions, clinicians taught him to use "What's happening?" to expand his verb use. To improve his attention-seeking strategies, clinicians taught him to say "Look!" and "Look, Mom, bubbles!" In order to provide a meaningful natural reward after this attention-seeking utterance, clinicians immediately rewarded him with the desired item he brought to another person's attention. His language was progressing nicely, and Anthony began learning his letters and numbers also using the motivational components of PRT.

When he began preschool at age 4, he was fully included and was provided with a one-to-one aide. He was ahead of the other children academically, but socially, he isolated himself and demonstrated behavior problems such as leaving the area and refusing to participate when asked to join circle time or go to his desk for a group activity.

Throughout elementary school, Anthony continued to excel academically and gradually improved socially, but he exhibited disruptive behavior when he was bored or the activity was too easy, which was frequently the case. Special education support staff partnering with the university autism center developed programs to decrease his disruptive behaviors, such as the use of self-management to decrease his behavior issues during nonpreferred activities, individualized instruction so that he would be challenged, priming (previewing the materials before they were presented) in areas that were highly verbal, and token economies used by the class for work completion and on-task behavior.

By middle school, he no longer needed assistance. He had friends and continued to excel academically. Anthony recently graduated from a 4-year university in engineering. The early intervention, parent education, full-inclusion with assistance, coordinated team efforts, and comprehensive intervention programs implemented across all of his environments resulted in a very positive outcome for Anthony.

Application to an Adult

Skyler was a freshman in college when he came into the university autism center with his family for treatment. He had a diagnosis of autism (Asperger type), and although he excelled academically, he struggled socially. Skyler began attending weekly 1-hour sessions with a trained PRT therapist. During baseline measurements, the therapist observed Skyler in his natural environment and had conversations with him to assess his current social-communication skills. He walked repetitively in circles, tossing a box of breath mints, keys, or any other small item he could find in his pocket into the air, catching it, and repeating this behavior again and again. Although this behavior was not a concern when he was in his room or a private location, in public areas it drew unwanted attention and stares from his peers. Further, because he appeared so preoccupied by this repetitive behavior, others seldom approached him. When clinicians discussed this behavior with Skyler, he shared that he would like to reduce the repetitive behavior in public settings. Thus, the first program they put into place was a self-management procedure to reduce the repetitive behavior that interfered with his making friends. Each day, he recorded whether or not he was able to engage in the behavior only in private settings and whether the repetitive behavior was self-controlled in public settings. If he successfully recorded doing this behavior only in private for 5 of 7 days per week, then he chose a reinforcer to earn (he chose getting a smoothie with his clinician). The self-management rapidly resulted in the elimination of the repetitive behavior in public.

Next, Skyler expressed concern that he did not go to any social events and spent most of his time alone in his dorm room and on the computer. He expressed a strong desire to have friends, participate in extracurricular activities, and enjoy the social side of campus. To help increase his socialization, he was first instructed to select three campus clubs around his interests (note the PRT motivational component of choice with a natural reward for attending the club). Skyler had a strong interest in art and dancing, and his clinician coached him in navigating the campus website to find clubs related to these hobbies. He discovered an art club, anime club, and swing and ballroom dance recreation class.

Skyler was then matched with a typical undergraduate student who served as a peer mentor and social coach. The peer mentor accompanied Skyler to the school clubs at least once a week and then provided feedback to Skyler's clinician regarding his social skills in these natural settings with peers. His peer mentor reported a few areas as challenging for Skyler. First, he was highly interested in the topic of the clubs, so he often talked nonstop to his peers. In order to decrease this monologuing, his clinician used video feedback to help him practice asking questions, listening to his peers, and balancing the conversation approximately 50/50. Next, his peer mentor mentioned that she saw him eating lunch alone each day in the large university cafeteria. She volunteered to sit with him and introduce him to other students at lunchtime. Her strategy worked well, and within a few weeks he was eating with a group of regulars in the dorm commons. During his one-to-one clinic sessions, his clinician practiced important social skills that he had never acquired, such as ways to ask for a phone number so that he could meet up with people outside of the club, greet and exit conversations, express empathy, use social media, and communicate with faculty.

After several months of attending the anime club, Skyler met a woman who had similar strong interests in the topic. They began dating and eventually he graduated from college and reported being satisfied with his social life. By meeting once a week with a therapist in the clinic and at least once a week with a peer mentor in various places on campus, Skyler received comprehensive support along with social opportunities that enhanced his success in college. Because of his strong desire to meet people and have a girlfriend, he was cooperative with intervention and willingly practiced self-management and other strategies to address deficit social areas. Receiving individualized programming for socialization is often critical for adults on the autism spectrum who struggle with making friends. A combination of explicit teaching of social areas that needed remediation, practice with feedback, video feedback, peer support, motivational components to encourage socialization in the context of his preferred activities, and self-management were instrumental in helping him successfully integrate with peers, succeed in college, and later find employment.

> **To review an extended application and implementation of this intervention, see Case 10 about a child with ASD in the companion volume *Case Studies for the Treatment of Autism Spectrum Disorder*.**

Future Directions

As a whole, most ASD intervention research has targeted young children, including PRT studies. Further research with other age groups, including infants, toddlers, adolescents, and adults, is warranted. Developing and refining interventions with infants may help young children get on a more favorable developmental trajectory earlier in life. Moreover, few parent education studies have been published regarding procedures to support parents with children on the spectrum beyond the elementary school years. Parent education programs for adolescents and adults are greatly needed, particularly using the motivational procedures or PRT. Research focusing on comorbidity (e.g., depression and anxiety) that is common in adolescence and beyond is important. Some preliminary studies have suggested that targeting socialization using PRT may have the serendipitous effect of reducing comorbid disorders and thus making such strategies worthy of future research (Ashbaugh et al., 2017; L. K. Koegel et al., 2016). In addition, as parents are an integral and critical component of the habilitation process, addressing their well-documented stress continues to be essential.

Studies focusing on predictors of positive outcomes would help us assess important variables that need to be targeted. For example, our retrospective study showing that children who initiated interactions had more positive long-term outcomes (L. K. Koegel, Koegel, Shoshan, & McNerney, 1999) led us to develop methodologies for teaching initiations. Understanding which behaviors lead to the most positive outcomes is vital in guiding treatment goals. Next, there are still some children with ASD who remain nonverbal throughout their lifespan. Although this number is decreasing with the development of improved interventions, further research is warranted in this area. Another area that warrants future research relates to the brain changes that occur after behavioral interventions. This area may provide a clearer understanding of the underlying neurological correlates of ASD, which in turn may suggest refinements to or new developments in treatment.

Methods to improve employment outcomes for individuals on the spectrum is yet another understudied topic. Too many adults with ASD have difficulty obtaining and maintaining employment. As the wave of children diagnosed with ASD reach adulthood, treatments and programs will be essential to help this population integrate into the workplace. Continuing to adapt PRT for adults in the workplace is an important future direction.

In short, as autism has become more prevalent, a critical and immediate need for intervention research has arisen. In the 1960s, ASD was considered a hopeless diagnosis. Research since that time has proven that this assumption is far from the truth, but science is cumulative, and further research should result in even more positive outcomes for individuals with ASD, their families, and the greater community.

Suggested Readings

1. Koegel, R. L., & Koegel, L. K. (2012). *The PRT pocket guide: Pivotal Response Treatment for autism spectrum disorders.* Paul H. Brookes Publishing Co. This pocket guide provides parents and professionals concise information about the basics of PRT, including the research behind PRT, what PRT looks like in practice, and examples of how to use PRT strategies.

2. Koegel, R. L., & Koegel, L. K. (2019). *Pivotal response treatments for autism spectrum disorder.* Paul H. Brookes Publishing Co. This comprehensive book covers how to use PRT strategies from infancy to adulthood as well as other important topics, including assessment, treatment options at home and school, self-management, training parents, and helping young adults succeed in college and the workplace.

3. Koegel, L. K., & LaZebnik, C. S. (2014). *Overcoming autism: Finding the answers, strategies, and hope that can transform a child's life.* Penguin. This inspiring book is coauthored by Lynn Koegel and Claire LaZebnik, a mother of a child with autism, and it provides practical advice on how to manage symptoms of ASD.

Learning Activities

1. How would you describe the six motivational components of PRT to a colleague versus to a parent?

2. What are other pivotal areas in addition to motivation? Discuss why they are considered pivotal in regard to the research and theoretical underpinnings.

3. What changes would you make to an analog session in order to better align it with PRT teaching strategies?

4. If your goal is to teach a child prepositions, what are some natural activities and rewards that may be good for teaching? Pick three other target behaviors and describe what natural activities and rewards you would use to teach.

5. What collateral areas have been shown to result in improved performance when motivational procedures are incorporated?

6. How are parents and other individuals incorporated into PRT programs?

7. How is FoI assessed for PRT?

8. Think about a child or adolescent with ASD with whom you work, identify appropriate goals for social communication and social interaction, and design an intervention plan based on the principles outlined for PRT.

Summary of Video Clip

*See the **About the Videos and Downloads** page at the front of the book for directions on how to access and stream the accompanying video to this chapter.*

This video clip shows a therapist working with a child with ASD during a Pivotal Response Training one-to-one session. The child is 2 years, 8 months old and is learning her first words. The child is playing with the therapist on the floor of the family's living room. Expressive language targets in this video are "fish" and "tickle." The therapist uses the child's interest (an inset puzzle and tickling game) to target these words and varies his prompting level. He uses silly sounds to gain her attention and to keep her engaged and interested in the puzzle. The therapist also contingently reinforces her word attempts. The child's responsivity and affect are high, suggesting high motivation for the activity with the therapist. Finally, the therapist does an excellent job following the child's lead when she appears to be no longer interested in tickles at the end of the video clip, especially when reinforcing her initiation for "tickles."

REFERENCES

Alpert, C. L., & Kaiser, A. P. (1992). Training parents as milieu language teachers. *Journal of Early Intervention, 16*(1), 31–52.

American Psychiatric Association. (2000). *Diagnostic and statistical manual of mental disorders fourth edition, text revision* (DSM-IV-TR).Author.

American Psychiatric Association. (2013). *Diagnostic and statistical manual of mental disorders, fifth edition* (DSM-5). Author.

Ashbaugh, K., Koegel, R., & Koegel, L. (2017). Increasing social integration for college students with autism spectrum disorder. *Behavioral Development Bulletin, 22*(1), 183–196.

Barnhill, G. P., & Myles, B. S. (2001). Attributional style and depression in adolescents with Asperger syndrome. *Journal of Positive Behavior Interventions, 3*(3), 175–182.

Bernheimer, L. P., Gallimore, R., & Weisner, T. S. (1990). Ecological theory as a context for the individual family service plan. *Journal of Early Intervention, 14*(3), 219–233.

Bozkus Genc, G., & Vuran, S. (2013). Examination of studies targeting social skills with Pivotal Response Treatment. *Educational Sciences: Theory & Practice, 13*(3), 1730–1742.

Bozkus-Genc, G., & Yucesoy-Ozkan, S. (2016). Meta-analysis of pivotal response training for children with autism spectrum disorder. *Education and Training in Autism and Developmental Disabilities, 51*(1), 13–26.

Bradshaw, J., Koegel, L. K., & Koegel, R. L. (2017). Improving functional language and social motivation with a parent-mediated intervention for toddlers with autism spectrum disorder. *Journal of Autism and Developmental Disorders, 47*(8), 2443–2458.

Brown, W., & Odom, S. (1995). Naturalistic peer interventions for promoting preschool children's social interactions. *Preventing School Failure, 39*(4) 38–43.

Buckley, T. W., Ente, A. P., & Ruef, M. B. (2014). Improving a family's overall quality of life through parent training in pivotal response treatment. *Journal of Positive Behavior Interventions, 16*(1), 60–63

Cadogan, S., & McCrimmon, A. W. (2015). Pivotal response treatment for children with autism spectrum disorder: A systematic review of research quality. *Developmental Neurorehabilitation, 18*(2), 137–144.

Coolican, J., Smith, I. M., & Bryson, S. E. (2010). Brief parent training in pivotal response treatment for preschoolers with autism. *Journal of Child Psychology and Psychiatry, 51*(12), 1321–1330.

Duifhuis, E. A., Den Boer, J. C., Doornbos, A., Buitelaar, J. K., Oosterling, I. J., & Klip, H. (2017). The effect of pivotal response treatment in children with autism spectrum disorders: A non-randomized study with a blinded outcome measure. *Journal of Autism and Developmental Disorders, 47*(2), 231–242.

Dunlap, G. (1984). The influence of task variation and maintenance tasks on the learning and affect of autistic children. *Journal of Experimental Child Psychology, 37*(1), 41–64.

Dunlap, G., & Koegel, R. L. (1980). Motivating autistic children through stimulus variation. *Journal of Applied Behavior Analysis, 13*(4), 619–627.

Ennis-Cole, D., Durodoye, B. A., & Harris, H. L. (2013). The impact of culture on autism diagnosis and treatment: Considerations for counselors and other professionals. *The Family Journal, 21*(3), 279–287.

Gengoux, G. W., Berquist, K. L., Salzman, E., Schapp, S., Phillips, J M, Frazier, T. W., Minjarez, M. B., & Hardan, A. Y. (2015). Pivotal response treatment parent training for autism: Findings from a 3-month follow-up evaluation. *Journal of Autism and Developmental Disorders, 45*(9), 2889–2898.

Gillett, J. N., & LeBlanc, L. A. (2007). Parent-implemented natural language paradigm to increase language and play in children with autism. *Research in Autism Spectrum Disorders, 1*(3), 247–255.

Hardan, A. Y., Gengoux, G. W., Berquist, K. L., Libove, R. A., Ardel, C. M., Phillips, J., Frazier, T. W., & Minjarez, M. B. (2015). A randomized controlled trial of Pivotal Response Treatment Group for parents of children with autism. *Journal of Child Psychology and Psychiatry, 56*(8), 884–892.

Harper, C. B., Symon, J. B. G., & Frea, W. D. (2008). Recess is time-in: Using peers to improve social skills of children with autism. *Journal of Autism and Developmental Disorders, 38*(5), 815–826.

Harrower, J. K., & Dunlap, G. (2001). Including children with autism in general education classrooms: A review of effective strategies. *Behavior Modification, 25*(5), 762–784.

Harry, B., Grenot-Scheyer, M., Smith-Lewis, M., Xin, F., & Schwartz, I. (1995). Developing culturally inclusive services for individuals with severe disabilities. *Journal of the Association for Persons with Severe Handicaps, 20*, 99–109.

Kaiser, A. P., & Trent, J. A. (2007). Communication intervention for young children with disabilities: Naturalistic approaches to promoting development. In S. Odom, R. Horner, M. Snell, & J. Blacher (Eds.), *Handbook of developmental disabilities* (pp. 224–245). Guilford Press.

Koegel, L. K. (2011). *Pivotal Response Treatment: Using motivation as a pivotal response.* UCSB Koegel Autism Center.

Koegel, L. K., Ashbaugh, K., Koegel, R. L., Detar, W. J., & Regester, A. (2013). Increasing socialization in adults with Asperger's syndrome. *Psychology in the Schools, 50*(9), 899–909.

Koegel, L. K., Ashbaugh, K., Navab, A., & Koegel, R. L. (2016). Improving empathic communication skills in adults with autism spectrum disorder. *Journal of Autism and Developmental Disorders, 46*(3), 921–933.

Koegel, L. K., Camarata, S. M., Valdez-Menchaca, M., & Koegel, R. L. (1998). Setting generalization of question-asking by children with autism. *American Journal on Mental Retardation, 102*(4), 346–357.

Koegel, L. K., Carter, C. M., & Koegel, R. L. (2003). Teaching children with autism self-initiations as a pivotal response. *Topics in Language Disorders, 23*, 134–145.

Koegel, L. K., Koegel, R. L., Green-Hopkins, I., & Barnes, C. C. (2010). Brief report: Question-asking and collateral language acquisition in children with autism. *Journal of Autism and Developmental Disorders, 40*(4), 509–515.

Koegel, L. K., Koegel, R. L., Harrower, J. K., Carter, C. M. (1999). Pivotal response intervention I: Overview of approach. *Journal of the Association for Persons with Severe Handicaps, 24*, 174–185.

Koegel, L. K., Koegel, R. L., Hurley, C., & Frea, W. D. (1992). Improving social skills and disruptive behavior in children with autism through self-management. *Journal of Applied Behavior Analysis, 25*(2), 341–353.

Koegel, L. K., Koegel, R. L., Shoshan, Y., & McNerney, E. (1999). Pivotal response intervention II: Preliminary long-term outcome data. *Journal of the Association for Persons with Severe Handicaps, 24*(3), 186–198.

Koegel, L. K., Koegel, R. L., & Smith, A. (1997). Variables related to differences in standardized test outcomes for children with autism. *Journal of Autism and Developmental Disorders, 27*(3), 233–243.

Koegel, L. K., Kuriakose, S., Singh, A. K., & Koegel, R. L. (2012). Improving generalization of peer socialization gains in inclusive school settings using initiations training. *Behavior modification, 36*(3), 361–377.

Koegel, L. K., Park, M. N., & Koegel, R. L. (2014). Using self-management to improve the reciprocal social conversation of children with autism spectrum disorder. *Journal of Autism and Developmental Disorders, 44*(5), 1055–1063.

Koegel, L. K., Singh, A. K., & Koegel, R. L. (2010). Improving motivation for academics in children with autism. *Journal of Autism and Developmental Disorders, 40*(9), 1057–1066.

Koegel, L. K., Singh, A. K., Koegel, R. L., Hollingsworth, J. R., & Bradshaw, J. (2014). Assessing and improving early social engagement in infants. *Journal of Positive Behavior Interventions, 16*(2), 69–80.

Koegel, R. L., Bimbela, A., & Schreibman, L. (1996). Collateral effects of parent training on family interactions. *Journal of Autism and Developmental Disorders, 26*(3), 347–359.

Koegel, R. L., Bradshaw, J. L., Ashbaugh, K., & Koegel, L. K. (2014). Improving question-asking initiations in young children with autism using pivotal response treatment. *Journal of Autism and Developmental Disorders, 44*(4), 816–827.

Koegel, R. L., Camarata, S., Koegel, L. K., Ben-Tall, A., & Smith, A. E. (1998). Increasing speech intelligibility in children with autism. *Journal of Autism and Developmental Disorders, 28*(3), 241–251.

Koegel, R. L., Dyer, K., & Bell, L. K. (1987). The influence of child preferred activities on autistic children's social behavior. *Journal of Applied Behavior Analysis, 20*(3), 243–252.

Koegel, R. L., & Egel, A. L. (1979). Motivating autistic children. *Journal of Abnormal Psychology, 88*(4), 418–426.

Koegel, R. L., Fredeen, R., Kim, S., Danial, J., Rubinstein, D., & Koegel, L. (2012). Using perseverative interests to improve interactions between adolescents with autism and their typical peers in school settings. *Journal of Positive Behavior Interventions, 14*(3), 133–141.

Koegel, R. L., Glahn, T., & Nieminen, G. (1978). Generalization of parent-training results. *Journal of Applied Behavior Analysis, 11*, 95–109.

Koegel, R. L., Kim, S., Koegel, L., & Schwartzman, B. (2013). Improving socialization for high school students with ASD by using their preferred interests. *Journal of Autism and Developmental Disorders, 43*(9), 2121–2134.

Koegel, R. L., & Koegel, L. K. (2006). *Pivotal response treatments for autism: Communication, social, & academic development.* Paul H. Brookes Publishing Co.

Koegel, R. L., & Koegel, L. K. (2019). *Pivotal response treatments for autism spectrum disorder.* Paul H Brookes Publishing Co.

Koegel, R. L., Koegel, L. K., & Surratt, A. (1992). Language intervention and disruptive behavior in preschool children with autism. *Journal of Autism and Developmental Disorders, 22*(2), 141–153.

Koegel, R. L., & Mentis, M. (1985). Motivation in childhood autism: Can they or won't they? *Child Psychology & Psychiatry & Allied Disciplines, 26*(2), 185–191.

Koegel, R. L., O'Dell, M. C., & Dunlap, G. (1988). Producing speech use in nonverbal autistic children by reinforcing attempts. *Journal of Autism and Developmental Disorders, 18*(4), 525–538.

Koegel, R. L., O'Dell, M. C., & Koegel, L. K. (1987). A natural language teaching paradigm for nonverbal autistic children. *Journal of Autism and Developmental Disorders, 17*(2), 187–200.

Koegel, R. L., Werner, G. A., Vismara, L. A., & Koegel, L. K. (2005). The effectiveness of contextually supported play date interactions between children with autism and typically developing peers. *Research and Practice for Persons with Severe Disabilities, 30*, 93–102.

Koegel, R. L., & Williams, J. (1980). Direct versus indirect response-reinforcer relationships in teaching autistic children. *Journal of Abnormal Child Psychology, 8*(4), 537–547.

Laski, K. E., Charlop, M. H., & Schreibman, L. (1988). Training parents to use the natural language paradigm to increase their autistic children's speech. *Journal of Applied Behavior Analysis, 21*(4), 391–400.

Lei, J., & Ventola, P. (2017). Pivotal response treatment for autism spectrum disorder: current perspectives. *Neuropsychiatric Disease and Treatment, 13*, 1613.

Maier, S. F., & Seligman, M. E. (1976). Learned helplessness: Theory and evidence. *Journal of Experimental Psychology: General, 105*(1), 3–46.

McGee, G., Krantz, P., & McClannahan, L. (1984). Conversational skills for autistic adolescents: Teaching assertiveness in naturalistic game settings. *Journal of Autism and Developmental Disorders, 14*(3) 319–330.

Miller, W. R., & Seligman, M. E. (1975). Depression and learned helplessness in man. *Journal of Abnormal Psychology, 84*(3), 228–238.

Minjarez, M. B., Williams, S. E., Mercier, E. M., & Hardan, A. Y. (2011). Pivotal response group treatment program for parents of children with autism. *Journal of Autism and Developmental Disorders, 41*(1), 92–101.

Mirenda-Linne, F., & Melin, L. (1992). Acquisition, generalization, and spontaneous use of color adjectives: A comparison of incidental teaching and traditional discrete-trial procedures for children with autism. *Research in Developmental Disabilities, 13*, 191–210.

Mohammadzaheri, F., Koegel, L. K., Rezaee, M., & Bakhshi, E. (2015). A randomized clinical trial comparison between pivotal response treatment (PRT) and adult-driven applied behavior analysis (ABA) intervention on disruptive behaviors in public school children with autism. *Journal of Autism and Developmental Disorders, 45*(9), 2899–2907.

Mohammadzaheri, F., Koegel, L. K., Rezaee, M., & Rafiee, S. M. (2014). A randomized clinical trial comparison between pivotal response treatment (PRT) and structured applied behavior analysis (ABA) intervention for children with autism. *Journal of Autism and Developmental Disorders, 44*(11), 2769–2777.

National Autism Center. (2015). *Findings and conclusions: National Standards Project, Phase 2.* Author

National Research Council. (2001). *Educating children with autism.* National Academy Press.

Nefdt, N., Koegel, R. L., Singer, G., & Gerber, M. (2010). The use of a self-directed learning program to provide introductory training in pivotal response treatment to parents of children with autism. *Journal of Positive Behavior Intervention, 12*(1), 23–32.

Pierce, K., & Schreibman, L. (1995). Increasing complex social behaviors in children with autism: Effects of peer-implemented pivotal response training. *Journal of Applied Behavior Analysis, 28*(3), 285–295.

Pierce, K., & Schreibman, L. (1997). Multiple peer use of pivotal response training to increase social behaviors of classmates with autism: Results from trained and untrained peers. *Journal of Applied Behavior Analysis, 30*(1), 157–160.

Ravindran, N., & Myers, B. (2012). Cultural influences on perceptions of health, illness, and disability: A review and focus on autism. *Journal of Child & Family Studies, 21*(2), 311–319.

Renshaw, T., & Kuriakose, S. (2011). Pivotal Response Treatment for children with autism: Core principles and applications for school psychologists. *Journal of Applied School Psychology, 27*(2), 181–200.

Seligman, M. E., & Maier, S. F. (1967). Failure to escape traumatic shock. *Journal of Experimental Psychology, 74*(1), 1–9.

Smith, A., & Camarata, S. (1999). Using teacher-implemented instruction to increase language intelligibility of children with autism. *Journal of Positive Behavior Interventions, 1*(3), 141–151.

Sparrow, S. S., Cicchetti, D. V., & Balla, D. A. (2005). *Vineland Adaptive Behavior Scales–Second edition.* Pearson.

Stahmer, A. C. (1995). Teaching symbolic play skills to children with autism using pivotal response training. *Journal of Autism and Developmental Disorders, 25*(2), 123–141.

Stahmer, A., Suhrheinrich, J., Reed, S., Schreibman, L., & Bolduc, C. (2011). *Classroom pivotal response teaching for children with autism.* Guilford Press.

Steiner, A. M., Gengoux, G. W., Klin, A., & Chawarska, K. (2013). Pivotal response treatment for infants at-risk for autism spectrum disorders: A pilot study. *Journal of Autism and Developmental Disorders, 43*(1), 91–102.

Thorp, D. M., Stahmer, A. C., & Schreibman, L. (1995). Effects of sociodramatic play training on children with autism. *Journal of Autism and Developmental Disorders, 25*(3), 265–282.

Venkataraman, A., Yang, D. Y. J., Dvornek, N., Staib, L. H., Duncan, J. S., Pelphrey, K. A., & Ventola, P. (2016). Pivotal response treatment prompts a functional rewiring of the brain amongst individuals with autism spectrum disorder. *Neuroreport, 27*(14), 1081.

Ventola, P., Yang, D. Y., Friedman, H. E., Oosting, D., Wolf, J., Sukhodolsky, D. G., & Pelphrey, K. A. (2015). Heterogeneity of neural mechanisms of response to pivotal response treatment. *Brain Imaging and Behavior, 9*(1), 74–88.

Vernon, T. W., Koegel, R. L., Dauterman, H., & Stolen, K. (2012). An early social engagement intervention for young children with autism and their parents. *Journal of Autism and Developmental Disorders, 42*, 2702–2717.

Verschuur, R., Didden, R., Lang, R., Sigafoos, J., & Huskens, B. (2014). Pivotal response treatment for children with autism spectrum disorders: A systematic review. *Review Journal of Autism and Developmental Disorders, 1*(1), 34–61.

Vismara, L. A., & Lyons, G. L. (2007). Using perseverative interests to elicit joint attention behaviors in young children with autism: Theoretical and clinical implications for understanding motivation. *Journal of Positive Behavior Interventions, 9*(4), 214–228.

Voos, A. C., Pelphrey, K. A., Tirrell, J., Bolling, D. Z., Vander Wyk, B., Kaiser, M. D., McPartland, J., Volkmar, F., & Ventola, P. (2013). Neural mechanisms of improvements in social motivation after pivotal response treatment: Two case studies. *Journal of Autism and Developmental Disorders, 43*(1), 1–10.

Weiss, M., & Harris, S. (2001). Teaching social skills to people with autism. *Behavior Modification, 25*(5), 785–802.

Wilczynski, S. M. (2010). Evidence-based practice and autism spectrum disorders: The National Standards Project. *Communique, 38*(5), 1, 24–25.

Wilder, L. K., Dyches, T. T., Obiakor, F. E., & Algozzine, B. (2004). Multicultural perspectives on teaching students with autism. *Focus on Autism and Other Developmental Disabilities, 19*(2), 105–113.

Williams, J. A., Koegel, R. L., & Egel, A. L. (1981). Response-reinforcer relationships and improved learning in autistic children. *Journal of Applied Behavior Analysis, 14*, 53–60.

Wong, C., Odom, S. L., Hume, K. A., Cox, A. W., Fettig, A., Kucharczyk, S., Brock, M. E., Plavnick, J. B., Fleury, V. P., & Schultz, T. R. (2015). Evidence-based practices for children, youth, and young adults with autism spectrum disorder: A comprehensive review. *Journal of Autism and Developmental Disorders, 45*(7), 1951–1966.

14

The SCERTS® Model: Social Communication, Emotional Regulation, and Transactional Supports

Amy C. Laurent, Emily Rubin, and Barry M. Prizant

INTRODUCTION

The SCERTS® Model is a comprehensive educational approach for young children and older individuals with autism spectrum disorder (ASD) and their families (Prizant et al., 2006b). It is an assessment and intervention framework that is grounded in developmental theory as well as evidenced-based research from the fields of child development, neuroscience, education, speech-language pathology, occupational therapy, psychology, and autism. Collectively, this knowledge base is integrated within the model to provide individuals with ASD with targeted educational support aimed at fostering meaningful long-term outcomes, such as the attainment of social-communicative competence, the ability to cope successfully with daily stressors, and a high quality of life (Prizant et al., 2006b).

The SCERTS Model comprises three high priority domains, which represent core challenges and areas often requiring support for individuals with ASD and their communication partners: Social Communication, Emotion Regulation, and Transactional Support. **Social Communication (SC)** encompasses skills and abilities supportive of the development of spontaneous initiated, functional communication, secure and trusting relationships with others, and an understanding of the expected conventions of different social situations. **Emotional Regulation (ER)** reflects capacities and skills necessary to facilitate the regulation of arousal and emotional states in order to be available for learning and interacting within the social and physical environment, to cope with everyday stress, and to utilize effective tools and strategies by oneself and in interactions with others to increase active engagement in daily routines. **Transactional Support (TS)** refers to the abilities of communication partners to develop and implement interactive and environmental supports to help individuals with ASD succeed in daily interactions and activities and develop new skills. The model provides processes and guidelines for both assessment and intervention in each of the three domains, which are consistent with a strengths-based educational philosophy as well as individual and family-centered practice (Prizant et al., 2006b).

The SCERTS Model curriculum for assessment and intervention is designed to help support individuals who demonstrate a broad range of developmental abilities across the lifespan. The use of a lifespan model derived from research and literature in human development is important because it is well documented that challenges in social communication, emotional regulation, and transactional support are persistent issues for individuals with ASD of all ages. The developmental age range of the model spans from approximately 8 months to 12 years of age. Therefore, it can be used to provide educational support for individuals with ASD ranging in chronological age from toddlerhood through adulthood. It can be used to effectively support individuals who are presymbolic in their communicative means, those who are early symbolic communicators, and those who are conversational in their interactions with others. Practical aspects of this chapter focus largely on application to school-age individuals with ASD.

The SCERTS Model is activity based and emphasizes an individual's abilities to demonstrate functional skills needed to navigate daily life. Therefore, assessment, intervention, and ongoing data collection are all accomplished within the natural environments, routines, and activities of the individual with ASD. Designed to be a cross-contextual model of intervention, transactional supports are embedded within naturally occurring activities in the individual's typical environments (e.g., home, school, community) and by all communication partners (e.g., educational team, family, and peers). These interpersonal and learning supports often augment naturally occurring learning opportunities within an activity or environment; however, the model is flexible to allow for direct teaching of a developmental skill or ability when appropriate. Given that SCERTS is a framework, it is structured such that strategies from a wide range of focused, evidenced-based educational and intervention methodologies can be incorporated as transactional supports to help address priorities in social communication and emotional regulation at the individual's developmental level (Prizant et al., 2006a).

The model's focus on learning within natural activities, as well as intervention occurring across environments and geared at promoting functional, spontaneous generalization of social-communicative and social interactive abilities, aligns with the National Research Council (NRC) (Lord & McGee, 2001) guidelines for effective educational practice in ASD. It incorporates additional NRC guidelines as critical priorities to be considered when designing intervention for individuals and students with ASD. These include 1) active engagement for 25 hours a week for the full year, 2) individualized programming and attention, 3) family involvement and support, 4) ongoing tracking and programmatic evaluation that facilitates adjustments in programming, 5) supporting the development of play skills with focus on peer interactions, 6) functional assessment and positive behavior support to address problem behaviors, and 7) facilitating functional academic skills as appropriate (Lord & McGee, 2001).

Table 14.1. Developmental partner stages within The SCERTS® Model

Partner stage	Social-communicative means
Social Partners	Individuals who use *only* presymbolic means of communication to connect to others (e.g., reenactment gestures, conventional gestures, facial expressions, body position, vocalizations, proximity)
Language Partners	Individuals who are at an emerging language stage and are early language learners. They regularly use simple symbolic means with communicative intent (e.g., single spoken words, sign language, pictures, other forms of augmentation). They may use echolalia.
Conversational Partners	Individuals who have robust vocabularies and are able to convey their own ideas using their own phrasing. They may use spoken language or augmentative means to communicate with others.

Source: Prizant, Wetherby, Rubin, & Laurent, (2003).

TARGET POPULATONS

The SCERTS Model was designed for and is implemented primarily in educational and intervention settings for individuals diagnosed with ASD. However, given that The SCERTS Model is developmental in nature, it can be used to assess and to scaffold development for any individual demonstrating challenges related to social communication and emotional regulation, regardless of chronological age and diagnosis. Clinically, the model has been used in educational settings for individuals with social-communication disorder, mixed expressive/receptive language disorder, nonverbal learning disorder, and attention deficit disorder, among others.

In the context of The SCERTS Model, all individuals or students with ASD are assigned communication partner stages based on their symbolic communicative abilities. This categorization is achieved during the first step of the SCERTS Assessment Process (SAP) and is critical to assessment and subsequent intervention planning. There are three partner stages in the model (see Table 14.1), which reflect the developmental sophistication of individuals' communicative abilities and start to inform clinicians' and educators' understanding of who the individuals are as learners. Chronological age is not a factor in making these determinations. These stages encompass a wide breadth of developmental abilities and are applicable to individuals with coexisting language and intellectual impairments.

THEORETICAL BASIS

The SCERTS Model is a transdisciplinary developmental model that incorporates research from a broad literature base. Recognizing that ASD is a developmental disorder, the model attempts to honor the complexity of child development as well as to address the challenges specifically associated with ASD. The SCERTS Model is based on several key assumptions that address the nature of ASD, the foundation of learning in relationship with others, the underlying components of social-communicative and social emotional competence that support positive outcomes and mental health, and the importance of functional assessment and intervention. This section explains the theoretical rationale, underlying assumptions, and functional outcomes of The SCERTS Model.

Theoretical Rationale

The theoretical rationale for The SCERTS Model is the transactional nature of development as well as family-centered practice.

Transactional Nature of Development   SCERTS is grounded in the transactional theory of development. This theory is rooted in the understanding that much of an individual's development and growth occurs within the context of relationship and interaction with others. In addition, a key underlying assumption in the theory is that children are active learners who seek out opportunities for learning and also integrate developmental experiences when acquiring new skills and abilities (Sameroff & Fiese, 1990). Therefore, efforts to support the development of an individual with ASD within The SCERTS Model occurs within the context of daily interactions with natural communicative partners in everyday routines. In keeping with the transactional nature of development, The SCERTS Model does not focus solely on developing the individual's skills; it also prioritizes developing supportive contexts and interactive partners who can help to facilitate an individual's social emotional and social-communicative competence. This relational approach is similar to cognitive and social models of language acquisition/development (Bates, 1976; Bloom, 2000) as well as, interactive models of emotional regulation development (Eisenberg & Sulik, 2012; Fox, 1994; Tronick, 2002).

To support the growth and development of individuals with ASD, the model targets the core challenges associated with difficulties in social-adaptive functioning (American Speech-Language-Hearing Association [ASHA], 2006; Lord & McGee, 2001). In accordance with the literature, the model prioritizes the SC, ER, and TS domains. These domains have strong correlations with long-term positive outcomes and high quality of life for all human beings, as they contribute to abilities to form relationships and to adapt to the demands of everyday social situations (Lord & McGee, 2001; Prizant et al., 2006b).

Social Communication   Social communication is a complex developmental capacity that includes an individual's abilities to initiate, respond to, and maintain interactions. It is the foundation of social engagement and participation where shared experiences support the development of meaningful relationships with others. The presentation of ASD is extremely heterogeneous, and this presentation changes with both maturation and development. However, individuals with ASD share common social-communication challenges that inhibit the development of critical social-communication skills, which in turn interfere with the development of the individual's social-communicative competence (ASHA, 2006). One diagnostically significant characteristic, regardless of an individual's cognitive abilities or learning style differences, is difficulty in establishing shared attention (i.e., joint attention). Challenges in joint attention and difficulties with social orienting, monitoring emotional states, considering another's intentions, and predicting the actions of others have been well documented (Gulsrud et al., 2010; Kasari et al., 2010; Tomasello et al., 2005; Wetherby et al., 2007). Joint attention difficulties have also been documented with respect to limitations in social reciprocity, such as challenges initiating bids for interactions, maintaining interactions by taking turns, and providing contingent responses to bids for interaction initiated by others (Kasari et al., 1988).

Symbol use or language abilities and related cognitive skills (e.g., understanding and using nonverbal and verbal communication, symbolic play, and the conventions and rules of social conversations in different situations) present additional social-communication challenges for individuals with ASD. Delays in the acquisition and use of symbols are associated with both expressive and receptive communication profiles in ASD (American Psychiatric Association, 2013). Collectively, joint attention and symbol use difficulties have far-reaching implications with respect to social-communicative competence for individuals with ASD, as they impact overall rate of communication for children with ASD and their abilities to glean information in social contexts (Kasari et al., 2008). Therefore, **joint attention** and **symbol use** are two critical capacities targeted within the SC domain of The SCERTS Model for skill development. Intervention in these areas is designed to help individuals develop the skills needed to establish and maintain satisfying relationships that contribute to success at home, at school, and in the community. It may reduce the risk for mental health conditions such as anxiety and depression often associated with social-communication and social-adaptive functioning difficulties (Tsatsanis et al., 2004). Clinicians and educators assess joint attention and symbol use skills and target them for intervention in developmentally sensible ways based on the individual's developmental stage. The SCERTS Model uses a three-stage developmental curriculum divided into the Social Partner, Language Partner, and Conversational Partner stages (see Table 14.1 for description). Within each stage, potential goals and objectives are delineated in a curriculum-based assessment tool to support the selection of targets and to measure progress over time that can be used from early intervention into adulthood.

Emotional Regulation   ER is a developmental domain that plays a significant role in fostering social-communicative competence. It is critical to the attainment and maintenance of arousal levels and emotional states that support active engagement in the social and physical environments (Tronick, 2002). Enhanced emotional regulation abilities have been correlated with the development of social relationships, behavioral adjustment, and academic success (Gulsrud et al., 2010; Jahromi et al., 2013; Mazefsky et al., 2013). The literature on ASD highlights regulatory difficulties as significant challenges for individuals with ASD (Mazefsky et al., 2013). Individuals with ASD have difficulty managing emotions, focusing attention, inhibiting reactions, delaying gratification, tolerating unexpected and unpredictable changes in their environment, and seeking comfort in conventional ways (American Psychiatric Association, 2013; Baron et al., 2006; DeGangi, 2000; Lord & McGee, 2001). Limitations in emotional regulation abilities are also correlated with higher levels of repetitive and restricted behaviors, arousal, anxiety, and challenging behaviors. Such behaviors can have a significant impact on individuals' access to educational and social opportunities (Koegel et al., 1996; Prizant & Laurent, 2012a; Walker et al., 2004).

The presentation of regulatory challenges for individuals with ASD is varied; however, difficulties in the capacity for mutual regulation are substantiated at all developmental levels among individuals with ASD. **Mutual regulation** is the ability to respond to and/or request assistance in regulating one's emotional state (Tronick, 2002). As individuals with ASD frequently misinterpret social cues, they often fail to recognize regulatory assistance that is offered by partners, such as parents, educators, service providers, and peers (Laurent & Rubin, 2004). For example, they may overlook a bid by a parent to offer a less stimulating environment. In addition, they may avoid initiating asking for assistance from others because of social-communicative challenges as well as social anxiety. Likewise, partners of individuals with ASD often miss opportunities to provide support because of the subtle and atypical signals of emotional distress in individuals with ASD (Prizant & Laurent, 2012b).

The capacity for self-regulation poses significant challenges for individuals with ASD across the developmental spectrum (Mazefsky, 2015; Mazefsky et al., 2013). **Self-regulation** is the developmental capacity to attain and maintain arousal and emotional states supportive of active engagement across one's day independently. Conventional behaviors associated with effective self-regulation vary with developmental age but include sensory motor actions such as fidgeting, expressing emotions, referring to schedules to organize oneself, and reflecting on the effectiveness of previously used strategies in similar circumstances. For individuals with ASD, challenges in imitating others, following instructions, and considering the perspective of others are correlated with difficulties in acquiring conventional or socially acceptable strategies for self-regulation (Gulsrud et al., 2010). As a result, an individual with ASD may use behaviors that are atypical, unconventional, or simply not based on an understanding of the perspective of others. As such, individuals with ASD often continue to use early developing and/or atypical strategies to regulate their emotions and arousal beyond early childhood. Behaviors such as insisting on specific routines, hoarding preferred items, and averting gaze may persist in older individuals with ASD. Unusual or ineffective patterns in self-regulation can lead to social isolation, as the negative perception of these behaviors can create barriers to building relationships and contribute to an increased risk for depression (Little, 2001; Tantam, 2000).

Given the prevalence of emotional regulatory challenges in individuals with ASD, clinicians and educators need to understand the nature of these challenges as well as to provide support and intervention that will minimize the far-reaching implications of such deficits. Therefore, **mutual regulation** and **self-regulation** are the two critical capacities targeted within the ER domain for skill development to help individuals develop needed skills to maintain active engagement and navigate their home, school, and community environments successfully; these skills serve as protective factors against mental health challenges. Skills and abilities in this domain are also assessed using the SAP according to the individual's communication partner stage (e.g., Social Partner, Language Partner, or Conversational Partner; Prizant et al., 2006b).

Transactional Support   Because The SCERTS Model is predicated on the transactional model of development (Sameroff & Fiese, 1990), addressing social communication and emotional regulation challenges cannot successfully occur in isolated teaching contexts such as one-to-one therapy or a social skills group. Rather, these developmental domains must be supported across social activities, social partners, and social contexts (e.g., home, school, and community). Many focused, evidenced-based intervention approaches to help support SC and ER skill development exist. However, a partner's ability to provide these supports in natural contexts is often compromised in part by the difficulty an individual with ASD may have in maintaining active engagement. In addition, partners may struggle in providing these accommodations, as the subtle and unconventional bids for interaction and displays of emotional distress of individuals with ASD can lead to frequent misinterpretations. Intervention research has demonstrated a strong correlation between how communication partners adapt their communicative styles (i.e., interpersonal supports) and modify the environment (i.e., through the provision of learning supports) and the social-communicative competence of an individual with ASD (ASHA, 2006; NRC, 2001). Therefore, **interpersonal support** and **learning support** are the two critical capacities targeted within the TS domain of The SCERTS Model for interactive partners. Prioritizing these areas is designed to ensure that communication partners use evidence-based interactive strategies and environmental arrangements to foster successful engagement in daily routines. Partners' skills and abilities in these two areas are assessed using the curricular framework as part of the individual's assessment and intervention planning process.

Family-Centered Practice   Finally, The SCERTS Model is grounded in the family-centered practice literature. Family-centered practice is recognized as an efficacious intervention model for young children diagnosed with ASD (Dunn et al., 2012; Wetherby et al., 2014). Less research is available related to its effectiveness for older individuals. However, a central tenet of family-centered practice is that the involvement of family members in all aspects of programming is linked to cross-contextual learning and generalization of learning. This level of family involvement in educational practice is consistent with recommendations from the National Research Council (Lord & McGee, 2001). Additional hallmarks of family-centered practices incorporated in The SCERTS Model include partnering with the family to identify the strengths of an individual and family, recognizing family members as experts with respect to their loved one's abilities and challenges, and educational support related to scaffolding development (McWilliam, 2010).

Underlying Assumptions

As a natural extension of its theoretical foundations in the developmental literature, The SCERTS Model embraces several basic tenets of recommended educational practice. These reflect the model's underlying assumptions regarding the nature of social-communicative impairment and treatment priorities. An educational approach should do the following (adapted from Prizant et al., 2006b, pp. 14–16):

- Directly address the core developmental challenges for individuals with ASD

- Be based on current knowledge of child development, which places learning within the context of the natural environments and is both child and family centered

- Be individualized to match a child's current developmental level and his or her profile of learning strengths and weaknesses

- Demonstrate a logical consistency between its long-term goals and teaching strategies to achieve those goals

- Be derived from a range of sources

- Develop and apply meaningful measures of progress and outcome

Likewise, The SCERTS Model has several core values and principles that guide educational and treatment efforts. These core values and guiding principles were developed to ensure that educational practices within the model focus on functional and meaningful goals while being respectful of individuals with ASD and their family members (adapted from Prizant et al., 2006b, p. 18):

1. The development of spontaneous, functional communication abilities and emotional regulatory capacities have the highest educational priorities because they support development and independence.

2. Principles and research on child development frame assessment and educational efforts. Goals and activities are developmentally appropriate and relevant to a child's life.

3. All domains of child development are viewed as interrelated and interdependent. Assessment and intervention must address these relationships.

4. All behavior is viewed as purposeful. For children who display unconventional and/or problem behaviors, there is an emphasis on determining the functions of the behaviors and supporting the children's development of more appropriate ways to accomplish those functions.

5. A child's unique learning profile of strengths and weaknesses is used to determine appropriate transactional supports for facilitating the development of social-communicative and emotional regulatory competence.

6. Natural routines across home, school, and community environments provide educational and treatment contexts for learning and the development of relationships. Progress is measured in relation to increasing competence and independence across these natural routines.

7. Professionals bear the primary responsibility for establishing and maintaining positive relationships with children and family members. All are treated with dignity and respect.

8. Family members are considered experts about their child. Assessment and educational efforts are collaborative processes.

Functional Outcomes

The overarching objective of The SCERTS Model is increased meaningful participation and active engagement in daily routines, activities, and relationships. Prioritization of the development of social-communication competence is critical to this objective. Therefore, the model emphasizes addressing the needs of individuals with ASD in domains that support social-communicative competence. As previously discussed, this translates to three developmental domains within the model, each of which comprises two capacities (see Table 14.2).

By selecting goals and objectives in core areas of challenge for individuals with ASD, team members implementing the model are able to target foundational skills critical to active engagement and meaningful relationships. The scope and sequence of goals and objectives within The SCERTS Model curriculum is not sequential in the sense that mastery of one skill must be demonstrated before moving to the next in a sequence. Rather, SCERTS expects teams to determine the appropriate steps for the individual as part of the assessment and intervention planning process. This is done based on three criteria: 1) student and family priorities, 2) developmental appropriateness, and 3) functionality.

Table 14.2. Domains and components of The SCERTS® Model

Domain	Component
Social Communication	Joint attention—the *why* of communication
	Symbol use—the *how* of communication
Emotional Regulation	Mutual regulation—the capacity to maintain well-regulated state with assistance of another person
	Self-regulation—the capacity to maintain active engagement without assistance
Transactional Support	Interpersonal support—adjustments in interactive style made by partners
	Learning support—modifications to activity and physical environment made by partners

Once the team selects goals and objectives for inclusion in the individual's educational plan, implementation of strategies and learning opportunities becomes focused on authentic progress. Authentic progress reflects the acquisition and use of functional skills and abilities in natural contexts for active engagement in roles, relationships, and activities, thereby supporting greater social-communicative competence (Prizant et al., 2006b).

Goals and objectives within The SCERTS Model are organized within the three-stage developmental curriculum. Tables 14.3, 14.4, and 14.5 provide a very brief

Table 14.3. Abbreviated scope and sequence of goals for social partner

Domain	Component	Goal area	Sample objective
Social Communication	Joint attention	Engage in reciprocal interaction	Responds to others
			Initiates with others
		Share attention	Shifts gaze
			Follows point
	Symbol use	Understands nonverbal communicative signals	Follows point
			Responds to distal point
		Uses gestures to engage	Uses proximity
			Uses contact gestures
Emotional Regulation	Mutual regulation	Responds to assistance	Soothes when comforted
			Engages when partners initiate
		Asks partners for assistance	Shares negative emotion for comfort
			Protests when upset
	Self-regulation	Uses behavioral strategies (e.g., sensory motor strategies) to regulate	Uses sensory motor strategies in solitary activities
			Uses sensory motor strategies in social routines
		Recovers from extreme dysregulation	Removes self from overwhelming activity
			Reengages in activity after recovery
Transactional Support	Interpersonal support	Fosters initiation	Waits and encourages initiations
			Offers choices visually
		Adjusts language input	Uses gestures to support understanding
			Uses simple repetitive phrases tied routines
	Learning support	Provides visual and organizational support	Uses objects to define steps within a task
			Uses objects to support smooth transitions
		Modifies learning environment	Adjusts sensory properties of environment
			Infuses motivating and meaningful materials

Adapted from Prizant, B. M., Wetherby, A. M., Rubin, E., Laurent, A. C., & Rydell, P. J. (2006). *The SCERTS Model: A comprehensive educational approach for children with autism spectrum disorders.* Baltimore, MD: Paul H. Brookes Publishing Co.

Table 14.4. Abbreviated scope and sequence of goals for language partner

Domain	Component	Goal area	Sample objective
Social Communication	Joint attention	Engages in reciprocal interaction	Initiates with others
			Participates in reciprocal interactions
		Shares attention	Monitors attentional focus of communicative partner
			Secures attention prior to initiating communication
	Symbol use	Uses words to express self	Uses personal, social words, actions, and modifiers
			Uses word combinations (e.g., agent + action)
		Understands variety of words without contextual cues	Responds to name
			Understands simple sentences without contextual cues
Emotional Regulation	Mutual regulation	Expresses emotions	Understands and uses symbols to express emotion
			Shares range of emotions
		Requests partner assist to regulate state	Uses language to request break
			Uses symbols to request regulating activity
	Self-regulation	Uses language strategies to regulate arousal	Uses language to regulate in extended activities
			Uses language to express range of emotions
		Regulates emotion during transitions	Uses sensory motor strategies to regulate in transitions
			Uses language strategies to regulate in transitions
Transactional Support	Interpersonal support	Responsive to individual	Offers breaks as needed
			Responsive to communicative initiations of individual
		Provides developmental support	Encourages interactions with peers
			Provides guidance on expressing emotions
	Learning support	Structures activity for participation	Creates clear beginning and end of activity
			Offers repeated learning opportunities
		Uses augmentative communication	Uses augmentative communication to support understanding
			Uses augmentative communication to facilitate expression

From Prizant, B. M., Wetherby, A. M., Rubin, E., Laurent, A. C., & Rydell, P. J. (2006). The SCERTS Model: A comprehensive educational approach for children with autism spectrum disorders. Baltimore, MD: Paul H. Brookes Publishing Co.

Table 14.5. Abbreviated scope and sequence of goals for conversational partner

Domain	Component	Goal area	Sample objective
Social Communication	Joint attention	Shares attention	Monitors attentional focus of partners
			Modifies communication based on partners' perspective
		Initiates for a variety of reasons	Communicates to protest and request
			Communicates to share information (e.g., commenting)
	Symbol use	Participates in play and recreation	Plays with other children
			Participates in rule-based recreation
		Uses creative language to express self	Understands and uses complex sentence structures
			Understands and uses pronouns
Emotional Regulation	Mutual regulation	Responds to regulatory assistance offered by partners	Responds to partners' expression of emotion
			Responds to regulatory strategies offered by partners
		Responds to partners' attempts to help recover from extreme dysregulation	Responds to partners' strategies and supports
			Reengages in activity with support of partners after recovery
	Self-regulation	Uses meta-cognitive strategies to regulate	Internalizes rules to guide behavior
			Uses self-monitoring to guide behavior
		Demonstrates availability for learning and interaction	Persists with tasks with reasonable demands
			Engages fully in reciprocal interactions
Transactional Support	Interpersonal support	Respects the individual's independence	Allows individual to move about as needed
			Honors protests as appropriate
		Adjusts language input	Uses nonverbal cues to support understanding
			Adjusts language for arousal level
	Learning support	Uses visual and organizational support	Uses visuals to define steps within a task
			Uses visuals to support engagement in group activities
		Modifies goals, activities, and environment	Adjusts social complexity to help support attention and engagement
			Provides activities that promote opportunities for extended interaction

Adapted from Prizant, B. M., Wetherby, A. M., Rubin, E., Laurent, A. C., & Rydell, P. J. (2006). The SCERTS Model: A comprehensive educational approach for children with autism spectrum disorders. Baltimore, MD: Paul H. Brookes Publishing Co.

overview of goals and objectives at the Social, Language, and Conversational Partner stages, respectively, targeted to increase social-emotional and social-communicative competence.

An expanded format of this structure functions as the curriculum-based assessment and intervention planning tool within The SCERTS Model. The scope and sequence of SC and ER goals and objectives is designed to scaffold typical developmental abilities while understanding, respecting, and working within the unique neurology of ASD. The scope and sequence of TS goals and objectives is designed to help teams select and implement evidence-based learning support and interpersonal support with fidelity in order to be responsive and supportive partners.

EMPIRICAL BASIS

In this age of evidence-based practice, clinicians who work with individuals with ASD are frequently asked to carefully evaluate the research base for well-designed intervention approaches and to implement therapeutic strategies and models with the strongest evidence. This edict calls into question what comprises the strongest evidence for behavioral intervention enacted in applied settings. One primary factor that is often considered germane to the level of evidence for any given study is the nature of the study's design (Courtemanche et al., 2011; Kazdin, 2003; Smith et al., 2007). However, it is important to consider that the level of evidence offered by a study is incumbent on more than its design. The fidelity of the study as well as the appropriate statistical analysis and the freedom from bias are all crucial to ensuring the validity of the evidence offered by a study (Black, 1996; Courtemanche et al., 2011).

In addition, evaluating research examining the effectiveness of educational approaches for individuals with ASD demands attention to the requirements of evidence-based practice. That is, it demands the integration of research findings with other critical factors, including the values and preferences of stakeholders and the ecological validity of intervention (e.g., its relevance to natural contexts and developmental level of the individual). In addition, it demands that the clinical team realistically examine its capacity to implement the evidence-supported approach with high fidelity (Rubin & Lewis, 2016). The SCERTS Model is designed with these considerations in mind, and many of the research designs exploring the efficacy of The SCERTS Model reflect this expanded view of evidence-based practice.

The SCERTS Model is considered to be a transdisciplinary developmental model. It is also often referred to as a Naturalistic Developmental Behavioral Intervention (Schreibman et al., 2015). Drawing from a transdisciplinary literature, The SCERTS Model has a strong empirical base supporting the prioritization of SC and ER as key areas for educational intervention. For example, there is a robust body of literature linking early social-communication milestones and symbolic language outcomes (Kasari et al., 1988; Mundy et al., 2007). In addition, there is a significant proliferation in the qualitative and quantitative literature identifying emotional regulation as a key challenge for individuals with ASD and correlating developmentally appropriate regulatory abilities with greater active engagement and social-communicative competence (Mazefsky et al., 2013). Collectively, these and other foundational research studies are incorporated into The SCERTS Model, which is designed to be a comprehensive educational framework consistent with recommendations to address the needs of children with social learning differences (Wong et al., 2014). The framework is designed to allow practitioners to utilize focused, evidence-based strategies at the correct developmental level to help individuals achieve SC and ER objectives. This incorporation of focused, evidence-based approaches as TS into the comprehensive framework bolsters the research base of the model.

In recent years a number of studies have been conducted and published that highlight the efficacy of the model as a whole beyond its empirical and theoretical foundations. Two randomized, controlled trials (RCTs) have been completed demonstrating the efficacy of The SCERTS Model in the home and classroom settings.

The first RCT adapted the SCERTS framework for delivery within the early intervention setting (Wetherby et al., 2014). Specifically, this study examined the effectiveness of the model when implemented by parents for toddlers with ASD within natural settings. Eighty-two children with ASD, age 19 months (SD = 1.93 months), participated in this 9-month longitudinal study with their primary caregiver. Children were randomized into two groups: an individual coaching format and a group coaching format, both focused on teaching parents how to support active engagement within natural contexts using the SCERTS framework. Individual coaching consisted of in-home support from an interventionist 2–3 times weekly using a collaborative coaching model to build parent capacity and independence in implementation of supports within natural routines geared at facilitating SC and ER development. Parents in this condition were encouraged to deliver intervention by embedding evidence-based strategies for their child's SC and ER targets in everyday activities for >25 hours per week. This dosing is consistent with The SCERTS Model recommendations. The group condition consisted of four to five families participating in clinician-led playgroups in the clinic once a week. These sessions were structured around monthly topics. Results found individual coaching was more efficacious than the group-based format. Common language effect sizes (CLES) were derived from g effect and represent the likelihood that a child in the individual coaching condition will demonstrate greater improvement than a child in the group coaching condition. Outcomes for social communication ($g = 0.76$, $p < .001$, CLES = 0.70), receptive language ($g = 0.41$, $p < .001$, CLES = 0.61), adaptive behavior ($g = 0.50$, $p < .001$, CLES = 0.64), and developmental level ($g = 0.54$, $p < .001$, CLES = 0.61) reached statistical significance (Wetherby et al., 2014).

The efficacy of The SCERTS Model in the classroom was the focus of another large longitudinal RCT. Morgan and colleagues (2018) conducted a cluster RCT for 197 diverse students with ASD in 129 classrooms across 66 schools. Mean age of the students was 6.76 years (SD = 1.05 years). Classrooms were randomly assigned to the Classroom SCERTS Intervention (CSI) or Autism Training Modules (ATM) condition. Special education and general education teachers assigned to the CSI condition in this study were trained on the model and provided coaching throughout the school year. ATM teachers engaged in usual school-based educational practices and had access to online training resources related to autism treatment practices. Notably, in this study, active engagement was used as an outcome measure and was measured by the Classroom Measure of Active Engagement (CMAE; Morgan et al., 2010). Additional outcome measures included the Vineland Adaptive Behavior Scales–Second Edition (VABS-II; Sparrow et al., 2005), the Social Skills Rating System (SSRS; Gresham & Elliot, 1990), and the Behavior Rating Inventory of Executive Functioning (BRIEF [Teacher form]; Gioia et al., 2000).

Results of Morgan and colleagues (2018) revealed that students in the CSI condition showed statistically significant better outcomes on observed measures of adaptive communication, social skills, and executive functioning than did students within the ATM condition. Effect sizes were reported using Cohen's d, where 0.2 is considered small effect, 0.5 is considered medium effect, and 0.8 is considered large effect. Specifically, findings supported improvement in active engagement ($F(1,49) = 6.24, p < .05, d = 0.34$), adaptive communication ($F(1,116) = 6.63, p < .05, d = 0.31$), executive functioning ($F(1,57) = 11.96, p < .001, d = 0.40$), and problem behaviors ($F(1,52) = 10.41, p < .01, d = 0.36$). These data demonstrate the positive impact of SCERTS within a natural environment, that is, the classroom setting, for a heterogeneous sample of students with ASD (Morgan et al., 2018). The Interagency Autism Coordinating Committee chose this study for its *2018 Summary of Advances in Autism Spectrum Disorder Research Report* as a key study addressing the question "Which treatments and interventions will help?" In its review, the committee highlighted that 70% of teachers trained in CSI implemented with fidelity, indicating scalability of the model and also reflecting feasibility with teacher commitment to the model. The committee also acknowledged that this is one of the largest studies to measure the effect of school-based active engagement intervention in children with ASD and that the results appear generalizable to a diverse population (Interagency Autism Coordinating Committee [IACC], 2019).

The prioritization of active engagement as a measure of effectiveness for educational programs for students with ASD aligns with work by Sparapani and colleagues (2015) that identifies the challenges students diagnosed with ASD face in terms of maintaining active engagement and the resulting impact on learning and educational outcomes. In fact, results suggest that students with ASD actively engage less than half of the time in the classroom (Sparapani et al., 2015). Consideration of this finding in the context of additional research suggests that increasing active engagement is critical to positive educational outcomes in ASD and reveals a clear need for approaches such as SCERTS that focus on active engagement (Lord & McGee, 2001).

The SCERTS Model has also been the object of international study. A pilot study was implemented in Hong Kong examining the effectiveness of The SCERTS Model for children with ASD (Yu & Zhu, 2018). This study examined the implementation of SCERTS for two different durations (5 months and 10 months) for children age 53.43 months (SD = 9.05 months) in preschool settings. Special education teachers, occupational therapists, speech pathologists, and physiotherapists were recruited from 10 special child care centers in Hong Kong. Participating professionals received initial training and then were provided coaching throughout the school year. Each participating special education teacher taught 5–7 children. Results showed that participating children improved significantly in their social communication and emotional behavior after intervention as measured by the Developmental Assessment Chart (DAC) and the Chinese Psychoeducational Profile–Third Edition (CPEP-3). Overall, mixed ANOVA results revealed that students in both intervention groups made significant gains between pre- and posttests in terms of social communication and emotional behavior as measured by the DAC, and in communication, motor abilities, and adaptive behaviors as assessed by the CPEP-3 ($p < .001$ for all). Partial η^2 for all scores was greater than 0.30, indicating large effect sizes. These robust findings existed for both intervention groups and were independent of treatment duration. Treatment duration had an effect for only 1 of the 15 outcome factors, social communication, ($F = 11.81, p < .01, \eta^2 = .09$). Therefore, length of intervention did not seem to influence effectiveness of the program.

As part of this same study, focus groups were conducted with educators who were implementing the project and parents of children enrolled in the study. These groups were analyzed qualitatively, and results yielded three key themes. First, participants perceived The SCERTS Model as a comprehensive and multidisciplinary model aimed at supporting children in their core areas of challenge. Second, participants recognized notable improvement in child social communication, indicated by the children paying more attention to others and initiating more frequently. Third, participants acknowledged changes in student emotional regulation, specifically, better understanding of basic emotions and use of behavioral strategies to express their emotions. In addition to these themes, study results included a shift in educator attitudes related to understanding appropriate supports for emotional regulation and no longer seeing problem behavior as noncompliant and willful as well as a shift in educator behaviors from being highly directive in instruction to more facilitative.

The SCERTS Model has also been the subject of a multiple case study design (O'Neill et al., 2010). Implementation of SCERTS in this study followed a multidisciplinary team training for the teams of four pupils (i.e., two Social Partners and two Language Partners). Measures of assessment included the VABS-II (Sparrow et al., 2005) and The SCERTS Model curriculum. All four pupils made progress in joint attention, symbol use, mutual regulation, and self-regulation as well as on the VABS-II Receptive Communication, Expressive Communication, Interpersonal, Play, and Coping Skills scales, according to raw score comparisons. Qualitative methods were used to gain insights from the staff related to their experiences in implementing SCERTS. Central findings from the focus groups with the multidisciplinary team members revealed increased understanding of emotional regulation as a developmental construct as well as increased clarity of team member roles in supporting children when dysregulated. Additional findings reflected team members acknowledging changes in their educational practice consistent with increasing learning support (e.g., greater use of visual supports, augmented communication, occupational therapy strategies). They also revealed changes in interpersonal support such that staff reported giving more wait time, modeling communication behaviors, recognizing dysregulation, and providing support. Staff also described students as happier, calmer, more focused on academic tasks, and ready to learn.

Researchers in the United Kingdom (Molteni et al., 2013) also examined the feasibility of implementing SCERTS as an ecologically valid model in an independent residential school. This research was undertaken under the premise that effective programs for students with ASD require the coordinated expertise of a team of professionals working in partnership with parents and family members (Molteni et al., 2013). This study aimed to understand how teams work together while learning to implement The SCERTS Model. Three teams of professionals (e.g., teachers, teaching assistants, care staff, therapists, heads of departments, and psychologists), each involved in supporting a student at one of the three partner stages, participated. Quantitative and qualitative analyses were conducted. At the conclusion of the study, 89% of the team members said they felt comfortable using SCERTS, and 78% said the framework helped in working with colleagues and provided an opportunity to exchange ideas. Qualitative themes revealed a recognition of a direct link between SCERTS and teamwork. Specifically, teams highlighted that the quality and accuracy of assessment enabled better working together and understanding of students and their environment. In addition, teams achieved consensus that the model provides a framework to support teams of professionals in implementing a plan that respects students and their families.

PRACTICAL REQUIREMENTS

SCERTS is predicated on a team-based approach with multiple disciplines contributing their perspectives. Given the comprehensive nature of the model, a commitment to continuing education and current knowledge of evidence-based practice, in addition to professional collaboration, are critical for implementation fidelity.

Team Approach

The SCERTS Model incorporates a transdisciplinary team-based approach. It is designed to include all members of an individual's educational or intervention team. Members include educational professionals, related services providers, family members, and whenever possible, the individual diagnosed with ASD. Teaming begins during assessment with all members contributing information and observations as data points to build a developmental profile of the individual with ASD as well as a profile of strengths and challenges for the team in terms of transactional support provision. These two profiles are then used as the foundation of a team-based conversation to determine appropriate goals and objectives for the individual and the transactional supports to be implemented by partners.

Once the team reaches consensus on goals and objectives, the members turn their attention to educational planning and infusing learning opportunities in the individual students' daily activities and routines. The team recognizes that the natural partner in those learning opportunities and activities should implement the interpersonal support and learning support and collect the data. So, in essence, all team members are responsible for the implementation of all goals, objectives, and transactional support. Some team members may have expertise in designing specific developmentally appropriate transactional support, and this expertise should be capitalized on (i.e., a speech-language pathologist (SLP) with knowledge of augmentative communication may create a communication system). However, once the support is created and other members of the team are trained within the context of The SCERTS Model, all team members across all contexts would be expected to utilize the support. Given this level of teaming and the transdisciplinary nature of SCERTS, opportunities to meet as a team to share ideas and collaborate are critically important to implementation with fidelity. Indeed, several qualitative research studies focusing on the implementation of SCERTS discuss teaming as a strength of the model but one that requires proactive planning.

Training

The SCERTS manuals published in 2006 are designed to stand alone, that is, they describe the entire model. It is conceivable that a team could purchase the manuals, engage in self-study, and begin to implement the model drawing on their professional expertise. Currently, there is not a formal training process that leads to certification in The SCERTS Model. However, the authors of the model do recognize that teams can often benefit from and expand their practice with additional guidance. Therefore, trainings focused on introduction to the model and implementation of the assessment process and program planning are offered. It should be noted that all research studies demonstrating efficacy of the model involved some form of initial team-based training which was followed up with ongoing mentorship. Within the context of formal trainings, teams are always encouraged to identify a point person within their ranks who can provide ongoing support and resources related to the model. Ideally, this person is well versed in The SCERTS Model and in a range of focused, evidence-based strategies that may be useful within the framework as transactional support to embed in natural activities and environments.

Materials Needed

Minimal materials are required to implement The SCERTS Model. However, access to SCERTS resources and the SCERTS manuals (Prizant et al., 2006a, 2006b) are critical for fidelity of assessment and educational planning. The manuals, a two-volume set, are detailed and comprehensive in an effort to ensure greater fidelity of practice, thereby improving the quality of programming. All assessment and program planning forms are included in the manuals and are reproducible.

Other practical considerations from a material standpoint will be variable and dependent on the individualized SCERTS education plan. Despite this anticipated variability, the commitment is critical to using transactional support to foster development. The nature of these supports will depend on the naturally occurring activities of the individual with ASD. Likewise, material requirements will change depending on the goals selected by teams. For example, if a team is targeting initiation for a Social Partner during play and choosing to do so by structuring the environment to encourage initiation (learning support), see-through containers with preferred toys that can be placed within sight, but out of reach, may be needed. In contrast, if a team is supporting a Conversational Partner's ability to use metacognitive strategies to regulate emotion during familiar and unfamiliar situations (e.g., an assembly at school), access to augmentative supports for emotional regulation (e.g., a feelings book; learning support) may be needed. Therefore, materials are individualized and entirely context dependent.

KEY COMPONENTS

The core values and guiding principles highlighted in the underlying assumptions portion of this chapter are considered to be foundational key components of the model. These serve as the contextual background for the practical key components discussed here.

Commitment to Collaboration

The SCERTS Model entails strong commitment to collaboration. The model is most effective when a team of knowledgeable professionals surrounds the individual and works in a careful and coordinated manner with parents and family members. Therefore, the team may include teachers, teaching assistants, occupational therapists, SLPs, psychologists, social workers, physical therapists, additional specialists, parents, family members, and whenever possible, the individual with ASD. This transdisciplinary approach supports intervention and programming intensity appropriate to an activity-based model that prioritizes intervention in natural contexts with natural partners.

Curriculum-Based Assessment

The core of The SCERTS Model is a developmentally based three-stage curriculum that serves as the foundation for both assessment and intervention planning as well as program implementation. The curriculum focuses on social communication

Table 14.6. Ten steps of The SCERTS® Assessment Process

Step 1	Determine communication stage (Table 14.1).
Step 2	SCERTS Assessment Process–Report (SAP-R) form
	Gather information from families and teachers or other caregivers using SAP-R data to be used in planning observation and building profile of student.
Step 3	SAP Map—Identify assessment team members and plan the SAP observation (natural contexts, length of observation, partners, group size, activity variables, transitions): Who will observe and take data during what naturally occurring activities and when.
Step 4	Team members conduct observations and complete SAP–Observation at appropriate partner stage form.
	Document observed behaviors and consider reported ones.
Step 5	Conduct behavior sampling if needed—not enough information gleaned from direct observations or parent report to inform scoring of goal areas.
Step 6	Compile and integrate information into SAP summary form, summarizing needs and strengths and family perception of SAP–Observation results and priorities.
Step7	Prioritize goals and objective based on developmental appropriateness, family priority, and functionality.
Step 8	Recommend further assessment if needed.
Step 9	Design SCERTS educational program.
Step 10	Continue ongoing tracking.

Source: Prizant et al (2006a).

and emotional regulation for individuals with ASD and transactional support for the partners.

The SAP is a 10-step sequence that is implemented by teams to establish a profile of developmental strengths and a profile of opportunities for growth (see Table 14.6). It also helps teams select motivating, meaningful, and developmentally appropriate social-communication and emotional-regulation goals as well as targeted evidence-based transactional support. Finally, it provides guidance to teams for embedding the individual's goals and the team's transactional support in natural activities as well as mechanisms for monitoring progress. Given the robust nature of the SAP, it is apparent that in addition to commitment to teaming, there is a need to allocate ample time to accomplish the process. As a point of reference, the length of observations for both Social Partners and Language Partners is 2 hours, whereas Conversational Partner observations are 4 hours.

Commitment to Intervention in Natural Routines

Once the SAP–Observation form is completed and reviewed, the team uses that information to select goals and objectives to be included in the student's educational plan. Goals and objectives are to be functional, developmentally appropriate, and responsive to a family's and/or individual's priority. They are then embedded across the entire day. This process involves creating a daily schedule for the student and identifying natural activities to imbed social-communication and emotional-regulation objectives for the child while identifying critical transactional supports to be implemented by partners. Partners implementing transactional support and helping to support student acquisition of social-communication and emotional-regulation skills may expand beyond the core team involved in the assessment to include siblings, peers, and community members. Activity planning grids (see Figures 14.1, 14.2, and 14.3)

Activity	Requests desired food or things	Uses giving or pointing gestures	Expresses negative emotion to seek comfort	Uses behaviors modeled by partners to self-soothe or focus self	Transactional supports
	Educational goals				Transactional supports
Transitions			X	X	Provide *concrete objects to hold related to upcoming activities* and *provide access to materials that serve as sources of regulation.* With each transition, *offer an object* that represents where child is going (e.g., water pail for garden, tray for cafeteria, shaving cream can for sensory room).
Mealtimes	X	X			*Offer choices* of desired food items in see-through containers with photo of family member on top to encourage a gaze shift and directed communication. *Respond to nonverbal signals* to foster sense of competence; be sure to follow child's gaze to specific materials and then model key language targets.
Play	X	X			Entice with developmentally appropriate *hands-on activities* such as cause–effect (e.g., blowing bubbles, wind-up toys, balloons), building, cooking, messy play, music, and art, and *encourage initiations* by giving numerous chances to communicate through choices of objects or see-through containers.
Music	X	X			*Provide objects to match each song* (e.g., scarf for "Ring Around the Rosie," a puppet for "Row, Row, Row Your Boat"). *Offer choices* of objects in see-through containers to allow child to request a preferred song.

Figure 14.1. Home-based activity planning grid sample for Annie, a 3-year-old Social Partner.

Activity	Initiates and maintains extended interactions	Uses a variety of developmental word combinations	Uses words or symbols to communicate emotion	Uses language to engage productively in extended activity	Transactional supports
	Educational goals				
Transitions			X	X	Provide *visuals for smooth transitions to upcoming activities* and *visuals to define steps within each task*; include a timetable for the sequence of activities across the day as well as visuals to mark steps toward completion of each activity (e.g., 3, 2, 1, . . . all finished). Provide *visuals for emotional expression* (John is [tired, excited, angry]) with *choices of how to cope* on the reverse of the visual (e.g., John can ask for help, John can cuddle).
Meal time	X	X			*Offer choices* of food item visuals with names, verbs, and color-coded sentence-building templates and *encourage initiations* by giving choices for actions related to the activity (e.g., Ms. Sarah, pour milk or Ms. Sarah, open chips); include his teachers' and peers' names to encourage sentences about both John and those he is playing with.
Reading	X	X			Provide pictures with a range of subject plus verbs and sentence-building templates to ensure that John has a visual to use to comment on books (e.g., Frog blow bubbles, Toad push wagon).

Figure 14.2. School-based activity planning grid sample for John, a 10-year-old Language Partner. *Source:* Adapted from Prizant, B. M., Wetherby, A. M., Rubin, E., Laurent, A. C., & Rydell, P. J. (2006). The SCERTS Model: A comprehensive educational approach for children with autism spectrum disorders. Baltimore, MD: Paul H. Brookes Publishing Co.

are used to visually operationalize programming decisions and promote fidelity of intervention. These grids are constructed so they reflect at least 25 hours of intervention. It is likely that teams will select a number of learning supports and interpersonal supports to help support skill development in any one activity. For example, at the Language Partner stage, partners would not simply implement one learning support, such as the use of augmentative communication (e.g., picture symbols), but would be encouraged to offer choices of desired items, to provide a balance

Activity	Uses language for greetings, turn taking, calling out for others	Uses appropriate volume and intonation for the context	Uses language to request help from others	Uses language to work out and think about coping strategies that may be helpful in future situations	Transactional supports
	Educational goals				Transactional supports
Transitions			X	X	Provide visuals to *define steps within each task* and visuals to *model appropriate coping strategies* for different emotional states and needs.
Language arts	X		X		*Provide guidance* for interpreting others' thoughts in literature using visuals to illustrate character thoughts. *Model language* for emotional expression, negotiation, and coping.
Science	X	X			Infuse *motivating topics* in activities and *provide visuals* for success in group activities (e.g., turn-taking dials, vocal volume meter, social narratives).
Math	X		X		*Provide visuals to define steps* within each task. Infuse *motivating topics* in activities and *provide visuals* for success in group activities (e.g., math strategy helper cards—using a ruler, protractor).

Figure 14.3. School-based activity planning grid sample for Stuart, a 16-year-old Conversational Partner.

between initiated and respondent turns, and to ensure that the individual is motivated to engage by modifying the environment to provide developmentally appropriate activities.

Figure 14.1 highlights SCERTS Model programming for Annie, a young Social Partner, in her home environment. Based on her SAP results and in collaboration with her parents, Annie's team selected four objectives as the focus of their interventions: supporting her ability to request desired food and objects, using conventional gestures, expressing negative emotions to seek comfort, and using behaviors modeled by others to self-soothe. When considering evidence-based, developmentally appropriate transactional supports to scaffold development in these areas within natural routines, the team agreed to use object-based representations of activities, to support initiation by implementing communicative temptations, and to infuse motivating and meaningful materials. Figure 14.1 illustrates the programming decisions made by the team to embed these goals and supports during specific activities in Annie's day.

Figure 14.2 highlights SCERTS Model programming for John, a 10-year-old Language Partner. Based on his SAP results and in collaboration with family members, John's team selected four objectives as the focus of their school-based interventions: initiating and maintaining extended interactions, using a variety of developmental word combinations, using symbols to communicate emotions, and using language to engage productively in extended activities. When considering evidence-based, developmentally appropriate transactional supports to scaffold development in these areas within natural routines, the team agreed to use visual schedules to support smooth transitions and understanding of flow within activities, visuals for emotional expression, and visual structures for creative language development. Figure 14.2 illustrates the programming decisions made by the team for embedding these goals and supports during specific activities in John's day.

Figure 14.3 highlights SCERTS Model programming for Stuart, a 16-year-old Conversational Partner. Based on his SAP results and in collaboration with family members, Stuart's team selected four objectives as the focus of their school-based interventions: using language to connect to others for social reasons, modifying volume and intonation based on social context, using language to request assistance, and using language to reflect on the effectiveness of coping strategies. When considering evidence-based, developmentally appropriate transactional supports to scaffold development in these areas within natural routines, the team agreed to provide visuals to define steps within activities, to model coping strategies and emotional expression, and to infuse motivating topics in activities. Figure 14.3 illustrates the programming decisions made by the team for embedding these goals and supports during specific activities in Stuart's day.

ASSESSMENT FOR TREATMENT
PLANNING AND PROGRESS MONITORING

As detailed in previous sections, The SCERTS Model is applicable to a wide range of individuals with ASD. There is no formal process for establishing whether the SCERTS Model is appropriate for a particular student because it is a developmental framework. Therefore, all students functioning within the age range covered by the curriculum can in theory be assessed using the curriculum to establish their profile of strengths and challenges. This is particularly true for children who are struggling with social communication and/or emotional regulation. However, the curriculum and the intervention process are most appropriate for children with ASD or those who have similar learning styles because the transactional support curriculum is geared to the neurologically based learning difference of individuals with ASD.

The SCERTS Model is designed to align with the recommendations of the National Research Council's *Educating Children with Autism* report (Lord & McGee, 2001), which suggests that progress toward objectives should be observable within 3-month periods of time. Therefore, SCERTS incorporates multiple options for collecting data to ensure the individual is making progress and that transactional supports are being implemented with fidelity. Specifically, forms for collecting data related to individual social-communication and emotional-regulation targets and transactional support are included in the SCERTS manual that allow data collection on an activity, daily, and/or weekly basis, with the choice of methods left to the discretion of the team. Regardless of basis on which teams choose to collect the data, the resulting data document the child's progress and also the fidelity of implementation of transactional support. If students are not making progress toward their goals and objectives, transactional support data can be used to determine if factors related to consistency of supports or the developmental level of the supports being provided may be the reason.

IMPLICATIONS FOR INCLUSIVE PRACTICE

The SCERTS Model is designed to align with the Individuals with Disabilities Education Act; free, appropriate public education; and least restrictive environment; therefore, it is designed to support learners in a variety of environments. It is used in early intervention settings (for a detailed description of home-based parent-implemented iteration of the model in early intervention, please see Chapter 11). In schools, SCERTS is implemented in a wide variety of settings, including special schools, special education classrooms, and general education settings. The research discussed earlier in the chapter on CSI, the classroom version of SCERTS, highlights the applicability of SCERTS in all of these settings. Specifically, CSI addresses implementation in both special education classrooms and general education classrooms (Morgan et al., 2018). The SCERTS Model is also designed to be implemented in community-based settings.

Regardless of the setting, the goals and objectives for both the individual with ASD and his or her communication partners are embedded in naturally occurring activities throughout the day. For a preschool-age Social Partner working on initiating interactions with others (joint attention), educational team members may build in opportunities during snack and free play to encourage interactions by offering nonverbal choices (e.g., interpersonal support: holding out two objects), waiting to encourage initiations (e.g., giving time to process without verbal directives; interpersonal support), and arranging the environment to encourage initiation (e.g., placing preferred items in see-through containers that are difficult to reach or out of reach; learning support). For a middle school–age Language Partner who is learning to use symbols to express emotions (self-regulation), educational team members may build in opportunities and supports during activities where the student has predictable emotional responses. For example, modeling the use of visually based emotion cards (learning support) for expression and also providing verbal models (interpersonal support) during lunch when the student is happy and also during math class when the student is regularly frustrated is warranted. For a Conversational Partner in high school who is learning how to collaborate and negotiate with peers in problem solving (symbol use), educational staff may prioritize embedding supports during partner-based science labs and physical education classes. These supports may range from creating clear roles for partners (interpersonal support) in activities to learning to use visuals such as Venn diagrams (learning support) to facilitate discussions and reach consensus.

As previously stated, The SCERTS Model is designed to be cross contextual—meaning that goals are targeted, and supports are shared with communication partners in different settings of the individual's life. Therefore, if placing objects out of reach is a successful strategy used to encourage spontaneous nonverbal initiations by an individual at the Social Partner level in the school setting, this strategy would be shared with the student's family members so that they might incorporate it in the child's day at home and foster generalization of skills and learning. These same strategies could then be carried out by family members or other caregivers in the child's life in the community environment. For example, if the child attends a community-based music group in the community, sharing the objective related to spontaneous nonverbal initiations with the group leader as well as the strategies to support the student doing so would provide additional opportunities for the student to learn, practice, and acquire that skill. In this instance having the teacher store preferred musical instruments out of reach but also in sight may accomplish this objective.

This type of cross-contextual transactional support is a goal within The SCERTS Model, as it supports the idea of robust skill acquisition and students truly understanding that they are competent communicators regardless of setting and partner. This leads to increased confidence, which opens students up to additional learning opportunities.

CONSIDERATIONS FOR CHILDREN FROM CULTURALLY AND LINGUISTICALLY DIVERSE BACKGROUNDS

The SCERTS Model is family centered. By definition, family-centered models prioritize sensitivity to family characteristics. These characteristics may include cultural and linguistic differences. By inviting the family to participate in several aspects of their child's assessment as well as in the intervention across contexts, educational staff implementing The SCERTS Model are in a unique position to learn a great deal about the family values, beliefs, and educational priorities for their child. Because The SCERTS Model does not follow a prescribed curriculum for therapeutic activities and lessons, practitioners are able to modify daily activities and routines in ways that reflect family priorities and cultural preferences.

The SCERTS Model also offers support plans for families focusing on both educational and emotional support. Within these plans, educational team members implementing SCERTS with a student are able to spend time educating family on the how and why of SCERTS. Educational support within the model may address the core challenges of the child's diagnosis and why certain educational priorities may lead to better outcomes. For example, if a child is often quiet and calm during his or her day (and the family's culture supports this), but that arousal state is actually not supportive of active engagement in a given environment, it may be important to educate the family on why initiation of interactions supports greater opportunities for social learning and consequently for language acquisition. In addition, the importance of matching arousal state to the context in order to support active participation may emerge as a valuable focus for family education. Therefore, in the context of such conversations, families and educational providers can reach agreements related to strategies that will meet the student's needs but also be consistent with family preferences and culture. Studies by both Wetherby and colleagues (2014) and Morgan and colleagues (2018) included relatively diverse samples, thereby suggesting efficacy across cultures. However, further study with additional diverse populations is needed.

Anecdotally, SCERTS is viewed as a culturally sensitive model that allows for cultural adaptation. For example, SCERTS Model trainings have occurred on five continents and in many countries. The feedback of these worldwide trainings is that practitioners are able to adapt The SCERTS Model in ways that makes sense within their cultures. By focusing on core challenges and learning differences characteristic of individuals with ASD, as well as on the notion that learning is a social construct and that partners have significant impact on learning, The SCERTS Model encourages cultural adaptation to support communicative competence in the individual's natural environments and routines. Currently, The SCERTS Model manuals have been translated into Korean and Japanese with additional translations being pursued.

Application to a Child

Sammi is a 6-year-old first-grade student who is a member of a general education class-room in her public school district. In addition to instruction in the first-grade classroom, she receives support from her special education teacher, her instructional assistant, her occupational therapist, and her SLP. Outside of school, Sammi's inner circle of communica-tion partners and support network include her parents, her older brother, and neighbors who frequently babysit her after school.

Sammi was diagnosed with ASD at 2 years of age and has been involved in edu-cationally based interventions since that time. In preparation for her first-grade year, Sammi's team used the Worksheet for Determining Communication Stage, the first step of the SAP. Using this form, the team, which included her parents, agreed that she was a Language Partner. She has a fairly robust spoken vocabulary but most frequently uses single words to express her wants and needs. When she does use longer phrases, they are often echolalic in nature and do not reflect her demonstrated abilities to creatively combine words to make comments or other communicative functions.

Sammi's educational team and family completed the full SAP to build a develop-mental profile for Sammi. Throughout the assessment, the team noted that Sammi had several communicative functions in her repertoire (joint attention). In particular, Sammi engaged in brief reciprocal interactions; frequently shared both positive and negative emotions; and protested and requested desired food, activities, and objects. However, her team noted that she was not yet consistently commenting on objects and that her rate of communication was typically low even in highly preferred activities. Similar pro-files of strengths and challenges were noted in symbol use. She was observed to spon-taneously imitate actions and words immediately after a model, she used at least 5–10 words and echolalic phrases independently, and she used several conventional gestures. However, the team also noted that she was not yet using a variety of developmental word combinations, nor was she consistently combining a variety of actions with objects in play. In terms of mutual regulation, her team noted that she was often able to be soothed by others but did not yet seek out others for assistance with regulating her emo-tional state. With respect to self-regulation, Sammi was noted to consistently use behav-ioral strategies (e.g., bouncing up and down on her toes, rubbing her hands together, and twirling her hair) to attempt to regulate her arousal and participate actively in both solitary and social activities; however, the team noted that she was not yet independently using language strategies that had been provided (e.g., break cards, personal schedules).

At the time of assessment, the team also created a combined profile of strengths and opportunities for growth. Specifically, the team recognized that between the home and school contexts, Sammi's communication partners were consistently using interpersonal supports such as offering her choices, using proximity to encourage interactions, getting down on her level when communicating, and recognizing signs of dysregulation and offering her support. They also recognized that there was room for the team to increase consistency in a few interpersonal support areas that would be key to the accomplishment of her goals and objectives. In particular, they noted that all of Sammi's communication partners could more frequently model a range of communica-tive functions, child perspective language, and constructive and symbolic play. Finally, with respect to learning supports, the team recognized that they consistently worked to define clear beginnings and ends of activities and frequently modified the sensory properties of the environment, but they also recognized that they were not consistently using supports to define steps within a task or to support smooth transitions between activities. They also agreed that they were not using augmentative communication to enhance Sammi's expressive communication consistently and that augmentative communication would be helpful in her acquisition of word types and in the development of word combinations.

Her team set initial goals: commenting on objects (joint attention), using word developmental word combinations (symbol use), using language to request a break (mutual regulation), and using language strategies modeled by partners to regulate arousal level (self-regulation schedules). In order to help achieve these goals and objectives, the team included the following transactional supports as critical accommodations within Sammi's IEP: modeling a range of communicative functions (interpersonal support), providing augmented and alternative communication supports for expressive language and providing augmentative support for emotional regulation (i.e., visual break cards; learning support), and modeling and providing access to supports that define the steps within an activity (e.g., schedules; learning support).

The educational team sat as a group and created activity planning grids for home and school contexts. They collected data on Sammi's progress toward her objectives and the consistency with which team members implemented supports. As Sammi demonstrated abilities in a variety of contexts with a variety of partners, the team targeted skills in additional activities to bolster her confidence and competence with the new skills prior to selecting new objectives.

Application to an Adolescent

Justin is a 17-year-old high school senior who is on target to graduate at the top of his class from his public high school. His educational team consists of his general education teachers, his special education case manager, as well as his school psychologist and SLP, who provide consultation as needed. Outside of school, Justin's regular communication partners include his parents, his twin younger brothers, and his grandparents.

In preparation for his senior year of high school, Justin's team conducted the SAP appropriate for the Conversational Partner stage with college preparation in mind. As a college-bound senior, Justin demonstrated many strengths in social communication, especially with regard to symbol use. His ability to understand and use generative language to express himself was very robust. However, he continued to struggle with understanding nonverbal cues and nonliteral meanings in conversations with others. From a joint attention standpoint, although Justin demonstrated reciprocity in the speaker and listener roles when interacting with others, he was challenged by the ability to gauge the length and content of turns based on partners. The team agreed that Justin's biggest challenges were not in the area of social communication but in regulation. In contrast to his advanced academic and linguistic abilities, Justin often struggled with maintaining active engagement and supporting his attention in conventional ways. Staff noted that he was meticulous at following his schedules, but he continued to struggle with using effective and efficient behavioral strategies that have been modeled by partners during classroom activities. He tended to pace about the room, asking frequent questions for clarification, and often sat perched in a chair, occasionally biting on his clothing. While his team recognized the functions of each of these behaviors for Justin, they also acknowledged that these behaviors, at times, interfered with both his focus and the learning environment as a whole. From a mutual regulatory standpoint, the team acknowledged that he often struggled with responding to information or strategies for regulation offered by partners.

During the course of the SAP, they recognized that there was room for the team to increase consistency in a few interpersonal support areas that would be key to the accomplishment of his goals and objectives. Specifically, team members could provide him with more direct teaching and modeling related to behavior strategies for regulation as well as with more guidance and feedback for improving his success in activities. Likewise, they agreed that providing visual supports to help Justin navigate challenges in emotional regulation was a priority, as was using visual supports to assist him in working in groups, promoting his extended interactions with others, and providing opportunities to bolster his functional social-communication abilities with his peers.

The team created initial goals as the result of collaboration with Justin, his parents, and his educational team. These included gauging length of conversational turns (joint attention), responding to assistance offered by others (mutual regulation), and using behavioral strategies modeled by partners to regulate arousal in activities (self-regulation). In order to help achieve these goals and objectives, staff members included the following transactional supports as potentially critical accommodations within his IEP: provide him with more direct teaching and modeling related to behavior strategies for regulation (interpersonal support) and provide guidance and feedback needed for success in activities (interpersonal support). They also agreed that providing visual supports to help Justin navigate challenges in emotional regulation was a priority, as was using visual supports (learning support) to assist him in group work that would promote his extended interactions with others and provide opportunities to bolster his functional social-communication abilities with his peers (learning support).

The staff sat as a group and created activity planning grids for both home and school contexts. They collected data on Justin's progress toward his objectives and on the consistency of the staff's implementation of supports. As Justin demonstrated abilities in a variety of contexts with a variety of partners, the team targeted skills in additional activities to bolster his confidence and competence with the new skills prior to selecting new objectives.

To review an extended application and implementation of this intervention, see Case 11 about a child with ASD in the companion volume *Case Studies for the Treatment of Autism Spectrum Disorder.*

Future Directions

Although The SCERTS model has a number of efficacy studies demonstrating its applicability and utility in a variety of settings, ongoing research in a variety of settings is warranted. Likewise, expansion of research to include a broader age range of participants and even more culturally diverse samples are appropriate next steps. It also is important to study SCERTS as a cross-contextual assessment and intervention model. To date, although SCERTS is designed to be utilized across contexts, studies exploring the efficacy of SCERTS have included observational measurement in a single context. and intervention priority has been placed on fidelity within that one context.

For SCERTS to expand its feasibility as a model of intervention within the public schools, continued research into effective dissemination and fidelity of implementation is warranted. Therefore, it is critical to identify the basic competencies for personnel training and for making sure that educational materials are easily accessible and comprehensible. Based on the existing efficacy research, it appears that ongoing training and mentorship opportunities may be very supportive of implementation fidelity. Research to understand those mechanisms as well as to develop consistent training and mentorship protocols will help with dissemination of the model and with the likelihood that practitioners can routinely develop high degrees of competence and confidence with implementation.

Suggested Readings

1. Prizant, B. M., Wetherby, A. M., Rubin, E., Laurent, A. C., & Rydell, P. J. (2006). *The SCERTS® Model: A comprehensive educational approach for children with autism spectrum disorders. Volume I: Assessment.* Paul H. Brookes Publishing Co. This volume serves as the comprehensive assessment resource.

2. Prizant, B. M., Wetherby, A. M., Rubin, E., Laurent, A. C., & Rydell, P. J. (2006). *The SCERTS® Model: A comprehensive educational approach for children with autism spectrum disorders. Volume II: Program planning and intervention.* Paul H. Brookes Publishing Co. This volume serves as the comprehensive intervention planning resource. It includes resources for linking transactional supports to individual objectives in social communication and emotional regulation.

3. Morgan, L., Hooker, J. L., Sparapani, N., Reinhardt, V. P., Schatschneider, C., Wetherby, A. M. (2018). Cluster randomized trial of CSI for elementary students with autism spectrum disorders. *Journal of Consulting and Clinical Psychology, 86*(7), 631–644. This article discusses the implementation of the model in public schools and demonstrates its efficacy.

4. Wetherby, A., Guthrie, W., Woods, J., Schatschneider, C., Holland, R, Morgan, L., & Lord, C. (2014). Parent implemented social intervention for toddlers with autism: An RCT. *Pediatrics, 134*(6), 1084–1093. This article discusses the implementation of the model in the home environment for children in early intervention services and demonstrates its efficacy.

5. SCERTS, www.SCERTS.com. This website is dedicated to the dissemination of information related to The SCERTS Model.

Learning Activities

1. Reflect on the nature of The SCERTS Model. What are some of the key defining characteristics? How are the theoretical foundations in person- and family-centered intervention reflected in the model? How is the developmental perspective infused throughout the model?

2. Consider a student on your caseload. What is his or her partner stage within the context of the model (see Table 14.1)?

3. For the same student, reflect on how the order of intervention priorities might be based on the developmental and intervention literature as well as on the student's daily schedule (see Tables 14.3, 14.4, and 14.5).

4. Using the information from Questions 2 and 3, map out a simple activity planning grid that starts to focus intervention for the student (see Figure 14.1 for example).

5. Jacob's educational team agrees that he is a Social Partner; however, they are struggling to figure out how best to support his communicative development. What do you suggest as top communication priorities? How will these best be accomplished? Who will be responsible for implementation on the team?

6. Suppose the family is thrilled with progress at school and the reports they receive from staff on a weekly basis, but they have seen little transference of learning to the home and are concerned that generalization of learning is not happening naturally. How might you support the family to support their child's use of skills at home?

Summary of Video Clip

*See the **About the Videos and Downloads** page at the front of the book for directions on how to access and stream the accompanying videos to this chapter.*

The series of two videos represents the observation and action planning of an educational team using The SCERTS framework. Jaron is a 6½-year-old Conversational Partner who is participating in a first-grade general education math lesson. The academic standard is focused on the students' learning how to identify the value of coins and trade up coins to those of higher value. The teacher has embedded this learning target into a dice game that gives students the opportunity to take turns with a peer rolling the dice, identify coins that match the value of the dice, and trade up their coins to those of higher value. This natural activity provides the context for SCERTS intervention. The team, however, will need to engage in SCERTS observation and action planning to ensure that social communication and emotional regulation are being addressed using both interpersonal supports and learning supports embedded in the lesson.

Before implementing SCERTS, the educational team had been focused on ensuring that Jaron was following the social rules of the classroom. In the first video (titled "Baseline"), an instructional assistant has provided a dry erase board with the instructions written to "sit nicely" and "sit quietly" (this support is not visible on the video). As the lesson progresses, Jaron is clearly referencing this visual and working to achieve these goals. He turns to his teacher and asks, "Am I doing a good job?" and appears to be hoping that he has achieved a reward for his nice sitting.

The educational team met and reviewed the key priorities of SCERTS and recognized a need to shift the focus to that of active engagement and participation (e.g., initiating with his peers and self-regulating by talking through the steps of the task). As far as transactional supports, the team appreciated those that were already in place in the lesson (e.g., a meaningful, hands-on task with frequent role modeling). Next, they collaborated to discuss how next steps accessible to the whole class could benefit Jaron as well as his peers. These transactional supports included a visual for each peer dyad to hold during group instruction to indicate the coin values and how to trade up as a means to foster their initiation as well as a to-do list for each step of the task to foster their self-regulation. The second video illustrates the impact of this shift in focus to that of active engagement and a planned discussion of which transactional supports to embed in the lesson. One can see how both Jaron and his peers are engaging in more sophisticated social communication and emotional regulation with these changes in place.

REFERENCES

American Psychiatric Association. (2013). *Diagnostic and statistical manual of mental disorders, Fifth edition* (DSM-5). Author.

American Speech-Language-Hearing Association. (2006). *Guidelines for speech-language pathologists in diagnosis, assessment, and treatment of autism spectrum disorders across the life span*. Retrieved on February 5, 2021 from, http://faculty.washington.edu /jct6/ASHAGuideLinesAutismAssessmentScreening.pdf

Baron, G., Groden, J., Groden, G., & Lipsitt, L. P. (2006). *Stress and coping in autism.* Oxford University Press.

Bates, E. (1976). *Language and context: The acquisition of pragmatics*. Academic Press.

Black, N. (1996). Why we need observational studies to evaluate the effectiveness of health care. *British Medical Journal, 312* (7040), 1215–1218.

Bloom, L. (2000). *The transition from infancy to language.* Cambridge University Press.

Courtemanche, A. B., Schroeder, S. R., & Sheldon, J. B. (2011). Designs and analyses of psychotropic and behavioral interventions for the treatment of problem behavior among people with intellectual and developmental disabilities. *American Journal on Intellectual and Developmental Disabilities, 116*(4), 315–328.

DeGangi, G. (2000). *Pediatric disorders of regulation in affect and behavior: A therapist's guide to assessment and treatment.* Academic Press.

Dunn, W., Cox, J., Foster, L., Mische-Laweson, L., & Tanquaray, J. (2012). Impact of an integrated intervention on parental competence and children's participation with autism. *American Journal of Occupational Therapy, 36*(5), 520–528.

Eisenberg, N., & Sulik, M. J. (2012). Emotion-related self-regulation in children. *Teaching of Psychology, 39*(1), 77–83.

Fox, N. A. (1994). The development of emotion regulation: Biological and behavioral considerations. *Monographs of the Society for Research in Child Development, 59*(2–3, Serial No. 240).

Gioia, G. A., Isquith, P. K., Guy, S. C., & Kenworthy, L. (2000). *BRIEF: Behavior Rating Inventory of Executive Function.* Psychological Assessment Resources.

Gulsrud, A. C., Jahromi, L. B., & Kasari, C. (2010). The co-regulation of emotions between mothers and their children with autism. *Journal of Autism and Developmental Disorders, 40*(2), 227–237.

Gresham, F. M., & Elliott, S. N. (1990). *Social Skills Rating System Manual.* American Guidance Service.

Interagency Autism Coordinating Committee (IACC). (2019). *2018 IACC summary of advances in autism spectrum disorder research.* U.S. Department of Health and Human Services Interagency Autism Coordinating Committee. https://iacc.hhs.gov/publications /summary-of-advances/2018

Jahromi, L. B., Bryce, C. I., & Swanson, J. (2013). The importance of self-regulation for the school and peer engagement of children with high-functioning autism. *Research in Autism Spectrum Disorders, 7*(2), 235–246.

Kasari, C., Paparella, T., Freeman, S., & Jahromi, L. B. (2008). Language outcome in autism: Randomized comparison of joint attention and play interventions. *Journal of Consulting and Clinical Psychology, 76*(1), 125–137.

Kasari, C., Sigman, M., Mundy, P., & Yirmiya, N. (1988). Caregiver interactions with autistic children. *Journal of Abnormal Child Psychology, 16*(1), 45–56.

Kasari, C., Gulsrud, A. C., Wong, C., Kwon, S., & Locke, J. (2010). Randomized controlled caregiver mediated joint engagement intervention for toddlers with autism. *Journal of Autism and Developmental Disorders, 40*(9), 1045–1056.

Kazdin, A. (2003). *Research design in clinical psychology* (4th ed.). Allyn & Bacon.

Koegel, R., Koegel, L., & Dunlap, G. (Eds.). (1996). *Positive behavioral support: Including people with difficult behavior in the community.* Paul H. Brookes Publishing Co.

Laurent, A., & Rubin, E. (2004). Challenges in emotional regulation in Asperger syndrome and high-functioning autism. *Topics in Language Disorders, 24*(4), 286–297.

Little, L. (2001). Peer victimization of children with Asperger spectrum disorders. *Journal of the American Academy of Child and Adolescent Psychiatry, 40*(9), 995–996.

Lord, C., & McGee, J. P., (Eds.). (2001). *Educating children with autism.* Committee on Educational Interventions for Children with Autism, Commission on Behavioral and Social Sciences and Education, National Research Council. National Academy Press.

Mazefsky, C. A. (2015). Emotion regulation and emotional distress in autism spectrum disorder: Foundations and considerations for future research. *Journal of Autism and Developmental Disorders, 45*(11), 3405–3408.

Mazefsky, C. A., Herrington, J., Siegel, M., Scarpa, A., Maddox, B. B., Scahill, L., & White, S. W. (2013). The role of emotion regulation in autism spectrum disorder. *Journal of the American Academy of Child and Adolescent Psychiatry, 52*(7), 679–688.

McWilliam, R. A. (2010). *Working with families of young children with special needs.* Guildford Press.

Molteni, P., Guldberg, K., & Logan, N. (2013). Autism and multidisciplinary teamwork through The SCERTS Model. *British Journal of Special Education, 40*(3), 137–145.

Morgan, L., Hooker, J. L., Sparapani, N., Rinehardt, V., Schatschneider, C., & Wetherby, A. (2018). Cluster randomized trial of the classroom SCERTS intervention for students with autism spectrum disorder. *Journal of Consulting and Clinical Psychology, 86*(7), 631–644.

Morgan, L., Wetherby, A., & Holland, R. (2010). *Classroom measure of active engagment and transactional supports* [Unpublished manuscript]. Florida State University.

Mundy, P., Block, J., Delgado, C., Pomares, Y., Van Hecke, A. V, & Parlade, M. V. (2007). Individual differences and the development of joint attention in infancy. *Child Development, 78*(3), 938–954.

O'Neill, J., Bergstrand, L., Bowman, K., Elliott, K., Mavin, L., Stephenson, S., & Wayman, C. (2010). The SCERTS model: Implementation and evaluation in a primary special school. *Good Autism Practice, 11*(1), 7–15.

Prizant, B. M., & Laurent, A. C. (2012a). *Preventing problem behavior for students with developmental challenges through an emotional regulation approach (ERA): Guide #1 Presymbolic Stage.* National Professional Resources.

Prizant, B. M., & Laurent, A. C. (2012b). *Preventing problem behaviors for students with developmental challenges through an emotional regulation approach (ERA): Guide #2 Symbolic Stage.* National Professional Resources.

Prizant, B. M., Wetherby, A. M., Rubin, E., & Laurent, A. C. (2003). The SCERTS Model: A transactional, family-centered approach to enhancing communication and socioemotional abilities of children with autism spectrum disorder. *Infants & Young Children, 16*(4), 296–316. https://doi.org/10.1097/00001163-200310000-00004

Prizant, B. M., Wetherby, A. M., Rubin, E., Laurent, A. C., & Rydell, P. J. (2006a). *The SCERTS Model: A comprehensive educational approach for children with autism spectrum disorders, Volume 1 Assessment.* Paul H. Brookes Publishing Co.

Prizant, B. M., Wetherby, A. M., Rubin, E., Laurent, A. C., & Rydell, P. J. (2006). The SCERTS® Model: A comprehensive educational approach for children with autism spectrum disorders. Volume II: Program planning and intervention. Paul H. Brookes Publishing Co.

Rubin, E., & Lewis, M. (2016). Issue editor foreword: A developmental framework for evidence-based practices for the autism spectrum. *Topics in Language Disorders, 36*(3), 194–197. https://doi.org/10.1097/TLD.0000000000000097

Sameroff, A. J., & Fiese, B. H. (1990). Transactional regulation and early intervention. In S. J. Meisels & J. P. Shonkoff (Eds.), *Handbook of early childhood intervention* (pp. 119–149). Cambridge University Press.

Schreibman, L., Dawson, G., Stahmer, A. C., Landa, R., Rogers, S. J., McGee, G. G., Kasari, C., Ingersoll, B., Kaiser, A., Bruinsma, Y., McNerney, E., Wetherby, A., & Halladay, A. (2015). Naturalistic developmental behavioral interventions: Empirically validated treatments for autism spectrum disorder. *Journal of Autism and Developmental Disorders, 45*(8), 2411–2428. https://doi.org/10.1007/s10803-015-2407-8

Smith, T., Scahill, L., Dawson, G., Guthrie, D., Lord, C., Odom, S., Rogers, S., & Wagner, A. (2007). Designing research studies on psychosocial interventions in autism. *Journal of Autism and Developmental Disorders, 37*(2), 354–366. https://doi.org/10.1007/s10803-006-0173-3

Sparapani, N., Morgan, L., Reinhardt, V. P., Schatschneider, C., & Wetherby, A. M. (2015). Evaluation of classroom active engagement in elementary students with autism spectrum disorder. *Journal of Autism and Developmental Disorders, 46*(3), 782–796. https://doi .org/10.1007/s10803-015-2615-2

Sparrow, S. S., Cicchetti, D. V., & Balla, D. A. (2005). *Vineland Adaptive Behavior Scales–Second edition.* American Guidance Service.

Tantam, D. (2000). Adolescence and adulthood of individuals with Asperger syndrome. In A. Klin, F. Volkmar, & S. S. Sparrow (Eds.), *Asperger syndrome* (pp. 367–399). Guilford Press.

Tomasello, M., Carpenter, M., Call, J., Behne, T., & Moll, H., M. (2005). Understanding and sharing intentions: The origins of cultural cognition. *Behavioral and Brain Sciences, 28,* 675–735.

Tronick, E. (2002). Emotions and emotional communication in infants. *American Psychologist, 44*(2), 112–119.

Tsatsanis, K. D., Foley, C., & Donehower, C. (2004). Contemporary outcome research and programming guidelines for Asperger syndrome and high functioning autism. *Topics in Language Disorders, 24*(4), 249–259.

Walker, H. M., Ramsay, E., & Gresham, F. M. (2004). *Antisocial behavior in school: Evidence-based practices.* Thomson Wadsworth.

Wetherby, A. M., Guthrie, W., Woods, J., Schatschneider, C., Holland, R. D., Morgan, L., & Lord, C. (2014). Parent-implemented social intervention for toddlers with autism: An RCT. *Pediatrics, 134*(6), 1084–1093. https://doi.org/10.1542/peds.2014-0757

Wetherby, A. M., Watt, N., Morgan, L., & Shumway, S. (2007). Social communication profiles of children with autism spectrum disorders late in the second year of life. *Journal of Autism and Developmental Disorders, 37*(5), 960–975. https://doi.org/10.1007 /s10803-006-0237-4

Wong, C., Odom, S. L., Hume, K., Cox, A. W., Fettig, A., Kucharczyk, S., Brock, M. E., Plavnick, J. B., Fleury, V. P., & Schultz, T. R. (2014). Evidence-based practices for children, youth, and young adults with autism spectrum disorder: A comprehensive review. *Journal of Autism and Developmental Disorders, 45*(7), 1951–1966. https://doi.org/10.1007/s10803 -014-2351-z

Yu, L., & Zhu, X. (2018). Effectiveness of a SCERTS model-based intervention for children with autism spectrum disorder (ASD) in Hong Kong: A pilot study. *Journal of Autism and Developmental Disorders, 48*(11), 3794–3807. https://doi.org/10.1007/s10803-018-3649-z

15

Social Skills Interventions

Patricia A. Prelock and Ashley Brien

INTRODUCTION

Autism spectrum disorder (ASD) is characterized by impairments in social interaction and social communication as well as restricted and repetitive patterns of
behavior and interests (American Psychiatric Association [APA], 2013). The social
impairments in ASD are at the core of many challenges faced by this population.
This core deficit impacts the ability of individuals with ASD to understand the social
world in which they live and to fully participate in their home, school, and community environments.

Several chapters in this book offer insights regarding evidence-based interventions designed to support social communication and social interaction in individuals with ASD, including but not limited to Social Stories, video modeling, peer
mediation, and Pivotal Response Treatment. This chapter focuses on social skills
intervention programs that support a child's appropriate use of gestures; eye gaze;
reciprocity; and initiating, sustaining, and closing an interaction in a meaningful
way. Most of the intervention programs reviewed here are manualized, following a
curriculum or systematic process for delivering activities that facilitate social skills
development.

There is good evidence that directly training social skills can be effective, and
increasing prosocial behaviors is typically a primary outcome in applied behavioral
analysis interventions. Both the National Professional Development Center (NPDC;
Wong et al., 2014) and the National Autism Center (NAC; 2009) consider the use of
social narratives/stories to be useful tools for social skills training (see Chapter 16).
The use of peer-mediated interventions to build social skills is well established;
these interventions are described in Chapter 12. There is evidence that specific
aspects of social interaction (e.g., eye contact, joint attention, verbal greetings) can
be learned with focused training. The NPDC analysis documents solid evidence for
the effectiveness of social skills training groups, although the NAC considered a

"social skills package" to be an emerging rather than well-established practice in its 2009 National Standards Project review of 14 articles. However, in the 2015 review, social skills moved to an established intervention with an additional 21 articles reviewed, emphasizing the social skills training of adolescents 13 to 18 years of age. Social skills typically trained in the research reviewed focused on a range of abilities such as using appropriate eye contact and gestures in conversation; engaging in reciprocal exchanges; and knowing how to initiate, maintain, and close an interaction or conversation. The overall goal of any social skills intervention is to provide individuals with ASD the skills they need to meaningfully participate in a variety of social environments, including home, schools, and the community.

Social skills interventions take on a variety of forms and often include an outline of skills that are specifically taught (e.g., turn taking, initiation, problem solving). Strategies such as modeling, prompting, and reinforcement are used to teach the targeted social skills. Social skills interventions can occur in small groups, one-to-one, or in a dyad with a peer.

TARGET POPULATIONS

Social skills interventions have been specifically designed for preschool and school-age children as well as adolescents and adults with social deficits, including those with ASD, attention deficit-hyperactivity disorder (ADHD), specific language impairments, and other neurodevelopmental disabilities. Children with Asperger disorder, pervasive developmental disorder-not otherwise specified, high-functioning autism, and classic autism without intellectual disabilities are those typically described in literature prior to the *Diagnostic and Statistical Manual of Mental Disorders, Fifth Edition* (DSM-5; APA, 2013) as benefitting from social skills interventions (as described throughout this chapter). Since the publication of the DSM-5 in 2013, all of these children fall under the ASD category. Students with a social-communication disorder would also likely benefit from these interventions, although there are not yet specific studies that describe the benefit to this population. Notably, students with comorbid conditions (e.g., ASD + ADHD), would also benefit from social skills intervention, although less improvement has been reported for group intervention (Gates et al., 2017). In addition, there are reports that typically developing children who participate in social skills intervention as peer mentors or peer models also benefit from the intervention (Szumski et al., 2016). Research suggests that the greatest benefit is seen for school-age children and adolescents who can manage the language and cognitive requirements of a social skills curriculum (Frankel & Myatt, 2003; Laugeson et al., 2014; Lopata et al., 2012; Stichter et al., 2010; Vernon et al., 2018).

THEORETICAL BASIS

Theoretical Rationale

Social skills interventions are designed to address both skills acquisition and performance deficits, one or both of which must be addressed in teaching social skills to children and adolescents with ASD. Typically, a skills acquisition deficit indicates that a particular social skill or behavior is absent. In contrast, a performance deficit suggests that a specific skill or behavior is present, but it is not demonstrated or being performed in a consistent manner during social encounters (Gresham et al., 2001; Lerner & Mikami, 2012). To be most impactful, social skills interventions must be implemented frequently and intensely, with sufficient opportunities to maintain and generalize learned social skills across settings and social situations with different social partners (Thomeer et al., 2019). Often, however, there is a mismatch between the social skill strategy being implemented and the actual social skill deficit displayed by the child or adolescent with ASD (Gresham et al., 2001). Further, early traditional social skills training programs have been minimally effective in teaching social skills to children and adolescents (Gresham et al., 2001), particularly to preschool children who may require a more structured intervention plan.

Several components have been identified to support children with social-communication and social-interaction challenges in achieving positive social encounters. Bellini and colleagues (2007) describe five major components of social skills interventions that are important to their effectiveness. The components address not just the child but the context in which the child will likely experience social encounters, providing some guidance on how to navigate these social situations. First, environmental modifications are often used to foster social interaction between children with ASD and their peers. This may mean setting up the physical environment and activities to support engagement around shared interests. Second, child-specific interventions are used to facilitate social engagement from direct teaching of initiating and responding to modeling reciprocal conversation and problem solving. Third, social skills interventions often include the facilitation of collateral skills such as play and enhanced language abilities. Fourth, peer mediation is frequently used in social skills interventions in which peers without disabilities are trained to guide and respond to the social behaviors of children with ASD. Fifth, using a variety of the strategies mentioned previously is a common approach when implementing a comprehensive approach to social skills interventions

Underlying Assumptions

Social skills interventions for children with ASD are primarily designed to address the social-interaction and social-communication deficits outlined as the primary criteria in the diagnosis of ASD (APA, 2013). Deficits that are addressed include engaging in social-emotional reciprocity, participating in the back-and-forth exchange typical in conversation, approaching a social exchange with another, initiating bids for interaction with another, responding to bids for engagement, and sharing interests and affective connections. In addition, interventions might address challenges in the use of nonverbal communication behaviors, including strategies to integrate verbal and nonverbal communication, establish appropriate eye contact and gestures when communicating, manage body language and nonverbal communication, and use facial expressions appropriate to the social context. Further, addressing deficits in developing relationships with others is a priority in social skills interventions, including teaching the ability to adjust social behavior across contexts, engage in imaginative play, show an interest in connecting with peers, and make friends.

Functional Outcomes

Typically, social skills interventions target a range of behaviors that support a child's social communication and/or social interaction from decreasing behaviors that interfere with social connections to increasing behaviors that facilitate those connections. The following behaviors are frequently reported in the social skills intervention literature as functional outcomes likely to follow from acquisition of particular social skills (note that many of the interventions in this chapter report multiple positive behavioral outcomes from the following list, and a comprehensive list of findings and associated references can be found in the tables associated with each intervention described in the Empirical Basis section):

- Decreased problem behaviors including aggression

- Increased self-control

- Improvement in assertiveness

- Increased self-esteem

- Improved likability

- Improved social competence, social interaction, and social awareness

- Increased adaptive skills

- Decreased anxiety and withdrawal

- Increased emotion recognition, **theory of mind,** and executive function

- Decreased autistic behaviors

- Increased language skills

- Increased motivation

Target Area of Treatment

Both social interaction and social communication are targeted areas of treatment in social skills interventions. Studies usually emphasize social etiquette or rules, friendship training, behavior, adaptive skills, nonliteral language, face and emotion recognition, and theory of mind. The language modality most often emphasized is verbal, although the focus is often alignment of enhanced verbal communication with the appropriate gesture use.

EMPIRICAL BASIS

The NAC (2015) recognizes social skills packages as an established intervention. Research supporting several social skills intervention programs is summarized in Table 15.1. The focus of this chapter is on selected social skills interventions that are frequently used, have been associated with some research support, and are manualized or have a clear curriculum associated with implementation. The 10 interventions selected include 1) Children's Friendship Training (CFT), 2) I Can Problem Solve (ICPS), 3) Mind Reading, 4) Play Time/Social Time (PT/ST), 5) Program for the Education and Enrichment of Relational Skills (PEERS®), 6) Improving Parents as Communication Teachers (Project ImPACT), 7) Skillstreaming, 8) Social Competence Intervention (SCI), 9) Social Tools and Rules for Teens (START), and 10) Virtual Reality-Social Cognition Training (VR-SCT). A brief description of these programs can be found in Table 15.1. For each of the interventions described in this chapter, we provide a table describing findings from selected research studies. Information about the number of participants in each study, their age range and diagnosis, the study design, the treatment targets of the intervention, the results of the study, and the effect sizes for significant findings are reported in each table.

Table 15.1. Description of social skills interventions for children and adolescents with autism spectrum disorder

Social skills intervention	Target population	Practical components	Key components	Assessment measures for treatment planning and progress monitoring	General findings
UCLA Children's Friendship Program	7- to 17-year-old children with ASD, ODD, ADHD, fetal alcohol syndrome	*Personnel:* School counselors, teachers, health care professionals in training (e.g., social worker, psychologist, psychiatrist) *Training and Materials:* Manual	*Goals:* Increase social etiquette enforced by peer group *Dosage:* 12 sessions *Activities:* Child didactic sessions, socialization homework, free-play coaching modules, parent involvement *Participants:* Parents, peers	SSRS–parent PEI–teacher PHS–child	Skill generalization
Skillstreaming	Preschool, school-age children, adolescents with behavioral challenges, social skills deficits, ASD	*Personnel:* Intervention leader (e.g., SLP, behavior interventionist, school counselor, social worker), program coordinator, intervention program coordinator, teachers, para-professionals *Training:* Manuals *Materials:* Skillstreaming manual, Skillstreaming student manual	*Goals:* Increase social skills and functioning through role play *Dosage:* 3–5 times per week *Activities:* Peer role playing, homework, parent involvement *Participants:* Parents, peers	Student Skillstreaming Checklist–Child ASC–parent/ teacher BASC-PRS–parent BASC-TRS–teacher	Increases in social and adaptive skills Decreases in withdrawal and problem behaviors

(continued)

Table 15.1. *(continued)*

Social skills intervention	Target population	Practical components	Key components	Assessment measures for treatment planning and progress monitoring	General findings
Program for the Education and Enrichment of Relational Skills (PEERS®)	Adolescents with developmental disorders, ASD, ADHD	*Personnel:* Teen group leader, parent group leader, one or two coaches, mental health professionals (e.g., social workers, psychologist, psychiatrists, marriage and family therapists), teacher/educator *Training:* Coaches (through activities such as demonstrating social skills, handling behavior), parent (educated in implementing psychoeducational approaches) *Materials:* Manual	*Goals:* Improve social functioning through making friends and maintaining good relationships *Dosage:* 90-minute weekly sessions for 14 weeks *Activities:* How to have a two-way conversation with peers, peer entry strategies, how to plan successful get-togethers *Participants:* Parents, adolescents	SRS-2 SCQ TASSK QPQ-A QPQ-P VABS-II CBCL DSRS-C SSRS Friendship Qualities Scale Piers-Harris Self Concept Scale-2 SRS SAS	Improvement in overall social functioning, including socialization, communication, knowledge of social skills, autistic mannerisms and behavioral and emotional problems; reduction of social anxiety
I Can Problem Solve (ICPS)	3–9 year olds with ASD and neurotypical children	*Personnel:* Teacher, parent *Training:* Manual; Center for Schools and Communities provides training and consultation *Materials:* Manual	*Goals:* Prevent and reduce early high-risk behaviors (e.g., impulsivity, social withdrawal) and promote prosocial behaviors (e.g., concern for others, positive peer relationships) *Dosage:* 59 lessons, one per day; session durations begin at 10 minutes and increase to 20 minutes	No data on assessment or treatment planning	Improvement in social competence, reduction in problems related to coping with difficult social situations, some promise for developing ToM

			Activities: School-based, structured lessons following a teacher script, learning essential ICPS vocabulary and concepts, problem-solving skills *Interaction in the classroom:* Communicate using ICPS dialoging *Integration into the curriculum:* Practice ICPS problem-solving concept as children work on academic subjects Parent Pages: Parent learns to use ICPS to improve family interaction and generalize children's learning *Participants:* Neurotypical children		
Play Time/Social Time (PT/ST)	3- to 5-year-old children with or at risk for disabilities enrolled in special education, general preschool, or child care center; children with social-interaction skill deficits; neurotypical children	*Personnel:* Peers who are developing normally or have higher levels of social competence, teacher *Training:* Manual *Materials:* Manual	*Goals:* Promote social interaction and development of social competence *Dosage:* 100 days, each weekday for 15–20 minutes; occurs over several phases *Activities:* Teach specific social-interaction skills during play-based tasks; teacher verbally prompts children to use social interaction skills; direct exchange of behavior between two or more children; children may talk to one another, exchange materials, or take turns in an activity *Participants:* Preschool children	VABS-II Preschool BDI-3 TIS Teacher Rating of Social Interaction Teacher Rating of Intervention Behavior	Increase in social skills for children with low social skills, those with disabilities, and children acting as role models Development of social skills, improvement in social-interaction skills, decrease in problems coping with difficult social situations

(continued)

Table 15.1. *(continued)*

Social skills intervention	Target population	Practical components	Key components	Assessment measures for treatment planning and progress monitoring	General findings
Social Tools and Rules for Teens (START)	12- to 17-year-old adolescents with ASD	*Personnel:* High-school and college-age peer mentors with a licensed clinical psychologist jointly conducting all training and supervision sessions *Training:* Currently finalizing training program *Materials:* Not yet manualized	*Goals:* Social readiness, motivation, and competence *Dosage:* 10 weeks immersive social intervention; 90-minute sessions *Activities:* Individual check-in sessions; free socialization time to work on individual targets; role-plays; videos and skill practice; structured group activities to work on communication and teamwork; check-out session; feedback; setting weekly goals *Participants:* Adolescents with ASD, parents	SSIS-RS SRS-2 SMCS Dynamic conversation probe	Improvement in social inquiries, reduction in negative statements, increased or decreased total verbal contributions during social exchanges, improvement in global social functioning, reduction in social vulnerabilities
Social Competence Curricula (SCI)	Elementary (6–10 years), adolescent (11–14 years), and high school (14–18 years) students with ASD; others with similar social skills deficits	*Personnel:* Project staff, teacher at participant's school *Training:* Curriculum purchased online *Materials:* Manual, online curriculum, parent resources coming soon	*Goals:* Enhance social competence needs of youth and adolescents *Dosage:* 20–32 lessons, 45 minutes, 2–3 times per week *Activities:* Sessions occur in classroom, schoolwide, home, and community; sessions follow a structure with a review, introduction, modeling, and opportunities to practice; practiced skills include problem solving, feelings, emotions, turn-talking in conversation; sharing ideas, facial expressions; skills are layered from one unit to the next; uses a feedback/token economy system and behavior system	SRS BRIEF-2 Sally-Anne false-belief task Smarties false-belief task Friends ABC Story Ice Cream Van Test Faux Pas Stories DANVA-2-CF Reading the Mind in the Eyes Test TOPS-3	Recognition of social faux pas, use of cognitive resources and ability to regulate behavior, overall social improvement and improvement in social communication and motivation, recognition of facial expressions and interpretation of emotional and mental states, increased ability to label emotional/mental states

| Improving Parents as Communication Teachers (Project ImPACT) | Up to 6 years of age | *Personnel:* Practitioner
Training: Manual, videos, PowerPoint presentations
Materials: Manual | *Goals:* Enhance social engagement, communication, imitation and play skills within meaningful activities and daily routines
Dosage: 24 sessions, 1 hour each
Activities: Modeling, practice of intervention strategies, homework assignments, practice during child's daily activities
Participants: Parents, children | Children spontaneous use of language; parent-selected goal and goal achievement; videos recorded and scored for social engagement, language, and play
SRS
MB-CDI
CES-D
PSI-SF
VABS-II | Gains in communication skills and parent intervention adherence, improvement in language and social engagement, reduction in severity of social impairment, increased expressive vocabulary |
| Virtual Reality Social Cognition Training (VR-SCT) | Pediatric group: 7 to 16 years old
Young adult group: 18 to 26 years old | *Personnel:* Coach, confederate clinician
Training: Emotion recognition in others, responding to others, self-assertion
Materials: Not manualized | *Goals:* Usage across ages and contexts with complexity adjusted for developmental age in everyday situations
Dosage: 10 sessions, 1 hour each, over 5 weeks
Activities: Social reasoning strategy-based training, real-time interaction, no scripted response, immediate clinician-directed feedback
Participants: Children and adults | ACS-SP
Ekman 60
Mind in the Eyes
Triangles Social Perception Task
SSPA
Follow-up survey (self-report) | Improvement in affect recognition, understanding intentions, social judgment |

(continued)

Table 15.1. *(continued)*

Social skills intervention	Target population	Practical components	Key components	Assessment measures for treatment planning and progress monitoring	General findings
Mind Reading	7 year olds to adults with ASD and theory of mind challenges	*Personnel:* None *Training: Teaching Children with Autism to Mind-Read: A Practical Guide for Teachers and Parents* *Materials:* Manual, DVD	*Goals:* Increase decoding skills and exploit the systemizing strengths of individuals with high-functioning ASD *Dosage:* Not defined *Activities:* Interactive software teaches facial expression and prosody decoding using visual and auditory lessons and stimuli; practice trials and computer-delivered reinforcement	CAM-C Face-Voice Battery Reading the Mind in the Eyes task (revised adult version) Reading the Mind in the Voice task (revised) Reading the Mind in the Film task SRS BASC-2-PRS	Improvement in emotion recognition skills for facial and vocal expressions; some reduction in ASD symptoms; improvement in recognition of mental states, eye contact, attention to faces and emotions

Key: ACS-SP, Advanced Clinical Solutions for WAIS-IV and WMS-IV Social Perception Subtest; ADHD, attention deficit-hyperactivity disorder; ASC, Adapted Skillstreaming Checklist; ASD, autism spectrum disorder; BASC-PRS, Behavior Assessment System for Children Parent Rating Scales; BASC-TRS, Behavior Assessment System for Children Teacher Rating Scales; BDI-3, Battelle Developmental Inventory–Third Edition, BRIEF-2, Behavior Rating Inventory of Executive Functions–Second Edition; CAM-C, Cambridge Mind Reading Face-Voice Battery for Children; CAM, Cambridge Mind Reading Face-Voice Battery; CBCL, Child Behavior Checklist; CES-D, Center for Epidemiological Studies–Depression Scale; DANVA-2-CF, Diagnostic Analysis of Nonverbal Accuracy–Second Edition—Child Facial Expressions Test; DSRS-C, Depression Self-rating Scale for Children; Ekman 60, Facial Expressions of Emotion Stimuli and Tests; MB-CDI, MacArthur-Bates Communicative Development Inventories; Facial Affect Recognition; ODD, oppositional defiant disorder; PEI, Pupil Evaluation Inventory; PHS, Pier-Harris Self-Concept Scale; PSI-SF, Parenting Stress Index–Short Form; QPQ-A, Quality of Play Questionnaire–Adolescent; QPQ-P, Quality of Play Questionnaire–Parent; SAS, Social Anxiety Scale; SCQ, Social Communication Questionnaire; SCS, Social Competence Scale; SMCS, Social Motivation & Competencies Scale; SRS, Social Responsiveness Scale; SRS-2, Social Responsiveness Scale–Second Edition; SSRS, Social Skills Rating System; SSIS-RS, Social Skills Improvement System Rating Scales; SSPA, Social Skills Performance Assessment; TASSK, Test of Adolescent Social Skill Knowledge; TIS, Teacher's Impression Scale; TOPS-3, Test of Problem Solving–Third Edition; VABS-II, Vineland Adaptive Behavior Scales–Second Edition.

Children's Friendship Training Program

The CFT program (Frankel & Myatt, 2003) is a manualized parent-assisted intervention used to support the social behavior of several clinical populations, including children with ADHD, fetal alcohol spectrum disorders, oppositional defiant disorder (ODD), childhood obesity, and ASD. Laugeson and colleagues (2009) examined the efficacy of an immediate compared to a delayed intervention friendship group focused on fostering friendship quality and social skills in 13- to 17-year-old students with ASD. The intervention program targets ways to have a conversation, how to enter and exit peer interactions, approaches to developing a network of friends, appropriate ways to approach sportsmanship and getting together with friends, how to manage reputational issues, and how to recognize differences between teasing and bullying and to address conflicts. Compared to the control group, those students receiving friendship training demonstrated greater improvements in their knowledge of social skills and increased the number of times they got together with friends. Parents, but not teachers, reported similar gains in social skills.

Frankel and colleagues (2010) examined the impact of the CFT program on the social behavior of children with ASD in second through fifth grades. They compared the CFT group with a delayed intervention group. Several social skills were taught, including how to have a conversation, how to enter an interaction with peers, ways to develop a network of friends, ways to approach sportsmanship, strategies to handle behavior during playdates, and ways to manage teasing. Following the intervention, the CFT group demonstrated greater changes than the delayed intervention group on several parent measures assessing social skills and behavior during playdates as well as child measures assessing levels of loneliness and popularity. Improvements continued at a 3-month follow-up visit. A detailed description of selected studies examining CFT can be found in Table 15.2.

I Can Problem Solve and Play Time/Social Time

ICPS (Shure, 2001) has been the subject of numerous research and evaluation studies over the last 30 years. Studies conducted by the developer of the program and independent researchers have reported a range of outcomes associated with ICPS for preschool, school-age, and adolescent populations who exhibit aggressive, social-emotional, substance abuse, attentional, and interpersonal problems. Some of these outcomes include improved ICPS skills (i.e., **perspective taking, alternative solution thinking, consequential thinking, recognizing mixed emotions, understanding motives,** and **means–end thinking;** Shure & Spivak, 1980; Vestal & Jones, 2004), decreased aggression and emotional intensity (Boyle & Hassett-Walker, 2008; Kurnpfer et al., 2002; Shure & Spivack, 1980), increased ability to cope with frustration (Shure & Spivack, 1980), and improved academic achievement (Ciancio et al., 2001; Hawkins et al., 1999).

A randomized controlled trial (RCT) was conducted comparing ICPS and PT/ST and a control group with 52 preschool children, including those with ASD, ages 3–7 years (Szumski et al., 2017). The researchers found positive improvements in children with ASD on a theory of mind task and found that ICPS led to improvements in social problem solving and that PT/ST positively influenced both interaction skills and social problem solving (Szumski et al., 2017).

Table 15.2. Summary of selected research on Children's Friendship Training

Study	Sample size	Grade or age range (years)	Diagnosis	Design	Targets of intervention	Outcome data			
						Significant findings	Trends	Nonsignificant findings	Effect size
Frankel et al. (2010)	68	Second to fifth grade	ASD	RCT	Popularity, loneliness, play date quality, social skills, peer relationships	**Child measures** *Loneliness Scale:* Lower loneliness ratings *PHS:* Increased popularity **Parent measures** *QPQ-P:* • Increased number of play dates hosted • Decreased disengaged behaviors during play dates *SSRS:* Improvement in self-control	—	**Teacher measure** *PEI:* No differences in withdrawal, likeability, aggression	Not reported
Laugeson et al. (2009)	33	13–17	ASD	RCT	Social skills (e.g., rules of social etiquette)	**Parent and teacher measures** *SSRS:* Improvement in parent-rated social skills **Child measures** *QPQ:* Increases in hosted get-togethers *FQS:* Better quality friendships compared to delated treatment group *TASSK:* Improvement in knowledge of social skills	—	**Child measures** *FQS:* No significant increases in friendship quality from pre- to postintervention	Not reported

Key: FQS, Friendship Qualities Scale; PEI, Pupil Evaluation Inventory; PHS, Piers-Harris Self-Concept Scale; QPQ, Quality of Play Questionnaire; QPQ-A, Quality of Play Questionnaire-Adolescent; QPQ-P, Quality of Play Questionnaire-Parent; SSRS, Social Skills Rating System; TASSK, Test of Adolescent Social Skills Knowledge

Szumski and colleagues (2016) investigated PT/ST with 150 preschoolers in three groups: children with autism, intellectual, physical, and sensory disabilities; children with low social skills but without disabilities; and typically developing children. They found that PT/ST was particularly effective in developing social skills of children with ASD and related disabilities as well as those with lower social skills. They emphasized the importance of providing the intervention to young children to maximize results. A detailed description of selected studies examining ICPS and PT/ST is presented in Table 15.3.

Mind Reading

Golan and colleagues (2006) examined complex emotions and mental state understanding in adults with Asperger syndrome (AS) using Mind Reading, a computer software intervention program (Baron-Cohen, 2004). Several tasks were used, including faces and voices, to assess the participants' recognition of 20 emotions and mental states. Both males and females with AS were included, as were two control groups: adults with AS and neurotypical controls who did not receive the intervention. Importantly, both AS groups performed less well than the neurotypical controls on the emotion recognition tasks for 12 of 20 emotions. Females displayed better face recognition than males with and without AS, and males with AS had more difficulty with faces than voices. The AS intervention group did show increases in emotion recognition compared to the AS control group.

Thomeer and colleagues (2015) examined the efficacy of Mind Reading in an RCT including 43 children with ASD, ages 7–12 years. The intervention group included 22 children who received a manualized intervention program over 12 weeks to facilitate their recognition and understanding of emotions and increase their social skills. Results indicated significantly better performance following intervention compared to the control group on three of the four measures of emotion recognition and understanding. These results were maintained at a 5-week follow-up. ASD symptoms were also lower at posttest and follow-up compared to prior to receiving the intervention. A detailed description of selected studies examining Mind Reading is presented in Table 15.4.

PEERS***

Laugeson and colleagues (2012) used PEERS (Laugeson, 2013) to improve the social skills of adolescents with ASD and high cognitive and linguistic abilities. They found significant improvement in the adolescents' social responsiveness and overall knowledge of social skills, including improvements in social cognition, social communication, motivation, and general social-awareness motivation. In addition, they saw improvements in the adolescents' ability to cooperate, assert themselves in social situations, and take responsibility for their own social behavior. With these improvements, they also reported decreases in ASD symptoms. The frequency of interacting with peers was also observed, and teachers reported similar improvements in the classroom following intervention, with gains maintained 14 weeks following the withdrawal of intervention.

Laugeson and colleagues (2014) studied the impact of PEERS intervention on 73 middle school children with ASD over a 14-week period. Children were assigned to the PEERS intervention group or an alternative social skills intervention curriculum with instruction provided by the teacher and instructional

Table 15.3. Summary of selected research on I Can Problem Solve and Play Time/Social Time

Study	Sample size	Age (years)	Diagnosis	Design	Targets of intervention	Outcome data			Effect size
						Significant findings	Trends	Nonsignificant findings	
Szumski et al. (2017)	52	Preschool (3.5–7.5)	ASD	*RCT:* Play Time/Social Time (PT/ST); I Can Problem Solve (ICPS); control group	Social skills and theory of mind	**Child measures** *Theory of Mind Chocolate Task:* • Positive improvements in children with ASD • PT/ST produces more general effect than ICPS • ICPS improves social problem solving • PT/ST influences interaction skills and social problem solving *PT/ST:* • Improves interaction skills by almost 1.5 SD • Problems in coping with difficult social situations decreased more than 1.5 SD • Moderate effects on social skills *ICPS:* • Improved social competence • Decreased problems in coping with difficult social situations (1 SD) • Promising ToM development	—	—	Not reported
Szumski et al. (2016)	Initial: 196 Final: 151	3–9	Children with low social skills, intellectual disabilities, physical sensory disabilities, and typically developing	Pretest–posttest repeated measures	Social skills	**Teacher measures** *TIS:* Social skills increased for children with disabilities and those with low social skills compared to those without disabilities	—	—	Teacher measures *TIS:* $\eta^2 = 0.32$

Key: ICPS, I Can Problem Solve; PEI, pupil evaluation inventory; PHS, Pier-Harris Self Concept Scale; PT/ST, Play Time/Social Time; TIS, Teacher Impression Scale; ToM, theory of mind.

Table 15.4. Summary of selected research on Mind Reading

Study	Sample size	Age (years)	Diagnosis	Design	Targets of intervention	Outcome data			
						Significant findings	Trends	Nonsignificant findings	Effect size
Golan & Baron-Cohen (2006) Experiment 1	AS/ASD: 19 ASD control: 22 Typical control: 28	Adults	Asperger syndrome, high-functioning ASD, and typical developing adults	Two RCTs with typical control group	Recognition of complex emotions in faces and voices	**Participant measures** *CAM:* Increases in emotion recognition in pictures and voice recordings for treatment group compared to control group	**Participant measures**	**Participant measures** *Reading the Mind in the Eyes task (revised adult version):* No differences found in emotion recognition in the eyes between groups *Reading the Mind in the Voice task (revised):* No differences found in emotion recognition between groups	**Participant measures** *CAM Faces:* $F = 11.82$ *CAM Voices:* $F = 7.51$
Golan & Baron-Cohen (2006) Experiment 2	AS/ASD: 13 ASD social skills course: 13 Typical control: 13	Adults	Asperger syndrome, high-functioning ASD, and typical developing adults	Two RCTs with typical control group	Recognition of complex emotions in faces and voices	**Participant measures** *CAM:* Increases in emotion recognition in pictures for treatment group compared to control group *Reading the Mind in the Eyes task (revised adult version):* Increases in emotion recognition	—	**Participant measures** *CAM:* No differences in emotion recognition for voices between groups *Reading the Mind in the Voice task (revised):* No differences found in emotion recognition between groups	**Participant measures** *CAM Faces:* $F = 11.82$ *Reading the Mind in the Eyes:* $F = 8.4$

(continued)

427

Table 15.4. *(continued)*

Study	Sample size	Age (years)	Diagnosis	Design	Targets of intervention	Outcome data			
						Significant findings	Trends	Nonsignificant findings	Effect size
Thomeer et al. (2015)	43	7–12	High-functioning ASD	RCT	Emotion decoding and encoding skills, autism symptoms, and social skills	**Child measures** CAM-C: Increases in emotion recognition skills for facial and vocal expressions for treatment group compared to control group and gain maintained at follow-up *ERDS-Receptive:* Increases in emotion decoding skills at follow-up **Child measures** *ERDS-Expressive:* Increases in emotion encoding at posttest and follow-up **Parent measures** *SRS:* Reduction in ASD symptoms at posttest and at follow-up	—	**Child measures** *ERDS-Receptive:* No changes in emotion decoding skills at post **Parent measures** *BASC-2 Social Skills:* No differences in social skills between groups	**Child measures** *CAM-C Faces:* Posttest: $d = 1.34$ Follow-up: $d = 0.86$ *CAM-C Voices:* Posttest: $d = 0.99$ Follow-up: $d = 0.66$ *ERDS-Receptive:* Follow-up: $d = 0.73$ *ERDS-Expressive:* Posttest: $d = 0.61$ Follow-up: $d = 0.85$ Parent measures *SRS:* Posttest: $d = 0.46$ Follow-up: $d = 0.45$

Key: BASC-2, Behavior Assessment System for Children-Second Edition; CAM, CAM-C, Cambridge Mindreading Face-Voice Battery for Children; ERDS, Emotion Recognition and Display Survey; SRS, Social Responsiveness Scale.

assistants. Children in the PEERS intervention group demonstrated greater improvement in social skills than did the control group, particularly in the areas of social motivation and awareness, as well as in social communication and responsiveness. The PEERS intervention group also demonstrated an overall reduction of autism symptoms. In fact, children with ASD reported their own improvement in social skills and an increase in the frequency with which they met with their friends.

In an RCT examining the efficacy of PEERS with adolescents with and without ASD, Dolan and colleagues (2016) examined the social behavior of adolescents with ASD and a neurotypical peer in 10-minute interactions before and immediately following the implementation of the PEERS social skills intervention program using the Contextual Assessment of Social Skills (CASS; Ratto et al., 2010). Participants in the PEERS intervention group increased their expressiveness with some improvement in rapport as compared to those in the waitlist control group.

Yamada and colleagues (2020) investigated a Japanese version of PEERS, emphasizing the ability of 28 adolescents (11–15 years of age) with ASD to gain social skills in building and maintaining peer relationships. With several cultural and language modifications made, positive results were found, including increased social skills knowledge, improved social communication, and decreased associated symptoms of autism and related behavioral challenges. These gains were maintained 3 months following the withdrawal of the intervention. A detailed description of selected studies examining PEERS can be found in Table 15.5.

PROJECT IMPACT

Project ImPACT is a social-communication intervention for young children with ASD implemented by parents (Ingersoll & Dvortcsak, 2019). It was developed for implementation in community settings to expand its use. Ingersoll and Wainer (2013) reported on a single-subject, multiple-baseline design with eight preschoolers with ASD and their mothers. The study was designed to facilitate a child's spontaneous language and parent fidelity when implementing the intervention. Multilevel modeling was the primary strategy used to support children's language and the parents' implementation of the intervention. Spontaneous language increases were seen for six of the eight children, with parents' strategy use positively impacting the children's improved language use.

Stadnick and colleagues (2015) compared child and parent outcomes for a 12-week Project ImPACT intervention group and a community comparison group for 30 young children with ASD. They found significant improvement in the children's communication skills on the Vineland Adaptive Behavior Scales–Second Edition (VABS-II, Sparrow et al., 2006) Communication subscale and parent adherence for the expected intervention strategies.

Ingersoll and colleagues (2017) investigated the social engagement, language, and play for nine young children with ASD using the Project ImPACT intervention program. Following intervention, children with ASD showed a decrease in their social impairment as measured on the Social Responsiveness Scale (SRS) and an increase in their expressive vocabulary using the MacArthur-Bates Communicative Development Inventories (MB-CDI; Fenson et al., 1993). A detailed description of selected studies examining Project IMPACT is presented in Table 15.6.

Table 15.5. Summary of selected research on Program for the Education and Enrichment of Relational Skills (PEERS)

Study	Sample size	Age (years)	Diagnosis	Design	Targets of intervention	Outcome data			
						Significant findings	Trends	Nonsignificant findings	Effect size
Dolan et al. (2016)	58	11–16	Autism spectrum disorder (ASD)	Randomized control trial	Social skills (e.g., making and keeping friends)	**Child measures** CASS: Vocal expressiveness greater for treatment group vs. wait control group TASSK: Significant improvement for treatment group	CASS: Overall rapport quality improves	—	CASS: Vocal expressiveness: $\eta^2 = 0.08$; observed power = 0.56 Rapport quality: $\eta^2 = 0.07$; observed power = 0.49
Laugeson et al. (2014)	73	12–14	ASD	Treatment vs. active treatment control	Social skills	**Teacher measures** SRS: Improvements in total social responsiveness greater for treatment group vs. control group **Child measures** QPQ: Increased frequency of hosted and invited get-togethers for treatment group compared to control group TASSK: Increased social skills knowledge for treatment group compared to control group	**Parent measures** SAS: Decreases in social anxiety for treatment group compared to control group **Teacher measures** SRS: Improvements in social motivation, social awareness, social communication; decreased autistic mannerisms for treatment group compared to the control group	**Teacher measures** SRS: No differences in social cognition	**Parent measures** SAS social anxiety: $d = 0.95$ **Teacher measures** SRS: $d = -0.63$ SRS social awareness: $d = -0.52$ SRS social cognition: $d = -0.42$ SRS social communication: $d = -0.57$ SRS social motivation: $d = -0.52$ SRS social mannerisms: $d = -0.59$ **Child measures** QPQ host: $d = 0.82$ QPQ guest: $d = 0.59$ TASSK: $d = 1.88$

	N				Parent measures / Child measures		Teacher measures	Parent measures
Laugeson et al. (2012)	28	ASD	RCT	Social skills (e.g., making and keeping friends)	**Parent measures** *QPQ-P:* Improvement in hosted get-togethers *SSRS-P:* Greater improvement in overall social skills for treatment group **Child measures** *TASSK-R:* Improvement in knowledge of social skills for treatment group *QPQ-A host:* Improved performance in teen hosted get-togethers for treatment group	—	**Teacher measures** SRS Total – No significant differences	**Parent measures** *QPQ-P:* $p < .001$ (posttreatment); $p < .01$ (follow-up) *SRS:* $p < .02$ (posttreatment); $p < .01$ (follow-up) *SSRS social skills:* $p < .0001$ (posttreatment); $p < .01$ (follow-up) **Child measures** *TASSK:* $p < .0001$, $p < .01$ *QPQ-A host:* $p < .015$; $p < .05$
Yamada et al. (2022)	28	ASD	Cross-cultural validation trial	Social skills (e.g., making and keeping friends, managing conflict and rejection)	**Parent measures** SRS-2 SCQ QPQ-P CBCL VABS-II **Child measures** TASSK QPQ-A DSRS-C	—	QPQ-P QPQ-A DSRS-C	TASSK, SRS-2 total, and VABS-II composite, large effect size: $\eta_p^2 = 0.28$–0.86 SCQ, middle effect size: $\eta_p^2 = 0.09$ *CBCL total:* $\eta_p^2 = 0.03$

Table 15.6. Summary of selected research on Project IMPACT

Study	Sample size	Age	Diagnosis	Design	Targets of intervention	Outcome data			Effect size
						Significant findings	Trends	Nonsignificant findings	
Ingersoll & Wainer (2013)	8	44–80 months	ASD	Single subject, multiple-baseline design	Child spontaneous language; Parent-child language	**Child measures** Children spontaneous use of language (scored using frequency counts): Increases in spontaneous language	—	—	**Child measures** Children spontaneous use of language (scored using frequency counts): d = 0.48; follow-up: d = 1.44
Ingersoll et al. (2017)	9	32–93 months	ASD	Pretest–posttest	Social engagement, language, and play	**Parent measures** SRS: Decrease in social impairment MCDI: Increase in expressive vocabulary	—	—	**Parent measures** SRS: d = 1.42 MCDI: d = –0.63
Stadnick et al. (2015)	30	1.5–8 years	ASD or at risk	Pilot study; treatment vs. community group	Parent factors associated with changes in child communication	**Child measures** VABS-II, Communication: Increase in communication skills for treatment vs. community control group	—	**Parent measures** CES-D: No changes in parent depression symptoms PSI-SF: No changes in parent stress **Child measures** VABS-II, Socialization: No changes in social skills for treatment vs. community control group	**Child measure** VABS-II, Communication: η² = 0.17

Key: CES-D, Center for Epidemiological Studies-Depression Scale; MCDI, MacArthur-Bates Communicative Development Inventory; PSI-SF, Parenting Stress Index-Short Form; SRS, Social Responsiveness Scale; VABS-II, Vineland Adaptive Behavior Scales, Second Edition.

Skillstreaming

A number of studies have been conducted on the Skillstreaming intervention (McGinnis, 2011; McGinnis & Goldstein 1997a; 2003; McGinnis & Simpson, 2017), and the evidence suggests that this intervention package "deserve[s] additional and ongoing research and clinical attention" (Kaat & Lecavalier, 2014, p. 22). Given the variability in treatment duration and intensity described in the studies conducted, as well as the omission of this information in a number of studies, the recommended dosage of Skillstreaming intervention is currently unavailable. Four studies have been conducted since the Kaat and Lecavalier (2014) review and provide further evidence for the use of Skillstreaming as part of a larger intervention (Lopata et al., 2015; Lopata, Lipinski et al., 2017; Lopata, Rodgers et al., 2017; Thomeer et al., 2019). Overall, children receiving Skillstreaming instruction tend to show improvements in social skills and decreases in ASD symptomology and withdrawal behaviors at the end of the intervention period compared to prior to the intervention as well as compared to a waitlist-control group (as reported by parents and staff working with the child). Many of these studies showed positive outcomes for children with ASD, demonstrating at least average cognitive and language abilities (often referred to as *high-functioning autism*) between the ages of 6 and 12 years. Findings were derived mainly from parent and teacher report measures administered pre- and postintervention.

One team of researchers (see Thomeer et al., 2019, for a review) completed a four-phase model for validating psychosocial treatment interventions for individuals with ASD. This series of intervention studies examined Skillstreaming intervention in the context of a larger intensive summer program designed to "improve the social-cognitive skills, social-communicative performance, and ASD symptoms of children with [high-functioning] ASD" (Thomeer et al., 2019, p. 2). In the final study of the four-phase series, the researchers make the case that children with ASD who receive this summer-intensive treatment program with Skillstreaming at its core demonstrate higher social and social-communicative skills, show reduced withdrawal behaviors and overall ASD symptoms, and gain an increased understanding of nonliteral language. Moreover, the authors make the case that "this series of clinical trials provides the level of replication needed (Kaat & Lecavalier, 2014; Smith et al., 2007) to validate the efficacy of the summerMAX program (under controlled-lab and real-world conditions) for children, 7–12 years of age with [high functioning ASD]" (p. 11). It should be noted that while Skillstreaming techniques were used during this intervention, the clinical efficacy trials were performed on a larger treatment program. Care should be taken in the interpretation of these findings as they relate to Skillstreaming instruction, as the effects found in these studies may not be replicated in a less intensive, Skillstreaming-only intervention. A detailed description of selected studies examining Skillstreaming is presented in Table 15.7, which is available with the text's online materials (see About the Videos and Downloads at the front of the book for information on how to access this table).

Social Competence Intervention

The SCI is designed to enhance the social competence of school-age children and adolescents. Stichter and colleagues (2010) used a pretest–posttest design to examine the impact of the SCI on the social competence skills of 27 adolescents with ASD, ages 11–14 years. They observed increases in parents' ratings of their children's social awareness, social cognition, and social communication and decreases in ASD behaviors on the Social Responsiveness Scale (SRS; Constantino, 2005). Stichter and colleagues (2010) also reported increases in behavior regulation and use of cognitive resources on the Behavior Rating Inventory of Executive Function–Second Edition (BRIEF-2; Gioia & Isquith, 2015). The children exhibited increases in their ability to make inferences about the reasons for problems and were able to identify solutions for problem situations on the Test of Problem Solving–Third Edition (TOPS-3; Bowers et al., 2018). Increases were also noted for recognizing a social faux pas (the Faux Pas Stories; Baron-Cohen et al., 1999), identifying emotional states (Diagnostic Analysis of Nonverbal Accuracy–Second Edition—Child Facial Expressions Test [DANVA-2-CF]; Nowicki & Duke, 2000), and labeling emotional and mental states following viewing a person's eyes (Reading the Mind in the Eyes Test; Baron-Cohen et al., 1997).

Schmidt and colleagues (2011) applied the SCI to six adolescents with ASD who had high cognitive and linguistic abilities and targeted social competence and theory of mind skills in educational settings. Following a pretest–posttest design, they found increases in teachers' perception of the adolescents' social motivation on the SRS with trends toward increased social communication as well as increases in executive function and metacognition on the BRIEF. Significant increases in emotion recognition for children's faces on the DANVA-2-CF was also reported with mixed results for other theory of mind measures.

In a quasi-experimental study, Schultz and colleagues (2012) examined parenting stress and sense of competence as well as children's social skills in 27 youth with ASD. Following the use of the SCI, Schultz and colleagues reported decreased parental stress for those adolescents in the treatment versus control group. There were positive trends for parents' reported sense of efficacy but no difference between groups was found for the adolescents' social skills on the SRS.

In a study of 20 children with ASD, ages to 6–10 years, Stichter and colleagues (2012) examined the impact of the SCI on social competence. Parent ratings revealed improvements in social abilities, as measured on the SRS, as well as gains in executive functioning, utilization of cognitive resources, and behavior regulation on the BRIEF. Teachers also rated positive changes in social abilities on the SRS following the SCI. Children demonstrated an increased ability to recognize a social faux pas but no significant improvement in emotion recognition on the Reading the Mind in the Eyes Test. Although the children showed some increased ability to recognize the chronology of events, they did not show improvements in making inferences and in problem solving on the TOP-3.

Stichter and colleagues (2013) also used the SCI for 11 students with ASD and a mean age of 12 years, targeting social competence using distance education and a virtual environment. Parent ratings indicated significant increases in social behaviors and interaction, and teacher ratings showed positive trends for social behaviors and social communication on the SRS. Parent ratings also indicated improvements in executive function and metacognition on the BRIEF. Student performance changes were noted for cognitive flexibility and generativity but not for inhibition or cognitive switching on the Delis-Kaplan Executive Functioning System (D-KEFS). No changes were noted for parental ratings for social awareness (SRS) and behavioral regulation (BRIEF) or teachers' assessment of executive function (BRIEF). Changes also were not seen in the children's performance on several advanced theory of mind measures. A detailed description of selected studies examining SCI is located in Table 15.8, which is available with the text's online materials (see About the Videos and Downloads at the front of the book for information on how to access this table).

Social Tools and Rules for Teens

START is an intervention program designed by researchers at the Koegel Autism Research Center (Vernon et al., 2016). START is a socialization intervention program with multiple components, including both didactic and experiential elements targeting deficits in motivation and social skills. It is most often used for adolescents with ASD who encounter social difficulties. In an initial study examining the START program, Vernon and colleagues (2016) saw improvements in social competence using survey and conversational measures for six adolescents with ASD. Specifically, adolescents with ASD increased their ability to make social inquiries and decreased their negative statements.

An RCT of the 20-week START program with 40 adolescents with ASD found significant differences in social skills between those in the START program and waitlist control groups (Vernon et al., 2018). Those in the START program showed a decrease in the overall severity of their ASD symptoms and an increase in their social skills. A detailed description of selected studies examining START is located in Table 15.9.

Virtual Reality Social Cognition Training

Few evidence-based social interventions exist for young adults with high-functioning autism, many of whom encounter significant challenges during the transition into adulthood. Kandalaft, Didehbani, Krawczyk, and colleagues (2012) investigated the feasibility of using the VR-SCT (https://brainhealth.utdallas.edu/more-information -about-charisma-virtual-social-learning) intervention program to facilitate the social skills, social cognition, and social functioning of eight young adults with ASD. The intervention was implemented for 10 sessions across 5 weeks. Results revealed significant increases on measures of emotion recognition and theory of mind following intervention, indicating promise for the use of a virtual reality platform to support social cognition in adults with ASD.

Didehbani and colleagues (2016) examined the impact of VR-SCT on 30 children with ASD, ages 7–16 years. The intervention was implemented across 5 weeks with ten 1-hour sessions. Using a pretest–posttest design, Didehbani and colleagues saw improvements in social attribution during a Social Attribution Task (Abell et al., 2000), increases in the Affect Recognition subscale of the Neuropsychological Assessment–Second Edition (Korkman et al., 2007), and increases in executive function on an Analogical Reasoning Task (Krawczyk et al., 2010). As in the previous study, these findings suggest the virtual reality platform can be effective for improving the social skills of children with ASD.

Yang and colleagues (2018) used a neuroimaging task to identify biomarkers that could predict young adults' responses to the VR-SCT program. In a pilot study of 17 young adults with high-functioning ASD, the researchers found neural predictors of change in emotion recognition following VR-SCT intervention. The predictors were characterized by the preintervention brain activations that support language comprehension, prosody, socioemotional affective information, and emotional regulation. Significant brain-behavior changes were identified and showed

Table 15.9. Summary of Selected Research on Social Tools and Rules for Teens (the START Program)

Study	Sample size	Age (years)	Diagnosis	Design	Targets of intervention	Outcome data				Effect size
						Significant findings	Trends	Nonsignificant findings		
Vernon et al. (2018)	40	12–17	ASD	RCT, treatment vs. waitlist control	Social functioning	**Parent measures** *SRS-2:* Decrease in ASD severity for treatment group compared to control group *SMCS:* Increase in social motivational factors and concrete skill competencies for treatment group compared to control group **Adolescent measures** *SISS:* Increase in social skills for treatment group compared to control group	—	**Parent measures** *SSIS:* No differences found between groups **Adolescent measures** *SMCS:* No differences found between groups		**Parent measures** *SRS-2, parent:* $\eta^2 = 0.189$ *SMCS, parent:* $\eta^2 = 0.287$ **Adolescent measures** *SSIS, teen:* $\eta^2 = 0.207$
Vernon et al. (2016)	6	12–17	ASD	Pretest–posttest	Socialization	**Parent and Adolescent Social Survey measures** *SSIS-RS:* Parent responses yielded increase in social skills; 4 of 6 adolescents showed increases in social skills	—	—		**Parent and adolescent social survey measures** *SSIS-RS, parent:* Adol Effect size (*d*)

SSIS-RS, parent:

Adol Effect size (*d*)

1	2.44
2	1.94
3	0.32
4	0.33
5	1.07
6	0.67

Adolescent:

Adol	Effect size (*d*)
1	20.21
2	0.68
3	−3.29
4	27.00
5	4.13
6	−1.91

SRS-2, parent (lower indicates improvement):

Adol	Effect size (*d*)
1	−1.36
2	−3.24
3	−0.25
4	NA
5	−3.57
6	−3.27

SMCS, parent total raw scores:

Adol	Effect size (*d*)
1	11.79
2	3.27
3	0.40
4	0.83
5	4.06
6	0.54

SMCS, adolescent total raw score:

Adol	Effect size (*d*)
1	13.14
2	−1.23
3	0.59
4	18.98
5	4.57
6	−0.74

SRS-2:
Parent responses showed a decrease in reported autism symptoms

SMCS:
Parents reported social increases pre to post-treatment; 4 of 6 adolescents showed social increases

Key. Adol, Adolescent; SMCS, Social Motivation and Competencies Scale; SSIS-RS, Social Skills Improve System Rating Scales; SRS-2, Social Responsiveness Scale, Second Edition.

increased brain activation in the right posterior superior temporal sulcus (important for social-cognitive processing) in response to social versus nonsocial stimuli
in those adults who showed gains on a theory of mind measure. Gains in emotion
recognition were observed for adults with decreased activation in the left inferior
frontal gyrus to social versus nonsocial stimuli. Significantly decreased activation
was also seen in the left superior parietal lobule to nonsocial versus social stimuli.
This is the first study to demonstrate neuroimaging-based biomarkers predictive of
treatment effectiveness in adults with ASD following 5 weeks of intervention with
ten 1-hour sessions. A detailed description of selected studies examining VR-SCT is
presented in Table 15.10.

PRACTICAL REQUIREMENTS

Generally speaking, the practical components for each social skills intervention
program requires trained personnel, including school counselors, teachers, and
a range of health care professionals (e.g., social workers, psychologists, psychiatrists, counselors, speech-language pathologists, behavior interventionists). Social
skills interventions implemented in schools often train paraprofessionals to support implementation. In addition, parents and neurotypical peers are often key participants and coaches in the intervention. Peers are usually neurotypical children
or those who demonstrate social skills beyond the skills of the child or adolescent
requiring intervention. Coaches are often used to model targeted social skills and
are typically high school or college-aged peer mentors. Most of the formalized social
skills interventions have a manual and related materials and activities including videos, DVDs, PowerPoint presentations, and training guides for parents and teachers.
Some materials are commercially available (e.g., Skillstreaming books and manuals), and others are available online (e.g., SCI) and through telehealth and boot
camps (e.g., PEERS). Some intervention programs (i.e., ICPS) offer trainings for
implementers, which include on-site and off-site coaching.

KEY COMPONENTS

Children's Friendship Program

The UCLA Children's Friendship Program (Frankel & Myatt, 2003) supports school-
age children who struggle making and keeping friends through skills building in
group sessions that are guided by licensed psychologists. Children who benefit most
are those who lack friends, are aggressive or shy with other children, have difficulty
managing conflicts, and are rarely included in the social activities of others (e.g.,
playdates, birthday parties). Using small-group sessions, children learn and practice
skills with other children and have weekly homework assignments to facilitate skills
application in their natural environment. Parents are key participants in the intervention and they are taught ways to support their children's social skills development. Parents often serve as coaches to remind children when and how they might
use their newly learned skills in real social situations. Children who participate in
this intervention learn several social skills, including the following:

- How to make a good first impression

- Ways to have conversations with other children

- Identification of common interests with other children

Table 15.10. Summary of Selected Research on Virtual Reality Social Cognition Training (VR-SCT).

Study	Sample size	Age (years)	Diagnosis	Design	Targets of intervention	Significant findings	Outcome Data Trends	Nonsignificant findings	Effect size
Didehbani et al (2015)	30	7–16	ASD	Pilot study with ASD compared to ASD + ADHD	Affect recognition, social attribution, executive function	**Participant measures** *NEPSY-II AR:* Increases in affect recognition *Triangles:* Increases in intentionality *Analogical Reasoning Task:* Significant increases in analogical reasoning	**Participant measures** *Ekman 60:* Increases in affect recognition *Triangles, total:* Increases in total score	**Participant measures** *NEPSY-II, AA and RSF:* No differences in selective attention or ability to maintain attention	
Kandalaft et al (2013)	8	18–26	High-functioning autism	Pilot study	• Investigate feasibility of intervention in adult with high-functioning autism • Qualify social change over time using social performance and skill measures and functional questionnaire	**Participant measures** *ACS-SP, total:* Increases in matching basic emotion words with pictures and auditory stimuli *ACS-SP-Prosody:* Increases in matching basic emotion words with auditory stimuli *Ekman 60:* Increases in emotion recognition for basic emotions *Triangles:* Increases in attributing intentionality to inanimate stimuli	**Participant measures** *SSPA:* Increases in conversational skills	**Participant measures** *ACS-SP-Pairs:* No differences in abilities deciphering nonliteral language or intention of speaker *ACS-SP-Affect Naming:* No differences in matching basic emotion words with pictures *Eyes:* No differences in matching photos of eyes to cognitive states	**Participant measures** *ACS-SP, total:* $\eta^2 = 0.53$ *SP-Prosody:* $\eta^2 = 0.6$ *Ekman 60:* $\eta^2 = 0.69$ *Triangles-Intentionality:* $\eta^2 = 0.63$

(continued)

Table 15.10. *(continued)*

Study	Sample size	Age (years)	Diagnosis	Design	Targets of intervention	Outcome Data			Effect size
						Significant findings	Trends	Nonsignificant findings	
Yang et al. (2018)	17	18–31	ASD	Pilot study	Language comprehension, emotion regulation; biomarkers predictive of treatment effectiveness	**Participant measures** *ACS-SP:* • Significant gains in emotion recognition with decreased activation in left inferior frontal gyrus to social vs. nonsocial stimuli • Significantly decreased activation to nonsocial vs. social stimuli in left superior parietal lobule	*Triangles:* Increased gains in theory of mind; brain activation to social vs. nonsocial stimuli in right posterior superior temporal sulcus	—	*ACS-SP: Hedges's g* = 0.53 *Triangles: Hedges's g* = 0.53

Key: ACS-SP, Advanced Clinical Solutions for WAIS-IV and WMS-IV Social Perception Subtest; Eckman 60, Facial expressions of emotion stimuli and tests; Eyes, Reading the Mind in the Eyes; NEPSY-II AR, Neuropsychological Assessment Second Edition, Affect Recognition; NEPSY-II AA, Neuropsychological Assessment Second Edition, Auditory Attention; NEPSY-II RSF, Neuropsychological Assessment Second Edition, Response Set F; SSPA, Social Skills Performance Assessment, Version 3.2(2); Triangles, Triangles social attribution task.

- Ability to play in a fair and gracious manner

- Conflict resolution

- Management of rejection, teasing, and bullying

- Engagement in play with other children

- Respect for other children and adults

This intervention is typically used for children in second through fourth grades with participation of their parents or primary caregivers. In some situations, first-graders may be considered (see https://www.semel.ucla.edu/sites/default/files/pdf/research/Children%27s%20Friendship%20Application%202017_0.pdf).

I Can Problem Solve

ICPS, an evidence-based intervention, is designed as a prevention program for children as young at 4 years old. The intervention emphasizes several theory of mind skills, including perspective-taking, alternative solution thinking, and consequential thinking. At age 8, more sophisticated theory of mind skills, such as recognizing mixed emotions, understanding motives, and means–end thinking, are highlighted.

ICPS has been implemented with a range of children from preschool through sixth grade, representing diverse populations, including Black, American Indian, Asian American/Pacific-Islander, Hispanic/Latino, and White, as well as an international population in Brazil, Chile, Greece, India, Israel, and Korea. The skills taught include learning vocabulary important to problem solving, identifying one's own and others' feelings, finding alternative solutions to problems, engaging in consequential thinking, understanding how one's own behavior impacts the behavior of others, and learning how to plan for a goal while managing the likely challenges to realizing that goal. Skills are sequentially presented to facilitate ease of acquisition and have differential expectations depending on the child's grade level. ICPS activities support social-cognitive problem solving through role play, puppet use, and games.

For preschool children (age 4 years), 59 lessons are delivered, and for early school-age children (kindergarten through second or third grade), 83 lessons are delivered two to three times weekly with an available script for teachers to follow. The training begins with 5- to 10-minute sessions, which gradually increases to 20 minutes over the course of 3–5 months. Typically, the sessions include small groups of 10 or fewer children. Several pre-problem-solving (e.g., vocabulary, feelings, preferences, listening, attending) and problem-solving (e.g., alternative solution, consequential thinking) skills are emphasized. Children are able to practice the concepts they learn as they work on academic tasks, and parents learn the skills to facilitate improved interactions at home while reinforcing the concepts taught. Both teachers and parents are also taught to use **ICPS dialoguing** that helps children connect what they do with how they think.

For elementary school children (third or fourth through sixth grade), 77 lessons are delivered with an available script for teachers. Sessions provide opportunities to learn targeted ICPS vocabulary, concepts, and problem-solving skills delivered two to three times weekly, building from 5- to 10-minute sessions to 20-minute sessions over 3–5 months. Problem-solving skills taught include the same as previously described with the addition of means–end thinking or sequential planning. ICPS dialoguing is also used with older elementary children.

PEERS

The PEERS is an internationally known evidence-based social skills intervention for preschoolers, adolescents, and young adults with ASD, ADHD, anxiety, depression, and other socioemotional problems. Developed by Dr. Elizabeth Laugeson, the program's popularity and success have expanded across the United States and internationally, with several translations, and PEERS is used in more than 80 countries.

When using PEERS with preschoolers, they must be between 4 and 6 years of age, speak in phrases or sentences of four or more words, and have a diagnosis of ASD or other social difficulties with no significant behavior problems. The targeted skills include listening and following directions, greeting, sharing, taking turns, asking friends their names and if they want to play, entering games, regulating emotions during play, being a good sport, transitioning across play activities, asking for or giving help, and using appropriate volume and body proximity. The intervention is designed to occur over 16 weeks with weekly 90-minute sessions.

Using PEERS for adolescents (i.e., middle and high school students) also involves weekly 90-minute group sessions with teens and their parents over the course of 16 weeks. Skills emphasized include developing and maintaining friendships, having a conversation, entering and exiting conversations, using electronic forms of communication, organizing get-togethers, being a good sport, managing disagreements, using humor, understanding teasing and bullying, and adjusting reputations. The weekly sessions usually involve didactic lessons in which skills are taught, and role play is used to apply newly learned skills for practice in real social situations. Parent participation is required, and teens must be interested in participating and must commit to attending the weekly program sessions.

For young adults, PEERS highlights many of the skills taught to adolescents, including ways to develop and maintain friendships, engage in conversation, enter and exit a conversation, use humor, manage electronic communication, and organize get-togethers. The additional skills include strategies for dating, managing bullying, and handling disagreements and dating pressures. PEERS for young adults is designed to support those interested in developing romantic relationships and making and keeping friends. Participants include individuals who have graduated from high school and are between the ages of 18 and 35. As described for the preschool and adolescent training, PEERS training for young adults includes sixteen 90-minute weekly sessions with didactic skills learning, role play, and practice. Social coaches are an added feature to the young adult training to help facilitate friendship-building and dating skills. To participate, young adults must commit to attending the program and have a social coach also willing to attend the training each week.

Mind Reading

The Mind Reading social skills training is used for individuals with ASD and those with theory of mind challenges. The primary focus is to increase decoding skills (making sense of what one sees and experiences) and capitalize on the systemizing strengths of individuals with ASD who have higher cognitive and linguistic abilities. The training uses interactive software to teach recognition of various facial expressions and prosodic cues, using both visual and auditory stimuli to practice with computer-delivered reinforcement. A manual and training guide, *Teaching Children with Autism to Mind-Read: A Practical Guide for Teachers and Parents,* is provided along with a DVD. Following implementation of Mind Reading, improvements have been seen in emotion recognition skills for facial and vocal expressions with some reduction in ASD symptoms. Other improvements have been reported in mental state recognition, greater attention to faces and emotions, and increased eye contact.

Play Time/Social Time

PT/ST is a manualized intervention program for 3- to 5-year-old children, with or at risk for disabilities, who exhibit social-interaction challenges, including those enrolled in special education programs, typical preschools, or child care centers. The goals of the program are to develop social competence and foster social interaction. Intervention occurs daily for 15 to 20 minutes over the course of 100 days in multiple phases. Activities range from play to prompted interactions to the social exchanges between two or more children whereby they learn to talk with one another, share ideas and materials, and engage in turn taking. The program includes the use of neurotypical peers to serve as social skills role models for those with ASD and other disabilities and associated social skills deficits. Training targets primarily include increasing social interaction and decreasing behavior challenges in problematic social situations.

Project ImPACT

Project ImPACT is a parent-based curriculum developed by Brooke Ingersoll and Anna Dvortcsak at Michigan State University to foster the social-communication skills of children with ASD (Ingersoll & Dvortcsak, 2019). In this social skills intervention, parents increase their understanding of ways to support the social skills of their children through daily activities and routines. Both behavioral and developmental strategies are incorporated to support the play, language, imitation, and social engagement of children with ASD. Parents are taught to implement social-communication strategies through videotaped viewings, coaching, and homework activities.

Skillstreaming

Skillstreaming is a manualized social skills intervention program designed to increase prosocial behaviors in young children, school-age children, adolescents, and children and youth with high-functioning autism (McGinnis & Goldstein, 1997a; 2003; McGinnis & Simpson, 2017; McGinnis et al., 2011) through planful, organized, and systematic instruction. This intervention is based on cognitive-behavioral techniques (Lopata et al., 2006), including the principles of modeling, role playing, feedback, and transfer of skills to various settings (McGinnis & Goldstein, 1997a). A variety of prosocial skills that vary in complexity and take into consideration the individual's age (i.e., young child, elementary-age child, adolescent) and whether he or she has a diagnosis of ASD are the focus of this intervention.

To enhance generalizability of skills, it is suggested that intervention take place in the child's classroom (if available). If this is not an option, treatment sessions can occur in a smaller room, such as the special educator's classroom or social worker's office. The authors suggest implementing Skillstreaming instruction three to five times a week for 25–40 minutes per session. Depending on the needs of the specific child, instruction can last for as short as 2 days or as long as multiple years. In a school setting, however, Skillstreaming instruction typically lasts the length of the school year. Prior to beginning the intervention, the leaders should explain the following to the group, as outlined in the clinician manual: the purpose, procedures, incentives, and rules for the group meetings. Each student in the group should receive a student manual in which descriptions of the teaching steps and social skills are outlined. This manual also includes examples of how the intervention might look in real life, as well as homework examples and templates (McGinnis & Goldstein, 1997b).

As highlighted in both the clinician and student manuals, nine steps are followed during each intervention session (McGinnis & Goldstein, 1997a):

1. Defining the skill

2. Modeling the skill

3. Establishing student skill need

4. Selecting a role player

5. Setting up the role player

6. Conducting the role play

7. Providing performance feedback

8. Assigning skill homework

9. Selecting next role player

Target skills should be selected on the basis of the individual's and/or group's needs. This should be determined through an interprofessional and family-centered approach, including collaboration with the child's team, observation of areas of social skills deficits for each child, and completion of the Student Skillstreaming Checklist (discussed further in the next section). Although the Skillstreaming manuals describe a number of social skills, the skills chosen should be specific to the target child(ren). The authors suggest practicing one skill until it becomes automatic before moving on to a second skill.

Because family involvement is paramount to successful treatment outcomes (Beatson, 2008; Beatson & Prelock, 2002; Prelock & Hutchins, 2008), Skillstreaming intervention encourages providing training and resources to the target individual's caregivers (e.g., through an orientation meeting or letter describing the intervention procedures). This affords caregivers an understanding of the intervention and can help increase skills generalization across the home and school environments. Group leaders are encouraged to send home videos of the child acting as the role player and to provide updates on the child's progress throughout the intervention.

Social Competence Intervention

The Social Competence Intervention (SCI) comes from the Center for Social and Behavioral Competence and is designed to support the development of social skills in children and youth from kindergarten through 12th grade. The SCI is a group-based program that draws from the principles of applied behavior analysis and cognitive-behavioral approaches. It was developed to address the social skills deficits of adolescents with ASD and higher cognitive and linguistic abilities. The SCI has three basic components: 20 hours of group lessons, personnel training to ensure knowledge of the curriculum and skills in supporting social skills generalization in educational settings, and strategy development for families to facilitate social skills generalization at home and in the community.

The SCI for elementary age children (6–10 years) and adolescents (11–14 years) incorporates several strategies, including modeling, direct instruction, and practice with and without support over the course of five sessions with sequenced lesson plans to scaffold learning. Skills emphasized include recognizing facial expressions, feelings, and emotions; turn taking; problem solving, and sharing ideas. For high school students (14–18 years), the strategies are similar, but the skills emphasized are a little different, including how to communicate ideas, have a conversation, collaborate, take the perspective of others, and problem-solve, as well as how to engage in interactions and apply the skills learned.

Social Tools and Rules for Teens

The START Program is a 10-week social skills intervention for adolescents with ASD that focuses on improving motivation, insight, and social skills. START highlights learning through social and experiential learning sessions. This program is designed for middle and high school students (12–17 years of age), focusing on experiential learning through a social club involving group activities with targeted social skills and peer mentors in high school or college. Each 90-minute session begins with individual check-ins, followed by socialization time to practice individual social skills, and then engagement in topical discussions using videos, practice, and role playing. Structured activities are included to facilitate the ability to work as a team and communicate effectively with one another. Each session ends in a check-out with the students' parents to provide feedback and review goals for the coming week.

START specifically targets social readiness in those with ASD, including **social motivation** and **social competence.** Social motivation involves the ability to experience pleasure in seeking out social interactions, and social competence includes the skills and insights necessary to engage in and manage various social encounters. Having these factors allows a person to engage with receptive social partners, become immersed in social interactions, benefit from experiential social learning, and ultimately strengthen existing social motivation and competencies. The START program was developed by the Koegel Autism Center, which offers 10-week group socialization programs for adolescents with ASD, ADHD, and other social challenges.

Virtual Reality Social Cognition Training

VR-SCT is designed to be used with children and youth (7–16 years) and young adults (18–26 years) to teach emotion recognition, responding to others, and asserting oneself across social contexts. The program includes ten 1-hour sessions over 5 weeks, with program complexity adjusted for developmental age. Training strategies support social reasoning with real-time nonscripted interaction, using a coach and confederate clinician with immediate feedback provided. The training is not manualized but has been shown to support improvements in emotion recognition, understanding the intention of others, and social judgment.

ASSESSMENT FOR TREATMENT PLANNING AND PROGRESS MONITORING

Across the several social skills intervention programs described here, a number of student-, parent-, and teacher-reported outcome measures were used to assess change in social skills and behavior following intervention. Individual assessments and observations of change were also developed for many programs and assessed at pre- and postintervention and often during a follow-up period to determine skills maintenance without ongoing intervention. Specific strategies used for each social skills intervention program are briefly summarized in the following sections.

Children's Friendship Training

The CFT program incorporates the Social Skills Rating System (SSRS; Gresham & Elliot, 1990), recently replaced with the Social Skills Improvement System Rating Scales (SSIS; Gresham & Elliot, 2008), as an assessment and progress monitoring tool for the program. The SSRS and SSIS examine children's (ages 3–18 years) social behaviors from the perspective of teachers, parents, and students. A range of social behaviors, particularly behavior and interpersonal skills (e.g., initiating conversations, making friends) that influence relationships between the child and the teacher as well as peers, are assessed. Parents and teachers rate both the perceived frequency of a particular behavior and the perceived importance of that behavior to a child's success. This assessment system helps clinicians identify those behaviors that should be targets for intervention and assists in planning the treatment approach. The CFT program primarily uses the parent rating scale.

The CFT program also includes the Pupil Evaluation Inventory (Pekarik et al., 1976) to assess the peer ratings of children's behavior in first through ninth grades, with three primary factors analyzed: aggression, withdrawal, and likeability. This inventory can be used as an outcome measure to examine behavior change once children have participated in the CFT program.

In addition, the CFT program uses the Piers-Harris Self-Concept Scale (Piers et al., 2018), now in its third edition, to examine self-concept. It is a self-report measure for individuals age 6 to 22 years, using a yes/no format, and it yields an overall self-concept score with items related to social isolation, body image, and bullying to facilitate more effective assessment of social acceptance and physical self-concept.

I Can Problem Solve and Play Time/Social Time

Assessment and progress monitoring activities for ICPS are not specifically reported. There are, however, a number of tools used to assess behavior change in PT/ST. The Vineland Adaptive Behavior Scales–Third Edition (VABS-3; Sparrow et al., 2016) is most often used to support the diagnosis of those with developmental and intellectual challenges, including those with ASD, from birth to 90 years of age. It includes an interview and parent/caregiver and teacher forms. The specific domains assessed include socialization, communication, and daily living skills. It is frequently used to qualify individuals for services, treatment planning, and progress monitoring, as well as for research. The Vineland Adaptive Behavior Scales Special Population (Carter et al., 1998) provides specific norms for four groups of individuals with ASD: those under 10 who are nonverbal, those under 10 who have some verbal skills, those 10 or older who are nonverbal, and those 10 or older who have some verbal skills.

The California Preschool Social Competency Scale (Flint et al., 1980; Julvez et al., 2008; Proger, 1974) is another measure used to assess behavior change in the PT/ST program; it examines the interpersonal skills of preschool children (ages 2–6 years) and how effectively young children assume responsibility for their behavior. It is a teacher informant measure that asks teachers to rate children's abilities to follow a routine, respond to unfamiliar situations, follow instructions, share, help others, provide explanations, initiate and direct activities, accept limits, and react to frustrating situations.

In addition, the Battelle Developmental Inventory–Third Edition (BDI-3; Newborg, 2019) is used in the PT/ST program to assesses the developmental skills of infants, toddlers, preschoolers, and school-age children through 7 years, 11 months. This assessment gathers input through a number of sources, including child observations, parent/caregiver interviews, a comprehensive developmental and social history, and interactions with the child incorporating a variety of tasks, toys, and games. It is often used as an initial assessment of function across several developmental domains but can be used to help develop a treatment plan and monitor progress over time.

The SSRS (Gresham & Elliot, 1990) is also used as an assessment and progress monitoring tool for PT/ST, as are several teacher rating scales, including the Teacher Impression Scale, the Teacher Rating of Social Interaction, and the Teacher Rating of Intervention Behavior.

Mind Reading

Assessing the outcomes of the Mind Reading intervention program includes the Reading the Mind in the Eyes task, as briefly described earlier; this also includes the voice element of the task, so individuals are asked to perceive emotion not only from examining the eyes of individuals but also from the tone of their voice. This is also true of the Cambridge Mindreading (CAM) Face-Voice Battery (Golan et al., 2006). This tool, comprising 54 video and audio clips of facial expressions and voices, is used to assess emotion recognition in adults with ASD who have higher cognitive and linguistic abilities. It was designed to assess the frequently reported challenges individuals with ASD have in emotion recognition and understanding, especially for more complex emotions. These emotion recognition challenges frequently influence social communication, so this tool can be an effective assessment and progress monitoring tool following intervention.

In addition, the SRS (Constantino, 2005) is used as a measure of social impairment for the Mind Reading intervention program. The tool is often used to assess change in an individual's social performance over time. Finally, the Behavior Assessment System for Children, Second Edition–Parent Rating Scales (BASC-2-PRS; Reynolds & Kamphaus, 2004) is an assessment approach with a variety of ways to gather information about a child. The Parent Report Scales of the BASC-2 requires parents to rate their child's behaviors as they have observed them in the home setting. Each of these tools is used to assess and monitor improvements in emotion recognition, decreases in ASD symptoms, increases in mental state recognition, attention to faces and emotions, and eye contact.

PEERS

Following implementation of the curriculum, several postintervention assessment methods are used to evaluate outcomes. The Test of Adolescent Social Skills Knowledge (TASSK; Laugeson & Frankel, 2006) and the Quality of Socialization

Questionnaire–Adolescent and Parent (Frankel & Mintz, 2008) versions are the most frequently used outcome measures in PEERS. In addition, students are asked to keep several logs to monitor their progress in homework completion, sportsmanship, and daily assignments.

Project ImPACT

To assess outcomes as a result of participating in the Project ImPACT intervention program, children's spontaneous language use is evaluated, as is their social engagement and play (as measured through a video analysis of their interactions). Formal tools, such as the SRS (Constantino, 2005), the MB-CDI (Fenson et al., 1993), the Center for Epidemiological Studies-Depression Scale (CES-D; Radloff, 1977), the Parent Stress Index–Short Form (PSI-SF; Abidin, 1995), and the VABS-II (Sparrow et al., 2016), are used to evaluate positive change in social skills knowledge and ability. These outcome measures are used to assess gains in communication, vocabulary, language, and social engagement.

Skillstreaming

Prior to beginning Skillstreaming sessions, areas of deficit should be determined to establish treatment goals. Assessment procedures include conducting observations of the child in a natural setting, completion of parent and teacher behavior rating scales, and completion of social skills checklists by parents, teachers, and the child. Some of the rating scales and checklists that have been used in research studies examining Skillstreaming include the Adapted Skillstreaming Checklist for parents and teachers (Lopata et al., 2008) and the Behavior Assessment System for Children, Third Edition–Parent Rating Scales (BASC-3-PRS) and Teacher Rating Scales (BASC-3-TRS; Reynolds & Kamphaus, 2015). Rating scales and social skills checklists offer valuable input from the child's teachers and caregivers regarding social and behavioral strengths and challenges. In addition, parent and teacher rating forms can be administered at various times throughout the intervention as a way to examine efficacy of the treatment and monitor the child's progress.

After a child has been selected to participate in treatment, he or she should complete the Student Skillstreaming Checklist (McGinnis & Goldstein, 1997b). This checklist provides the team with the child's perspective of his or her own skills and challenges. Bringing awareness to the child's own challenges in this way may help the child to see the importance of the skill(s) as it relates to everyday life and thus increase buy-in to the intervention (McGinnis & Goldstein, 1997a).

In addition to conducting observations and completing rating scales, another component of data collection includes reviewing the child's completed homework assignments. As previously mentioned, Skillstreaming homework should be assigned at the end of each treatment session. This allows the child the opportunity to practice the skills outside of the group setting. While not explicitly stated in the Skillstreaming manual, reviewing the child's completed homework assignments at the beginning of each session allows opportunity for discussion regarding practice of the social skill. These discussions could include 1) what went well, 2) what made practicing the skill challenging, 3) supports used, and 4) what the child might do differently next time. Furthermore, the clinician is discouraged from progressing through the skills too quickly. Sufficient time for the child to master a skill should be given before a new skill is introduced.

Social Competence Intervention

The SCI uses a variety of research-based tasks (e.g., Sally-Anne false belief [Baron-Cohen et al., 1985], Smarties false belief [Perner et al., 1989], Faux Pas Stories [Baron-Cohen et al., 1999]) to determine baseline understanding of various elements of theory of mind. These tasks are frequently used as outcome measures to assess change following intervention. To assess adolescents' and adults' ability to mentalize or discriminate different emotions by looking at the eyes of particular faces, the Reading the Mind in the Eyes Test is administered (Baron-Cohen et al., 1997). The SRS is also used as an outcome measure for the SCI.

To assess children's executive functions and self-regulation, BRIEF-2 (Gioia & Isquith, 2015) is used in the SCI. The BRIEF-2 is designed as a parent, teacher, and self-report measure for children five to 18 years of age. It is often used as a tool to assess working memory, the ability to think flexibly, and the ability to self-regulate or exhibit self-control. These are important skills for individuals with ASD to help manage their daily activities, as those with executive functioning challenges find themselves having difficulty focusing, following directions, and managing their emotions sufficiently to learn, work, and manage daily life. The BRIEF-2 is frequently used as an outcome measure following intervention.

In addition, the DANVA-2 (Nowicki & Duke, 1994, 2000), which measures an individual's ability to recognize emotions by reading facial expressions and listening to different voices and vocal tones, is also used as part of this curriculum assessment. The DANVA-2 includes four subtests with child and adult faces and child and adult paralanguage. Basic emotions (i.e., happiness, sadness, fear, anger) are probed with both high and low emotional intensity. This measure can be used to probe changes in affect recognition.

The final tool used for assessment and progress monitoring in the SCI program is the TOPS-3 (Bowers et al., 2018). The elementary version of the TOPS-3 assesses the ability of children 6–12 years of age to integrate linguistic information with an ability to reason, using picture stimuli to prompt verbal responses. It is used to assess an overall ability to problem-solve, and performance on this tool often guides intervention, identifying areas of particular challenge for students with ASD, especially when attempting to problem-solve in complex social situations.

Social Tools and Rules for Teens

Similar to the CFT and PT/ST programs, START uses SSRS and SSIS rating scales to examine the social behaviors of teens prior to and following intervention. The SSIS rating scales are appropriate measures to identify intervention targets and monitor behavior change over time.

The SRS (Constantino, 2005) or the Social Responsiveness Scale–Second Edition (SRS-2; Constantino, 2012) is frequently used to measure the social impairment in individuals with ASD from 4 to 18 years of age. The SRS is a parent and teacher rating scale that can be used to monitor positive change in the social impairment of individuals with ASD following intervention. The SRS-2 expands the age range from 2.5 years to adulthood and adds a self-report measure for adults 19 and older. Both can be used as outcome measures to detect change in social impairment following intervention.

Among other tasks, the START program probes several aspects of conversation (e.g., verbal contributions, social inquiries, negative statements) for those participating in the intervention program to obtain a sense of how an individual dynamically engages in conversation with others, using these probes to measure change over time.

Virtual Reality Social Cognition Training

VR-SCT also uses both standardized and research measures to assess positive change in social skills knowledge and use. The Wechsler Advanced Clinical Solutions Social Perception (ACS-SP; Wechsler, 2009) subtest is used as a measure of social cognition. This subtest focuses on functional deficits examining skills related to understanding social communication (Kandalaft, Didehbani, Cullen, et al., 2012). The Ekman 60 Faces Test, a neuropsychological assessment using facial expressions to measure emotion recognition (Dodich et al., 2014), is also used as an outcome measure for research examining neurological and psychiatric disorders. To assess adolescents' and adults' abilities to mentalize or discriminate different emotions by looking at the eyes of particular faces, the Reading the Mind in the Eyes Test is administered (Baron-Cohen et al., 1997). The Triangles Task, also known as the Social Attribution Task (Abell et al., 2000), also measures an individual's ability to mentalize and to understand social intentions.

In addition to the previously mentioned outcome measures, the Social Skills Performance Assessment (SSPA) is a performance-based measure of the social skills of adults with ASD, which takes approximately 12 minutes to complete and includes role playing and ratings of the role plays (Bellack et al., 1990; Patterson et al., 2001). As a direct assessment of social behavior, it is likely to provide a more accurate assessment of an individual's social functioning. Follow-up self-report surveys are also included to assess the individual's perceived improvement in emotion recognition, understanding the intentions of others, and making social judgments.

IMPLICATIONS FOR INCLUSIVE PRACTICE

Social skills interventions support social understanding and appropriate behavior across a wide range of social environments, including home, school, work, and community settings. Their practical components are foundational to inclusive practice, as each program reviewed in this chapter works to generalize skills in the school or academic environments. The programs are also designed to facilitate a skillset that has broad implications for the social success of individuals with ASD when interacting at home and in social situations within the community.

CONSIDERATIONS FOR CHILDREN FROM CULTURALLY AND LINGUISTICALLY DIVERSE BACKGROUNDS

Regardless of the size of the social skills intervention group, it is likely that members of the group will come from different cultural backgrounds. Culture is not limited to race and ethnicity but also includes age, socioeconomic status, gender, sexual orientation, geographic region, social class, and other factors. For social skills interventions to be successful, students must have an opportunity to recognize and understand the cultural differences of others, and instructors must be mindful of cultural differences when choosing intervention targets. It is paramount that instructors for social skills interventions fundamentally understand the difference between social skills *deficits* and social skills *differences* due to cultural influences (Cartledge & Leo, 2001). Social skills deficits can be addressed; however, cultural differences should never be the focus of intervention. Social skills interventions require users to understand that the skills taught are not designed to create a middle-class example of how one should act in a social context. Instead, culturally mindful social skills instruction expects instructors to respect the various cultural values while helping students to learn new behaviors that may be deemed appropriate by a given social situation (Cartledge & Johnson, 1997, as cited in McGinnis & Goldstein, 2003).***

Applications to Children, Adolescents, and Adults

As described in this chapter, a number of manualized social skills intervention packages exist to help increase social skills functioning in children, adolescents, and adults with ASD. Clinicians should carefully consider the available options, the evidence base of those options, and the specific social skills taught before deciding on which intervention best suits the needs of a particular child, adolescent, or adult. When deciding on a social skills intervention program, considerations should include the following:

- Is this intervention program appropriate for the individual's language and/or cognitive abilities?
- Does this intervention program demonstrate evidence for individuals similar to the target individual's age?
- Are there pertinent intervention requirements and/or resources (e.g., materials, training, personnel, time) that are unavailable or cannot be acquired?
- Is the intervention program manualized?
- Does the intervention program use a family-centered approach?
- Does the intervention program have a generalization plan?
- Does the intervention program involve peers?
- Does the intervention program have a family component?
- How does the intervention program support success across environments, including home, school, and the community?

   Decisions about the best social skills intervention programs to use across the lifespan are highly dependent on the unique social challenges of the individual with ASD, the available training and staff fidelity with implementing the intervention program, and the likelihood that the intervention can be supported across environments.

To review an extended application and implementation of Skillstreaming, see Case 12 about an older elementary student in the companion volume *Case Studies for the Treatment of Autism Spectrum Disorder*.

Future Directions

Much work has been done to examine the social skills of persons with ASD from childhood through adulthood. Efforts to research the effectiveness of manualized programs or systematic curricula focused on increasing social knowledge and social skills are showing promising results.

   Engagement with families appears to be a key ingredient to success, as does access to socially competent peers and thoughtful ways to measure behavior change. In addition, there are opportunities to increase access and adaptation of the social skills intervention programs so that more diverse populations might benefit. Clinicians should note, however, that competence in social skills development appears to be a more achievable goal than social skills performance, as not all social skills intervention programs demonstrate the same level of sustained performance and social validity once intervention is no longer being implemented. Clinicians should continually examine and monitor the outcomes targeted in any social skills intervention program to ensure these goals are appropriate for the individual with ASD.

Suggested Readings

1. McGinnis, E. (2011). *Skillstreaming the adolescent: A guide for teaching prosocial skills* (3rd ed.). Research Press. This guide describes the training approach used to teach adolescents key prosocial skills using a variety of strategies such as modeling, role play, feedback, and generalization. It describes the Skillstreaming program and provides instructions for teaching 50 different social skills. Some of the skills taught are friendship-making, dealing with feelings, managing aggression, dealing with stress, and surviving classroom expectations. One-page summaries are provided for each skill, giving suggestions, instructions, and ways to model expected behavior. Appendices are available with program forms, as are checklists to ensure intervention fidelity.

2. Shure, M. B. (2001). *The "I Can Problem Solve" Program.* Research Press. In this book, Dr. Myrna B. Shure demonstrates applications of the ICPS strategies that are relevant to parents and children from preschool to early adolescence. Including problem-solving scenarios, this book provides meaningful ways parents can help their children learn how to think.

3. Laugeson, E. A. (2013). *The PEERS® Curriculum for School-Based Professionals: Social Skills Training for Adolescents with Autism Spectrum Disorders.* Taylor & Francis. The PEERS manual for school-based professionals describes an evidenced-based 14-week intervention program to improve the social skills and social interactions of teens with ASD. The manual provides details for each intervention session, including homework assignments, review plans, activities to apply learning, and parent handouts. The manual serves as a guide for professionals with ideas for implementing lessons and ways to problem-solve when activities do not go as expected.

Learning Activities

1. Describe a preschool child, school age child, and adolescent with ASD, highlighting the social skills that are most interfering with their ability to have a conversation and engage with peers. For each individual complete the following:

   a. Identify the most appropriate social skills intervention program to implement with this individual.

   b. Explain why you chose this program.

   c. Describe the social skills you will target for each individual.

   d. Determine the outcome measure you will use to assess behavior change for each individual.

2. Compare and contrast the Skillstreaming and PEERS social skills intervention programs. Describe their strengths, appropriateness for a population of children with ASD, and ease of implementation.

3. Describe two social skills intervention programs you would select to target the theory of mind deficits in a school-age child or adolescent.

4. Which social skills intervention program would you choose to support a culturally diverse group of children with ASD? What modifications would you make to ensure the curriculum is accessible to the children and their families and the activities are appropriate to their culture.

REFERENCES

Abell, F., Happé, F., & Frith, U. (2000). Do triangles play tricks? Attribution of mental states to animated shapes in normal and abnormal development *Cognitive Development, 15* (1), 1–16.

Abidin, R. R. (1995). *Parenting Stress Index (PSI) manual* (3rd ed.). Pediatric Psychology Press.

American Psychiatric Association. (2013). *Diagnostic and statistical manual of mental disorders, fifth edition* (DSM-5). Author.

Antshel, K. M., Polacek, C., McMahon, M., Dygert, K., Spenceley, L., Dygert, L., Miller, L., & Faisal, F. (2011). Comorbid ADHD and anxiety affect social skills group intervention treatment efficacy in children with autism spectrum disorders. *Journal of Developmental & Behavioral Pediatrics, 32*(6), 439–446.

Baron-Cohen, S. (2004). Mind reading: An interactive guide to emotions. Jessica Kingsley Publishers.

Baron-Cohen, S., Jolliffe, T., Mortimore, C., & Robertson, M. (1997). Another advanced test of theory of mind: Evidence from very high-functioning adults with autism or Asperger Syndrome. *Journal of Child Psychology and Psychiatry, 38*, 813–822.

Baron-Cohen, S., Leslie, A. M., & Frith, U. (1985). Does the autistic child have a "theory of mind"? *Cognition, 21*, 37–46.

Baron-Cohen, S., O'Riordan, M., Stone, V., Jones, R., & Plaisted, K. (1999). A new test of social sensitivity: Detection of faux pas in normal children and children with Asperger syndrome. *Journal of Autism and Developmental Disorders, 29*, 407–418.

Beatson, J. (2008). Walk a mile in their shoes: Implementing family-centered care in serving children and families affected by autism spectrum disorder. *Topics in Language Disorders, 28*(4), 309–322.

Beatson, J., & Prelock, P. (2002). The Vermont Rural Autism Project: Sharing experiences, shifting attitudes. *Focus on Autism and Other Developmental Disabilities, 17*(1), 48–54.

Bellack, A., Morrison, R., Wixted, J., & Mueser, K. (1990.) An analysis of social competence in schizophrenia. *British Journal of Psychiatry, 156*, 809–818.

Bellini, S., Peters, J. K., Benner, L., & Hopf, A. (2007). A meta-analysis of school-based social skills interventions for children with autism spectrum disorders. *Remedial and Special Education, 28*, 153–162.

Bowers, L., Huisingh, R., & LoGiudice, C. (2018). *Test of Problem Solving-third edition* (TOPS-3). Western Psychological Services.

Boyle, D., & Hassett-Walker, C. (2008). Reducing overt and relational aggression among young children: The results from a two-year outcome evaluation. *Journal of School Violence, 7*(1), 27–42.

Cartledge, G., & Leo, S. (2001). Cultural diversity and social skill instruction. *Exceptionality, 9*, 33–46.

Carter, A. S., Volkmar, F. R., Sparrow, S. S., Wang, J.-J., Lord, C., Dawson, G., Fombonne, E., Loveland, K., Mesibov, G., & Schopler, E. (1998). The Vineland Adaptive Behavior Scales: Supplementary norms for individuals with autism. *Journal of Autism and Developmental Disorders 28*, 287–302.

Ciancio, D., Rojas, A. C., McMahon, K., & Pasnak, R. (2001). Teaching oddity and insertion to head start children: An economical cognitive intervention. *Journal of Applied Developmental Psychology, 22*(6), 603–621.

Constantino, J. N. (2005). *Social Responsiveness Scale.* Western Psychological Publishing.

Constantino, J. N. (2012). *Social Responsiveness Scale–Second edition.* Western Psychological Publishing.

Didehbani, N., Allen, T., Kandalaft, M., Krawczyk, D., & Chapman, S. (2016). Virtual reality social cognition training for children with high functioning autism. *Computers in Human Behavior, 62,* 703–711.

Dodich, A., Cerami, C., Canessa, N., Crespi, C., Marcone, A., Arpone, M., Realmuto, S., & Cappa, S. F. (2014). Emotion recognition from facial expressions: a normative study of the Ekman 60-Faces Test in the Italian population. *Neurological Science, 35*(7), 1015–1021.

Dolan, B., Van Hecke, A. V., Carson, A. M., Karst, J. S., Stevens, S. J., Schohl, K. A., Potts, S., Kahne, J., Linneman, N., Remmel, R., & Hummel, E. (2016). Assessment of intervention effects on in vivo peer interactions in adolescents with autism spectrum disorders (ASD). *Journal of Autism and Developmental Disorders, 46*(6), 2251–2259.

Feis, C. L., & Simons, C. (1985). Training preschool children in interpersonal cognitive problem-solving skills: A replication. *Prevention in Human Services, 3*(4), 59–70.

Fenson, L., Dale, P. S., Reznick, J. S., Thal, D., Bates, E., Hartung, J. P., Pethick, S., & Reilly, J. S. (1993). MacArthur Communicative Development Inventories: User's guide and technical manual. Singular Publishing Group.

Flint, D. L., Hick, T. L., Horan, M. D., Irvine, D. J., & Kukuk, S. E. (1980). Dimensionality of the California Preschool Social Competency Scale. *Applied Psychological Measurement, 4*(2), 203–212.

Frankel, F., & Mintz, J. (2008). Measuring the quality of play dates. Available from UCLA Parenting and Children's Friendship Program, 300 Medical Plaza, Los Angeles.

Frankel, F., & Myatt, R. (2003). *Children's Friendship Training.* Brunner-Routledge.

Frankel, F., Myatt, R., Sugar, C., Whitham, C., Gorospe, C., & Laugeson, E. (2010). A randomized controlled study of parent-assisted Children's Friendship Training with children having autism spectrum disorders. *Journal of Autism and Developmental Disorders, 40*(7), 827–842.

Gates, J., Kang, E., & Lerner, M. (2017). Efficacy of group social skills interventions for youth with autism spectrum disorder: A systematic review and meta-analysis. *Clinical Psychological Review, 52,* 164–181.

Gioia, G. A., & Isquith, P. S. (2015). *Behavior Rating Inventory of Executive Function–Second Edition (BRIEF-2).* Western Psychological Services.

Golan, O., & Baron-Cohen, S. (2006). Systemizing empathy: Teaching adults with Asperger syndrome or high-functioning autism to recognize complex emotions using interactive multimedia. *Development and Psychopathology, 18*(2), 591–617.

Golan, O., Baron-Cohen, S. & Hill, J. (2006). The Cambridge Mindreading (CAM) Face-Voice Battery: Testing complex emotion recognition in adults with and without Asperger syndrome. *Journal of Autism and Developmental Disorders 36*(2),169–183.

Gresham, F., & Elliot, S. N. (1990). *Social Skills Rating System.* Pearson.

Gresham, F., & Elliot, S. N. (2008). *Social Skills Improvement System Rating Scales.* Pearson.

Gresham, F., Sugai, G., & Horner, R. H. (2001). Interpreting outcomes of social skills training for students with disabilities. *Exceptional Children, 67*(3), 331–344.

Hawkins, J. D., Catalano, R. F., Kosterman, R., Abbot, R., & Hill, K. G. (1999). Preventing adolescent health-risk behaviors by strengthening protection during childhood. *Archives of Pediatric and Adolescent Medicine, 153*(3), 226–234.

Ingersoll, B., & Dvortcsak, A. (2019). *Teaching social communication to children with autism and other developmental delays* (2nd ed.). Guilford Press.

Ingersoll, B., & Wainer, A. (2013). Initial efficacy of Project ImPACT: A parent-mediated social communication intervention for young children with ASD. *Journal of Autism and Developmental Disorders, 43*(12), 2943–2952.

Ingersoll, B. R., Wainer, A. L., Berger, N. I., & Walton, K. M. (2017). Efficacy of low intensity, therapist-implemented Project ImPACT for increasing social communication skills in young children with ASD. *Developmental Neurorehabilitation, 20*(8), 502–510.

Julvez, J., Forns, M., Ribas-Fitó, N., Mazon, C., Torrent, M., Garcia-Esteban, R., Ellison-Los-chmann, L., & Sunyer, J. (2008). Psychometric characteristics of the California Preschool Social Competence Scale in a Spanish population sample. *Early Education and Development, 19*(5), 795–815.

Kandalaft, M. R., Didehbani, N., Cullum, C. M., Krawczyk, D. C., Allen, T. T., Tamminga, C. A., & Chapman, S. B. (2012). The Wechsler ACS Social Perception Subtest: A preliminary comparison with other measures of social cognition. *Journal of Psychoeducational Assessment, 30*(5), 455–465.

Kandalaft, M. R., Didehbani, N., Krawczyk, D. C., Allen, T. T., & Chapman, S. B. (2012). Virtual Reality Social Cognition Training for young adults with high-functioning Autism. *Journal of Autism and Developmental Disorders, 43*(1), 34–44.

Kaat, A., & Lecavalier, L. (2014). Group-based social skills treatment: A methodological review. *Research in Autism Spectrum Disorders, 8*, 15–24.

Korkman, M., Kirk, U., & Kemp. S. (2007). *NEPSY-Second Edition* (NEPSY-II). Harcourt Assessment.

Krawczyk, D. C., Hanten, G., Wilde, E. A., LI, X., Schnelle, K. P., Merkley, Tl. L., Vasquez, A. C., Cook, L. G., McClelland, M., Chapman, S. B., & Levin, H. S. (2010). Deficits in analogical reasoning in adolescents with traumatic brain injury. *Frontiers in Human Neuroscience, 4*, 62.

Kurnpfer, K. L., Alvarado, R., Tait, C., & Turner, C. (2002). Effectiveness of school-based family and children's skills training for substance abuse prevention among 6-8-year old rural children. *Psychology of Addictive Behaviors, 16*(4S), S65–S71.

Laugeson, E. A. (2013). *The PEERS® curriculum for school-based professionals: Social skills training for adolescents with autism spectrum disorder*. Taylor & Francis.

Laugeson, E. A., Ellingsen, R., Sanderson, J., Tucci, L., & Bates, S. (2014). The ABC's of teaching social skills to adolescents with autism spectrum disorder in the classroom: The UCLA PEERS® Program. *Journal of Autism and Developmental Disorders, 44*(9), 2244–2256.

Laugeson, E. A., & Frankel, F. (2006). Test of Adolescent Social Skills Knowledge. Available from UCLA Parenting and Children's Friendship Program, 300 Medical Plaza, Los Angeles.

Laugeson, E. A., Frankel, F., Gantman, A., Dillon, A. R., & Mogil. C. (2012). Evidence-based social skills training for adolescents with autism spectrum disorders: The UCLA PEERS program. *Journal of Autism and Developmental Disorders, 42*(6), 1025–1036.

Laugeson, E. A., Frankel, F., Mogil, C., & Dillon, A. R. (2009). Parent-assisted social skills training to improve friendships in teens with autism spectrum disorders. *Journal of Autism and Developmental Disorders, 39*, 596–606.

Lerner, M. D., & Mikami, A. Y. (2012). A preliminary randomized controlled trial of two social skills interventions for youth with high-functioning autism spectrum disorders. *Focus on Autism and Other Developmental Disabilities, 27*(3), 147–157.

Lopata, C., Lipinski, A. M., Thomeer, M. L., Rodgers, J. D., Donnelly, J. P., McDonald, C. A., & Volker, M. A. (2017). Open-trial pilot study of a comprehensive outpatient psychosocial treatment for children with high-functioning autism spectrum disorder. *Autism, 21*(1), 108–116.

Lopata, C., Rodgers, J., Donnelly, J., Thomeer, M., McDonald, C., & Volker, M. (2017). Psychometric properties of the Adapted Skillstreaming Checklist for high-functioning children with ASD. *Journal of Autism and Developmental Disorders, 47*, 2723–2732.

Lopata, C., Thomeer, M. L., Volker, M. A., Lee, G. K., Smith, T. H., Smith, R. A., McDonald, C. A., Rodgers, J. D., Lipinski, A. M., & Toomey, J. A. (2012). Feasibility and initial efficacy of a comprehensive school-based intervention for high-functioning autism spectrum disorders. *Psychology in the Schools, 49*(10), 963–974.

Lopata, C., Thomeer, M. L., Volker, M. A., & Nida, R. E. (2006). Effectiveness of a cognitive-behavioral treatment on the social behaviors of children with Asperger disorder. *Focus on Autism and Other Developmental Disabilities, 21*(4), 237–244.

Lopata, C., Thomeer, M. L., Volker, M. A., Nida, R. E., & Lee, G. K. (2008). Effectiveness of a manualized summer social treatment program for high-functioning children with autism spectrum disorders. *Journal of Autism and Developmental Disorders, 38*(5), 890–904.

Lopata, C., Thomeer, M. L., Volker, M. A., Toomey, J. A., Nida, R. E., Lee, G. K., Smerbeck, A. M., & Rodgers, J. D. (2010). RCT of a manualized social treatment for high-functioning autism spectrum disorders. *Journal of Autism and Developmental Disorders, 40*(11), 1297–1310.

Lopata, C., Toomey, J. A., Thomeer, M. L., McDonald, C. A., Fox, J. D., Smith, R. A., Meichenbaum, D. L., Volker, M. A., Lee, G. K., & Lipinski, A. M. (2015). Community trial of a comprehensive psychosocial treatment for HFASDs. *Focus on Autism and Other Developmental Disabilities, 30*(2), 115–125.

McGinnis, E. (2011). *Skillstreaming the adolescent: A guide for teaching prosocial skills* (3rd ed.). Research Press.

McGinnis, E., & Goldstein, A. (1997a). *Skillstreaming the elementary school child: New strategies and perspectives for teaching prosocial skills* (rev. ed.). Research Press.

McGinnis, E., & Goldstein, A. (1997b). *Skillstreaming the elementary school child: Student manual.* Research Press.

McGinnis, E., & Goldstein, A. (2003). *Skillstreaming in early childhood: New strategies and perspectives for teaching prosocial skills.* Research Press.

McGinnis, E. & Simpson, L. (2017). *Skillstreaming children and youth with high-functioning Autism: A guide for teaching prosocial skills.* Research Press.

McGinnis, E., Sprafkin, R. P., Gershaw, N. J., & Klein, P. (2011). *Skillstreaming the adolescent: New strategies and perspectives for teaching prosocial skills* (3rd ed.). Research Press.

National Autism Center. (2009). *Findings and conclusions: National Standards Project, Phase 1.* Author.

National Autism Center. (2015). *Findings and conclusions: National Standards Project, Phase 2.* Author.

Newborg, J. (2019). *Battelle Developmental Inventory–Third Edition* (BDI-3). Riverside Insights.

Nowicki, S., & Duke, M. P. (1994). Individual differences in the nonverbal communication of affect: The Diagnostic Analysis of Nonverbal Accuracy Scale. *Journal of Nonverbal Behavior, 18,* 9–35.

Nowicki, S., & Duke, M. P. (2000). Nonverbal receptivity: The Diagnostic Analysis of Nonverbal Accuracy (DANVA). In J. A. Hall & F. Bernieri (Eds.), *Interpersonal sensitivity: Theory and measurement* (pp.183–198). Erlbaum.

Patterson, T. L., Moscona, S., McKibbin, C. L., Davidson, K., & Jeste, D. V. (2001). Social skills performance assessment among older patients with schizophrenia. *Schizophrenia Research, 48*(2–3), 351–360.

Pekarik, E. G., Prinz, R. J., Liebert, D. E., Weintraub, S., & Neale, J. M. (1976). The pupil evaluation inventory. *Journal of Abnormal Child Psychology, 4,* 83–97.

Perner, J., Frith, U., Leslie, A. M., & Leekam, S. R. (1989). Exploration of the autistic child's theory of mind: Knowledge, belief, and communication. *Child Development, 60,* 689–700.

Piers, E. V., Shemmassian, S. K., & Herzberg, D. S. (2018). *The Piers-Harris Self Concept Scale.* Western Psychological Services.

Prelock, P., & Hutchins, T. (2008). The role of family-centered care in research: Supporting the social communication of children with autism spectrum disorder. *Topics in Language Disorders, 28*(4), 323–339.

Proger, B. B. (1974). Test Review No. 17: California Preschool Social Competency Scale. *Journal of Special Education, 8*(4), 391–395.

Punia, D., Balda, S., & Punia, S. (2004). Training disadvantaged rural children for interpersonal cognitive problem-solving skills. *Studies of Tribes and Tribals, 2* (1), 9–13.

Radloff, L. S. (1977). The CES-D scale: A self-report depression scale for research in the general population. *Applied Psychological Measurement, 1,* 385–401.

Ratto, A. B., Turner-Brown, L., Rupp, B. M., Mesibov, G. B., & Penn, D. L. (2010). Development of the Contextual Assessment of Social Skills (CASS): A role play measure of social skill for individuals with high-functioning autism. *Journal of Autism and Developmental Disorders, 41*(9), 1277–1286.

Reynolds, C. R., & Kamphaus, R. W. (2004). *Behavior Assessment System for Children, Second Edition–Parent Rating Scales (BASC-2-PRS).* Pearson.

Reynolds, C., & Kamphaus, R. (2015). *BASC-3: Behavior Assessment System for Children–Third Edition.* Pearson.

Schmidt, C., Stichter, J. P., Lierheimer, K., McGhee, S., & O'Connor, K. V. (2011). An initial investigation of the generalization of a school-based social competence intervention for youth with high-functioning autism. *Autism Research and Treatment.* https://doi.org/10.1155/2011/589539

Schultz, T. R., Stichter, J. P., Herzog, M. J., McGhee, S. D., & Lierheimer, K. (2012). Social Competence Intervention for Parents (SCI-P): Comparing outcomes for a parent education program targeting adolescents with ASD. *Autism Research and Treatment.* https://doi.org/10.1155/2012/681465

Sheridan, B. A., Macdonald, D. A., McGovern, K., Donlon, M., Kuhn, B., & Friedman, H. (2011). Evaluation of a social skills program based on social learning theory, implemented in a school setting. *Psychological Reports, 108*(2), 420–436.

Shure, M. B. (2001). *I Can Problem Solve: An interpersonal cognitive problem-solving program.* Research Press.

Shure, M. B., & Spivack, G. (1980). Interpersonal problem solving as a mediator of behavioral adjustment in preschool and kindergarten children. *Journal of Applied Developmental Psychology, 1*, 29–44.

Smith, T., Scahill, L., Dawson, G., Guthrie, D., Lord, C., Odom, S., Rogers, S., & Wagner, A. (2007). Designing research studies on psychosocial interventions in autism. *Journal of Autism and Developmental Disorders, 37*(2), 354–366.

Sparrow, S. S., Chicchetti, D. V., & Balla, D. A. (2006). *Vineland Adaptive Behavior Scales – Second Edition (Vineland-II).* Pearson.

Sparrow, S. S., Cicchetti, D. V., & Saulnier, C. A. (2016). *Vineland Adaptive Behavior Scales–Third Edition (Vineland-3).* Pearson.

Stadnick, N. A., Stahmer, A., & Brookman-Frazee, L. (2015). Preliminary effectiveness of Project ImPACT: A parent-mediated intervention for children with autism spectrum disorder delivered in a community program. *Journal of Autism and Developmental Disorders, 45*(7), 2092–2104.

Stichter, J. P., Herzog, M. J., Visovsky, K., Schmidt, C., Randolph, J., Schultz, T., & Gage, N. (2010). Social competence intervention for youth with Asperger Syndrome and high-functioning autism: An initial investigation. *Journal of Autism and Developmental Disorders 40*(9), 1067–1079.

Stichter, J. P., Laffey, J., Galyen, K., & Herzog, M. (2013). ISocial: Delivering the Social Competence Intervention for Adolescents (SCI-A) in a 3D virtual learning environment for youth with high functioning autism. *Journal of Autism and Developmental Disorders, 44*(2), 417–430.

Stichter, J. P., O'Connor, K. V., Herzog, M. J., Lierheimer, K., & McGhee, S. D. (2012). Social Competence Intervention for elementary students with Asperger's syndrome and high functioning autism. *Journal of Autism and Developmental Disorders, 42*, 354–366.

Szumski, G., Smogorzewska, J., Grygiel, P., & Orlando, A. (2017). Examining the effectiveness of naturalistic social skills training in developing social skills and theory of mind in preschoolers with ASD. *Journal of Autism and Developmental Disorders, 49*(7), 2822–2837.

Szumski, G., Smogorzewska, J., & Karwowski, M. (2016). Can play develop social skills? The effects of "Play Time/Social Time" programme implementation. *International Journal of Developmental Disabilities, 62*(1), 41–50.

Thomeer, M. L., Lopata, C., Donnelly, J. P., Booth, A., Shanahan, A., Federiconi, V., McDonald, C. A., & Rodgers, J. D. (2019). Community effectiveness RCT of a comprehensive psychosocial treatment for high-functioning children with ASD. *Journal of Clinical Child & Adolescent Psychology, 48*(Suppl. 1): S119–S130.

Thomeer, M. L., Lopata, C., Volker, M. A., Toomey, J. A., Lee, G. K., Smerbeck, A. M., Rodgers, J. D., McDonald, C. A., & Smith, R. A. (2012). Randomized clinical trial replication of a psychosocial treatment for children with high-functioning autism spectrum disorders. *Psychology in the Schools, 49*(10), 942–954.

Thomeer, M. L., Smith, R. A., Lopata, C., Volker, M. A., Lipinski, A. M., Rodgers, J. D., McDonald, C. A., & Lee, G. K. (2015). Randomized controlled trial of mind reading and in vivo rehearsal for high-functioning children with ASD. *Journal of Autism and Developmental Disorders, 45*(7), 2115–2127.

Thomeer, M. L., Lopata, C., Donnelly, J. P., Booth, A. J., Shanahan, A., Federiconi, V., McDonald, C. A., & Rodgers, J. D. (2016). Community effectiveness RCT of a comprehensive psychosocial treatment for high-functioning children with ASD. *Journal of Clinical Child and Adolescent Psychology.* https://doi.org/10.1080/15374416.2016.1247359.

Tse, J., Strulovitch, J., Tagalakis, V., Meng, L., & Fombonne, E. (2007). Social skills training for adolescents with Asperger Syndrome and high-functioning autism. *Journal of Autism and Developmental Disorders*, *37*(10), 1960–1968.

Vernon, T. W., Miller, A. R., Ko, J. A., Barrett, A. C., & McGarry, E. S. (2018). A randomized controlled trial of the Social Tools and Rules for Teens (START) Program: An immersive socialization intervention for adolescents with autism spectrum disorder. *Journal of Autism and Developmental Disorders*, *48*(3), 892–904.

Vernon, T. W., Miller, A. R., Ko, J. A., & Wu, V. L. (2016). Social Tools and Rules for Teens (the START Program): Program description and preliminary outcomes of an experiential socialization intervention for adolescents with autism spectrum disorder. *Journal of Autism and Developmental Disorders*, *46*(5), 1806–1823.

Vestal, A., & Jones, N. (2004). Peace building and conflict resolution in preschool children. *Journal of Research in Childhood Education, 19*, 131–142.

Wechsler, D. (2009). *Advanced Clinical Solutions for WAIS-IV and WMS-IV.* Pearson.

Wong, C., Odom, S. L., Hume, K. Cox, A. W., Fettig, A., Kucharczyk, S., Brock, M. E., Plavnick, J. B., Fleury, V. P., & Schultz, T. R. (2014). *Evidence-based practices for children, youth, and young adults with autism spectrum disorder. Journal of Autism and Developmental Disorders*, *45*(7), 1951–1966.

Yamada, T., Miura, Y., Oi, M., Akatsuka, N., Tanaka, K., Tsukidate., Yamamoto, T., Okuno, H., Nakanishi, M., Taniike, M., Mohri, I., & Laugeson, E. A. (2020). Examining the Treatment Efficacy of PEERS in Japan: Improving social skills among adolescents with autism spectrum disorder. *Journal of Autism and Developmental Disorders, 50*, 976–997.

Yang, D. Y. J., Allen, T., Abdullahi, S. M., Pelphrey, K. A., Volkmar, F. R., & Chapman, S. B. (2018). Neural mechanisms of behavioral change in young adults with high-functioning autism receiving virtual reality social cognition training: A pilot study. *Autism Research, 11*, 713–725.

16

Social Stories™

Tiffany L. Hutchins

INTRODUCTION

Autism spectrum disorder (ASD) is characterized by impairments in social, behavioral, and communicative functioning (American Psychiatric Association, 2013), although tremendous variation in these abilities is evident. Related deficits in **social cognition**—the process by which people make sense of the self and others and acquire, use, and understand social knowledge—also are considered a universal feature of ASD. As a result, individuals with ASD often have difficulty identifying relevant and meaningful social information and interpreting this information accurately. These difficulties may, in turn, lead to behaviors that limit the individual's ability to participate in family, school, and community life (Crozier & Tincani, 2005; Dunlap & Fox, 1999). Thus, strategies to enhance social understanding and reduce challenging behaviors have the potential to significantly improve quality of life and facilitate access to educational opportunities among individuals with ASD (Carr et al., 2002; Crozier & Tincani, 2005).

Social Stories™ represent one of the most popular intervention strategies for use with ASD (Hess et al., 2008; Reynhout & Carter, 2009). Introduced in 1993 by Carol Gray, an educational consultant and former teacher, Social Stories are carefully written, individualized stories designed to facilitate social understanding among individuals with autism by providing what Gray and Garand (1993) described as "direct access to social information" (p. 2). According to Gray (1998), Social Stories adhere to a "specific format and guidelines to objectively describe a person, skill, event, concept, or social situation" (p. 171). They typically follow a storybook format and are composed of simple sentences and a title. Key messages conveyed in text in a Social Story are often, but not always, reinforced using visual supports (e.g., line drawings, icons, photographs, videos, actual objects) or other media (e.g., audiotapes). A frequent goal of Social Stories has been to share relevant information in the context of a challenging situation. This information often includes a description of where and when a situation takes place, who is involved, what is happening, and why (Gray, 1998) as well as suggestions for expected behaviors.

TARGET POPULATIONS

Social Stories have been used to facilitate a wide range of social, behavioral, and communicative functions in preschool and school-age children and adolescents with ASD who vary widely in their cognitive and linguistic profiles. Although Social Stories originally were developed for individuals with ASD, some studies have found support for their use with individuals with learning disability (Kalyva & Agaliotis, 2009; Moore, 2004), dyslexia (Haggerty et al., 2005), hearing loss (Richels et al., 2014), language impairment (Schneider & Goldstein, 2010), fragile X syndrome (Kuttler et al., 1998), and hyperlexia (Soenksen & Alper, 2006).

Gray and Garand (1993) proposed early on that Social Stories were most likely to benefit individuals with intellectual disabilities who had basic language skills. In line with this supposition, their early reports focused on how to construct effective Social Stories for individuals with high-functioning autism and Asperger syndrome. Subsequently, Gray (1998) suggested that, with slight modification, Social Stories can be helpful for those with ASD and more severe challenges. Several studies have found support for the effectiveness of Social Stories not only for individuals with autism with high language and intellectual abilities (e.g., Bledsoe et al., 2003; Rogers & Myles, 2001; Sansoti et al., 2004; Scattone, 2008), but also those with pervasive developmental disorder-not otherwise specified (PDD-NOS; e.g., Dodd et al., 2008; Ivey et al., 2004; Kuoch & Mirenda, 2003), and ASD (e.g., Lorimer et al., 2002; Mancil et al., 2009; Norris & Datillo, 1999). However, investigations of the efficacy of Social Stories for individuals with ASD who have severe intellectual impairment or very limited language skills are rare, and the evidence is mixed (see Barry & Burlew, 2004; Hutchins & Prelock, 2013a, 2013b; Quirmbach et al., 2009; Swaggart et al., 1995). As such, the efficacy of Social Stories for individuals with ASD with the most severe challenges remains an open question (Scattone et al., 2006; Walton & Ingersoll, 2013).

THEORETICAL BASIS

The theoretical bases of Social Stories are varied and include theory of mind, executive function, weak central coherence, schemata, and episodic memory. Each is described next.

Theoretical Rationale

> *"It's hard for me to understand some*
> *things. . . . I just don't have that social link in my brain."*
> —*Steven (pseudonym), 11-year-old boy diagnosed with ASD*

Steven's lucid description of his challenges involving social understanding underscore what is considered a universal feature of ASD. The premise underlying the use of Social Stories is that they facilitate the development of social understanding through the sharing of meaningful information (e.g., Gray, 1998, 2010, 2015; Gray & Garand, 1993). Gray has emphasized that Social Stories are not intended as a direct tool for behavior change. Instead, "the theory is that the improvement in behavior that is frequently credited to a Social Story is the result of improved understanding of events and expectations" (Gray, 2010, p. xxxi).

Four (closely related) mechanisms—*theory of mind, executive functions, weak central coherence, schemata,* and *episodic memory*—may separately or in combination be responsible for affecting social understanding through the use of Social Stories. Gray (1998) implicated **theory of mind** as a factor that contributes to the success of this intervention. In its broadest application, theory of mind is used interchangeably with terms like s*ocial cognition, mind reading*, and *perspective taking* and may be defined here as the ability to reason about the inner mental worlds of self and others and to understand that others may have perspectives that differ from our own. As Gray (1998) argued, "Theory of mind provides most people with access to a 'secret code': a system of unspoken communication that carries essential information; a system that eludes individuals with [ASD]" (p. 160).

More recently, Reynhout and Carter (2011a) proposed that Social Stories may be effective because they support **executive functions.** Executive functions are a set of cognitive processes and resources that operate to control and guide behavior. They include, for example, working memory, inhibition, focused attention, attention shifting, and planning. Social Stories make explicit key elements of an event and often teach appropriate responses to perform in specific situations. This may increase predictability and assist with planning. Moreover, because Social Stories are "concrete, easily referred to and consistent, [they] would seem to have the potential to both reduce the need to hold information on-line in working memory and facilitate self-monitoring" (Reynhout & Carter, 2011a, p. 372).

In addition, Gray (1998) invoked the notion of **weak central coherence** as a factor in the social cognition difficulties of persons with ASD. Weak central coherence is a cognitive style, believed to be present in ASD, in which the processing of parts takes precedence over the processing of wholes (Frith, 1989; Happe, 1999). Indeed, making accurate social judgments requires, among other things, the ability to read social cues in context and relate them to the physical and social environment in order to extract meaningful and relevant information.

Yet another cognitive mechanism was proposed by Rowe (1999), who invoked the notion of **schemas** to explain the success of Social Stories for enhancing social understanding. Rowe described a schema as a mental representation of what things are and how individuals deal with them: "You have schemas for eating with a knife and fork, crossing the road and buying things in shops. We don't all have schemas for eating with chopsticks, swimming, or being a shop assistant" (p. 14). More recently, Hutchins and Prelock (2018) argued that the success of Social Stories is largely attributable to their ability to support **episodic memory.** While often able to recall autobiographical *facts* (e.g., my birthday is August 31, I live in Vermont), the accuracy and richness of recollections for *personally experienced events* (i.e., episodic memories) in ASD is poor, even in older individuals with high language and intellectual abilities (Bowler et al., 2000; Lind & Bowler, 2010). Episodic memory is a special kind of autobiographical memory crucial for healthy social cognition that has been traditionally overlooked as a promising treatment target. As Hutchins and Prelock (2018) explained, Social Stories "may be effective because they recount historical events, relate past experience to future planning, and adopt a first-person perspective, all of which are relevant to the development of episodic memory" (p. 129)

Underlying Assumptions

One important assumption underlying the use of Social Stories is that the social impairments of ASD do not lie solely within the affected individual but rather in the social space between people. Gray (1998) argued that people make a variety of assumptions based on a common social understanding that, when applied to someone who perceives the world differently, can be wrong: "The result is a shared social impairment: two parties responding with equally valid but different perceptions of the same event" (p.168). Thus, it is through abandonment of the assumptions that people make in most social situations that they may develop the most meaningful interventions. To accomplish this, interventionists need to have a good understanding of social cognition in ASD (Gray, 1998). Social Stories are written from the perspective of the audience (i.e., the individual for whom the story is written) after thoughtful consideration of how a social situation is experienced and interpreted by that person.

Social Stories may be effective not only because they are individualized and personally relevant but also because the activities, by nature, are in accord with certain practices identified as especially useful for individuals with ASD (Hutchins & Prelock, 2006, 2013a, 2013b; Smith, 2001). As Smith (2001) recounted, Social Stories capitalize on the strengths of individuals with ASD, which often include a preference for visually cued instruction. Because they are permanent, Social Stories can be shared with important others (e.g., parents, teachers, members of the community), who can read or revisit the story across settings. Social Stories are written in simple language that is sensitive to the child's language level and vocabulary. They are situation specific and written in a predictable style using prescribed conventions. They are factual and accurate yet unusual in that they focus directly on how people think. Social Stories are also inherently family centered in that they should be developed through careful observations of the child, discussions with the child, and information gathered from those who know the child best: the parents.

Targets of Treatment

Social Stories are not intended to *directly* target any functional limitation but do *indirectly* address a range of functional outcomes through enhanced social understanding. The range of such outcomes that has been addressed in practice and research has been truly remarkable (see Table 16.1 for a list of targets). They have included the reduction of disruptive behaviors, including tantrums, aggression, and self-injurious acts. Social Stories have also been used to establish more appropriate behavioral routines and self-care living skills and to introduce changes in routines and acquaint the individual with an unfamiliar event. They have been used to promote social skills, such as getting a peer's attention, making choices and playing independently, and increasing peer engagement and participation. They have also been used to remediate communicative deficits in ASD, such as to reduce echolalia and interrupt and address physical inactivity, sleep disturbances, and sensory issues, and to provide sexual education. Other applications suggested by Gray (1998, 2010) include teaching academic skills and acknowledging the individual's achievements; however, these remain largely unexplored in the literature (Kokina & Kern, 2010). Thus, Social Stories have been used to address a range of social, communicative, and behavioral outcomes and theoretically could be used for any developmentally appropriate outcome that would benefit from enhanced social cognition. In a

Table 16.1. Summary of peer-reviewed single-subject studies (dissertations and case studies utilizing anecdotal data are not included)

Study	Sample size	Age (years)	Diagnosis	Design	Targets of intervention	Outcome data	Other instructional strategies	Result
Adams et al. (2004)	1	7	ASD	ABAB	Crying, falling, hitting, screaming	Tallies of target behaviors during homework sessions, parent and teacher survey	Verbal cueing	+
Barry & Burlew (2004)	2	7, 8	ASD	Multiple baseline across participants	Choice making, appropriate play in classroom, how to play with a peer	Level of prompting for choices, duration of appropriate play, anecdotal teacher report	Photographs, corrective feedback, prompting, peer modeling, teacher-led instructional phase	+
Bernad-Ripoll (2007)	1	9	Asperger syndrome	AB	Detecting and understanding emotions in self, identifying appropriate response	Percentage accuracy of identifying emotion, explaining emotion, and giving appropriate response	Photographs, videotapes, reinforcers	+
Bledsoe et al. (2003)	1	13	Asperger syndrome and ADHD	ABAB	Decreasing food spilling, increasing mouth wiping	Frequency of behaviors during lunchtime	None	+
Brownell (2002)	4	6–9	ASD	ABAB	TV talk, following directions, using a quiet voice	Tallies of target behaviors during 60-minute observation sessions	Mayer-Johnson picture symbols, verbal prompting, musical (song) format	+
Chan & O'Reilly (2008)	2	5, 6	ASD	Multiple probe across behaviors	Inappropriate social interactions, appropriate hand raising, inappropriate vocalizations, appropriate social initiations	Frequency and percentage of opportunities for target behaviors during 60-minute observation sessions	Verbal prompts, comprehension questions, role play	+
Chan et al. (2011)	3	8	ASD	Multiple baseline across participants	Sitting, attending teacher during group lessons, working independently	Percentage of 10 sec. intervals during 30-minute session with performance of target behavior	Comprehension questions	+
Crozier & Tincani (2005)	1	8	ASD	ABAC	Talking disruptively during classroom activities	Percentage of talk-outs during 30-minute observation	Comparison between Social Stories™ with and without prompting	+

(continued)

Table 16.1.　(continued)

Study	Sample size	Age (years)	Diagnosis	Design	Targets of intervention	Outcome data	Other instructional strategies	Result
Crozier & Tincani (2007)	3	3, 3, 5	ASD	ABAB	Appropriate sitting, talking with peers, appropriate play with peers	Number and duration of target behavior in 10-minute session	Comprehension questions, verbal prompting, color icons	+
Delano & Snell (2006)	3 6	6, 6, 9	ASD Typically developing peers	Multiple probe across participants	Appropriate and inappropriate social engagement with peer, absence of engagement	Number and duration of target behavior in 10-minute session	Comprehension questions, play with peer, verbal prompting	+
Dodd et al. (2008)	2	9, 12	PDD-NOS	Multiple baseline across behaviors/ participants	Decrease excessive directions to others; increase compliments	Frequency of target behaviors during play session	Comprehension questions, photographs, clip-art	±
Graetz et al. (2009)	3	12, 12, 13	ASD	Multiple baseline across participants	Standing independently during gym class, appropriate voice pitch, hands down, materials away from lips	Percentage of time doing inappropriate behavior during either 45-minute observations or 15-second intervals during 20-minute observations	Photographs with callouts (speech bubbles), comprehension questions and/or comments	+
Grigore & Rusu (2014)	3	7, 7, 8	ASD	ABAC	Greeting, introducing oneself	Frequency of target behavior, level of prompt required, frequency of social initiations in 15-minute observation sessions	Social Story + therapy dog (Phase C)	+
Hagiwara & Myles (1999)	3	7, 7, 9	ASD	Multiple baseline across settings	Washing hands, on-task behavior	Percentage completion of hand-washing steps; average duration per occurrence of on-task behavior in 20-minute observation	Video self-modeling presented on computer, verbal prompting	±
Halle et al. (2016)	4	12, 13, 13, 13	ASD (3 with intellectual disability)	ABA Multiple baseline across participants	Greeting	Number of appropriate behaviors recorded "by way of event-recording" (p. 49)	Stories delivered via video modeling format + use of trained peer helpers	+

Study	N	Age	Diagnosis	Design	Target behaviors	Frequency of target behaviors	Comprehension questions	
Hanler-Hochdorfer et al. (2010)	4	6, 9, 11, 12	Asperger syndrome (3) ASD (1)	AB	Verbal initiations, contingent responses to peers	Frequency of target behaviors during 15-minute lunch period	Comprehension questions	−
Hutchins & Preloct (2013a)	17	4–12; mean age = 7;3	ASD	ABA Multiple baseline across participants	A range of social behaviors (e.g., taking turns, playing nicely with others)	Subjective caregiver ratings and reports of behavior change in the form of daily diaries	Family-centered approach to intervention + Comic Strip Conversations	±
Hutchins & Prelock (2013b)	20	4–12; Mean age = 7;3	ASD	ABA Multiple baseline across participants/behaviors	A range of communication (e.g., greeting, eye contact) and behavior targets (tantrums, transitions)	Subjective caregiver ratings and reports of behavior change in the form of daily diaries	Family-centered approach to intervention	±
Hutchins & Prelock (2006)	2	6, 12	ASD	AB	Reduce negative behavior toward sibling, increase ability to cease a preferred activity	Maternal subjective daily diary data	Comic Strip Conversations	±
Hutchins & Prelock (2008)	1	5	ASD	ABA	Staying calm, using words to talk about situation, taking others' perspectives	Maternal subjective daily diary data	Comic Strip Conversations	+
Iskander & Rosales (2013)	2	8, 11	PDD-NOS + ADHD	ABC Multiple baseline across behaviors	Decrease disruptive behaviors (e.g., interrupting, out of seat)	Frequency of target behavior in a 10-minute session	Differential reinforcement of zero behavior procedure	+
Ivey et al. (2004)	3	5, 7, 7	PDD-NOS	ABAB	Remaining on-task, following directions/rules, using provided materials, using target vocabulary	Tally of target behaviors during 10-minute observations	Photographs, illustrations, verbal and gestural prompting, behavior modeling	+
Kagohara et al. (2014)	2	10, 10	Asperger syndrome + ADHD	ABCA Multiple baseline across participants	Greeting	Cumulative number of greetings across sessions and study phases	Video modeling	+

(continued)

Table 16.1. (continued)

Study	Sample size	Age (years)	Diagnosis	Design	Targets of intervention	Outcome data	Other instructional strategies	Result
Karayazi et al. (2014)	1	22	ASD	AB	Greeting, nose-wiping	Percentage of appropriate target behavior during 15-minute observational sessions	None	+
Kassardjian et al. (2014)	3	5, 5, 5	ASD	ABA	Social skills (e.g., showing appreciation, giving a compliment)	Percentage of correct steps observed across performance probes	Teaching interaction procedure (questions, teacher demo, role play)	+
Klett & Turan (2012)	3	9, 11, 12	ASD	ABCA	Menstrual care	Task analysis for 11 steps required for successful behavior during 2-minute observation periods	Parent-implemented intervention + comprehension checks	+
Kuoch & Mirenda (2003)	3	3, 5, 6	ASD (2), PDD-NOS (1)	ABA (n = 2) ACABA (n = 1)	Aggression, tantrums, eating problems, touching self inappropriately, game-playing skills	Tally of responses per minute (varying lengths of observation)	Cartoon pictures, verbal prompting, verbal corrective feedback	+
Kuttler et al. (1998)	1	12	ASD, fragile X, and Intermittent explosive disorder	ABAB	Reducing precursors to tantrum behavior	Tally of precursors to tantrum behavior in classroom and at lunch	Mayer-Johnson pictures, token economy	+
Lorimer et al. (2002)	1	5	ASD	ABAB	Reducing precursor to tantrum behavior	Tally of interrupting vocalizations and frequency of tantrums/day	Mayer-Johnson line drawings	+
Mancil et al. (2009)	3	6, 7, 8	ASD	ABABCBC	Pushing (grabbing, touching, shoving) peers	Mean frequency of pushing per 5-minute session	Verbal prompts, pictures of peers, interactive text in PowerPoint version	+
Marr et al. (2007)	4	4, 4, 4, 5	ASD	ABA	Remaining in assigned seat, reducing stereotypical behaviors	Percentage of observation sessions with targeted behavior	Sensory story Illustrations, verbal and physical cues	±

Study	N	Ages	Diagnosis	Design	Target behavior	Dependent measure	Intervention components	Outcome
Norris & Dattilo (1999)	1	8	ASD	AB	Reducing inappropriate social behaviors (talking or singing to herself), increasing appropriate alternative behaviors	Percentage of 10-second intervals during 8-minute observation with inappropriate, appropriate, or no social interactions with peers during lunch	Picture symbols, behavior management systems, comprehension questions	±
Ozdemir (2008)	3	7, 8, 9	ASD	Multiple baseline across participants	Disruptive behaviors (using a loud voice, chair tipping, cutting in line)	Percentage of 15-second partial intervals of disruptive behavior during 20-minute observations	Illustrations of stick figures with callouts, photo of aide	+
Pane et al. (2015)	2	10, 15	ASD and language and learning disabilities	Alternating treatments design	Decrease inappropriate behaviors (e.g., facial grimacing), increase functional communication (e.g., requests)	Percentage of intervals with target behavior	FBA, comprehension checks, functional communication training	+
Pasiali (2004)	3	7, 8, 9	ASD	ABAB	Aberrant vocalizations during meals, increasing appropriate use of VCR, decreasing rummaging	Daily tallies of target behaviors	Listening to music, playing rhythmic instruments, singing, picture schedule	±
Samuels & Stansfield (2011)	3	Adults	ASD and learning disability	ABA	More appropriate behaviors and social interactions	Behavior count data during "specific settings, situations, and times" (p. 40)	Individual with ASD collaborated in production of story	+
Sansosti & Powell-Smith (2006)	3	9, 10, 11	Asperger syndrome	Multiple baseline across participants	Sportsmanship, maintaining conversations with peers, joining in play	Percentage of 15-second partial intervals with target behavior during 15-minute observation	Social Story journal	±
Scattone (2008)	1	9	Asperger syndrome	Multiple baseline across behaviors	Eye contact, smiling, initiations	Percentage of 10-second intervals with target behavior during 5-minute observations	Video modeling (by two adults), comprehension questions	±
Scattone et al. (2002)	3	7, 7, 15	ASD	Multiple baseline across participants	Chair tipping, staring at girls, shouting	Percentage of 10-second partial intervals with target behavior during 20-minute observation	Comprehension questions, verbal prompting	+

(continued)

Table 16.1. *(continued)*

Study	Sample size	Age (years)	Diagnosis	Design	Targets of intervention	Outcome data	Other instructional strategies	Result
Scattone et al. (2006)	3	8, 8, 13	ASD (2), Asperger syndrome (1)	Multiple baseline across participants	Increase appropriate social interactions	Percentage of 10-second partial intervals of appropriate social interactions during 10-minute observation	Comprehension questions, verbal prompting	±
Schneider & Goldstein (2010)	3	6, 6, 9	Language and social impairment	Multiple baseline across participants	Following directions, completing work, making eye contact, raising hand	Percentage of time intervals with on-task behavior with varying observation length	Mayer-Johnson pictures, comprehension questions	+
Swaggart et al. (1995)	3	11, 7, 7	ASD (2), PDD-NOS (1)	AB	Greeting, reducing aggression, sharing toys	Number of aggressions/day, mean percentage of sessions with target behaviors	Illustrations, response cost, prompting	+
Thiemann & Goldstein (2001)	5	6, 7, 8, 11, 12	ASD (4), Language and social impairment (1)	Multiple baseline across skills and participants	Contingent responses, securing attention, initiating comments, initiating requests	Number of behaviors recorded during 15-second intervals of a 10-minute session, teacher and graduate student subjective ratings of social behaviors	Comprehension checks, role play, pictorial and written cues, verbal cues, video feedback, token economy	±
Thompson & Johnston (2013)	3	3, 3, 5	ASD	ABA Multiple baseline across participants	Tolerating sand-type textures during play, remaining seated during snack time and circle time	Percent of 30-second intervals during observation sessions (range 7–15 minutes) where target behavior occurred	Sensory integrative-based strategies to increase self-regulation	+
Toplis & Hadwin (2006)	5	Mean age = 7;5	Behavioral difficulties	ABAB	Decreasing disruptive behavior during lunch time	Tally of appropriate/inappropriate behaviors	Illustrations, picture icons, verbal/physical prompting	±
Vandermeer et al. (2015)	3	4, 4, 4	ASD	AB (*n* = 2) ABA (*n* = 1)	Increasing on-task behavior	Observational count data using time-event sampling	Social Stories presented using iPad	±
Wright & McGathren (2012)	4	4, 4, 4, 5	ASD	ABA Multiple baseline across participants	Increase prosocial behavior and reduce problem behavior	Behavior ratings during free play	Comprehension checks, Social Stories revised if no improvement in first half of B phase of study	±

Key: +, denotes effect associated with treatment; –, denotes null results; ±, denotes mixed results; A, baseline; B, treatment phase. ADHD, attention-deficit/hyperactivity disorder; ASD, autism spectrum disorder; FBA, functional behavioral assessment; PDD-NOS, pervasive developmental disorder–not otherwise specified.

meta-analysis, Kokina and Kern (2010) suggested that Social Stories targeting the reduction of problem behaviors may be more effective than those that teach appropriate social skills; however, researchers have rarely considered whether and which prerequisite skills or social understandings are needed to achieve social interaction goals (Kokina & Kern, 2010)—an important direction for future research that will be described more fully later in the chapter.

EMPIRICAL BASIS

Efficacy studies, those that illustrate the usefulness of an intervention under conditions that allow for rigorous experimental control, are typically performed prior to studies of effectiveness, which illustrate the usefulness of an intervention under the conditions of everyday practice (Robey & Schultz, 1998). Because Social Stories are intended as a personalized instructional strategy, they are well suited to the needs of individuals with ASD across a range of settings and service delivery models. As a result, studies on the effectiveness of Social Stories are plentiful, whereas studies of efficacy are lacking. Table 16.1 summarizes the peer-reviewed single-subject studies conducted to date.

Single-Subject Designs

As inspection of Table 16.1 reveals, a handful of studies have used a pre-experimental AB design. The remainder used more rigorous designs (e.g., ABA, ABAB, multiple-baseline designs), although some of these utilized a single participant, which limits the ability to draw causal conclusions and evaluate the generalizability of results. The majority of studies (31 of 47) yielded positive results, an additional 15 studies yielded mixed results (i.e., treatment was associated with positive outcomes for some individuals or behaviors but not for others), and one study (i.e., Hanley-Hochdorfer et al., 2010) yielded null results only. Thus, a review of the single-subject literature suggests that intervention using Social Stories is a promising approach; however, considerable variation in outcome exists (Rhodes, 2014). In a related vein and despite being addressed in the quantitative reviews (described next), it is noteworthy that effect size data are rarely reported in the single-subjects' studies on Social Stories. One reason involves the theoretical and statistical challenges surrounding the interpretation of traditional effect size measures for single-subjects' data (i.e., percent non-overlapping data points [PND] and mean difference between phases). Yet, advances in the operations to estimate effect size for complex single-subjects designs (e.g., Tau-U; Lee & Cherney, 2018; Parker et al., 2011) are beginning to be employed to evaluate behavior change associated with this intervention (Hutchins & Prelock, 2013a, 2013b) and are promising for examining between- and within-groups variability and identifying factors that predict success.

Crucially, the literature is replete with examinations of Social Stories when combined with other instructional methods, making it difficult to determine their effects when used in isolation. As Table 16.1 indicates, these have included video modeling, visual schedules, Comic Strip Conversations, token economies, prompting, role playing, and music therapy, among others. In light of the tremendous methodological variation across studies, it is not surprising that systematic reviews are inconclusive with regard to the value of using Social Stories in combination with other instructional strategies (e.g., Reynhout & Carter, 2006; Whalon et al., 2015).

What is clear is that research is needed to examine the relative contribution of Social Stories versus a wide range of additional supports that are used in practice.

Until recently, the Social Story literature was routinely criticized for a lack of data on generalizability, maintenance, and social validity (e.g., Nichols et al., 2006; Reynhout & Carter, 2006). Although it is still true that examinations of *generalizability* remain relatively infrequent, some studies now demonstrate generalization to untrained settings (e.g., Hagiwara & Myles, 1999; Hutchins & Prelock, 2008; Kuttler et al., 1998; Mancil et al., 2009), materials (e.g., Klett & Turan, 2012), activities (Thompson & Johnston, 2013), and behaviors (e.g., Hutchins & Prelock, 2006; Theimann & Goldstein, 2001).

Although a few studies report a notable lack on *maintenance of skills* following Social Story intervention (e.g., Samuels & Stansfield, 2011; Theimann & Goldstein, 2001), other research has documented convincing evidence for maintenance (Chan & O'Reilly, 2008; Hutchins & Prelock, 2013a, 2013b; Klett & Turan, 2012; Wright & McCathren, 2012). Consequently, one fruitful direction for research involves the identification of factors that predict maintenance of skills following Social Story intervention.

Social validity data for Social Stories have been collected in the form of interviews, questionnaires, and formal and informal rating scales to assess the feasibility and perceived effects of treatment among parents and professionals. When data for social validity are available, the results have been quite positive (e.g., Cihak et al., 2012; Klett & Turan, 2012; Pane et al., 2015). For example, in a study of caregivers' impressions of the effectiveness of Social Stories, Hutchins and Prelock (2013a, 2013b) reported that caregivers overwhelmingly held positive impressions of child behavior change for a variety of treatment targets. Similarly, Reynhout and Carter (2009) surveyed 45 teachers working with children with ASD. Teachers agreed that

> Social Stories™ are an acceptable (100%) and effective intervention (93%), appropriate for a wide variety of children (78%), behaviors and skills (93%), that can be easily implemented in a wide variety of settings (93%), and that are complementary to other interventions (100%). In contrast a minority of teachers (45%) agreed that Social Stories™ result in generalized behavior change and only 53% agreed that Social Stories maintain well. (p. 241)

Group Designs

Few peer-reviewed group studies have been conducted to examine the efficacy of Social Stories. To address the need for a large, experimentally controlled group study, Quirmbach and colleagues (2009) examined the efficacy of Social Stories for 45 children with ASD who varied widely in cognitive and language skills. They used a standard Social Story (i.e., it was the same for all children) without photographs or icons to address communication in the context of game play, including how to greet and initiate appropriate interactions (e.g., saying, "Hello," and "Do you want to play with me?"). Results indicated that improved game-play skills generalized to a similar game-play context and were maintained 1 week postintervention. Verbal comprehension skills contributed the greatest amount of variance in predicting success, leading the authors to conclude that individuals with very low verbal comprehension may not benefit from Social Stories without supporting pictures. On the other hand, Quirmbach and colleagues recognized that the targets of intervention may have been too advanced and therefore inappropriate for children with low verbal comprehension. Moreover, their stories were lengthy and contained many complex sentences (e.g., "When I am finished playing my game, it makes other people happy if I ask, 'What game do you want to play?'"). Thus, the findings of Quirmbach and colleagues (2009) cannot be taken as indisputable evidence for a lack of efficacy of Social Stories when used with children with the most limited receptive language. Rather, the findings may underscore the importance of tailoring interventions to the child's developmental level.

More recently, Golzari and colleagues (2015) examined the use of Social Stories for enhancing the social skills of males ($n = 30$; ages 6–12) with ASD using a randomized experimental group and a no-treatment control group. Improvements were most evident for measures of social understanding, perspective taking, and the ability to initiate and maintain social interactions. These findings are consistent with the theoretical bases of Social Stories. Golzari colleagues explained, "If children are better able to understand others' perspectives, and predict how, where, and when behavior will occur, they are more motivated to interact with others and maintain communication" (2015, p. 6).

Descriptive and Quantitative Reviews

Several common themes have emerged from descriptive (Ali & Frederickson, 2006; Karkhaneh et al., 2010; Nichols et al., 2006; Qi et al., 2018; Rhodes, 2014; Rust & Smith, 2006; Sansoti et al., 2004) and quantitative reviews (Kokina & Kern, 2010; Reynhout & Carter, 2006, 2011b; Test et al., 2010; Whalon et al., 2015) of the Social Story literature. Most authors agree that Social Stories are a promising intervention while acknowledging a number of serious methodological limitations in the research base. These include confounding treatment variables and lack of experimental control, weak designs, and small or highly variable treatment effects. Thus, some critics have concluded it would be premature to recognize Social Stories as an evidence-based practice (Bozkurt & Vuran, 2014; Kokina & Kern, 2010; Leaf et al., 2015; Test et al., 2010; Whalon et al., 2015).

The conclusions of other reviewers have been more positive. For example, Ali and Frederickson (2006) noted that although single-case designs, such as those used in support of Social Stories, have traditionally been considered to occupy a lower level of evidence, methods exist to establish internal and external validity within and across studies, especially when consistent findings are obtained across a number of single-case design. This approach to the evidence is consistent with the recent conclusions of the National Standards Project, Phase 2 (NSP2; National Autism Center, 2015), which has identified Social Story intervention as an established treatment. The National Standards Project concluded that there is sufficient quality, quantity, and consistency in the evidence base to assert that the treatment produces beneficial effects for some individuals with autism.

PRACTICAL REQUIREMENTS

Gray has created a website (https://carolgraysocialstories.com) that offers information, resources, and training opportunities to support effective strategies for developing Social Stories that adhere to Gray's guidelines. In addition, *The New Social Story Book: 15th Anniversary Edition* (Gray, 2015) describes Gray's most recent guidelines for writing Social Stories. This book includes a series of tutorials to gain practice writing Social Stories and more than 150 standard Social Stories that may be borrowed or adapted. The premade stories that Gray and others (e.g., Ghanouni et al., 2018; Gray, 2000, 2010, 2015; Gray & White, 2002) have made available for purchase may seem to violate the recommendation that Social Stories use individualized information, yet their use seems reasonable if they are selected after careful review and are subsequently adapted to meet the needs of the individual (Ali & Fredrickson, 2006; Gray, 2010, 2015).

Generally, the materials required to construct a Social Story are readily available and inexpensive. Social Stories were traditionally written on paper; however, a variety of innovative additions can be used appropriately (Test et al., 2010), including the use of video and audio recordings, photographs, and illustrations. The most widely used visual supports are photographs and illustrations such as Picture Communication Symbols (PCS), also referred to as Mayer-Johnson or Boardmaker pictures, which require a computer and word processing software. Social Stories can also take the form of computer-assisted stories (Mancil et al., 2009) and iPad apps and may involve other technological enhancements to make delivery and development more flexible and interesting (Doyle & Arnedillo-Sanchez, 2011; Vandermeer et al., 2015; see also Constantin et al., 2013, who discuss the use of popular social story applications, including Story Builder, Story2Learn, Sandbox Learning, Pictello, StoryMaker).

KEY COMPONENTS

Gray has described the characteristics of Social Stories and processes for developing and implementing them. Gray's (2010, 2015) most recent criteria represent adjustments of previous versions (e.g., Gray, 1995, 1998; Gray & Garand, 1993). Moreover, researchers and practitioners (e.g., Nichols et al., 2006; Scott et al., 2000; Swaggart et al., 1995; Tarnai & Wolfe, 2008) have offered their own recommendations for implementing Social Stories intervention. As a result, guidelines for Social Stories have been continuously evolving for approximately 30 years. A synthesis of the most common and salient elements and recommendations for practice is offered next.

Determine a Topic

Review of the literature and practical experience suggest that Social Stories topics are most often identified by looking at situations that result in challenging behaviors. Salient topics may also be identified through an examination of situations that continue to present difficulty after implementation of a social skills curriculum or other positive interventions to address the problem have been deemed unsuccessful (Gray, 1995). Authors may also anticipate how novel situations or changes in routine might be experienced to support the individual with accurate information in advance of when it is needed (Gray, 1998). Although often overlooked, Social Stories should acknowledge success, for example, as an excellent topic for a "first story" (Gray, 1998, p. 174), to establish a positive introduction to this instructional strategy. In a related vein, when problem behaviors demonstrate improvement through the use of Social Stories, they may be adapted to acknowledge success and foster confidence. In fact, Gray (2010) recommends that no less than 50% of Social Stories applaud what the individual is doing well. Gray explained, "The rationale is simple. Given that Social Stories are helpful in teaching new concepts and skills, they may also be just as powerful in adding meaning and detail to praise" (2010, p. xxxv).

Gather Individualized Information

Once a topic is identified, it is necessary to gather detailed, relevant, and individualized information—an important process that is often overlooked (Gray, 2010, 2015). Several examples in the literature can be turned to as illustrations of appropriately rich data collection practices (Crozier & Tincani, 2005, 2007; Delano & Snell, 2006; Hutchins & Prelock, 2008, 2013a, 2013b; Lorimer et al., 2002). For example, Hutchins and Prelock (2008) used a collaborative, family-centered approach to gather information from parents to determine appropriate intervention targets and content. Cozier and Tincani (2005) completed teacher interviews, child observation, and the Motivational Assessment Scale (MAS; Durand & Crimmins, 1992) to understand behaviors (their frequency, context, precursors, antecedents, sequalae, causes, and underlying motivations) and ensure that their Social Story would accurately address the target behavior. Indeed, the authors of Social Stories are encouraged to look beyond behaviors and to use a variety of techniques to better understand their purpose. Ideally, a team may conduct observations, interviews with relevant others, and, when resources allow, a **functional behavioral assessment (FBA)**, a problem-solving process designed to identify the purpose of a behavior and strategies to address it (e.g., see Pane et al., 2015). In support of this recommendation, a meta-analysis concluded that studies that used some form of FBA yielded higher effect sizes than those that did not (Kokina & Kern, 2010).

Develop the Social Story

Careful consideration of the gathered information guides the writing of the Social Story. Social Stories are typically written in the first person to reflect the perspective of the individual, but third-person narratives, called *Social Articles* (Gray, 2010), are recommended for an older or more advanced audience. They often incorporate a newspaper format to minimize what Gray calls "any 'babyish' or insulting quality in the text" (2010, p. xlvii). By contrast, younger individuals or those who occupy a less advanced developmental level are believed to benefit from shorter narratives with larger font, where each page contains only one or two simple sentences (e.g., Swaggart et al., 1995). The length and complexity of Social Stories (and font and formatting choices) should be guided by individual factors such as age, verbal comprehension, reading level, and attention span (Attwood, 1998).

As a positive behavior intervention, clinicians should state the content of Social Stories in positive terms. Thus, a sentence such as "I will try to remember to stay calm" is preferable to "I will not hit and scream," which clinicians should avoid. The Social Story should be written using vocabulary that is meaningful to the individual and language that is developmentally appropriate. In addition, the use of flexible language (e.g., *sometimes, usually*) is preferred to inflexible language (e.g., *always, never*) because the former is more likely to be literally accurate.

Gray (2010, 2015) recommends that Social Stories be composed of a title and three basic parts: an introduction that clearly identifies the topic, a body that adds relevant detail, and a conclusion that summarizes the story and reinforces key messages. Gray proposed that Social Stories be composed of specific types of sentences, although the number and kind of sentences has changed over the years. Individuals familiar with the evolution of Social Stories guidelines will be familiar with descriptive, perspective, directive, affirmative, control, and cooperative sentences.

Table 16.2. Social Story™ sentence types

Sentence type	Description
Descriptive sentences	Factual, objective, assumption- and debate-free statements that describe context and/or the relevant but often unspoken aspects of a situation, person, activity, skill, or concept
Perspective sentences	Statements that accurately refer to or describe a person's internal state or his or her knowledge, thoughts, feelings, beliefs, opinions, motivation, or physical condition or health
Sentences that coach the audience	Statements that gently guide the behavior or the audience by describing a suggested response or a choice of responses
Sentences that coach the team	Statements that guide behavior of the audience or members of his or her team and describe a suggested response, a choice of responses, or self-coaching strategies
Self-coaching sentences	Statements written by the audience to identify a personal strategy to recall and apply its content in practice
Affirmative sentences	Statements that enhance the meaning of surrounding statements and often express a commonly shared value or opinion within a given culture
Partial sentences	Fill-in-the-blank statements that check for comprehension and encourage the audience to make guesses regarding the next step in a situation, the response of another individual, or his or her own response

Source: Gray (2010, 2015).

(*Note:* In the re-release of Gray's *The New Social Stories Book* [2015], mention of perspective, affirmative, and partial sentences is omitted and appears to be collapsed under the category of descriptive sentences.) A description of each of Gray's (2010) sentence types, which are conceptually similar to their predecessors, is presented in Table 16.2.

Gray (2010) states that the sentences in a Social Story must adhere to a ratio such that the total number of descriptive, perspective, affirmative, and partial sentences divided by the total number of sentences that coach the audience, team, or the individual is equal to or greater than 2. Gray explained that this ratio (which has also changed over the years) is driven by the notion that Social Stories should "*describe more than direct*" (italics in original, Gray, 1998, p. 179). Although this reflects the goal and theoretical bases of Social Stories as an instructional strategy that aims to enhance social understanding, the ratio lacks empirical support, and many have questioned its utility and appropriateness. For the time being, one defensible proposal is that authors avoid preoccupation with the Social Story ratio. Hutchins and Prelock (2006) suggested a primary focus on content that is "responsive to the specific contexts and targets of intervention may be more appropriate" (p. 49).

Gray's ideas about the value of visual supports that may accompany a Social Story have also undergone revision over the years. The use of visual graphics in a Social Story was initially discouraged on the grounds that they may distract or lead to inaccurate interpretation (Gray & Garand, 1993). This is an especially important consideration given the tendency of individuals with ASD to interpret information (including images) literally. Gray and Garand (1993) explained,

> For example, if an illustration depicts a child tying his shoe, seated next to a cat on a blue carpet, the student may interpret this to mean that shoes should be tied only when seated, next to a cat, on a blue carpet. (p. 4)

Gray now emphasizes the importance of the appropriateness of visual stimuli, which can take many different forms, including "actual objects, photos, video, drawings, PowerPoint, figures, charts, and diagrams" (Gray, 2015, p. xliii). Whatever the choice, the goal of visual supports should be to highlight or summarize information, capture interest, and improve comprehension (Gray, 2010, 2015). Gray (2010, 2015) offers several questions to consider when making decisions about whether and which visual supports will be effective. These include 1) Does the audience have the prerequisite skills to use this form of illustration? 2) Has the audience previously demonstrated interest in this type of illustration? and 3) Would a combination of two or more forms of illustration work best?

Authors of Social Stories need to be as thoughtful about the use of visual supports as they are about the content of a story's text and must consider any potential negative influence of images: The images selected for inclusion in a Social Story must both emotionally safe (i.e., respectful to the audience) and physically safe (i.e., never seeming to condone an unsafe behavior).

Consider Additional Supports

The use of additional supports is widely advised in the Social Stories literature as a means to promote good outcomes (Gray, 2010, 2015; Nichols et al., 2006; Tarnai & Wolfe, 2008). Social Story authors should consider strategies that have been successful with an individual in the past or otherwise have the potential to improve comprehension, participation, or interest (e.g., picture schedules, prompting, modeling, role playing, token economies, multimedia presentations, video modeling; see Iskander & Rosales, 2013; Kagohara et al., 2013).

Critically Review and Share the Social Story

Before the Social Story is introduced, a draft is shared with parents, teachers, or others who have direct contact with the individual and knowledge of the topic. Ideally, these individuals will have participated in the information-gathering process and are situated to provide critical review of content. The goal is to catch inaccuracies or missing details that should trigger revision (Gray, 1998).

The Social Story may then be distributed to relevant others along with an implementation plan that outlines review schedules (who, when) and any additional instructional strategies to be used (Gray, 1998). This process has the potential to foster shared responsibility and the involvement of a team (Gray, 1998). Moreover, it may help reinforce key messages across contexts by demonstrating to the individual that multiple people have the same social information (Gray, 1995).

Introduce the Social Story

Social Stories should be introduced in a relaxed and nonthreatening manner (Gray, 1998, 2010, 2015). Often, a simple statement such as "Here is a story that I wrote for you" is sufficient, but the complexity and content of the introduction will vary with circumstance. The audience can be encouraged to turn pages or read independently if appropriate, and there is some evidence that Social Stories intervention is more effective when the individual is responsible for reading the story independently (Kokina & Kern, 2010). A priming procedure is often employed in which the Social Story is read immediately prior to a novel or challenging situation (Scattone, 2007).

Social Stories may be introduced to address single or multiple targets of intervention. When multiple targets are identified, they have been introduced simultaneously (Kokina & Kern, 2010) and sequentially (e.g., Gray, 2010, 2015). It is possible that new skills and understandings may be taught in a single exposure (e.g., Gray, 2010, 2015) or after several repetitions (e.g., Hutchins & Prelock, 2006, 2008; Norris & Datillo, 1999). Thus, the number of presentations required to effect change (if change occurs) is expected to vary considerably. Because Social Stories are a personalized intervention, Gray recommends the reading schedule be "read frequently enough to provide review without needless repetition" (1995, p. 229).

Complete Comprehension Checks and Revise as Necessary

Closely monitoring the individual's response to the Social Story (Gray, 1995, 1998, 2010, 2015; Tarnai & Wolfe, 2008) will promote modifications when aspects of the story lack meaning or are misconstrued. Comprehension checks can be conducted in a variety of ways, including the use of comprehension checklists (Gray, 1998) and written or spoken question/answer or fill-in-the-blank activities (Tarnai & Wolfe, 2008). Recent meta-analyses (Kokina & Kern, 2010; Reynhout & Carter, 2006) have concluded that Social Stories procedures that incorporate comprehension checks yield better outcomes than those that do not.

Implement Generalization Training, Maintenance, and Reading

When gains are demonstrated, a common recommendation is to implement procedures designed to promote the generalization of skills (Nichols et al., 2006; Swaggart et al., 1995; Tarnai & Wolfe, 2008). Efforts have focused on including peers in the intervention, reading of the Social Story by other people in a wider variety of settings, and expanding Social Story content to include other situations where newly acquired skills are relevant. As Gray (2010, 2015) argued, there may be no such thing as a retired Social Story because previously used stories can be updated to share new and related information.

Another common recommendation for practice is that successful Social Stories be maintained following gains but systematically faded by extending the time periods between readings or by shifting more responsibility to the individual for independent reading when appropriate (Swaggart et al., 1995). At this phase, new topics for Social Stories intervention are often considered.

ASSESSMENT FOR TREATMENT PLANNING AND PROGRESS MONITORING

Clinicians and educators have experienced increasing pressure from consumers, professional organizations, legislatures, and courts to be accountable for their practices and have been asked to provide objective data to support and guide their decision making for intervention (Gast, 2010). Because Social Stories are tailored interventions that have been administered by a variety of professionals across a range of settings, many different ways to evaluate their effectiveness have been employed. Table 16.1 reveals the variability evident in the research methods used to assess outcomes. These include simple frequency tallies of behaviors during an activity (e.g., recess, circle time) or fixed period of time, the percentage of time engaged in an activity, the percentage of accurate responses given in semistructured tasks, the number of steps in a behavioral routine completed, subjective daily ratings of behavior, the number of prompts needed to facilitate a desired behavior, time/event sampling (e.g., the percentage of 10-second intervals in which a behavior occurs), and various methods to assess social validity (e.g., interviews, questionnaires). There has also been some discussion in the Social Stories literature surrounding whether the most appropriate outcomes focus on decreasing undesirable behaviors, increasing desirable behaviors, or both (Nichols et al., 2006; Rust & Smith, 2006). In short, the nature of the data and its appropriateness as evidence to guide decision making may follow from the intervention target and goals, the individuals and setting, and practical considerations related to resources. In any event, what is taken as the index of success should be clearly operationalized and personalized to reflect what is functional and meaningful in the life of the individual (Ali & Fredrickson, 2006).

In research and practice, baseline and intervention phase data are often gathered to evaluate the treatment, frequently in the form of an AB (A = baseline, B = treatment phase) or simple time-series design. Only correlational conclusions are possible given this design (Gast, 2010). However, in educational and clinical settings, simple AB designs may be preferable to more extensive experimental designs (e.g., ABA, ABAB, multiple-baseline designs), which are difficult or impossible to implement in such settings. Practitioners might also consider the use of simple probes (maintenance, generalization) across baseline, intervention, and withdrawal phases to monitor the effectiveness of intervention.

Gray and Garand (1993) noted that when Social Stories treatment is effective, results are often dramatic and apparent within 1 week. Swaggart and colleagues (1995) recommended that if desired behavioral changes fail to occur after 2 weeks, program alterations should be made. Hutchins and Prelock (2013b) reported that when positive outcomes were detected, an average of eight intervention sessions (the range was 1 to 14 sessions) were required to secure a reliable therapeutic effect. These data make sense given the dynamic nature of Social Stories intervention, and so there is no single criterion or time-interval that can be offered to facilitate decisions regarding treatment. This is important considering that the number of times a Social Story must be read to reach a desired level of functioning (if this indeed occurs) is expected to vary significantly across individuals and behaviors, and for many, any effect of treatment will be gradual (Gray, 1998).

If Social Stories intervention is not deemed effective, authors should consider the possibility that lack of success may be due to several factors (Gray & Garand, 1993), including the reading schedule, accuracy and content (words and images) of the Social Story, the complexity of the language used, the motivation of the individual, and the appropriateness of the intervention target. Consequently, it is advisable to monitor, rethink, and revise a Social Story or its plan for implementation prior to abandonment, as adjustments or additional supports may be needed to secure desirable outcomes (Gray, 1995).

IMPLICATIONS FOR INCLUSIVE PRACTICE

Social Stories are used to support social understanding and more appropriate behavior across a wide range of situational and physical environments, including home, school, work, clinic, residential, and community settings. In a related vein,

Social Stories are flexible in that they can be developed using a variety of materials and media (e.g., iOS apps) and may be delivered using variable schedules of administration by different individuals (e.g., parents, service providers) including, when appropriate, the individual with ASD. Moreover, Social Stories can be developed on any topic of interest or concern (see Table 16.1 to review a wide range of topics that have been addressed in the literature) and can be used to augment or support access to other interventions that can be administered jointly (e.g., Halle et al., 2016; Grigore & Rusu, 2014). Finally, Social Stories have been employed in a range of service delivery models (e.g., pull-out, classroom based, community based, and self-contained special education classrooms) as well as parent-training and telepractice models (Lewandowski et al., 2014; Vivian et al., 2012) and may be particularly useful for facilitating inclusion of students with ASD in general education classrooms (Chan & O'Reilly, 2008; Gray & Garand, 1993; Greenway, 2000; Swaggart et al., 1995).

CONSIDERATIONS FOR CHILDREN FROM CULTURALLY AND LINGUISTICALLY DIVERSE BACKGROUNDS

Macrolevel and microlevel cultural and linguistic differences underscore the importance that Social Stories be developed in close collaboration with families who know the child best. The goal of Social Stories is to share relevant social information, the content of which can be expected to vary among individuals from culturally and linguistically diverse backgrounds. Members of different cultures often differ with regard to the importance they place on self-reliance and social conformity and how they construe appropriate social interaction. For instance, reduced eye contact is considered to be part of the impaired nonverbal behavior in ASD; however, direct eye contact with authorities may be considered a sign of disrespect in Asian culture (Bernier et al., 2010) as well as other cultures. Thus, it is essential to consider differences in how families prioritize various developmental skills to ensure that the goals of treatment are consistent with the culturally relevant goals of the family. In fact, professionals may find it useful to focus on improving the specific impairments about which the family is most concerned (Mandell & Novak, 2005).

Of course, the structure and explicit nature of Social Stories (e.g., "My mom likes it when I brush my teeth") may seem strange to some members of culturally and linguistically diverse backgrounds as well as to families who are not familiar with this intervention. For this reason, the rationale behind Social Stories should be made clear and adjustments in literary style should be considered with the proviso that the accuracy of all statements is preserved. Appropriate visual supports should also be used that draw on the relevant people and objects in the individual's life. When using Boardmaker (Mayer-Johnson Co.), a variety of symbols is available that can be appropriate for individuals from a wide range of racial and ethnic backgrounds.

Application to a Child

The stories help him think through problems. They really work for him.
I've been telling everyone at his school to just "go wild with Social Stories!"
—Mother of a 5-year-old boy diagnosed with ASD

Clinicians met Zach and his mother when they participated in a study examining the effectiveness of Social Stories for facilitating social cognition and remediating challenging behaviors (Hutchins & Prelock, 2008). At the time, Zach was 5 years old with a recent diagnosis of ASD. He was enrolled in a general education classroom and was receiving services from a school-based speech-language pathologist (SLP) and special educator. As a first step in developing the intervention, clinicians engaged in an information-gathering process that included child observation; joint interviews with Zach's mother and teacher; the administration of standardized measures to assess social, communicative, and theory of mind functioning; and a record review (i.e., individualized education program and diagnostic evaluations). Clinicians' goals were to understand Zach's strengths and challenges and to identify an intervention target that would be both responsive to parental priorities and sensitive to Zach's linguistic and social cognitive developmental level.

They learned that Zach was a sensitive, affectionate child who strived to please his parents. He demonstrated good receptive language skills and emerging theory of mind capacities, including the ability to engage in sustained episodes of joint attention, recognize facial expressions, and understand desire-based emotion (e.g., that people are happy when they get what they want). Clinicians planned to capitalize on these strengths to support development of enhanced social understanding and more appropriate behaviors. In particular, the sources of information that they consulted converged to identify "willful," "oppositional," and "explosive" aggressive acts that usually occurred in situations requiring adjustment and making transitions.

Based on the information gathered, a small research team developed the Social Story. The team members took care to ensure that the language level was appropriate, the words chosen would be meaningful to Zach, and all statements were accurate. They then asked Zach's mother to review and edit the Social Story for language level and accuracy of content.

They collected subjective data in the form of behavior ratings and daily diaries over baseline, intervention, and withdrawal phases of study. Zach's mother rated Zach's ability to stay calm and use words to talk in the context of the challenging situation. During the intervention phase (5 weeks, three times per week), clinicians read the Social Story to Zach in his home 15 times. Each Social Story was preceded by a Comic Strip Conversation (a related story-based intervention procedure that uses visual supports during conversation; see Gray, 1994) during which Zach drew and talked about a recent challenging event requiring adjustment. The subjective maternal ratings of Zach's behaviors across ABA phases of study are presented in Figure 16.1. Zach's mother also provided a number of comments describing Zach's behavior at home and school (see Hutchins & Prelock, 2008, for more detail). For example, she said, "He comes to me now when he gets upset and says, 'I'm angry,' and asks for help."

This example illustrates several important features of Social Stories intervention. First, as review of the literature reveals, Social Stories are often combined with other instructional strategies. In this case, Social Stories were combined with Comic Strip Conversations, an effective companion strategy to enhance social cognition (Gray, 1998). The example also underscores the importance of information gathering and describes one way in which researchers, families, and educators can collaborate to develop effective intervention strategies for use in the home or other settings. This example also highlights

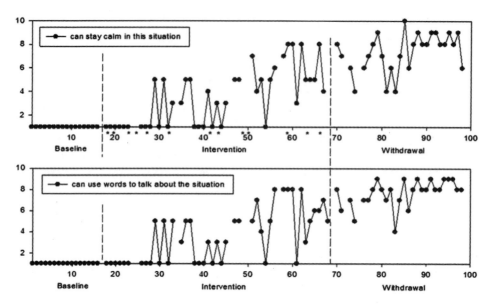

Figure 16.1. Maternal subjective ratings of Zach's ability to stay calm and use words to talk during a challenging situation (asterisks denote the days on which the Social Story was read). (From Hutchins, T. L., & Prelock, P. A. [2008]. Supporting theory of mind development: Considerations and recommendations for professionals providing services to individuals with autism spectrum disorder. *Topics in Language Disorders,* *28*(4), 340–364; Retrieved from https://journals.lww.com/topicsinlanguagedisorders/Abstract/2008/10000 /Supporting_Theory_of_Mind_Development_.5.aspx

the variety of data-collection techniques that have been used to evaluate Social Stories. Although a number of evaluative methods were available, the subjective maternal daily diary (both quantitative and qualitative data) was chosen because it was feasible, gathered relevant and personalized information, and was socially valid. As expected (e.g., Hutchins & Prelock, 2013b; Norris & Datillo, 1999), several repetitions of the story were needed before change was detected, and a positive effect of treatment was maintained following treatment withdrawal.

Application to an Adolescent

"Jacob needs a specific visual cognitive prosthesis to understand the who,
what, where, when, how, and why of our culture and how he fits and belongs."
—Mother of a 17-year-old boy diagnosed with PDD-NOS

Jacob was enrolled in a general education classroom and was receiving services from an SLP, special education teacher, case manager, and paraeducator at his local high school. Jacob was a sensitive young man who had an especially deep connection with his mother. He loved wind chimes and music and could play a variety of instruments in a truly gifted manner. Previous assessments indicated that oral language comprehension was an area of impairment for Jacob, productive language was limited to two- to five-word sentences, and reading and writing were areas of great strength. To enhance Jacob's communication, one important goal involved his voice, which was often soft, whispered, and trailed into silence. Following an examination that revealed normal structure and function of the larynx, Jacob began voice therapy with a university-based SLP. Jacob worked hard over the course of several weeks to find what he called his "excellent voice," which was louder and easier to understand, but gains failed to generalize to other settings.

Because clinicians knew that Jacob could produce an excellent voice, they decided to develop a Social Story with two objectives in mind. One objective was to enhance Jacob's understanding of the social importance of using his excellent voice. Another objective was to recruit the participation of those who had frequent contact with Jacob. They collaborated with Jacob, Jacob's mother, and his university SLP to learn about the who, what, when, where, and why of his different voices. The use of the Motivation Assessment Scale (MAS; Durand & Crimmins, 1992) and clinicians' previous observations of Jacob facilitated this effort.

Clinicians drafted a Social Story titled "Using My Excellent Voice" and revised it in adherence with Gray's 2010 recommendations, with input from Jacob's mother to ensure accuracy of content. When asked about pictures, Jacob noted that he would like Boardmaker pictures in his story so clinicians added PCS. They incorporated particular font and formatting choices to highlight key messages. They then introduced the story to Jacob and followed this with brief comprehension checks of the text and images. Jacob's Social Story is presented in Figure 16.2.

Clinicians shared hard and electronic copies of the Social Story with Jacob, Jacob's mother, and Jacob's school-based SLP, paraeducator, special educator, and case manager, all of whom agreed to read the Social Story across contexts to facilitate acquisition and generalization of skills. The electronic version of the Social Story was deemed particularly important for Jacob, who enjoyed using his iPod touch. All participants (including Jacob) agreed to read the Social Story once or twice a week for several weeks to ensure familiarity. The school team developed an ABA data-collection plan to track Jacob's use of an excellent voice over several weeks.

This example of Social Story development underscores the nature of this intervention as a collaborative process. The team identified a topic deemed critical to Jacob's success as a communication partner. Through testing and discussion, clinicians identified the target as an area of some competency, thereby increasing the likelihood it was a developmentally appropriate target; identified other possible supports; and developed treatment and data-collection schedules. In particular, they learned that Jacob was more likely to use his excellent voice when others spoke to him using short sentences and gave him more time to respond. In summary, the collaborative process helped clinicians refine their thinking, coordinate workable plans, and develop shared responsibility for supporting Jacob's success.

To review an extended application and implementation of this intervention, see Case 13 about a child with ASD in the companion volume *Case Studies for the Treatment of Autism Spectrum Disorder.*

Future Directions

The Social Stories literature has raised a number of questions representing important directions for future research (see also Ali & Fredrickson, 2006; Nichols et al., 2006; Sansoti et al., 2004). Based on scant or mixed evidence in the Social Stories

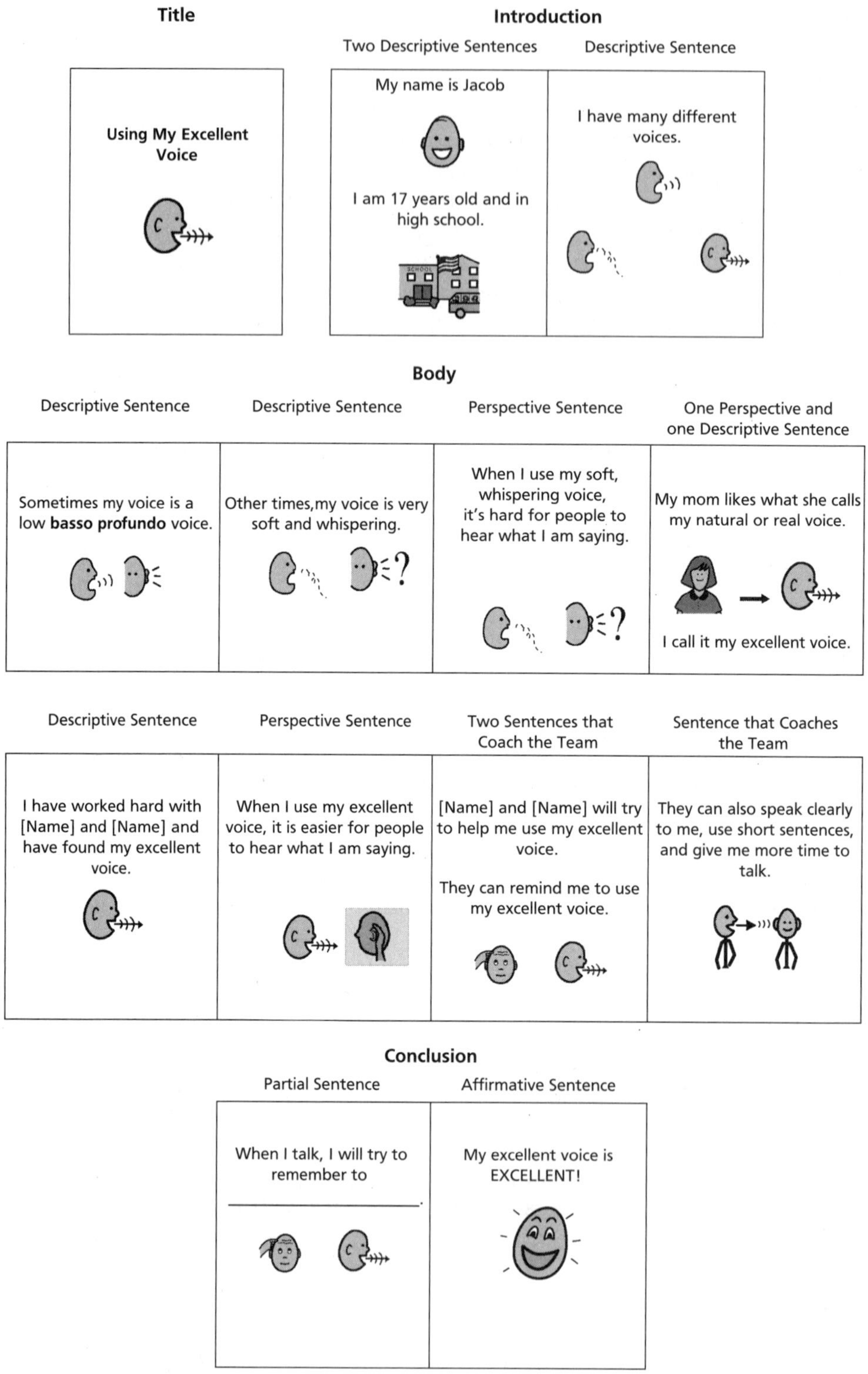

Title

Using My Excellent Voice

Introduction

Two Descriptive Sentences

My name is Jacob

I am 17 years old and in high school.

Descriptive Sentence

I have many different voices.

Body

Descriptive Sentence

Sometimes my voice is a low **basso profundo** voice.

Descriptive Sentence

Other times, my voice is very soft and whispering.

Perspective Sentence

When I use my soft, whispering voice, it's hard for people to hear what I am saying.

One Perspective and one Descriptive Sentence

My mom likes what she calls my natural or real voice.

I call it my excellent voice.

Descriptive Sentence

I have worked hard with [Name] and [Name] and have found my excellent voice.

Perspective Sentence

When I use my excellent voice, it is easier for people to hear what I am saying.

Two Sentences that Coach the Team

[Name] and [Name] will try to help me use my excellent voice.

They can remind me to use my excellent voice.

Sentence that Coaches the Team

They can also speak clearly to me, use short sentences, and give me more time to talk.

Conclusion

Partial Sentence

When I talk, I will try to remember to
_____.

Affirmative Sentence

My excellent voice is EXCELLENT!

Figure 16.2. Jacob's Social Story. Symbols from PCS® and Boardmaker by Tobii Dynavox® All rights reserved. Used with permission.

literature, some of the more salient research directions could address the following questions:

- Do intervention procedures that involve multiple readers across contexts result in better outcomes or more generalizable outcomes?

- Which individual characteristics (e.g., age, verbal ability, reading level) predict success with Social Stories?

- What is the effect of stories that praise or applaud what the individual has achieved or is already doing well?

- Do particular schedules of review (e.g., number of presentations, intensity and duration of treatment) predict success, and how might these vary with individual characteristics?

Determining whether certain targets of intervention are more amenable or resistant to change is also needed. Kokina and Kern (2010) suggested that Social Stories targeting the reduction of problem behaviors may be more effective than those teaching social skills. Yet, the success of a particular target is likely contingent on the individual's motivation, strengths, and challenges (Kokina & Kern, 2010). Although researchers and professionals have acknowledged the importance of developmentally appropriate language within Social Stories, very few have considered whether a particular social-cognitive understanding is a developmentally appropriate goal (Hutchins & Prelock, 2008). Examining the importance of developmental appropriateness in the selection of social-cognitive goals seems crucial given that the theoretical basis of Social Stories is to enhance social understanding.

This raises a related question regarding the need to test the theoretical assumptions of Social Stories. When Social Stories are deemed effective, good outcomes may result from more advanced social understanding or from the use of a nonepistemic strategy in which solutions are derived from logic or rote learning. Differentiating between these alternative explanations has important implications for maintenance and generalizability. If Social Stories have the potential to remediate a core deficit in social understanding as opposed to a behavioral symptom, then shifts in understanding should lead to sustained and positive changes across the range of behaviors and situations for which that understanding is relevant. In contrast, if behavioral learning is all that is occurring, evidence should show reduced generalizability and perhaps reduced maintenance. Thus, there is a need to develop sensitive ways of assessing whether Social Stories lead to meaningful changes in affect and social cognition, as much of the research has focused on behavior (Ali & Fredrickson, 2006).

Suggested Readings

1. Hutchins, T. L., & Prelock, P. A. (2018). Using story-based interventions to improve episodic memory in autism spectrum disorder. *Seminars and Speech and Language, 39*(2), 124–143. This article describes the theoretical importance of Social Stories for supporting episodic memory and social cognition in children with ASD and offers specific recommendations for practice.

2. Rust, J., & Smith, A. (2006). How should the effectiveness of Social Stories™ to modify the behavior of children on the autistic spectrum be tested? *Autism,*

10(2), 125–138. This article recounts the variability evident in the Social Stories literature, focusing on factors that should be considered when evaluating the effectiveness of Social Stories.

Learning Activities

1. Read *The New Social Story Book* (Gray, 2015), which offers a series of tutorials and exercises to develop competency with writing Social Stories. Complete the activities in the book.

2. Vincent is a 6-year-old African American boy who is verbal. He was diagnosed with ASD and is enrolled in a general education classroom. Vincent's SLP is concerned with behaviors—especially loud talking and interrupting others—that limit Vincent's ability to engage in appropriate social interaction. What kinds of information would you collect to determine whether these are appropriate targets for intervention? To understand the behaviors better?

3. Stuart is a 6-year-old boy of European descent who was diagnosed with PDD-NOS. Formal testing revealed significant cognitive and receptive and expressive language impairments. Stuart's level of reading comprehension is unclear, but writing is a relative strength, and he seems to enjoy writing, doodling, and looking at books. Stuart's special educator believes he engages in behaviors that may stigmatize him, namely, picking at his nose and ears, because of sensory issues. Would Stuart be a good candidate for Social Stories intervention? If you decide to pursue Social Stories intervention, what strategies could you use to ensure that the Social Story is presented in a way that preserves Stuart's self-esteem and is a positive behavioral intervention? Identify one way to evaluate the effect of intervention, making sure that the outcome is clearly operationalized and personally relevant and meaningful in the child's life.

Summary of Video Clip

*See the **About the Videos and Downloads** page at the front of the book for directions on how to access and stream the accompanying video to this chapter.*

The video shows Jacob's first introduction to his Social Story, which is also illustrated in Figure 16.2. In the video, Jacob attends to the images as the clinician reads the story at a leisurely pace. The clinician also uses significant pauses after each sentence to ensure that Jacob has adequate time to process the words and images.

REFERENCES

Adams, L., Gouvousis, A., VanLue, M., & Waldrom, C. (2004). Social Story intervention: Improving communication skills in a child with an autism spectrum disorder. *Focus on Autism and Other Developmental Disabilities, 19(*2), 87–94.

Ali, S., & Fredrickson, N. (2006). Investigating the evidence base of Social Stories. *Educational Psychology in Practice, 22*(4), 355–377.

American Psychiatric Association. (2013). *Diagnostic and statistical manual of mental disorders, fifth edition* (DSM-5). Author.

Attwood, T. (1998). *Asperger's syndrome: A guide for parents and professionals*. Jessica Kingsley.

Barry, L. M., & Burlew, S. B. (2004). Using social stories to teach choice and play skills to children with autism. *Focus on Autism and Other Developmental Disabilities, 19*(1), 45–51.

Bernad-Ripoll, S. (2007). Using a self-as-model video combined with Social Stories™ to help a child with Asperger syndrome understand emotions. *Focus on Autism and Other Developmental Disabilities, 22*(2), 100–108.

Bernier, R., Mao, A., & Yen, D. (2010). Psychopathology, families, and culture: Autism. *Child and Adolescent Psychiatric Clinics of North America, 19*, 855–867.

Bledsoe, R., Smith, B. S., & Simpson, R. (2003). Use of social story intervention to improve mealtime skills of an adolescent with Asperger syndrome. *Autism: The International Journal of Research and Practice, 7*, 289–295.

Bowler, D., Gardiner, J., & Grice, S., (2000). Episodic memory and remembering in adults with Asperger's syndrome. *Journal of Autism and Developmental Disorders, 30*(4), 295–304.

Bozkurt, S., & Vuran, S. (2014). An analysis of the use of social stories in teaching social skills to children with autism spectrum disorders. *Educational Sciences: Theory & Practice, 14*(5), 1875–1892.

Brownell, M. D. (2002). Musically adapted social stories to modify behaviors in students with autism: Four case studies. *Journal of Music Therapy, 39*(2), 117–144.

Carr, E. G., Dunlap, G., Horner, R. H., Koegel, R. L., Turnbull, A. P., Sailor, W., Anderson, J. L., Albin, R. W., Koegel, L. K., & Fox, L. (2002). Positive behavior support: Evolution of an applied science. *Journal of Positive Behavior Interventions, 4*(1), 4–6.

Chan, J. M., & O'Reilly, M. F. (2008). A Social Stories™ intervention package for students with autism in inclusive classroom settings. *Journal of Applied Behavior Analysis, 41*, 405–409.

Chan, J. M., O'Reilly, M. F., Lang, R. B., Boutot, E. A., White, P. J., Pierce, N., & Baker, S. (2011). Evaluation of Social Stories™ intervention implemented by pre-service teachers for students with autism in general education settings. *Research in Autism Spectrum Disorders, 5*, 715–721.

Cihak, D., Kildare, L., Smith, C., McMahon, D., & Quinn-Brown, L. (2012). Using video Social Stories™ to increase task engagement for middle school students with autism spectrum disorders. *Behavior Modification, 36*(3), 399–425.

Constantin, A., Pain, H., & Waller, A. (2013). Informing design of an authoring tool for developing social stories. *INTERACT. Part II*, 546–553.

Crozier, S., & Tincani, M. J. (2005). Using a modified Social Story to decrease disruptive behavior of a child with autism. *Focus on Autism and Other Developmental Disabilities, 20*(3), 150–157.

Crozier, S., & Tincani, M. J. (2007). Effects of social stories on prosocial behavior of preschool children with autism spectrum disorders. *Journal of Autism and Developmental Disorders, 37*, 1803–1814.

Delano, M., & Snell, M. E. (2006). The effects of social stories on the social engagement of children with autism. *Journal of Positive Behavior Interventions, 8*(1), 29–42.

Dodd, S., Stephen, D., Hupp, A., Jewell, J. D., & Krohn, E. (2008). Using parents and siblings during a social story intervention for two children diagnosed with PDD-NOS. *Journal of Developmental and Physical Disabilities, 20*, 217–229.

Doyle, T., & Arnedillo-Sanchez, I. (2011). Using multimedia to reveal the hidden code of everyday behavior to children with autism spectrum disorders (ASDs). *Computers & Education, 56*, 357–369.

Dunlap, G., & Fox, L. (1999). A demonstration of behavioral supports for young children with autism. *Journal of Positive Behavioral Interventions, 1*(2), 77–87.

Durand, V. M., & Crimmins, D. B. (1992). *The Motivation Assessment Scale.* Monaco & Associates.

Frith, U. (1989). *Autism: Explaining the enigma.* Blackwell.

Gast, D. L. (2010). *Single subject research methodology in behavioral sciences.* Taylor Francis.

Ghanouni, P., Jarus, T., Zwicker, J., Lucyshyn, J., Mow, K., & Ledingham, A. (2018). Social stories for children with autism spectrum disorder: Validating the content of a virtual reality program. *Journal of Autism and Developmental Disorders.* https://doi.org/10.1007/s10803-018-3737-0

Golzari, F., Alamdarloo, G., & Moradi, S. (2015). The effect of a Social Stories intervention on the social skills of male students with autism spectrum disorder. *SAGE Open.* https://doi .org/10.1177/2158244015621599

Graetz, J., Mastropieri, M., & Scruggs, T. (2009). Decreasing inappropriate behaviors for adolescents with autism spectrum disorders using modified social stories. *Education and Training in Developmental Disabilities, 44*(1), 91–104.

Gray, C. (1994). *Comic Strip Conversations.* Future Horizons.

Gray, C. (1995). Teaching children with autism to "read" social situations. In K. A. Quill (Ed.), *Teaching children with autism: Strategies to enhance communication and socialization* (pp. 219–241). Delmar Publishers.

Gray, C. (1998). Social Stories and Comic Strip Conversations with students with Asperger syndrome and high-functioning autism. In E. Schopler (Ed.), *Asperger syndrome or high-functioning autism?* (pp. 167–194). Plenum Press.

Gray, C. (2000). *The new Social Story book: Illustrated edition.* Future Horizons.

Gray, C. (2010). *The new Social Story book.* Future Horizons.

Gray, C. (2015). *The new Social Story book: Revised and expanded 15th anniversary edition.* Future Horizons.

Gray, C., & Garand, J. D. (1993). Social Stories: Improving responses of students with autism with accurate social information. *Focus on Autistic Behavior, 8*(1), 1–10.

Gray, C., & White, A. L. (2002). *My Social Stories book.* Jessica Kingsley.

Greenway, C. (2000). Autism and Asperger syndrome: Strategies to promote prosocial behaviors. *Educational Psychology in Practice, 16*(3), 469–486.

Grigore, A., & Rusu, A. (2014). Interaction with a therapy dog enhances the effects of social story method in autistic children. *Society and Animals*, 241–261.

Hagiwara, T., & Myles, S. B. (1999). A multimedia social story intervention: Teaching skills to children with autism. *Focus on Autism and Other Developmental Disabilities, 14*, 82–95.

Haggerty, N. K., Black, R. S., & Smith, G. J. (2005). Increasing self-managed coping skills through Social Stories and apron story-telling. *Teaching Exceptional Children, 37*, 40–47.

Halle, S., Ninness, C., Ninness, S., & Lawson, D. (2016). Teaching social skills to students with autism: A video modeling Social Stories approach. *Behavior and Social Issues, 25*, 42–63.

Hanley-Hochdorfer, K., Bray, M. A., Kehl, T. J., & Elinoff, M. J. (2010). Social Stories to increase verbal initiation in children with autism and Asperger's disorder. *School Psychology Review, 39*(3), 484–492.

Happe, F. (1999). Autism: Cognitive deficit or cognitive style? *Metaphor and Symbolic Activity, 10*, 275–295.

Hess, K. L., Morrier, M. J., Heflin, L. J., & Ivey, M. L. (2008). Autism treatment survey: Services received by children with autism spectrum disorders in public school classrooms. *Journal of Autism and Developmental Disorders, 38*, 961–971.

Hutchins, T. L., & Prelock, P. A. (2006). Using social stories and comic strip conversations to promote socially valid outcomes for children with autism. *Seminars in Speech and Language, 27*(1), 47–59.

Hutchins, T. L., & Prelock, P. A. (2008). Supporting theory of mind development: Considerations and recommendations for professionals providing services to individuals with autism spectrum disorder. *Topics in Language Disorders, 28*(4), 340–364.

Hutchins, T. L., & Prelock, P. A. (2013a). Parents' perceptions of their children's social behavior: The social validity of Social Stories™ and Comic Strip Conversations. *Journal of Positive Behavior Interventions, 15*(3), 156–168.

Hutchins, T. L., & Prelock, P. A. (2013b). The social validity of Social Stories™ for supporting behavioral and communicative function in autism spectrum disorder. *International Journal of Speech-Language Pathology, 15*(4), 383–395.

Hutchins, T. L., & Prelock, P. A. (2018). Using story-based interventions to improve episodic memory in autism spectrum disorder. *Seminars in Speech and Language, 39*(2), 124–143.

Iskander, J., & Rosales, R. (2013). An evaluation of the components of a Social Stories™ intervention. *Research in Autism Spectrum Disorders, 7*, 1–8.

Ivey, M. L., Heflin, J., & Alberto, P. (2004). The use of Social Stories to promote independent behaviors in novel events for children with PDD-NOS. *Focus on Autism and Other Developmental Disabilities, 19,* 164–176.

Kagohara, D., Achmadi, D., van der Meer, L., Lancioni, G., O'Reilly, M., Lang, R., Marschik, P. B., Sutherland, D., Ramdoss, S., Green, V. A., & Sigafoos, J. (2013). Teaching two students with Asperger syndrome to greet adults using Social Stories™ and video modeling. *Journal of Developmental and Physical Disabilities, 25,* 241–251.

Kalyva, E., & Agaliotis, I. (2009). Can social stories enhance the interpersonal conflict resolution skills of children with LD? *Research in Developmental Disabilities, 30,* 192–202.

Karayazi, S., Kohler Evans, P., & Filer, J. (2014). The effects of a social story intervention on the pro-social behaviors of a young adult with autism spectrum disorder. *International Journal of Special Education, 29*(3), 126–133.

Karkhaneh, M., Clary, B., Ospina, B. M., Seida, J. C., Smith, V., & Hartling, L. (2010). Social Stories™ to improve social skills in children with autism spectrum disorder: A systematic review. *Autism, 14*(6), 641–662.

Kassardjian, A., Leaf, J., Ravid, D., Leaf, J., Alcalay, A., Dale, S., Tsuji, K., Taubman, M., Leaf, R., McEachin, J., & Oppenheim-Leaf. (2014). Comparing the teaching interaction procedure to social stories: a replication study. *Journal of Autism and Developmental Disorders, 44,* 2329–2340.

Klett, L., & Turan, Y. (2012). Generalized effects of social stories with task analysis for teaching menstrual care to three young girls with autism. *Sexuality and Disability, 30,* 319–336.

Kokina, A., & Kern, L. (2010). Social Story™ interventions for students with autism spectrum disorders. *Journal of Autism and Developmental Disabilities, 40,* 812–826.

Kuoch, H., & Mirenda, P. (2003). Social story interventions for young children with autism spectrum disorders. *Focus on Autism and Other Developmental Disabilities, 18,* 219–227.

Kuttler, S., Myles, B. S., & Carlson, J. K. (1998). The use of social stories to reduce precursors to tantrum behavior in a student with autism. *Focus on Autism and Other Developmental Disabilities, 13,* 176–182.

Leaf, J., Oppenheim-Leaf, M., Leaf, R., Taubman, M., McEachin J., Parker, T., Waks, A., & Mountjoy, T. (2015). What is the proof? A methodological review of studies that have utilized social stories. *Education and Training in Autism and Developmental Disabilities, 50*(2), 127–141.

Lee, J., & Cherney, L. (2018). Tau-U: A quantitative approach to analysis of single-case experimental data in aphasia. *American Journal of Speech Language Pathology, 27,* 495–503.

Lewandowski, J., Hutchins, T., Prelock, P., & Murray-Close, D. (2014). Examining the benefit of including a sibling in story-based interventions with a child with Asperger syndrome. *Contemporary Issues in Communication Sciences and Disorders, 41,* 179–195.

Lind, S., & Bowler, D. (2010). Episodic memory and episodic future thinking in adults with autism spectrum disorder. *Journal of Abnormal Psychology, 119*(4), 896–905.

Lorimer, P. A., Simpson, R. L., Myles, B. S., & Ganz, J. B. (2002). The use of social stories as a preventative behavioral intervention in a home setting with a child with autism. *Journal of Positive Behavioral Interventions, 4,* 53–60.

Mancil, R. G., Haydon, E., & Whitby, P. (2009). Differentiated effects of paper and computer-assisted Social Stories™ on inappropriate behavior in children with autism. *Focus on Autism and Other Developmental Disabilities, 24*(4), 205–215.

Mandell, D. S., & Novak, M. (2005). The role of culture in families' treatment decisions for children with autism spectrum disorders. *Mental Retardation and Developmental Disabilities, 11,* 10–115.

Marr, D., Mika, H., Miraglia, J., Roerig, M., & Sinnott, R. (2007). The effects of sensory stories on targeted behaviors in preschool children with autism. *Physical and Occupational Therapy in Pediatrics, 27*(1), 63–79.

Moore, P. S. (2004). The use of social stories in a psychology service for children with learning disabilities: A case study of a sleep problem. *British Journal of Learning Disabilities, 32,* 133–138.

National Autism Center. (2015). *National Standards Project, Phase 2.* https://www.nationalautismcenter.org

Nichols, S. L., Hupp, S. D., Jewell, J. D., & Zeigler, C. S. (2006). Review of Social Story™ interventions for children diagnosed with autism spectrum disorders. *Journal of Evidence-Based Practices for Schools, 6*(1), 90–120.

Norris, C., & Dattilo, J. (1999). Evaluating effects of a social story intervention on a young girl with autism. *Focus on Autism and Other Developmental Disabilities, 14,* 180–186.

Ozdemir, S. (2008). The effectiveness of social stories on decreasing disruptive behaviors of children with autism: Three case studies. *Journal of Autism and Developmental Disorders, 38,* 1689–1696.

Pane, H., Sidener, T., Vladescu, J., & Nirgudkar, A. (2015). Evaluating function based Social Stories™ with children with autism. *Behavior Modification, 39*(6), 912–931.

Parker, R., Vannest, K., & Davis, J. (2011). Effect size in single-case research: A review of nine nonoverlap techniques. *Behavior Modification, 35*(4), 303–322.

Pasiali, V. (2004). The use of prescriptive therapeutic songs in a home-based environment to promote social skills acquisition by children with autism: Three case studies. *Music Therapy Perspectives, 22*(1), 11–20.

Qi, C., Barton, E., Collier, M., Lin, Y., & Montoya, C. (2018). A systematic review of effects of Social Stories interventions for individuals with autism spectrum disorder. *Focus on Autism and Developmental Disabilities, 33*(1), 25–34.

Quirmbach, L. M., Lincoln, A. J., Feinberg-Gizzo, M. J., Ingersoll, B. R., & Andrews, S. M. (2009). Social stories: Mechanisms of effectiveness in increasing game play skills in children diagnosed with autism spectrum disorders using a pretest posttest repeated measures randomized control group design. *Journal of Autism and Developmental Disorders, 39*(2), 299–321.

Reynhout, G., & Carter, M. (2006). Social Stories™ for children with disabilities *Journal of Autism and Developmental Disorders, 36,* 445–469.

Reynhout, G., & Carter, M. (2009). The use of Social Stories by teachers and their perceived efficacy. *Research on Autism Spectrum Disorders, 3,* 232–251.

Reynhout, G., & Carter, M. (2011a). Social Stories™: A possible theoretical rationale. *European Journal of Special Needs Education, 26*(3), 367–378.

Reynhout, G., & Carter, M. (2011b). Evaluation of the efficacy of Social Stories™ using three single subject metrics. *Research in Autism Spectrum Disorders, 5,* 885–900.

Rhodes, C. (2014). Do social stories help to decrease disruptive behavior in children with autistic spectrum disorder? A review of the published literature. *Journal of Intellectual Disabilities, 18*(1), 35–50.

Richels, C., Bobzien, J., Raver, S., Schwartz, K., Hester, P., & Reed, L. (2014). Teaching emotion words using social stories and created experiences in group instruction with preschoolers who are deaf or hard of hearing: An exploratory study. *Deafness & Educational International, 16*(1), 37–58.

Robey, R. R., & Schultz, M. C. (1998). A model for conducting clinical-outcomes research: An adaptation of the standard protocol for use in aphasiology. *Aphasiology, 12*(9), 787–810.

Rogers, M. G., & Myles, B. S. (2001). Using social stories and comic strip conversations to interpret social situations for an adolescent with Asperger syndrome. *Intervention in School and Clinic, 38,* 310–313.

Rowe, C. (1999). Do social stories benefit children diagnosed with autism in mainstream primary schools? *British Journal of Special Education, 26,* 12–14.

Rust, J., & Smith, A. (2006). How should the effectiveness of Social Stories to modify the behavior of children on the autistic spectrum be tested? *Autism, 10*(2), 125–138.

Samuels, R., & Stansfield, J. (2011). The effectiveness of Social Stories™ to develop social interactions with adults with characteristics of autism spectrum disorder. *British Journal of Learning Disabilities, 40,* 272–285.

Sansoti, F. J., & Powell-Smith, K. A., (2006). Using social stories to improve the social behavior of children with Asperger syndrome. *Journal of Positive Behavior Interventions, 8*(1), 43–57.

Sansoti, F. J., Powell-Smith, K. A., & Kincaid, D. (2004). A research synthesis of social story interventions for children diagnosed with autism spectrum disorders. *Focus on Autism and Other Developmental Disabilities, 19,* 194–204.

Scattone, D. (2008). Enhancing the conversation skills of a boy with Asperger's disorder through Social Stories™ and video modeling. *Journal of Autism and Developmental Disorders, 38,* 395–400.

Scattone, D. (2007). Social skills interventions for children with autism. *Psychology in the Schools, 44*(7), 717–726.

Scattone, D., Tingstrom, D. H., & Wilczynski, S. M. (2006). Increasing appropriate social interactions of children with autism spectrum disorders using Social Stories™. *Focus on Autism and Other Developmental Disabilities, 21*(4), 211–222.

Scattone, D., Wilczynski, S. M., Edwards, R. P., & Rabian, B. (2002). Decreasing disruptive behaviors of children with autism using social stories. *Journal of Autism and Developmental Disorders, 32*(6), 535–543.

Schneider, N., & Goldstein, H. (2010). Social Stories improve™ the on-task behavior of children with language impairment. *Journal of Early Intervention, 31*(3), 250–264.

Scott, J., Clark, C., & Brady, M. (2000). *Students with Autism: Characteristics and instructional programming for special educators.* San Diego, CA: Singular.

Smith, C. (2001). Using Social Stories to enhance behavior in children with autistic spectrum difficulties. *Educational Psychology in Practice, 17*(4), 337–345.

Soenksen, D., & Alper, S. (2006). Teaching a young child to appropriately gain attention of peers using a social story intervention. *Focus on Autism and Other Developmental Disabilities, 21*(1), 36–44.

Swaggart, B. L., Gagnon, E., Bock, S. J., Earlies, E. L., Quinn, C., Myles, B. S., & Simpson, R. L. (1995). Using social stories to teach social and behavioral skills to children with autism. *Focus on Autistic Behavior, 10*, 1–15.

Tarnai, B., & Wolfe, P. S. (2008). Social Stories for sexuality education for persons with autism/pervasive developmental disorder. *Sexual Disability, 26*, 29–36.

Test, D. W., Richter, S., Knight, V., & Spooner, F. (2010). A comprehensive review and meta-analysis of the Social Stories™ literature. *Focus on Autism and Other Developmental Disabilities*, 1–14. https://doi.org/10.1177/1088357609351573

Theimann, K. S., & Goldstein, H. (2001). Social stories, written text cues, and video feedback: Effects on social communication of children with autism. *Journal of Applied Behavior Analysis, 34*(4), 425–446.

Thompson, R., & Johnston, S. (2013). Use of social stories to improve self-regulation in children with autism spectrum disorders. *Physical & Occupational Therapy in Pediatrics, 33*(3), 271–284.

Toplis, R., & Hadwin, J. A. (2006). Using social stories to change problematic lunchtime behavior in school. *Educational Psychology in Practice, 22*(1), 53–67.

Vandermeer, J., Beamish, W., Milford, T., & Lang, W. (2015). Ipad-presented social stories for young children with autism. *Developmental Neurorehabilitation, 18*(2), 75–81.

Vivian, L., Hutchins, T., & Prelock, P. (2012). A family-centered approach for training parents to use Comic Strip Conversations with their child with autism. *Contemporary Issues in Communication Sciences and Disorders, 30*, 30–42.

Walton, K., & Ingersoll, B. (2013). Improving social skills in adolescents and adults with autism and severe to profound intellectual disability: A review of the literature. *Journal of Autism and Developmental Disorders, 43*, 594–615.

Whalon, K., Conroy, M., Martinez, J., & Werch, B. (2015). School-based peer-related social competence interventions for children with autism spectrum disorder: A meta-analysis and descriptive review of single case research design studies. *Journal of Autism and Developmental Disorders, 45*, 1513–1531.

Wright, L., & McCathren, R. (2012). Utilizing Social Stories to increase prosocial behavior and reduce problem behavior in young children. *Child Development Research*, Article ID 357291, 1–13. https://doi.org/10.1155/2012/357291

17

Video Modeling for Persons With ASD

Tom Buggey

INTRODUCTION

Students with autism spectrum disorder (ASD) can present parents and educators with a quandary. How do you educate children who often have difficulty attending to a task and who sometimes engage in behaviors seemingly intended to avoid the people instructing them? This challenge can result in a large proportion of instructional time spent providing models of appropriate behaviors and progressively more complex academic skills. Unless parents and educators can penetrate the social barriers presented by individuals with autism, the effects of instruction will be muted. One way around such barriers may be to use video models as a medium of instruction.

Television and computer screens act as magnets to many children and youth. The medium alone is a powerful attractor; yet, in addition to this widespread appeal, there may be reasons why video-based instruction holds special promise for people with autism. Video modeling has been developed with this possibility in mind. It is defined as an instructional method in which an individual develops a skill or behavior by viewing images of someone demonstrating the same skill or behavior. The model may be a peer, an adult, an animation, or, in the case of video self-modeling, the viewer him- or herself.

Video modeling can be used to teach new skills or behaviors, to improve a skill or behavior, or to replace or extinguish maladaptive behavior. A salient feature of all video-modeling formats is that demonstrated behavior is always positive. These methods address what to do versus what *not* to do by avoiding negative imagery. There is another form of video instruction, typically referred to as **self-observation** (Piersel & Kratochwill, 1979), in which raw video is analyzed so that observers can learn from mistakes as well as from successes. Sports teams often watch videos of past games to analyze performance by using self-observation. In contrast, in video-modeling movies, all evidence of inappropriate behavior, prompting of behaviors, and any errors made while recording are removed (Dowrick, 1983). Dowrick suggests that viewing mistakes in order to correct them is fine for someone with high self-confidence; however, if viewers lack self-confidence, seeing themselves commit mistakes can reinforce feelings of low self-esteem. That is why self-observation is not recommended for individuals who have any history of low academic performance or inappropriate behavior. Thus, video modeling and its inherent positive message makes it the preferred method for those at risk for learning difficulties. Video modeling also provides a good fit for behavior support plans because of its positive connotations and the uniformity of message that is conveyed.

Video modeling seems to be effective across all age ranges, with the possible exception of very young children from birth to 2½ years old. There is simply no research available on which to base claims about this entire age group, although a project carried out by the Early Intervention Division of the Minnesota Department of Education provided evidence that children as young as 2 years can benefit from **video self-modeling (VSM).** The type of behavior addressed and age-appropriateness were seen as critical factors for success, as major improvements were seen in functional skills such as bike pedaling and eating and with language skills (Grove & Buggey, 2014). In addition, some evidence suggests that people with severe autism who also have severe cognitive disabilities may not benefit from video modeling (Buggey, 2009); however, ample evidence suggests that video modeling can be effective with children who are classified in the moderate and severe range of the spectrum (e.g., Bellini et al., 2007; Buggey et al., 1999; LeBlanc et al., 2003). The essential factor of whether video modeling will be effective appears to be the viewer's ability to attend to the video (Buggey, 2009).

Video modeling can be used to supplement other methods or can be used as the main intervention. Anyone with knowledge of developmental sequences who has some basic skills with a video camera and access to video editing software can produce videos appropriate for use in video modeling. Production of the videos varies in complexity across the three main types of video modeling: **video peer modeling (VPM), point-of-view (PoV) modeling,** and VSM. The actual editing of video footage is the same across the various methods, but the strategy for arranging and composing the scenes to be shot is very different. Adult and peer modeling videos are relatively simple to create because the movies' stars are handpicked and are typically cooperative and easily coached. PoV modeling is also fairly simple to carry out. One needs to task-analyze a behavior and walk through the sequence of steps with the camera held at a child's eye level. The view from the camera, simulating the child's viewpoint, becomes the central instructional component. Self-modeling is more complicated because one must manipulate the recording and editing of the video footage to make it appear that learners are exhibiting more advanced behaviors than they typically are. This task can be challenging if the model tends to shy away from social interaction or has difficulty following directions.

Because video modeling is a relatively new methodology, there is little written about its delivery. The norm seems to be adapted from research studies where a static, controlled method is implemented. Video modeling has relevance in occupational, physical, and speech-language therapies; in homes; and in psychological and vocational counseling and training. It has also been used effectively for academic instruction. The critical factor in determining which form of video modeling is used, where it is used, and who is responsible for creating videos seems to be available time for the process. A video using PoV modeling can probably be produced in under an hour. Adult and peer modeling videos take somewhat longer and require more coordination and participants. Self-modeling videos can be produced in the same amount of time as the other methods under ideal conditions and with a cooperative star, but they usually take longer than the other forms, especially in the editing phase.

The time commitment necessary for producing modeling videos puts some constraints on who is likely to create them. Classroom teachers may not have the time or the flexibility in scheduling their time to devote to video modeling. In contrast, counselors, therapists, and parents are more likely to have the time and resources to devote to creating videos.

TARGET POPULATIONS

Video modeling has been successfully applied to people with autism across the full range of the spectrum from mild autism (formerly Asperger syndrome and often stated as such in some studies; e.g., Delano, 2007; Sansosti & Powell-Smith, 2008; Scattone, 2008) to severe autism (e.g., Buggey et al., 2011; Lee et al., 2017). Research has not been carried out with people with similar yet neurologically differentiated conditions such as Rett syndrome and childhood disintegrative disorder, probably because of the small numbers of children with these disorders.

Little has been written on who could most benefit from video modeling, nor is there any research concerning client attributes that would preclude the use of video-modeling intervention. It is logical to assume there is a bottom age limit or a threshold of cognitive ability needed for success with video modeling. The few instances in the literature in which video modeling has been unsuccessful have tended to involve preschool children for whom age or developmental levels may have been a deciding factor (i.e., Buggey et al., 2011; Clark et al., 1993). A prerequisite skill often ascribed to self-modeling is self-recognition (Dowrick, 1983). This claim becomes questionable when one considers the success of other forms of modeling. It may be that self-recognition, which typically develops between 18 and 24 months (Lewis & Brooks-Gunn, 1979), occurs at the same time as many other developmental milestones, and it is these other areas of development that are the critical factors. There is also some evidence that self-recognition is delayed in children with autism in terms of recognizing self and using personal pronouns (Carmody & Lewis, 2011); however, much more research is needed to better understand this issue.

There are no norm-referenced or criterion-referenced tests that can be used to determine whether video modeling might be effective with any given person. Much of the evaluation prior to implementation of video modeling takes the form of direct observation. A key observation is whether television attracts an individual's attention. Although video seems to attract most people and some people with autism can even exhibit selective attention to video, this is not always the case. The only direct research conducted in this area (Williamson et al., 2013) was carried out with three adolescents with severe autism and cognitive disabilities using VSM. Only one person showed improvement in initiating greetings. The other two had difficulty attending to the video. An anecdote from another study may provide a hint to how development might be linked to a child's ability to attend to a video (Buggey, 2012). During this study, where the goal was to encourage three typically developing 3 year olds to interact with their peers with autism, one little girl left the viewing of her video, stating, "Pretty flowers." The video was shown in a frame on the teacher's computer, which had a field of tulips as the background image. Apparently, the main memory the child had of this event was the still photo of flowers rather than the video. Interestingly, there were no observable effects on any of the children in this study, indicating that successful implementation of video modeling may require a higher level of cognitive development than exhibited by this small group of 3 year olds. Other studies conducted by the same author indicated strong positive results for children 4 and 5 years of age at the same site and targeting the same behavior (e.g., Buggey et al., 2011; Buggey et al., 2018).

THEORETICAL BASIS

Video modeling, in general, is supported by several lines of research (e.g., Dowrick, 1983; Smith et al., 2007) and theory (Bandura, 1969, 1997). Many researchers (e.g., Buggey, 2005; Hine & Wolery, 2006; Nikopoulos & Keenan, 2007) have focused on the use of video modeling with people with autism. Additional support has come from anecdotal evidence for the method provided by families who are using similar approaches to teach their children (Neumann, 2004; J. Benkert, personal communication, March 3, 2009) and from testimonials provided by people with autism. For example, the testimonial offered by Temple Grandin has had great influence in creating widespread interest in the approach. Dr. Grandin is a professor at Colorado State University in the field of animal husbandry who has autism. In her book *Thinking in Pictures*, Grandin (2006) offers at least two reasons why video modeling may be particularly effective with people with autism. The first is that video images are not socially threatening. Emotional barriers often seen in people with autism during human interactions are not necessarily present when two-dimensional video images are involved: There are no social obligations (or penalties) in the context of video characters.

A second reason Grandin offers for why video modeling may be effective involves the tendency for some people with autism to be visual- rather than language-based thinkers (Bauman, 1999; Bryan & Gast, 2000). Grandin described her thinking process as follows:

> I think in pictures. Words are like a second language to me. I translate both spoken and written words into full-color movies, complete with sound, which run like a VCR tape in my head. When somebody speaks to me, his words are instantly translated into pictures. (2006, p. 1)

If this visual mode of thinking is the case with a significant number of individuals with autism, then video modeling may present a particularly potent method of instruction.

There are several additional reasons why self-modeling might be particularly effective and appropriate for use with people with autism. The fact that the child serves as his or her own model has important implications. Bandura (1969, 1997) carried out extensive studies on the influence of specific models used. He found that the most effective models were those who had attributes that were most similar to the viewer. This included traits such as gender, age, race, and—interestingly—abilities. The best models were not the paragons of success but those who were only slightly more advanced than the observer. These findings indicate two advantages that VSM and PoV modeling may have over other forms of modeling. First, it would be impossible to find anyone more similar to the observer than the observer him- or herself. Second, and related to the first, the model would be only slightly more advanced than the observer. Even though the model and observer are the same person, the model would be pictured as more advanced in the targeted skill. In Bandura's later writings (1997), he addressed self-modeling as possibly the purest form of modeling. Following Bandura's line of logic here, it would seem that adults would serve as the weakest of the model types when children are the observers, peers would be better, and the individual him- or herself would be the best. (PoV modeling presents video from the child's eye level. While no models are actually visible, the task is seen from their perspective, possibly making PoV a form of self-modeling.). However, the research comparing others and self as models tends to demonstrate mostly comparable results (Bellini & Akullian, 2007; McCurdy & Shapiro, 1988; Schunk & Hanson, 1989). The video medium may make results across model types more equivalent to one another, but clearly this is another area in which more research is needed.

Another aspect of Bandura's research dealt with **self-efficacy,** or the confidence felt by people regarding their ability to successfully carry out a task (Bandura, 1997). A person's feeling of self-efficacy is often directly related to his or her success. Providing direct evidence of the potential for success by showing the child succeeding may have a strong impact on the person's feeling of self-efficacy. Bandura attributes self-efficacy to be a main component of behavior change.

Some research in sports physiology indicates that visually imaging performance may do more than raise feelings of self-efficacy or provide information: It may change physiology. Smith and colleagues (2007) conducted a study in which they compared five different strength-training regimens on bicep development. One group did a set of two exercises on a curl machine, one group used conventional mental imagery of arm curls, and a third group worked on the curl machine for one exercise set and watched videos of themselves doing curls for a time equivalent to that required for completion of another set (each 15 minutes). The other two groups consisted of one that used self-modeling only and another control group that neither exercised nor used self-modeling. After 6 weeks, it was found that the only groups that gained strength were the physical exercise only and the physical exercise/self-modeling groups. Particularly surprising, not only was the group that included some exercise and some self-modeling more effective than the control group and the self-modeling only group, but also, no significant difference was found between these two groups, although the combined group (VSM and exercise) gained 28% in strength and the exercise group gained 25%. Further validation needs to be done with this research, and it is ongoing; however, if the findings are replicated, it would suggest that self-modeling may facilitate changes in physiology. The fact that self-modeling alone caused no changes in strength indicates that a functional component is probably needed to promote improvement, at least when it comes to motor learning.

One last factor that should be considered is how self-modeling affects memory and how this in turn can affect habits. Kehle and his colleagues addressed this possibility after working with children with emotional disturbance (Kehle et al., 2002). They hypothesized that by having children view themselves performing positive, adaptive behaviors, this new memory would not only be implanted but also might supplant memories of the maladaptive behavior. Their findings confirmed this hypothesis. This would go a long way in explaining why behavior change is so rapid in some cases and why self-modeling has been shown to be effective in changing habitual behaviors that have been resistant to other forms of intervention. Consider a child who exhibits tantrums. The tantrum may become a habitual behavior related to a specific environmental demand (e.g., being asked to do an undesirable task, receiving negative feedback). Being able to visualize (remember) an alternative response in this context (e.g., compliance; the person saying, "I can do better") could result in the display of the new, alternative response, especially if the habitual response memory is suppressed. This is yet another area in need of further research.

The forms of modeling—self, adult, PoV, and peer—may seem roughly equivalent, with the primary difference being the person featured as the model. However, there is strong evidence that indicates that the brain processes images of self and images of others in different areas and that physiological reactions to these images are different (Kircher et al., 2000). Viewing images of oneself produces stronger galvanic skin responses and heart rates than viewing peers or strangers. This heightened physical sense may translate to higher and more sustained interest, yet there is little evidence addressing this possibility, and the stronger physiological reaction may not hold true for children with autism.

There are few limitations on what can be addressed with video modeling. If it is observable and measurable, it can be depicted in video format. Much of the research on the use of video modeling with people with autism has focused on social skills training, including recognition of emotions on faces (e.g., Akmanoglu, 2015; Golan & Baron-Cohen, 2006), expanding time engaged in play (Bellini et al., 2007; Bellini et al., 2016; Jung & Sainato, 2013), and training social language skills (e.g., Buggey, 2005; Charlop et al., 2010; Litras et al., 2010; Maione & Mirenda, 2006; Scattone, 2008; Wert & Neisworth, 2003). A somewhat smaller body of work has focused on attempts to train academic skills using video modeling (e.g., Decker & Buggey, 2014; Delano, 2007; Leach & Rodecki, 2013; Yakubova et al., 2016).

EMPIRICAL BASIS

The research base for the use of video modeling with people with autism is growing rapidly. A concise summary of recent video modeling research conducted between 2008 and 2018 is included in Tables 17.1–17.4. This is the most thorough summary to date. There are too many studies to cover in detail in this chapter, so only the most relevant research has been included here. Many of the studies include **percentage of non-overlapping data (PND)** as a measure of effect size (Scruggs et al., 1987). This statistic is designed to measure the percentage of times an individual's scores are higher during the intervention and maintenance phases of a study than the highest baseline score. This can be useful when comparing behaviors one is trying to reduce, such as tantrums or pushing. However, it can be questionable when the skills being trained are not meant to replace the original behavior. For example, when trying to teach social and/or verbal initiations, clinicians should encourage social interactions, but they should not target the elimination of solo play. Many researchers use timed intervals to record behavior to obtain a snapshot of children's activity. A child may increase his or her social interactions drastically, but if the researchers observe when the child is engaged in solo play several times, PND can drop off significantly. It is possible to see a mean improvement of 1000% and still have a PND score of 50 or lower, indicating weak or no effects of intervention. Scrugg and colleagues suggested the following ratings for PND scores: scores above 90 represented very effective treatments, scores from 70 to 90 represented effective treatments, scores from 50 to 70 were questionable, and scores below 50 were ineffective.

Table 17.1. Levels of evidence for studies of treatment efficacy for adult/peer video modeling carried out from 2008 through 2018

Level	Design type	References supporting adult/peer video modeling	References that do not support adult/peer video modeling
Ia	Meta-analysis of >1 randomized controlled trial	—	—
Ib	Randomized controlled study	—	—
IIa	Controlled study without randomization (including single case experimental designs)	Akmanoglu (2015) Akmanoglu et al. (2014) Bennett et al. (2017) Charlop et al. (2010) Dupere et al. (2013) Ergenekon (2012) Genc-Tosun & Kurt (2017) Halle et al. (2016) Jung & Sainato (2013) Kleeberger & Mirenda, (2010) Lee et al. (2014) Morlock et al. (2015) Ozen et al. (2012) Plavnick & Ferren (2011) Plavnick et al. (2015) Rex et al. (2018) Sancho et al. (2010) Scheflen et al. (2012) Smith et al. (2013) Taylor et al. (1999) Tereshko et al. (2010) Yakubova et al. (2016)	—
IIb	Quasi-experimental study	Alzyoudi et al. (2015) Hochhauser et al. (2015)	—
III	Nonexperimental studies (i.e., correlational and case studies)	—	—
IV	Expert committee report, consensus conference, clinical experience of respected authorities	—	—

Most video-modeling studies use a multiple-baseline design across persons or behaviors and are aimed at measuring effects of video-modeling methods. Results indicate nearly unanimous positive outcomes across a range of behaviors and ages. One of the difficulties in evaluating the efficacy of video modeling in some of these studies is that it is often paired with another teaching strategy, such as applied behavior analysis (ABA), prompting and cueing, or live modeling (e.g., Charlop-Christy et al., 2000; Dauphin et al., 2004; Gena et al., 2005). Consequently, although video modeling was used in all of the studies it is difficult to determine exactly what contributed to the changes reported in these studies, and it is necessary to use a critical eye when evaluating results.

Table 17.2. Levels of evidence for studies of treatment efficacy for video self-modeling carried out from 2008 through 2018

Level	Design type	References supporting video self-modeling	References that do not support video self-modeling
Ia	Meta-analysis of >1 randomized controlled trial	—	—
Ib	Randomized controlled study	—	—
IIa	Controlled study without randomization (including single case experimental designs)	Bellini et al. (2016) Boudreau & Harvey (2013) Buggey et al. (2018) Buggey et al. (2011) Burton et al. (2013) Cihak et al. (2010) Diorio et al. (2018) Kurnaz & Yanardag (2018) Lang et al. (2009) Lee et al. (2017) Litras et al. (2010) McCoy et al. (2017) O'Handley & Allen (2017) Schatz et al. (2016) Schmidt & Bonds-Raacke (2013) Smith et al. (2014) Victor et al. (2011) Williamson et al. (2013)	Buggey (2012); 3 year olds
IIb	Quasi-experimental study	Hart & Whalon (2012)	—
III	Nonexperimental studies (i.e., correlational and case studies)	Crandell & Johnson (2009)	—
IV	Expert committee report, consensus conference, clinical experience of respected authorities	—	—

Table 17.3. Levels of evidence for studies of treatment efficacy for point-of-view video modeling carried out from 2008 to 2018

Level	Design type	References supporting point-of-view video modeling	References that do not support point-of-view video modeling
Ia	Meta-analysis of >1 randomized controlled trial	—	—
Ib	Randomized controlled study	—	—
IIa	Controlled study without randomization (including single case experimental designs)	Kim (2018) Shrestha et al. (2013) Tetreault & Lerman (2010)	—
IIb	Quasi-experimental study	—	—
III	Nonexperimental studies (i.e., correlational and case studies)	—	—
IV	Expert committee report, consensus conference, clinical experience of respected authorities	—	—

Table 17.4. Summary of research that has compared two different types modeling carried out from 2008 through 2018

Level	Design type	References/types of modeling compared	Results
Ia	Meta-analysis of >1 randomized controlled trial	—	—
Ib	Randomized controlled study	—	—
IIa	Controlled study without randomization (including single case experimental designs)	Cihak & Schrader (2009)/VSM and VM (adult)	Three of the four made better progress with VSM.
		Ergenekon et al. (2014)/VM and LM	Two children made equivalent gains w/VM and LM. One did better with LM.
		Marcus & Wilder (2009)/VM and VSM	All three participants met mastery criterion in VSM condition. Only one met mastery criterion in peer-modeling condition.
		Wilson (2013)/VM and LM	No significant differences between methods
IIb	Quasi-experimental study	—	—
III	Nonexperimental studies (i.e., correlational and case studies)	—	—
IV	Expert committee report, consensus conference, clinical experience of respected authorities	—	—

Key: LM, live modeling; VM, video modeling; VSM, video self-modeling.

Another shortcoming of the research on all forms of video modeling is that most studies rely on single-participant designs that typically have between one and three participants. Despite the value of such research, relatively few children have been involved in the research; thus, information about the generalizability of these findings is limited. Despite such shortcomings, the results are encouraging. Bellini and Akullian (2007) confirmed the overall positive results achieved using video modeling. They conducted a meta-analysis of studies involving children with autism that addressed both video modeling using adults and peers and VSM. Twenty-three such studies were analyzed, 15 of which dealt with video modeling with peers and adults and 8 of which involved self-modeling. Moderate treatment effects were found for both techniques. Overall, the mean PND across all studies was 81% for peer and adult modeling and 77% for self-modeling. The difference between the modeling conditions was not statistically significant. Likewise, the results for maintenance and generalization effects in these studies were positive; yet, there were no significant differences between the modeling conditions. Consequently, Bellini and Akullian suggested that video modeling using self or others was successful in training social, language, and functional skills in children with autism. These authors also stated that both forms of video modeling met the Council for Exceptional Children's (2014) criteria for research-based practices. Finally, they cautioned that the sample size for video-modeling studies is small and that more research is needed. More recent meta-analyses studies have confirmed the results of Bellini and Akullian (e.g., Hong et al., 2016; Mason et al., 2013). Also, professional sites such as the National Autism Center at May Institute (2019) and the National Clearinghouse on Autism Evidence and Practice at the University of North Carolina at Chapel Hill (2019) have done extensive reviews of video-modeling research and concluded that all forms of video modeling represent established, evidence-based methods (Wong et al., 2015).

The following review of the research addresses video-modeling use in various formats with people on the autism spectrum.

Adult Models

Although adults, according to Bandura's theories, would not make the most ideal models, positive results have been obtained when they are depicted on video. A summary of video modeling studies used with adults and peers is shown in Table 17.1.

Charlop-Christy and Daneshvar (2003) attempted to train three boys, ages 6–9, in perspective-taking skills. They made short videos of adults simulating a perspective-taking task and showed them to the children. They used a multiple-baseline design across individuals to evaluate results. Two of the three participants made substantial improvements in their perspective taking.

In another study that examined teaching perspective-taking skills to three boys with autism, ages 7–13 years (LeBlanc et al., 2003), the authors arranged three perspective-taking tasks for the children to complete. The tasks involved puppets hiding objects (e.g., a bean) and having the children identify where a particular puppet should look for it. Clinicians used a multiple-baseline design across two tasks for evaluation purposes. The third task was not trained and served as an indicator of generalization. None of the children responded correctly to any of these tasks during baseline. Clinicians made videos of adults completing the tasks. The videos showed the models but also zoomed in on salient clues to help the child. After watching the videos, the children mastered the two trained tasks but did not transfer their skill to the untrained task. Two of the three participants needed repeated trials on the first trained task (three and four sessions) before improvement was seen. Although clinicians did not observe generalization to the selected task during the study, all three children learned it almost immediately when taught.

Another study that addressed video modeling by adults and had positive acquisition outcomes but poor generalization outcomes was conducted by D'Ateno and colleagues (2003). Both verbal and physical interaction increased in scripted play sessions (PND = 92%) following the viewing of adults modeling appropriate behaviors; however, responses in novel play situations did not change (PND = 22%). A similar outcome was found in another study that investigated scripted play sessions. MacDonald and colleagues (2005) used adult models and a multiple-baseline design across children to teach two boys, ages 4 and 7, pretend play using play scripts. The children improved at scripted play but showed no changes in other forms of play, despite that PND effect sizes for intervention and maintenance were almost 100%.

Maione and Mirenda (2006) were more successful when they used adults to model verbal initiations in social settings for a 5-year-old boy with autism. They used a multiple-baseline design across behaviors (play scenarios) for evaluation. They made videotapes of two adults playing and talking in three play scenarios. The boy then played with one of two peers known to him in the same settings and with the same materials. In two of the three activities, the boy increased his social language use. In the third activity, the video modeling alone was not effective, although gains were seen when video feedback (videos of the previous play sessions with the peer) and verbal prompting were applied.

Conversational skill was also the dependent variable in a study by Scattone (2008). The researcher used two adults to model appropriate conversation skills based on passages created using Social Stories™. The single participant, a 9-year-old child with Asperger syndrome, viewed videos of two adults interacting using social conversation skills such as eye contact, smiling, and initiations. Following introduction of the video modeling, rapid improvement was seen in eye contact and initiations in sessions with the researcher, but little gain was seen in smiling. The pairing of video modeling and Social Stories in the manner done in this study precludes analysis of the relative contribution of these two intervention methods.

Sansosti and Powell-Smith (2008) conducted a similar study involving Social Stories and computer-based modeling. They showed three children with Asperger syndrome (mild autism), ages 6–10, movies of adults modeling Social Stories that were prescribed to meet each child's individual social and communication needs. Clinicians collected data on the children's specific skill performance on the playground during recess and at other times when unstructured activities occurred. They used a multiple-baseline design across participants for evaluation purposes. The authors found that the students' rates of social communication increased following their viewing the videos; however, a social reinforcement system had to be initiated for two of the participants in order to reach criterion. A 2-week follow-up indicated that all three students maintained their increased performance.

Peers and Siblings as Models

Several studies have incorporated the use of age-similar peers and/or siblings as models. A common dependent variable in several of these studies was verbalization during play. Charlop and Milstein (1989) worked with three young children to facilitate their conversation skills using a multiple-baseline across participants design. The three individually watched videos of two other children of similar age having a conversation about toys with which they were playing. The results were positive and indicated that the new skills generalized across related situations (mean PND = 87%). Clinicians monitored the children's progress for 15 months following the end of the intervention, and children maintained all behaviors over that time (PND = 100%).

Reagon and colleagues (2006) also used a sibling as a model for a 4-year-old child with autism. In the baseline phase of this study, clinicians gave the participant and his sibling play equipment for four scenarios—cowboy, firefighter, teacher, and doctor—and told them to play without further instruction. Clinicians used a multiple baseline design across the scenarios for evaluation. They took videos of the sibling engaged in play with a typically developing peer in the same situations, then showed it to the child with autism. In play sessions in a university preschool setting, the child and sibling successfully engaged in pretend play across all four scenarios. Clinicians conducted probes in the home to test for generalization and maintenance, with positive outcomes for both. Because the baseline score was zero in all four scenarios, clinicians did not use PND in this study.

Nikopoulos and Keenan (2003) also used a peer interacting with an adult during play to create videos aimed at stimulating verbal behavior in seven children with autism (ages 9–15). The children individually watched videotapes depicting a peer interacting with one of the experimenters in a simple play activity. The results of the multiple-baseline design across participants revealed that four of the seven students increased their rate of social interaction during play. The new behavior generalized across various settings, peers, and toys and was maintained at a 2-month reevaluation session. When all students were evaluated, the effect size for the intervention stage was not strong (PND = 29%); however, maintenance and generalization had better effect sizes (PND = 80% and 100%, respectively). Nikopoulos and Keenan (2004) authored another study in which video modeling was used with three children with autism to stimulate social initiations and play behaviors. The methods used were very similar to those of the study described previously (Nikopoulos & Keenan, 2003). The authors found that all three children made gains in reciprocal play and social initiations (PND = 71% during intervention and PND = 100% during maintenance).

The authors completed a third study (Nikopoulos & Keenan, 2007) in which they tried to train more complex social initiations with three children with autism ages 6.5–7 years. Along with the video modeling, clinicians also used verbal instructions and behavior rehearsing. The results replicated the 2003 study; however, all three children made substantial gains in engagement, social initiations, and responding in this study, generating a PND effect size of greater than 80%. As in the first study, the children maintained the changes in behavior over a 2-month span.

Apple and colleagues (2005) worked with two 5-year-old children with high-functioning autism to teach compliment giving and responding. Children watched three videos with peers modeling responses to compliments and one in which the peers modeled compliment initiations. Adults narrated the video and embedded rules for giving and responding to compliments within it. The researchers found that video modeling alone was effective (PND = 71%) in training responses to compliments; however, the addition of reinforcement contingencies was needed for one of the children to produce initiations. More modest results were found for maintenance (PND = 58%).

Much of the research on video modeling deals with facilitating social skills. Little research exists that addresses academic or functional skill instruction. Haring and colleagues (1987) looked at three 20-year-old adults (two male, one female) with autism and their ability to generalize purchasing skills from a classroom environment to three stores located in the surrounding area. The participants were trained using conventional techniques and were evaluated during trips to the store. The young adults acquired the skill successfully during instruction; however, there was no evidence of generalization to the stores. The initial training was supplemented by the introduction of 1- to 3-minute peer modeling videos that illustrated a complete purchasing sequence. Following the viewing of the videos, the participants increased their purchasing skills in terms of the social interactions and the actual transactions (PND = 97% during intervention; PND =100% during maintenance).

One further study of note (Bennett et al., 2017) compared video modeling to video modeling with narration. The participants were four elementary students with ASD. The dependent variables addressed were conversational turn taking and conversational posture. Clinicians used an alternating treatment design to determine the efficacy of both methods. The students improved on both skills during both treatments; however, gains when narration was used were considerably better. The results of this study indicate the need for more research on how to maximize results for video-modeling interventions. Additions such as self-talk and self-congratulations, or the inclusion of background music, titles, credits, and so on, have not been addressed in the research to this point.

Self-Models

VSM differs from other forms of modeling in that the observer and the model are the same person. A summary of research using VSM is presented in Table 17.2. What causes self-modeling to be slightly more technologically challenging than other forms of modeling is that the models have to be seen as having more advanced skills or more appropriate behavior than they regularly demonstrate. Videos must be creatively edited so that children appear to be functioning beyond present levels or in a more adaptive manner. In the past, the editing demands of this type of modeling probably served as a deterrent to both research and practical applications. However, with the advent of user-friendly video editing software, such as iMovie for Mac and Movie Maker for PC, editing videos has become a relatively simple process. Collecting footage to use in the editing process does require some creative thinking; however, footage can be obtained by having children imitate or role-play behaviors or situations. For people with autism who do not comply with requests or demands, it might be necessary to film over time in order to capture rare behaviors or to employ peers to elicit behaviors.

Dowrick (1983) defined two forms of self-modeling: 1) feed-forward and 2) positive self-review. In the **feed-forward** method of VSM, a person is shown video of him- or herself performing a new, yet developmentally appropriate behavior. Feed-forward allows children to see themselves as they have the potential to be at some time in the future. It is hoped that this vision of the future serves as a magnet accelerating the growth toward that future skill level. It is important to be very careful not to project too far ahead so that the images represent reasonable expectations for the child.

The second form of VSM defined by Dowrick (1983) is positive self-review. This method involves watching videos of oneself to build fluency or proficiency in a skill already learned. Some top athletes like Laura Wilkinson, a U.S. gold medal winner in platform diving, use this method for training, but it has not been used in research with persons with disabilities.

VSM has been slowly growing in popularity as an intervention since the early 1970s. The use of VSM has expanded more rapidly as video-editing software has become more available and user friendly. Likewise, research into the effects of self-modeling has also accelerated, especially with children with autism.

The bulk of the research in video modeling seems aimed at some form of social skill, often in the areas of play or language use. In one of the few studies addressing academic skills (Delano, 2007), written language skills were the focus with three students ages 13, 15, and 17—all with Asperger syndrome. Specifically, the writing rate, or fluency, and the number of elements (e.g., introduction, conclusion, topic sentences) contained in an essay were measured. A multiple-baseline design across responses was used to evaluate results. Clinicians found that both number of words and number of essay elements increased for all students. All students maintained the word-writing gains as measured on follow-up probes administered 1 week and 3 months following withdrawal of the videos. However, they did not note maintenance for the essay elements.

In a study involving three adolescents with moderate to severe autism (Buggey et al., 1999), the researchers focused on teaching verbal responding during play sessions. They used a multiple-baseline across individuals to analyze results. Researchers asked a list of 10 play-related questions. Although responses were rare, with the play sessions occurring two nights a week for more than a month, researchers collected a sufficient number of responses to make 2-minute videos. All of the children increased their responses after watching videos of themselves responding appropriately and often. Analysis by question revealed that two of the participants went from never responding to a specific question during baseline to 100% responding during intervention. Because these questions did not appear in the movies, it indicated strong generalization effects. Students maintained gains for a month after the videos were withdrawn. The authors stated that the time commitment for capturing rare behaviors might make this form of VSM too cumbersome for teachers and therapists and suggested that direct question/answer sessions conducted by multiple individuals, including parents and siblings may be more appropriate.

Diorio and colleagues (2018) investigated whether VSM could be used to increase compliance to requests in a classroom using a multiple-baseline design across participants. Three children with ASD, ages 5, 6, and 9, served as participants in the study. These children were selected because of compliance issues they were having in the classroom. All three children exhibited increased compliance following viewing their videos. Social validity analysis revealed that teachers and assistants believed that VSM was workable and desirable in school situations.

An area that has received much attention in the research has been using VSM to work with preschoolers with autism. The author of this chapter conducted several studies with preschoolers who ranged in age from 3.5 to 5 years old. One study involved a boy with autism who had just turned 4 (Buggey, 2005). A multiple-baseline design across three behaviors, namely, pushing, verbal responding, and initiating conversation without prompting, was used in this study. The pushing behavior virtually ceased following the student viewing a tape showing positive interactions and appropriate touching. The two language behaviors also showed significant improvement following viewing of the tapes. The PND for each of the behaviors was 88% for pushing, 90% for responding, and 100% for verbal initiations. The language movies were created by filming individual words spoken by the child and editing them into multiword sentences.

Buggey and colleagues (2018) conducted a study with four preschoolers, three with autism and one with Down syndrome, to determine if social initiations could be facilitated using VSM. The 4 year olds had not responded to Social Stories and a buddy system introduced in their classrooms aimed at promoting social interactions. Clinicians took the participants, along with one or two peers, to the playground for filming. They coached and prompted the peers to interact with the children with autism during filming. They extracted segments of the video illustrating the best examples of social interactions and combined them into 3-minute videos. The children watched their movies in the morning for five successive days, and data were recorded when they went onto the playground about an hour later. Clinicians used a multiple-baseline design across individuals to determine results. Three of the four children made substantial gains in social initiations with peers, and two displayed a variety of new behaviors such as swinging, sliding, and verbalizing to adults. One child exhibited no gains, although he watched his videos with enthusiasm. This child was slightly younger than the others, raising the question of whether age or maturity was a critical factor in this case. The age at which self-modeling begins to be effective is unknown. Although the effect of age is likely to depend on a child's development and type of disability, very little is known about the effect of VSM with children under age 4.

Wert and Neisworth (2003) used VSM to teach spontaneous requesting in four preschoolers with autism. They used a multiple-baseline design across children to evaluate results. They trained the children to request items via a discrete trial method; however, the resulting requests were rote, and there was no generalization to spontaneous requesting. The prompted requests were included in the VSM tapes with the prompts and any negative behaviors edited out. Results for all four participants showed substantial gains. The gains in mean production of spontaneous requests ranged from 800% to 1,200%.

In another study that examined the effect of VSM in preschoolers with ASD, Bellini and colleagues (2007) addressed social engagement skills with the children while simultaneously evaluating teachers' ability to implement the intervention. The two 4 year olds in the study had sufficient social skills to establish a baseline and to permit direct filming of the children at play without any undue manipulation of events. Clinicians cut and pasted scenes of the children engaged in play into 2-minute videos. The dependent variable in this study was the percentage of time the children spent engaged in play with others. The children watched the videos in a private setting just before free-play time and then returned to the classroom to play. The results indicated a steep increase in the percentage of time the children spent engaged in play. The teachers found VSM to be easy to implement and reported little disruption to regular classroom routines. Measures of maintenance over several weeks indicated that engagement did not decrease over time.

In a similar study addressing social engagement with preschoolers Bellini and colleagues (2016) worked with three boys with ASD, between the ages of 4 and 5, to increase social engagement time. Two of the children had extremely limited engagement time during baseline, while the other had shown a severe drop in engagement when his preferred play partner transferred from the school. After watching VSM videos showing the participants playing with peers, their engagement time increased rapidly and strongly. A peer-training component was added following the intervention phase but was shown to be ineffective. The gains made were maintained across participants over a 2-week period.

Most of the preschool studies addressing social skills were carried out with children ages 4 and 5 years. Those including children with ASD younger than 4 showed mixed results (Clark et al., 1993) or no gains (Buggey, 2012). There seems to be a lack of development related to the behaviors selected or a problem with the research methodology that works against successful use of VSM with children under 4 years of age in the area of social skills training.

Point-of-View Modeling

There is a form of video modeling that is just beginning to be researched. PoV modeling takes people through a task as seen from their vantage point. This is accomplished by holding the camera at the eye level of the observer and navigating through a task. This method is related to self-modeling; however, it differs in that the children never see themselves. Rather, they must imagine that what they are seeing is viewed from their vantage point. This requirement may negate some of the positive aspects of self-modeling addressed previously regarding self-efficacy and the excitement generated from seeing oneself as the star of a video.

PoV modeling does have the advantage of not requiring the model to be manipulated and filmed. This advantage would be very useful when working with children who do not readily imitate. Hine and Wolery (2006) used this method to teach toy-play skills to two young girls with autism. The ages of the children were 30 and 43 months, making them some of the youngest to participate in a video-modeling study. Researchers chose gardening and cooking tasks as the dependent variables. They broke these down into six and five action steps, respectively, and the evaluation consisted of determining how many of the steps were exhibited during observation sessions. They used a multiple-probe single case experimental design to evaluate results. The children showed considerable improvement in the number of actions during each play session, except for the second child on the cooking task. Here, prompting and reinforcement were subsequently used, and results improved to the level of the other child.

Schreibman and colleagues (2000) used what they termed "video priming" to facilitate appropriate transition behaviors with three children with autism who were described as being severely disruptive during transitions. In video priming, children were shown PoV movies of task-analyzed transitions prior to similar transitions taking place. Researchers used a multiple-baseline design across the participants to evaluate results. The authors reported that, following the viewing of videos, the students' disruptive behaviors were significantly reduced or completely eliminated. Researchers observed and evaluated transitions other than those depicted in the video, and the improvement in behavior had generalized across situations.

Kim (2018) used PoV modeling to teach three male adolescents with autism gardening skills (i.e., weeding and watering) using a multiple-probe design across participants. It was shown to be effective in training both on-task behavior and independent task performance. For example, watering skills increased dramatically for all three: Participant 1, mean of 5% baseline to 90% during intervention and maintenance with a PND of 92%; Participant 2, >1% baseline to 90% during intervention and maintenance with a PND of 97%; and Participant 3, 0% baseline to 65% during intervention and maintenance with a PND of 100%. Gains in weeding were similar. In addition, the new skills maintained after instruction for 1 month and generalized to similar skills.

The only other study that addressed children with autism using PoV modeling was carried out by Shipley-Benamou and colleagues (2002) to teach functional living skills to three 5-year-old children with autism. Clinicians showed the children PoV videos related to community outings that had proven difficult for them in the past, including trips to the mall, pharmacy, and grocery store. They included verbal instruction at the beginning of the video. Only the hands of the individual filming were visible. Clinicians directed the children to watch what their "friends" were doing. In addition, clinicians placed a short clip of the child's favorite cartoon at the front of the video to attract attention. The authors concluded that this form of video modeling was effective in promoting the acquisition of the target skills, which were maintained upon withdrawal of videos and at a 1-month follow-up assessment.

Because of the ease of filming and the minimal editing necessary using PoV modeling, this method warrants additional research. It would also seem to warrant trials with children with autism at school, home, and in a clinical setting. Most applications of video modeling have potential to achieve gains in targeted behavior with little chance of adverse results if no behavior change is realized.

Comparison Studies

It is somewhat surprising that there is not more research comparing modeling formats. In one of the only such studies, Sherer and colleagues (2001) attempted to compare peer and self-modeling strategies with five children with autism between 4 and 11 years of age. The dependent variable was responding to a series of verbal questions. A combination of multiple-baseline and alternating treatment designs was used for the evaluation. Three of the five children reached 100% accuracy on the task, while the other two children exhibited very limited improvement. When the rate of acquisition was evaluated across methods, it was determined that there were no differences between self- and peer modeling. The authors stated that the three children who made the greatest gains were those considered to be strong visual learners.

Marcus and Wilder (2009) also compared peer and self-modeling with three young children with autism, ages 4, 9, and 9. They used a combination multiple-baseline design and multielement design to compare the two types of video modeling. Their target task was the identification novel alphabet letters. They found that all three children met criterion of 80% correct identification under the VSM condition, whereas only one was successful with peer modeling. The participant who met criterion using peer modeling took longer than the others to meet criterion.

In the only other study comparing two video modeling procedures, Gena and colleagues (2005) sought to compare the effects of peer video modeling with traditional teacher modeling in training affective skills with three preschoolers (ages 3; 11, 4;4, and 5;7) with autism. The two methods were supplemented with verbal praise and tokens for correct responding and a correction protocol that differed between treatments. The in vivo (live) modeling required a therapist to model the correct behavior and issue verbal prompts. The video-modeling procedure made use of videos of peers exhibiting the correct response and of therapist prompts. Researchers used a multiple-baseline design across participants for evaluation purposes. The researchers found that both treatment methods were equally well suited for promoting affective responses and that these results generalized to different situations and across people.

Charlop-Christy and colleagues (2000) attempted to compare video modeling to live modeling in teaching functional, social, and language skills to five children with ASD. They chose targeted behaviors on the basis of each child's needs. A multiple-baseline design across participants and within participants across behaviors addressed the two conditions. The authors found that the behaviors taught using video modeling were acquired more rapidly and that these learned behaviors generalized across similar conditions (as measured on specific generalization probes). Generalization did not occur with the live models. The PND rate for video modeling was 82% for intervention and 100% for generalization. The dearth of comparative studies shows there is still much to learn about the relative efficacy across these methods.

PRACTICAL REQUIREMENTS

The practical requirements needed to implement video modeling have changed drastically since its first use in the early 1970s. In the early 1990s when this author began research using video, tape-to-tape splicing using cumbersome equipment was needed to produce movies of sometimes dubious quality. Then came VHS, camcorders, computer-editing software, and now, tablets and cellphones that provide everything necessary to film, edit, and view videos in one user-friendly platform. Thus, the equipment needed to create and edit videos is now accessible to the majority of the population. The time needed to create all forms of video modeling has also improved greatly. The manual technical skills needed have been reduced to finger swipes and touch and drag on phones and tablets. Online resources such as YouTube, Instagram, and Facebook allow for instant sharing of videos to the public or to private users.

The most time-consuming aspect of video modeling is now the planning and filming process. Video modeling also requires accurate, coordinated communication among schools, therapists, and caregivers. Because teachers have relatively less planning time throughout the day, the coordination of video-modeling activities might best be carried out by therapists or school guidance counselors (although busy, they may have more flexibility in scheduling). Caregivers in the home may also have the necessary time if they are provided training.

Careful attention needs to be paid to school district and clinic rules regarding the filming of students. Likewise, parents need to be assured that videos will be handled with utmost care and with the highest ethical standards in place. This is why coordination and communication are so important.

Because of the ease of use of video modeling, it can be easily mastered by parents, teachers, and clinicians. However, it is important to include professionals with knowledge of child development in planning, especially with the selection of developmentally appropriate behaviors. Video modeling will not be effective if the chosen behavior it too advanced for the individual. A professional experienced with video modeling should also be available for training in the methods and data collection techniques.

KEY COMPONENTS

The possible behaviors that can be addressed with video modeling are almost limitless. Any skills or behaviors that are observable can be addressed through video modeling. Of course, if the person will not or cannot attend to a video, video modeling will not be effective. The following steps could be used for creation of a movie for modeling:

1. *Select the behavior:* This should be done with all caregivers, especially parents and the participant when appropriate. We often ask parents for the behavior they would most like to see change.

2. *Define the behavior:* Make sure that the behavior is observable and easy to evaluate.

3. *Determine evaluation method and who will be recording progress:* A simple form for recording occurrences or timing of events can be used (a sample duration form is provided in Figure 17.1).

4. *Observe behavior to determine baseline rates or durations:* It is best to use multiple observers and then compare, discuss, and collate forms for accuracy.

Duration Data Form

Child _____ Dates: from_____to _____

Observer _____

Specific behavior: _____

_____

_____

Monday	Tuesday	Wednesday	Thursday	Friday
Date: _____	Date: _____	Date: _____	Date: _____	Date: _____
Start: End: Duration	Start: End: Duration	Start: End: Duration	Start: End: Duration	Start: End: Duration
Start: End: Duration	Start: End: Duration	Start: End: Duration	Start: End: Duration	Start: End: Duration
Start: End: Duration	Start: End: Duration	Start: End: Duration	Start: End: Duration	Start: End: Duration
Start: End: Duration	Start: End: Duration	Start: End: Duration	Start: End: Duration	Start: End: Duration
Start: End: Duration	Start: End: Duration	Start: End: Duration	Start: End: Duration	Start: End: Duration
Start: End: Duration	Start: End: Duration	Start: End: Duration	Start: End: Duration	Start: End: Duration
Start: End: Duration	Start: End: Duration	Start: End: Duration	Start: End: Duration	Start: End: Duration
Daily events _____	Daily events _____	Daily events _____	Daily events _____	Daily events _____
Total duration_____ min.	Total duration_____ min.	Total duration_____ min.	Total duration_____ min.	Total duration_____ min.
Average duration____ min.	Average duration____ min.	Average duration____ min.	Average duration____ min.	Average duration____ min.

Weekly total events: _____

Weekly total time: _____

Figure 17.1. Duration of behaviors form for data collection.

5. *Plan the video:* Choose the main elements to include in the video—location, participants, time, and scenes if more than one. A storyboard can be helpful, as shown in Figure 17.2.

6. *Film:* Capture as much footage as possible. It is easy to delete unwanted content.

7. *Edit:* Use editing software to download the video and remove unwanted content. Remember to include only footage that appropriately illustrates the desired behavior. Reduce the length of the video to approximately 2–3 minutes (Dowrick, 1983).

8. *View:* Select a safe, secluded spot for viewing that will have limited distractions.

9. *Ongoing evaluation:* Watch for positive changes in behavior. If not successful, examine the video to see if there are changes that could be made or whether the desired target behavior is clear to the viewer. If successful, watch for other positive changes in related behavior. Move on to another behavior.

Skills typically taught or learned in sequences, such as math computation, can be addressed by a sequence of videos. PoV modeling could be especially useful to instruct viewers on all newly introduced arithmetic computations. Self-modeling would be particularly useful in teaching morphemes a child has not used or mastered

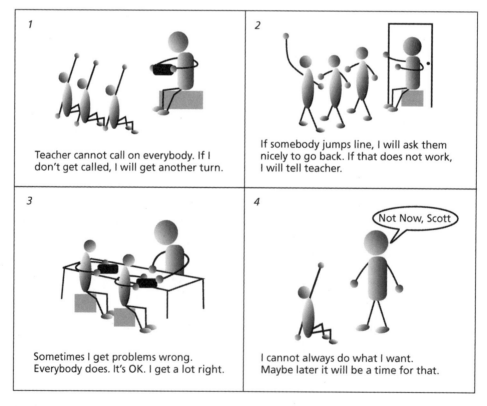

Figure 17.2. Storyboard for Scott's movie of good behavior. Text under the frames is for the child's self-narration that occurs after each scene.

but are deemed developmentally appropriate. Simply film the child imitating words with the desired morphemes, and combine these into a short movie.

Maladaptive social skills can be addressed in similar manner. A child with multiple behavior challenges could be shown video models of people performing adaptive behaviors in situations that typically trigger his or her negative ones. If the child can role-play these situations, the child can once again serve as his or her own model. Because of the dearth of research, it is not known whether children would reach a saturation point with these videos beyond which the method was ineffective nor whether the novelty of the intervention (especially VSM) wears thin.

ASSESSMENT FOR TREATMENT PLANNING AND PROGRESS MONITORING

Data collection for video modeling interventions should follow the same format as that used in single-participant designs (Kazdin, 1982) and curriculum-based measurements (Salvia & Hughes, 1990). Both of these types of data collection require the establishment of baseline rates or durations of behaviors, tracking these rates or durations through the intervention phase, and monitoring maintenance. This type of data collection is also often used with functional behavioral assessments, with various members of a team recording data to establish baselines, and with some team members carrying through with data collection to measure the efficacy of intervention. If this process of data collection is already in place, it would be sufficient to measure the impact of the video modeling intervention. Graphic representations can provide visual evidence of the effect and communicate progress to other stakeholders. In curriculum-based measurement, the child is often tasked with charting progress. This would be unacceptable in a research project, because one would be trying to control the variables that might be affecting behavior; however, it might serve as an effective supplement in practical applications. Clinicians should be aware at all times of other variables that might be affecting behavior, such as medical issues, the presence of other instruction, and changes in environmental conditions, so that these factors can be considered during data interpretation.

Parents can be instrumental in data collection and may need to be the primary recorders if intervention is carried out in the home. If the intervention is carried out at school, the parents can still collect data to determine whether effects are generalizing across settings.

To summarize, measure the pretreatment behavior in terms of duration (e.g., length of tantrum) or rate (e.g., number of pushes in a 30-minute period), compare this measure to the behavior after beginning treatment, and measure behavior occasionally once treatment is completed to determine if it is maintaining. The key measures will occur during intervention. Changes in behavior are typically seen early during intervention, so the efficacy of the videos can readily be determined. Check the video for possible edits if changes in behavior are not seen. If this still does not improve behavior, stop the intervention. Children who show interest in the videos typically do well with video-modeling interventions, but there are always exceptions.

IMPLICATIONS FOR INCLUSIVE PRACTICE

Acceptance of children with autism within general education programs can be complicated for several reasons. First, by definition, children with autism have some form of problem with socialization (American Psychiatric Association, 2013).

Second, they must also exhibit some form of repetitive behavior that would be different than is typical among children. Third, there is no apparent evidence that the child with autism has a disability. Thus, children with autism will often need additional supports and transitional plans for entering the general education setting (Crosland & Dunlap, 2012).

All types of video modeling can be applied to make the inclusion of a child on the autism spectrum successful. The first step of this process is for educators and parents to meet to determine what behaviors may be most problematic for inclusion and to determine how to communicate the child's differences to the peers. Certainly, if the child exhibits aggressive behaviors, these should be addressed first. Any direct threats or violent behaviors demonstrated within classrooms can be terms for dismissal or reassignment (Center for Parent Information and Resources, 2017). As stated previously in this chapter, all forms of video modeling may be useful in moderating the potentially dangerous behaviors. On the other hand, it is best to ignore repetitive behaviors such as hand flapping because such behaviors may represent an important coping mechanism for the person with autism. This should be explained to peers so that they expect it to occur and know how to respond (or not respond). The main goal of using video modeling would be to decrease negative behaviors and/or find suitable replacement behaviors to make inclusion easier using methods explained elsewhere in this chapter.

Video-modeling techniques can also be used as needed once the child is present in the inclusive setting and new obstacles are experienced. Teachers in Australia reported successful results for using video modeling for priming children for transitions (A. Naylor, personal communication, May 2019). Priming involved showing a 20-second clip of the children in the upcoming environment or activity prior to transitioning. Transitions can be particularly problematic for most children but especially for those on the autism spectrum. Reports from teachers indicated that the priming solved many problems related to transitions, saving valuable instructional time.

CONSIDERATIONS FOR CHILDREN FROM CULTURALLY AND LINGUISTICALLY DIVERSE BACKGROUNDS

Because sensitivity to cultural and language diversity is almost inherent in video modeling, little adaptation should be necessary. This is especially true with self-modeling, for the obvious reason that the child serves as his or her own model. For peer or adult modeling, it will be necessary to choose models who are as close as possible to the observer in terms of culture and language. This approach not only is sensitive to cultural diversity but aligns with Bandura's (1969) findings on who makes the best models. Clinicians should also take into account cultures where direct eye contact is not acceptable in general, is not appropriate across social classes, or is not recommended across generations (Uono & Hietanen, 2015). This chapter cannot go into great detail about eye-gaze norms across cultures. Suffice it to say that differences do exist, and clinicians working with individuals from another culture should be aware of social-interaction nuances that do exist. This would be important if the video modeling required direct eye contact, such as in a PoV job interview. Interestingly, there is little research into how cultural mores related to social interaction translate to viewing videos. Also note that in the Amish communities of North America, photography of individuals is prohibited, as photographs and video recordings are seen as graven images. The bottom line is that practitioners should consult with parents and receive informed consent prior to any attempts to use visual imagery.

Application to a Child

In this case example, self-modeling was chosen as the intervention to provide an example of video modeling in its most complex context. Scott, who is 8 years old, was diagnosed with Asperger syndrome by school district personnel at the age of 5. Scott perseverated on some tasks and tended to be distractible and sometimes disruptive during academics. He was an avid *Star Trek* fan and could talk about any of the episodes. He often tried to steer conversation to *Star Trek*. The principal arranged a meeting with Scott's parents to find a solution to one of his disruptive behaviors. Scott's parents and teachers noted tantrums, which occurred both at school and home when he was faced with criticism and frustration, as his most serious challenge. This disruptive behavior often took the form of loud and lengthy tantrums in which he would flail his arms and legs. These full-blown episodes could last for half an hour, followed by pouting that lasted up to half a school day. There was a progression of escalating behaviors, or warning, prior to the tantrum beginning, which consisted of Scott folding his arms and looking downward. A behavior modification plan to address this challenging behavior was practiced at home and school for several months with little effect.

The team agreed to collaborate in carrying out a functional behavioral assessment (FBA) to determine exactly what triggered the tantrums and to make some hypotheses regarding why they occurred. This assessment was to precede the development of a positive behavioral support plan. All members of the team were charged with collecting data on the tantrums, including time of onset, duration, and environmental antecedents that might be related to the behavior. After a week of observation, the team members met again to review the results. The team decided to focus first on school-specific behavior and, if improvements were seen, to then turn their attention to the home. Several specific events were found to trigger Scott's tantrums in school: 1) not being called on when he knew an answer, 2) another child jumping in line, 3) missing items on his homework or on seatwork when working in small groups, and 4) not receiving permission to do something when he asked. These four situations were depicted in a **storyboard** composed with the cooperation of Scott, who was told that he would be starring in a movie about good behavior. The four frames of the storyboard (illustrated in Figure 17.2) would serve as the scenes in the movie.

Two of Scott's classmates were asked to costar in the movie. For the filming of the video, the students and their teacher came to the classroom while their classmates were at the library. The guidance counselor, who was trained in VSM, served as the producer and cameraperson. The students and teacher followed the storyboard and were given lines and direction by the counselor. Similarly, Scott was fed a line to say concerning each situation. Everyone enjoyed the filming, although at one point Scott began his tantrum aura. When he was reminded that they were making a movie, he stopped. The teacher and counselor collaborated in making the movie using the Apple iMovie software. The footage was downloaded from the camera into iMovie. Because role playing had been used, little editing was needed. Transitions were put in between the scenes, and a still frame showing Scott smiling and raising his hand was added to the beginning. The counselor added her own voice, labeling the behavior ("Here's Scott's movie. Let's watch Scott handle these tough situations"). This introduction was followed by children cheering (a sound clip included in the iMovie software). The same cheering was added to the end of the movie, along with the counselor saying, "Good job, Scott!"

Because Scott was participating in a study, there was a delay before he was allowed to watch the video so that it could be determined if the role playing and filming had any effect on behavior. Scott averaged about 20 minutes per day in tantrums prior to watching his video. Following his first viewing of the tape, which took place upon his arrival at school and before classes began, he never had another tantrum during that school year—a follow-up period of 6 months. Interestingly, he did begin his tantrum aura on several occasions, but in each of these instances, he seemed to control himself and stopped short of a tantrum. According to Scott's teacher, "I've never used the term *life-changing* about any type of treatment or instruction.. until now. It hit me at the end of the day after he started watching his tape: No tantrums today . . . hmm. The second day, I was quietly shouting for joy."

Application to an Adult

Video modeling is also an appropriate intervention strategy for an adult with ASD. Sara was a 19 year old with more severe autism. She used picture symbols for most of her communication. She was verbal, but most of her expressive language was echolalic. She was being educated in functional life skills as part of her transition plan. One of her objectives was to learn how to perform at a job interview. Sara's teacher and parents decided to use a peer-modeling video to train this skill. One of Sara's classmates who was typically developing served as the model, and a teacher at the school served as the interviewer. The interview was task-analyzed and broken down into eight steps, including preparation (grooming and dressing), greetings, choosing appropriate picture symbols, and farewell. The classmate and interviewer were filmed in an office at school. She was also prompted during the filming on what picture symbols to use for each scripted question. Sara watched the movie upon returning home from school. She was also allowed to watch it if she indicated a desire to do so.

After 3 days of watching the video, Sara had her first interview. Sara's classmate sat behind her and was told that she could prompt her if she ran into difficulty. The first interview required two prompts by the classmate regarding the proper picture symbols. An additional interview was conducted every 3 days with the same interviewer until no prompts were needed (three interviews). A fourth interview was conducted with a different interviewer who asked two additional questions. Sara needed no prompts during this interview. Sara enjoyed the video and watching her friend and continued requesting to view the video for several weeks. After she lost interest in the video and stopped viewing it. Sara's parents decided to try video modeling to address other skills.

To review an extended application and implementation of this intervention, see Case 14 about a child with moderate to severe ASD in the companion volume *Case Studies for the Treatment of Autism Spectrum Disorder.*

Future Directions

Video modeling in all its forms has great potential for use with children with autism and other developmental disabilities. It is a ripe area for research because there is still much researchers do not know about the method and its applications. For example, when in a child's development does video modeling emerge as an effective strategy, and when does video modeling become developmentally appropriate across different skills and behaviors? What are the barriers to video modeling being implemented in real-life settings? (In particular, more information about the social validity of video modeling is needed.) What are the differences among the video modeling categories in terms of efficacy, and are there certain populations who would benefit more from a particular form of video modeling? These questions and many others remain unanswered. As awareness of video modeling grows and as people become more familiar with the technology needed for implementation, it will be receiving more attention in the research community and will be coming into more mainstream use by professionals and parents.

New technologies like virtual reality (VR) provide a three-dimensional world with the capacity to add interaction through the use of hand movement add-ons. This provides PoV modeling that could be used in training many social and functional skills. However, the software needed is just beginning to be developed, and the ability to create VR movies is not readily available to consumers. Good VR cameras with six or more lenses presently cost in the tens of thousands of dollars, but like most new technology, prices may drop significantly in the future.

Video modeling has the potential to be used with many viewers simultaneously. Sarah Spence and Anthea Naylor (2009, personal communication), working in the Victoria, Australia, Schools, have begun a TV channel called MeTV that is broadcast districtwide. These educators use self-modeling videos extensively in their own school for children with special needs. After gaining parent permission, they use videos with wide applicability, such as following school rules, manners, and other social skills as peer-modeling videos in their broadcasts. Students are also involved in production and serve as hosts for shows. The channel has been picked up by other districts in Australia and is now in use across the state of Victoria.

Overall, the advances in technology that can be applied to video modeling are developing so fast that it is hard to imagine what possibilities the future holds. As an example, during my research on self-modeling, I always wondered how VSM could be packaged to reach a larger population rather than one child at a time. I had no answers. However, I was contacted by Lois Brady (personal communication), a speech-language pathologist who had developed a product called INNERVOICE. She saw an application that used mouth and eye replacement to create funny videos of users on which you could dub in sound and voice. She recognized the potential for her clients and created an augmentative and alternative communication (ACC) device that featured the client as his or her own avatar. It looks like a typical ACC device; however, the clients speak for themselves through their voices or the voices of others who provide the audio. The lips and eyes move in conjunction with the words, and it looks very natural. Only a photo is needed, and the application animates the head to produce a three-dimensional view of the person. People can choose their own photo, or they can use someone famous, an animal or pet, or family member as their avatar. Thus, INNERVOICE can be used for self-modeling, peer modeling, and something entirely original: net-modeling. In 2019, artificial intelligence was added to this product, making voice and images even more accurate.

Other researchers in the field of occupational therapy have used cell phones containing video modeling movies to serve as prompts and refreshers for training and maintaining functional skills for youth (Campbell et al., 2015). The portability of the devices makes them easy to carry and use in locations where the skill is applied in natural settings.

The future holds many surprises, and researchers, with input from users, will continue to expand applications and technology for the use of video modeling for persons with autism.

Suggested Readings

1. Dittoe, C., & Bridgeman, H. (2017). *Show me: A teacher's guide to video modeling.* AAPC Publishing. This award-winning book provides an overview of video-modeling techniques and a step-by-step guide for implementing video modeling in the classroom.

2. Buggey, T. (2009). *Seeing is believing: Video self-modeling for people with autism and other developmental disabilities.* Woodbine House. This 200-page how-to book is presently out of print but can be found online in various locations in a PDF version for free. It is a good introduction to self-modeling but does not contain information on the use of cell phones and tablets.

3. National Professional Development Center on Autism Spectrum Disorder. (n.d.). *Evidence-based practice brief: Video modeling.* https://autismpdc.fpg.unc.edu/evidence-based-practices. This brief focuses on peer video modeling and presents useful resources, including research by age levels and checklists for evaluation and implementation.

4. Wilson, K. P. (2013). Incorporating video modeling into a school-based intervention for students with autism spectrum disorders. *Language, Speech, and Hearing Services in Schools, 44,* 105–117. Kaitlyn Wilson provides a tutorial on implementing video modeling for SLPs in school settings. She uses reviews and meta-analyses of the research in compiling a list of steps for implementation that includes preparation, creating the videos, showing the movies, monitoring progress, and designing next steps. This article is available in PDF format from ASHA.org.

Learning Activities

1. *Play and experiment with video editing software.* Basic programs like iMovie and MovieMaker are more than sufficient for creating a good video. Deleting unwanted video is the most used editing tool, and this task is easily mastered. On most phone or tablet apps, it is often done by swiping the section with a finger, touching the footage to be deleted, and pressing delete. Practice making a 3-minute music video of a vacation or reunion. Note that you will not lose any of the original footage when creating a new movie.

2. *Gauge interest and abilities of children.* Arrange a situation in which a child can observe videos of children playing. Make sure it is not disrupting an activity in which the child is presently engaged. Note how much time the child can sus-

tain attention. This will give a general indication of whether the child can attend to a 2- to 3-minute video. Also, interact with the child to determine whether he or she can 1) imitate, 2) role-play a situation, and/or 3) follow simple directions. This information will be helpful to determine what type of techniques can be used for collecting footage for a VSM movie.

3. *Familiarize children to the camera.* Use it in the classroom for other activities, like making a movie of art projects. Remember to follow school or agency policies on confidentiality and get informed consent from parents even when taking pictures of student work.

4. *Begin to create a library of PoV movies.* Because only the hands and arms should be visible in this type of modeling, you can serve as a model. You can also choose a peer who would have more age-appropriate hand size. A good way to begin would be by creating short videos depicting sequential arithmetic operations. These can be used to introduce new concepts to the class and thus not single out the person with autism. You could also create a video on classroom rules or steps in the transition process (e.g., pick up books, push in chair, line up, walk to next class, put books under chair, and sit down).

Summary of Video Clip

*See the **About the Videos and Downloads** page at the front of the book for directions on how to access and stream the accompanying video to this chapter.*

The video clip associated with this chapter stars Lillian, a 4 year old with ASD. The target behavior for her is social initiations on the playground. The beginning of the video is raw footage from the filming. Lillian can be seen playing on the playground. Three peers are also on the playground and act as costars in the movie. Lillian can be clearly seen having difficulty with social skills, and teachers and therapists can be clearly heard prompting peers to interact with Lillian. This footage is provided for contrast to the finished video. The self-modeling video viewed by Lillian begins with the music overlay and the title *Lillian's Movie.* The footage was clearly edited to make it appear that Lillian is actively and enthusiastically engaged in play, and adult prompting was removed.

REFERENCES

Akmanoglu, N. (2015). Effectiveness of teaching naming facial expression to children with autism via video modeling. *Educational Sciences: Theory and Practice, 15*, 519–537.

Akmanoglu, N., Yanardag, M., & Batu, E. (2014). Comparing video modeling and graduated guidance together and video modeling alone for teaching role playing skills to children with autism. *Education and Training in Autism and Developmental Disabilities, 49*(1), 17–31.

Alzyoudi, M., Sartawi, A. A., & Almuhiri, O. (2015). The impact of video modelling on improving social skills in children with autism. *British Journal of Special Education, 42*, 53–68.

American Psychiatric Association. (2013). *Diagnostic and statistical manual of mental disorders, fifth edition.* Author.

Apple, A. L., Billingsley, F., Schwartz, I. S., & Carr, E. G. (2005). Effects of video modeling alone and with self-management on compliment-giving behaviors of children with high-functioning ASD. *Journal of Positive Behavior Interventions, 7*(1), 33–46.

Bandura, A. (1969). *Principles of behavior modification.* Holt, Rinehart & Winston.

Bandura, A. (1997). *Self-efficacy: The exercise of control*. Freeman.

Bauman, M. L. (1999). Autism: Clinical features and neurobiological observations. In H. Tager-Flusberg (Ed.), *Neurodevelopmental disorders* (pp. 383–399). MIT Press.

Bellini, S., & Akullian, J. (2007). A meta-analysis of video modeling and video self-modeling interventions for children and adolescents with autism spectrum disorders. *Exceptional Children, 73*, 261–284.

Bellini, S., Akullian, J., & Hopf, A. (2007). Increasing social engagement in young children with autism spectrum disorders using video self-modeling. *School Psychology Review, 36*, 80–90.

Bellini, S., Gardner, L., Hudock, R., & Kashima-Ellingson, Y. (2016). The use of video self-modeling and peer training to increase social engagement in preschool children on the autism spectrum. *School Psychology Forum: Research to Practice, 10*, 207–209.

Bennett, K. D., Crocco, C., Loughrey, T. O., & McDowell, L. S. (2017). Effects of video prompting without voice-over narration among students with autism spectrum disorder. *Behavioral Development Bulletin, 22*(1), 147–158.

Boudreau, J., & Harvey, M. T. (2013). Increasing recreational initiations for children who have ASD using video self-modeling. *Education and Treatment of Children, 36*, 49–60.

Bryan, L. C., & Gast, D. L. (2000). Teaching on-task and on-schedule behaviors to high-functioning children with autism via picture activity schedules. *Journal of Autism and Developmental Disorders, 30*(6), 553–567.

Buggey, T. (2005). Applications of video self-modeling with children with autism in a small private school. *Focus on Autism and Other Developmental Disabilities, 20*, 180–204.

Buggey, T. (2009). *Seeing is believing: Self-modeling applications with children with autism and other developmental disabilities*. Woodbine House.

Buggey, T. (2012). Effectiveness of video self-modeling to promote social initiations by 3-year-olds with autism spectrum disorders. *Focus on Autism and Other Developmental Disabilities, 27*(2), 102–110.

Buggey, T., Crawford, C., & Rogers, C. L. (2018). Self-modeling to promote social initiations with young children with developmental disabilities. *Focus on Autism and Other Developmental Disabilities, 33*(2), 111–119.

Buggey, T., Hoomes, G., Sherberger, M. E., & Williams, S. (2011). Facilitating social initiations of preschoolers with autism spectrum disorders using video self-modeling. *Focus on Autism and Other Developmental Disabilities, 26*(1), 25–36.

Buggey, T., Toombs, K., Gardner, P., & Cervetti, M. (1999). Self-modeling as a technique to train response behaviors in children with autism. *Journal of Positive Behavior Intervention, 1*, 205–214.

Buggey, T. & Grove, V. (2014). The Minnesota Project VSM use in Early Intervention. The Division of Early Childhood (DEC) Annual Conference. Oct. 8, St. Louis, Mo.

Burton, C. E., Anderson, D. H., Prater, M. A., & Dyches, T. T. (2013). Video self-modeling on an iPad to teach functional math skills to adolescents with autism and intellectual disability. *Focus on Autism and Other Developmental Disabilities, 28*(2), 67–77.

Campbell, J. E., Morgan, M., Barnett, V., & Spreat, S. (2015). Handheld devices and video modeling to enhance the learning of self-help skills in adolescents with autism spectrum disorder. *OTJR: Occupation, Participation & Health, 35*(2), 95–100.

Carmody, D. P., & Lewis, M. (2011). Self-representation in children with and without autism spectrum disorders. *Child Psychiatry and Human Development, 43*, 227–237.

Center for Parent Information and Resources. (2017). Placement and school discipline. https://www.parentcenterhub.org/disciplineplacements

Charlop, M. H., & Milstein, J. P. (1989). Teaching autistic children conversational speech using video modeling. *Journal of Applied Behavior Analysis, 22*(3), 275–285.

Charlop, M. H., Dennis, B., Carpenter, M. H., & Greenberg, A. L. (2010). Teaching socially expressive behaviors to children with autism through video modeling. *Education & Treatment of Children, 33*, 371–393.

Charlop-Christy, M., & Daneshvar, S. (2003). Using video modeling to teach perspective taking to children with autism. *Journal of Positive Behavior Interventions, 36*(2), 12–21.

Charlop-Christy, M., Le, L., & Freeman, K. (2000). A comparison of video modeling with in vivo modeling for teaching children with autism. *Journal of Autism and Developmental Disorders, 30*, 537–552.

Cihak, D. F., & Schrader, L. (2009). Does the model matter? Comparing video self-modeling and video adult modeling for task acquisition and maintenance by adolescents with autism spectrum disorders. *Journal of Special Education Technology, 23*, 9–20.

Cihak, D. F., Wright, R., & Ayres, K. M. (2010). Use of self-modeling static-picture prompts via a handheld computer to facilitate self-monitoring in the general education classroom. *Education and Training in Autism and Developmental Disabilities, 45*, 136–149.

Clark, E., Beck, D., Sloane, H., Goldsmith, D., Jenson, W., Bowen, J., & Kehle, T. (1993). Self-Modeling with preschoolers: Is it different. *School Psychology International, 14*, 83–89.

Council for Exceptional Children. (2014). *Standards for evidence-based practices in special education.* Retrieved on February 11, 2021 *from* https://journals.sagepub.com/doi/10.1177/0040059914531389

Crandell, S., & Johnson, C. E. (2009). The impact of video instruction: A case study of a student with Asperger syndrome. *Teaching Exceptional Children Plus 5*(6), Article 1.

Crosland, K., & Dunlap, G. (2012). Effective strategies for the inclusion of children with autism in general education classrooms. *Behavior Modification, 36*(3), 251–269.

D'Ateno, P., Mangiapanello, K., & Taylor, B. A. (2003). Using video modeling to teach complex play sequences to a preschooler with autism. *Journal of Positive Behavior Interventions, 5*(1), 5–11.

Dauphin, M., Kinney, E. M., Stromer, R., & Koegel, R. L. (2004). Using video-enhanced activity schedules and matrix training to teach sociodramatic play to a child with autism. *Journal of Positive Behavior Interventions, 6*(4), 238–250.

Decker, M. M., & Buggey, T. (2014). Using video self-and peer modeling to facilitate reading fluency in children with learning disabilities. *Journal of Learning Disabilities, 47*(2), 167–177.

Delano, M. E. (2007). Improving written language performance of adolescents with Asperger syndrome. *Journal of Applied Behavior Analysis, 40*(2), 342–351.

Diorio, R., Bray, M., Sanetti, L., & Kehle, T. (2018). Using video self-modeling to increase compliance to classroom requests in students with autism spectrum disorder. *International Journal of School & Educational Psychology.* https://doi.org/10.1080/21683603.2018.1443857

Dowrick, P. W. (1983). Self-modeling. In P. W. Dowrick & J. Biggs (Eds.), *Using video: Psychological and social applications* (pp. 105–124). Wiley.

Dupere, S., Macdonald, R. P., & Ahearn, W. H. (2013). Using video modeling with substitutable loops to teach varied play to children with autism. *Journal of Applied Behavior Analysis, 46*, 662–668.

Ergenekon, Y. (2012). Teaching basic first-aid skills against home accidents to children with autism through video modeling. *Educational Sciences: Theory and Practice, 12*, 2759–2766.

Ergenekon, Y., Tekin-Iftar, E., Kapan, A., & Akmanoglu, N. (2014). Comparison of video and live modeling in teaching response chains to children with autism. *Education and Training in Autism and Developmental Disabilities, 46*, 200–213.

Gena, A., Couloura, S., & Kymissis, E. (2005). Modifying the affective behavior of preschoolers with autism using *in-vivo* or video modeling and reinforcement contingencies. *Journal of Autism and Developmental Disorders, 35*(5), 545–546.

Genc-Tosun, D., & Kurt, O. (2017). Effects of video modeling on the instructional efficiency of simultaneous prompting among preschoolers with autism spectrum disorder. *Education and Training in Autism and Developmental Disabilities, 52*, 291–304.

Golan, O., & Baron-Cohen, S. (2006). Systemizing empathy: Teaching adults with Asperger syndrome or high-functioning autism to recognize complex emotions using interactive multimedia. *Development and Psychopathology, 18*(2), 591–617.

Grandin, T. (2006). *Thinking in pictures and other reports from my life with autism.* Vintage Books.

Halle, S., Ninness, C., Ninness, S., & Lawson, D. (2016). Teaching social skills to students with autism: a video modeling social stories approach. *Behavior and Social Issues, 25*, 42–53.

Haring, T. G., Kennedy, C. H., Adams, M. J., & Pitts-Conway, V. (1987). Teaching generalization of purchasing skills across community settings to autistic youth using videotape modeling. *Journal of Applied Behavior Analysis, 20*(1), 89–96.

Hart, J., & Whalon, K. (2012). Using video self-modeling via iPads to increase academic responding of an adolescent with autism spectrum disorder and intellectual disability. *Education and Training in Autism and Developmental Disabilities, 47*(4), 438–446.

Hine, J. F., & Wolery, M. (2006). Using point-of-view video modeling to teach play to preschoolers with autism. *Topics in Early Childhood Special Education, 26*(2), 83–93.

Hochhauser, M., Gal, E., & Weiss, P. L. (2015). Negotiation strategy video modeling training for adolescents with autism spectrum disorder: A usability study. *International Journal of Human–Computer Interaction, 31,* 472–480.

Hong, E. R., Ganz, J. B., Mason, R., Morin, K., Davis, J. L., Ninci, J., Neely, L. C., Boles, M. B., & Gilliland, W. D. (2016). The effects of video modeling in teaching functional living skills to persons with ASD: A meta-analysis of single-case studies. *Research in Developmental Disabilities, 57,* 158–169.

Jung, S., & Sainato, D. M. (2013). Teaching play skills to young children with autism. *Journal of Intellectual and Developmental Disability, 38*(1), 74–90.

Kazdin, A. E. (1982). *Single-case research designs: Methods for clinical and applied settings.* Oxford University Press.

Kehle, T. J., Bray, M. A., Margiano, S. J. S., Theodore, L. A., & Zhou, Z. (2002). Self-modeling as an effective intervention for students with serious emotional disturbance: Are we modifying children's memories? *Psychology in the Schools, 39,* 203–207.

Kim, J. (2018). Effects of point-of-view video modeling for Korean adolescents with autism to improve their on-task behavior and independent task performance during vegetable gardening. *International Journal of Developmental Disabilities, 64,* 306–317.

Kircher, T. T., Senior, C., Phillips, M. L., Benson, P. J., Bullmore, E. T., Brammer, M., Simmons, A., Williams, S. C., R., Bartels, M., & David, A. S. (2000). Towards a functional neuroanatomy of self-processing: Effects of faces and words. *Cognitive Brain Research, 10,* 133–144.

Kleeberger, V., & Mirenda, P. (2010). Teaching generalized imitation skills to a preschooler with autism using video modeling. *Journal of Positive Behavior Interventions, 12*(2), 116–127.

Kurnaz, E., & Yanardag, M. (2018). The effectiveness of video self-modeling in teaching active video game skills to children with autism spectrum disorder. *Journal of Developmental and Physical Disabilities, 30,* 455–469.

Lang, R., Shogren, K. A., Machalicek, W., Rispoli, M., O'Reilly, M., Baker, S., & Regester, A. (2009). Video self-modeling to teach classroom rules to two students with Asperger's. *Research in Autism Spectrum Disorders, 3,* 483–488.

Leach, D., & Rodecki, J. (2013). Literacy based behavioral interventions and video self-modeling with students with autism spectrum disorder (ASD). *Journal of the American Academy of Special Education Professionals,* 1–9.

LeBlanc, L. A., Coates, A. M., Daneshvar, S., Charlop-Christy, M. H., Morris, C., & Lancaster, B. M. (2003). Using video modeling and reinforcement to teach perspective-taking skills to children with autism. *Journal of Applied Behavior Analysis, 36,* 253–257.

Lee, C. Y. Q., Anderson, A., & Moore, D. W. (2014). Using video modeling to toilet train a child with autism. *Journal of Developmental and Physical Disabilities, 26,* 123–134.

Lee, S. Y., Lo, Y.-Y., & Lo, Y. (2017). Teaching functional play skills to a young child with autism spectrum disorder through video self-modeling. *Journal of Autism Development Disorder, 47,* 2295–2306.

Lewis, M., & Brooks-Gunn, J. (1979). *Social cognition and the acquisition of self.* Plenum Press.

Litras, S., Moore, D. W., & Anderson, A. (2010). Using video self-modelled social stories to teach social skills to a young child with autism. *Autism Research and Treatment,* Article ID 834979. https://doi.org/10.1155/2010/834979

MacDonald, R., Clark, M., Garrigan, E., & Vangala, M. (2005). Using video modeling to teach pretend play to children with autism. *Behavioral Interventions, 20*(4), 225–238.

Maione, L., & Mirenda, P. (2006). Effects of video modeling and video feedback on peer-directed social language skills of a child with autism. *Journal of Positive Behavior Interventions, 8*(2), 106–118.

Marcus, A., & Wilder, D. A. (2009). Comparison of peer video modeling and self-video modeling to teach textual responses in children with autism. *Journal of Applied Behavior Analysis, 42,* 335–341.

Mason, R. A., Davis, H. S., Boles, M. B., & Goodwyn, F. (2013). Efficacy of point-of-view video modeling: A meta-analysis. *Remedial and Special Education, 34*(6), 333–345.

McCoy, D. M., Morrison, J. Q., Barnett, D. W., Kalra, H. D., & Donovan, L. K. (2017). Using iPad tablets for self-modeling with preschoolers: Videos versus photos. *Psychology in the Schools, 54*, 821–836.

McCurdy, B. L., & Shapiro, E. S. (1988). Self-observation and the reduction of inappropriate classroom behavior. *Journal of School Psychology, 26*, 371–378.

Morlock, L., Reynolds, J. L., Fisher, S., & Comer, R. J. (2015). Video modeling and word identification in adolescents with Autism Spectrum Disorder. *Child Language Teaching and Therapy, 31*(1), 101–111.

National Autism Center at May Institute. (2019). *National Standards Project–Phase 2.* http://www.nationalautismcenter.org/national-standards-project/phase-2

National Clearinghouse on Autism Evidence and Practice. (2019). *Bridging science and practice.* https://ncaep.fpg.unc.edu

Neumann, L. (2004). *Video modeling: A visual teaching method for children with autism* (2nd ed.). Willerik.

Nikopoulos, C. K., & Keenan, M. (2003). Promoting social initiation in children with autism. *Behavioral Interventions, 18*(2), 87–108.

Nikopoulos, C. K., & Keenan, M. (2004). Effects of video modeling on training and generalisation of social initiation and reciprocal play by children with autism. *European Journal of Behaviour Analysis, 5*(1), 1–13.

Nikopoulos, C. K., & Keenan, M. (2007). Using video modeling to teach complex social sequences to children with autism. *Journal of Autism and Developmental Disorders, 37*(4), 678–693.

O'Handley, R. D., & Allen, K. D. (2017). An evaluation of the production effects of video self-modeling. *Research in Developmental Disabilities, 71*, 35–41.

Ozen, A., Batu, S., & Birkan, B. (2012). Teaching play skills to children with autism through video modeling: Small group arrangement and observational learning. *Education and Training in Autism and Developmental Disabilities, 47*(1), 84–96.

Plavnick, J. B., & Ferren, S. J. (2011). Establishing verbal repertoires in children with autism using function-based video modeling. *Journal of Applied Behavior Analysis, 44*(4), 747–766.

Plavnick, J. B., MacFarland, M. C., & Ferreri, S. J. (2015). Variability in the effectiveness of a video modeling intervention package for children with autism. *Journal of Positive Behavior Interventions, 17*(2), 105–115.

Piersel, W. C., & Kratochwill, T. R. (1979). Self-observation and behavior change: Applications to academic and adjustment problems through behavioral consultation. *Journal of School Psychology, 17*(2), 151–61.

Reagon, T. S., Higbee, K. A., & Endico, K. (2006). Teaching pretend play skills to a student with autism using video modeling with a sibling as model and play partner. *Education and Treatment of Children, 29*(3), 1–12.

Rex, C., Charlop, M. H., & Spector, V. (2018). Using video modeling as an anti-bullying intervention for children with autism spectrum disorder. *Journal of Autism and Developmental Disorders, 48*(8), 2701–2713.

Salvia, J., & Hughes, C. A. (1990). *Curriculum-based assessment: Testing what is taught.* Macmillan.

Sancho, K., Sidener, T. M., Reeve, S. A., & Sidener, D. W. (2010). Two variations of video modeling interventions for teaching play skills to children with autism. *Education & Treatment of Children, 33*(3), 421–442.

Sansosti, F. J., & Powell-Smith, K. A. (2008). Using computer-presented social stories and video models to increase the social communication skills of children with high-functioning autism spectrum disorders. *Journal of Positive Behavior Interventions, 10*(3), 162–178.

Scattone, D. (2008). Enhancing the conversation skills of a boy with Asperger's disorder through social stories and video modeling. *Journal of Autism and Developmental Disorders, 38*(2), 395–400.

Schatz, R. B., Peterson, R. K., & Bellini, S. (2016). The use of video self-modeling to increase on-task behavior in children with high-functioning autism. *Journal of Applied School Psychology, 32*(3), 234–253.

Scheflen, S., Freeman, S., & Paparella, T. (2012). Using video modeling to teach young children with autism developmentally appropriate play and connected speech. *Education and Training in Autism and Developmental Disabilities, 47*(3), 302–318. www.jstor .org/stable/23879967

Schmidt, C., & Bonds-Raacke, J. (2013). The effects of video self-modeling on children with autism spectrum disorder. *International Journal of Special Education, 28*(3), 121–132.

Scruggs, T. E., Mastropieri, M. A., & Casto, G. (1987). The quantitative synthesis of single-subject research: Methodology and validation. *Remedial and Special Education, 8*(2), 24–43.

Schreibman, L., Whalen, C., & Stahmer, A. C. (2000). The use of video priming to reduce disruptive transition behavior in children with autism. *Journal of Positive Behavior Interventions, 2*(1), 3–11.

Schunk, D. H., & Hanson, A. R. (1989). Self-modeling and children's cognitive skill learning. *Journal of Educational Psychology, 81*, 155–163.

Sherer, M., Pierce, K. L., Paredes, S., Kisacky, K. L., Ingersoll, B., & Schreibman, L. (2001). Enhancing conversation skills in children with autism via video technology: Which is better, "self" or "other" as a model? *Behavior Modification, 25*(1), 140–158.

Shipley-Benamou, R., Lutzker, J. R., & Taubman, M. (2002). Teaching daily living skills to children with autism through instructional video modeling. *Journal of Positive Behavior Interventions, 4*(3), 166–177.

Shrestha, A., Anderson, A., & Moore, D. W. (2013). Using point-of-view video modeling and forward chaining to teach a functional self-help skill to a child with autism. *Journal of Behavioral Education, 22*(2), 157–167.

Smith, J., Hand, L., & Dowrick, P. W. (2014). Video feedforward for rapid learning of a picture-based communication system. *Journal of Autism and Developmental Disorders, 44*(4), 926–936.

Smith, M., Ayres, K., Mechling, L., & Smith, K. (2013). Comparison of the effects of video modeling with narration vs. video modeling on the functional skill acquisition of adolescents with autism. *Education and Training in Autism and Developmental Disabilities, 48*(2), 164–178.

Smith, D., Wright, C., Allsopp, A., & Westhead, H. (2007). It's all in the mind: PETTLEP-based imagery and sports Performance. *Journal of Applied Sport Psychology, 19*, 80–92.

Taylor, B. A., Levin L., & Jasper S. (1999). Increasing play-related statements in children with autism toward their siblings: Effects of video modeling. *Journal of Developmental and Physical Disabilities, 11*(3), 253–264.

Tereshko, L., MacDonald, R., & Ahearn, W. H. (2010). Strategies for teaching children with autism to imitate response chains using video modeling. *Research in Autism Spectrum Disorders, 4*(3), 479–489.

Tetreault, A. S., & Lerman, D. C. (2010). Teaching social skills to children with autism using point-of-view video modeling. *Education & Treatment of Children, 33*(3), 395–419.

Uono, S., & Hietanen, J. K. (2015). Eye contact perception in the West and East: A cross-cultural study. *PLoS ONE, 10*(2): e0118094. https://doi.org/10.1371/journal.pone.0118094

Victor, H., Little, S. G., & Akin-Little, A. (2011). Increasing social engaged time in children with autism spectrum disorders using video self-modeling. *Journal of Evidence-Based Practices for Schools, 12*(1), 105–124.

Wert, B. Y., & Neisworth, J. T. (2003). Effects of video self-modeling on spontaneous requesting in children with autism. *Journal of Positive Behavior Interventions, 5*, 300–305.

Williamson, R. W., Casey, L. B., Robertson, J. S., & Buggey, T. (2013). Video self-modeling in children with autism: A pilot study validating prerequisite skills and extending the utilization of VSM across skill sets. *Journal of Assistive Technology, 25*, 63–71.

Wilson, K. P. (2013). Incorporating video modeling into a school-based intervention for students with autism spectrum disorders. *Language, Speech, and Hearing Services in Schools, 44*, 105–117.

Wong, C., Odom, S. L., Hume, K. A., Cox, A. W., Fettig, A., Kucharczyk, S., Brock, M. E., Plavnick, J. B., Fleury, V. P., & Schultz, T. R. (2015). Evidence-based practices for children, youth, and young adults with autism spectrum disorder: A comprehensive review. *Journal of Autism and Developmental Disorders, 45*(7), 1951–1966.

Yakubova, G., Hughes, E. M., & Shinaberry, M. (2016). Learning with technology: Video modeling with concrete-representational-abstract sequencing for students with autism spectrum disorder. *Journal of Autism and Developmental Disorders, 46*, 20349–20362.

18

Future Directions

Rebecca J. McCauley and Patricia A. Prelock

The purpose of this book has been to provide information about communication and social-interaction interventions for a wide-ranging readership—including researchers, professionals, people with autism spectrum disorder (ASD) and their families, as well as students and their professors. Whereas the intervention chapters (4–17) primarily address the current state of practice, this chapter focuses on the future. The first major section of this culminating chapter offers suggestions about future directions for researchers—some of it derived from intervention chapter authors and the remainder from our own investigation of current trends. The last three sections of the chapter describe additional resources that groups of readers can consult to advance their learning and decision making.

FUTURE DIRECTIONS FOR RESEARCH

Knowing what researchers are thinking about future research can benefit not just current and upcoming researchers but also individuals with ASD and their families, professionals, students, and professors. It can clarify potential contributions that can be made by each of these groups, whether they become active researchers, participants without whose help research is impossible, or others who promote research to make it possible. Such knowledge can also help explain why interventions for communication and social interaction are not yet as universally effective and efficient as we all want them to be.

The model in Figure 18.1 represents one way to think about the factors contributing to the best intervention outcomes—in this case, the best outcomes of communication and social interaction interventions for people with ASD. Essentially, the idea captured in the model is that the best outcomes result when well-equipped interventionists choose and effectively use the most well-developed treatments in places and situations that can best facilitate that treatment given

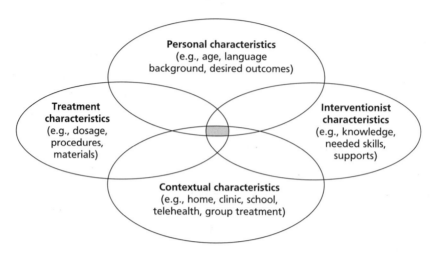

Figure 18.1. The factors contributing to intervention outcomes.

the particular strengths, difficulties, and interests of the person receiving it. The shaded center of the model represents an optimal situation where all four major components of the model work together in harmony to create the best possible outcomes.

This model highlights four major components and acknowledges their deep interconnections. *Personal characteristics* of the individual receiving an intervention, the first component, appears at the top of the model because the outcomes for which an intervention might be used are intended to improve communication, social interactions, and, explicitly or implicitly, quality of life while responding to the current and evolving characteristics of that person and their family. The age, language level, and cultural background of the individual will certainly influence the selected outcomes and the approach to intervention. *Treatment characteristics* are the specific procedures, activities, dosage, and so on, that distinguish one intervention from another and that are designed to produce particular changes in the person being treated, that person's environment, or both. Although these characteristics may seem singularly important to making an intervention work, developments occurring over the past few decades suggest that for interventions to be used most effectively and efficiently in real-world settings, their characteristics must mesh seamlessly with characteristics of the other three components. The term *interventionist characteristics*, rather than a more specific term like *clinician characteristics*, is used for the next component because collaborative teams as well as individual speech-language pathologists (SLPs), teachers, caregivers, and peers are just some of the intervention agents who play very active roles in treatment. This component of the model appears at the same level as treatment characteristics because it is through the professional, caregiver or team that treatments are actually realized. Among the characteristics of individual interventionists and teams that will affect the quality of the treatment they provide are not only their existing knowledge and skills but also their access to additional learning and ongoing supports (e.g., fidelity checklists, coaching, specialty training). Finally, *contextual characteristics* might simply be thought of as the location and delivery mode through which the treatment is administered. Locations include the home, the clinic, or school. Delivery modes include interventionists working in person, singly or as part of a team, with the client in a one-to-one context, within a group of other clients, or through telehealth. Rather than viewing these characteristics as simple givens, a brief review of recent trends in research suggests that context can play a critical role in producing positive outcomes. Alternatively, if overlooked or inadequately addressed, context can contribute to the underuse or misuse of interventions, regardless of how much research support the intervention has garnered in the laboratory or when studied in small community-based studies (e.g., Dingfelder & Mandell, 2011).

Considering each component of the model in turn, we argue that greater understanding of each component's characteristics allows researchers to respond to or shape them to improve outcomes. We draw on examples from the intervention chapters in this book as well as from broader research and practical efforts. For readers less accustomed to professional and research jargon, more esoteric terms are bolded to indicate their presence in the glossary, which follows this chapter.

Personal Characteristics

Identifying personal characteristics that could help how that person will respond to the intervention or how the intervention could be tailored to meet their needs is a common concern among intervention researchers both within and beyond the realm of autism. After looking at how autism researchers consider this issue, we address larger trends affecting how this work is likely to be carried out.

Researchers' Perspectives on Personal Characteristics   Each of the preceding chapters in this book has touched upon the many differences among people with autism and their families that help determine what goals and interventions might be most appropriate. Specific themes that emerged across the Future Directions sections of earlier chapters were the need to tailor interventions to better meet individual needs; to serve a broader age range than they do currently; to address differences in languages, cultures, sex, and gender; and to expand the variety of outcomes being sought.

Tailoring Interventions to Address Individual Needs   Tailoring treatments to meet the needs of individuals with autism as a means of improving outcomes was a theme in the discussion of future directions in several chapters. The two major strategies that emerged for achieving those ends were 1) paying attention to co-occurring difficulties and 2) identifying variables that could predict success or suggest additional strategies to increase the likelihood of success.

Suggested methods for addressing co-occurring difficulties included modifying existing interventions to mitigate the effects of those difficulties or adding a second intervention expressly designed to address them. For example, Howard and Dawson, writing about the Early Start Denver Model (ESDM, Chapter 5), describe an ongoing project to determine whether concurrent pharmacological intervention for children with ASD who also have attention deficit-hyperactivity disorder can improve social-communication skills when a parent-implemented version of ESDM is used. In a discussion of future directions for Pivotal Response Treatment (PRT, Chapter 13), Koegel, Strong, and Ponder stress the importance of studying the comorbidities of depression and anxiety among adolescents and adults with ASD, citing research suggesting that improved socialization, a goal of PRT, may also lead to reductions in co-occurring problems.

Looking at the broader autism intervention literature, however, it seems that co-occurring conditions are not even being universally acknowledged. In a 2020 study of intervention studies conducted between 1990 and 2017, Steinbrenner and colleagues found that only 55% reported on the co-occurring conditions of participants, with the most commonly reported condition being intellectual disability, which was identified in about 25% of those studies reporting co-occurring features. Given that most children and adults experience at least one and usually more than one co-occurring difficulty (Lever & Geurts, 2016; Soke et al., 2018), identification of co-occurring conditions in participants is crucial.

Further, research to examine the potential benefits of tailoring interventions to address particularly prevalent co-occurring difficulties represents an exciting future direction for intervention research. Difficulties that tend to occur more frequently in older individuals with ASD (e.g., depression; Lever & Geurts, 2016) might be mitigated or avoided altogether through effective interventions earlier in life. For example, by helping the person with ASD stay employed, make friends, and so on, the social risk factors associated with those later challenges could be reduced. At the very least, positive benefits of addressing co-occurring difficulties might be achieved for one or both current challenges (e.g., social interaction and anxiety during childhood).

Several chapter authors mentioned the identification of predictors of a person's response to intervention as a means of helping researchers develop additional or altered strategies and helping clinicians make better choices about which intervention is likely to be effective. For example, in response to studies suggesting better long-term outcomes in children who more regularly initiated communicative interactions, Koegel and her colleagues (Chapter 13 on PRT) developed methods to help increase such initiations. In Chapter 16, Social Stories™, Hutchins points to the need to identify predictors of success with that intervention and suggests age, verbal ability, and reading level as possible variables to investigate.

Addressing a Broader Age Range   Research that helps expand the age ranges for which an intervention might be appropriate is widely recognized as an important direction for future research (e.g., Maglione et al., 2012). Although this research direction could probably have been addressed under the previous heading, it is separated here to emphasize the point that many age groups are *dramatically* underrepresented. Examining 972 autism intervention studies conducted between 1990 to 2017, Steinbrenner and his colleagues (2020) found that only about 7.5% of the studies included children from birth to 35 months and only 5% included participants from the oldest age group they studied—young adults from 19 to 22 years. Further, although the percentage of studies including 12 to 18 year olds grew substantially from 1990 to 2017, by far the majority of studies over that timeframe focused on children between 3 and 11 years old. Two recent systematic reviews further underscore the scarcity of psychosocial intervention research including older adults with ASD (Bishop-Fitzpatrick et al., 2013; Pallathra et al., 2019). Examining psychosocial intervention research from 1950 to mid-2011 that included adults with ASD 18 years or older, Bishop-Fitzpatrick and colleagues (2013) found only 13 studies that met their inclusion criteria. Examining studies conducted from 1980 to 2017, Pallathra and colleagues (2019) found only 41 peer-reviewed studies that focused on psycho-social interventions targeting social function, included participants who were 16 or older (with at least 50% of participants 18 years or older) and included a majority of participants without a diagnosis of intellectual disability. Clearly, more autism treatment research is needed to begin to address the needs of persons with autism across the lifespan.

Not surprisingly, therefore, the need for future research into interventions for older individuals was mentioned in the Future Direction sections of several intervention chapters. For example, in Chapter 12, Peer-Mediated Support Interventions for Students With ASD, Carter identifies the potential value of expanding the use of that treatment to individuals in inclusive college programs and integrated workplaces. In Chapter 13, Koegel and her colleagues propose expanding the use of PRT to adolescents and adults for whom outcome measures would be related to employment. Writing about The SCERTS® Model (Chapter 14), which has primarily been studied for preschoolers, Laurent, Prizant, and Rubin discuss the need to broaden the age ranges included in their research. More specifically, they note that although SCERTS is designed to be used in multiple contexts, additional research is needed to confirm its viability in public schools. Chapter 15, Social Skills Interventions (Prelock and Brien), does address the importance of social-communication strategies for adolescents and young adults, with Skillstreaming and the START programs addressing 13 to 18 year olds and more computer-based programs, such as Virtual Reality-Social Cognition Training and Mind Reading, addressing the social cognition needs of adults 18 to 35 year olds, with more research needed on the long term effects for adults.

The need for future research into interventions for younger individuals is also mentioned frequently. Kasari and Sterrett describe research on JASPER (Chapter 9) as beginning to focus on clients who are minimally verbal or very young (12–21 months). Woods and colleagues describe continuing efforts to support Early Social Interaction (ESI; Chapter 11) as a preventative intervention for children whose behavior demonstrates multiple red flags by age 12–18 months. As a part of their First Words project, these researchers are working to produce tools to make identification and diagnosis of at-risk children more accurate and reliable at these younger ages (e.g., Guthrie et al., 2013). Research to support earlier identification of at-risk status and earlier diagnosis of ASD is likely to further increase attention to interventions designed for younger age groups, given expectations that brain plasticity at younger ages may reshape the trajectory of later development in powerful ways. Discussing future directions for PRT (Chapter 13), Koegel and colleagues indicate the desire for that intervention to be further developed for use with infants and toddlers. Taking a slightly different but related tack in regard to video modeling, Buggey (Chapter 17) identifies the need to determine when that intervention is developmentally appropriate for targeting specific skills and behaviors, a goal that will likely promote earlier and more effective interventions for younger children.

Addressing Differences in Language, Culture, Sex, and Gender The authors of four chapters mention the need to acknowledge differences in culture and language that help shape one's life in powerful ways. Howard and Dawson (Chapter 5) describe ongoing research designed to validate the use of ESDM intervention in underrepresented cultures, especially those with limited resources and low literacy levels (viz., a study being conducted in South Africa). Similarly, Kaiser and Heidlage (Chapter 10) point to the need to examine the effectiveness of Enhanced Milieu Teaching (EMT) for dual language learners, and Laurent and her colleagues, writing about SCERTS (Chapter 14), mention the need to broaden research populations to include more culturally diverse groups. Prelock and Brien (Chapter 15) highlight some social skills interventions that are intended to address the needs of diverse populations and the importance of continuing to investigate the effectiveness of these interventions across underrepresented populations. They point out that social skills instruction must accommodate the individual's cultural values while providing the individual with new ways to interact in a given social situation no matter what cultural context is represented.

The need to broaden autism interventions to serve individuals across more diverse languages and cultures is well recognized by many researchers and clinicians (e.g., Benevides et al., 2019; Dyches et al., 2004; Lim et al., 2018; Richmond, 2011; Wang et al., 2018); however, much remains to be done. For example, the Steinbrenner and colleagues (2020) review of 972 studies from 1990 to 2017 reported that very few intervention studies either described or compared participants on the basis of their racial or ethnic identity, language preference, or language context (monolingual, multilingual). Specifically, only 30% of 972 intervention studies examined by those researchers even reported on the race, ethnicity, and nationality of participants.

In the United States and Canada, the urgency for attention to language and culture in ASD interventions is growing because approximately 20% of children in those countries live in bilingual homes (Wang et al., 2018). Empirically based recommendations are needed for children with ASD and their families that speak to the benefits or risks of continued use of one or more home languages alongside exposure to the language of the majority community. In the United States, the language used by the broader community (usually English) is also the language predominantly used in intervention research. Further, English is the *only* language that most certified SLPs in the United States believe they are competent to use professionally, with fewer than 7% identifying as bilingual service providers (American Speech-Language-Hearing Association [ASHA], 2020). In an international survey conducted by Gillon and colleagues (2017), the majority of respondents indicated that they worked with children with ASD from a different cultural background than their own, suggesting that even countries that are less homogeneously monolingual than the United States may benefit from more information guiding work with people with diverse language and cultural backgrounds.

A recent **scoping review** (Zhou et al., 2019) suggests that the continuing use of more than one language does not necessarily present a barrier to either social interaction or language outcomes. In fact, effects on language development of multilingual environments have also been found to be benign or actually beneficial for children with ASD (Hambly & Fombonne, 2012; Zhou et al., 2019); for example, use of more than one language may afford advantages in nonverbal intelligence, adaptive functioning, and expressive vocabulary (Wang et al. 2018), not to mention the advantages that a shared language and culture bring to any child and family. Nonetheless, it seems that families are regularly being advised to use one language only (Lim et al., 2018) and that very little intervention research has thus far been done to further the development and support of multilingual interventions. Another important topic related to people with ASD from racial and ethnically diverse groups is the nature of stressors they experience (Benevides et al., 2019) and how those stressors differ from those of majority culture families dealing with autism (Hayes & Watson, 2013).

Sex and gender as personal characteristics are also of growing interest. A current estimate of the ratio of males to females diagnosed with ASD is about four to one at age 8 (Maenner et al., 2020). The predominance of boys being affected by autism may be the reason that sex differences in response to intervention were not mentioned by authors in this book. That topic has only recently been raised as an important topic for consideration in autism research overall (e.g., Lai et al., 2015; Wong et al., 2015). Nonetheless, sex differences between females and males affect core symptoms (e.g., ASD-restricted interests tend to involve people and animals among girls and women versus objects among boys and men) as well as comorbidities (e.g., eating disorders for women and girls with ASD more than for men and boys). Such differences may require not only special treatment consideration to address the separate needs of these populations but additions to the roster of available assessments for arriving at accurate diagnoses and effective treatment planning (e.g., Thompson et al., 2003; Van Wingaarden-Cremers et al., 2014).

Similarly, people with ASD whose gender identities differ from their sex assignment at birth are another group that may present personal characteristics warranting special attention in the intervention research. Although the gender identity of participants in the autism intervention literature is rarely described (Steinbrenner et al., 2020), a history of ASD is reported by as many as 8% of individuals with gender dysphoria (de Vries et al., 2010). (Gender dysphoria is the designation for a mismatch between physical characteristics and gender identity [American Psychiatric Association, 2013]). Although 8% may seem to be a relatively small percentage, it still hints that gender dysphoria may more frequently affect individuals with ASD than their peers. Fortunately, a recent systematic review by Øien and colleagues (2018) and a follow-up report on that study (Nordahl-Hansen et al., 2019) indicate that studies on gender dysphoria and autism represent a fast-growing field, a development that may eventually lead to its consideration in intervention studies for ASD.

Expanding Outcome Measures   Although outcome measures may not immediately strike some readers as related to personal characteristics, they are considered under this heading because of the universal recognition that intervention outcomes should squarely address the needs of the individual person being treated. In addition, as the diversity of populations being served increases, so does the likelihood that additional outcomes will be pursued, whether that diversity is based in linguistic, cultural, and socioeconomic factors; age, sex, and gender; or specific comorbid conditions.

Five intervention chapters speculate about future research designed to explore outcomes beyond those for which the intervention is commonly being used and studied. These range from examination of longer-term outcomes as well as changes in brain physiology (Chapter 5, Howard & Dawson) to the acceptability of behaviors intended to replace challenging behaviors (Chapter 8, on functional communication training [FCT], Durand & Moskowitz). Expansions of outcomes beyond those currently being targeted are proposed in three other chapters: using peer-mediated support strategies (Chapter 12, Carter) to address communication and language in addition to social-interaction skills, using Social Stories

(Chapter 16, Hutchins) to achieve social-cognitive goals in addition to reductions in problem behaviors, and using video modeling (Chapter 17, Buggey) to address a wider range of skills and problem behaviors. Given the diverse needs that any person with ASD may experience, expanding the range of needs an intervention might address could greatly simplify demands on the persons receiving the intervention if they have already experienced some success with the intervention as well as demands on the interventionist, who may have one less intervention to learn to use.

Larger Trends Affecting Attention to Personal Characteristics   Evidence-based practice and the application of the *International Classification of Functioning, Disability, and Health* (ICF; World Health Organization [WHO], 2001) provide influential frameworks shaping how researchers and clinicians view personal characteristics.

Evidence-Based Practice   Numerous, slightly different definitions of evidence-based medicine (EBM; Sackett et al., 1997) and, later, **evidence-based practice** (EBP) provide valuable guidance for SLPs and others (e.g., Dollaghan, 2007; Gillam & Gillam, 2006; Johnson, 2006). The website of the American Speech-Language-Hearing Association (ASHA) provides a serviceable definition of the three main components of EBP. They are 1) clinical expertise and expert opinion, 2) evidence that is obtained both from the research literature and from data collected for an individual client, and 3) client/patient/caregiver perspectives. Of particular importance to any discussion of personal characteristics is the third component, client/patient/caregiver perspectives, which is described as "the unique set of personal and cultural circumstances, priorities and expectations identified by your client and their caregivers" (ASHA, n.d.-a).

An initial purpose behind EBM and later EBP was to address the underuse of new, relevant, and better-quality research evidence by clinicians (Sackett et al., 1997). This concern certainly continues (e.g., Hoffman et al., 2013) despite that many clinicians referred only to the use of research findings in their definitions of EBP (Fulcher-Rood et al., 2020). Nonetheless, forces such as movements toward family-centered and patient-centered care (Committee on Hospital Care and Institute for Patient- and Family-Centered Care, 2012; Prelock & Hutchins, 2008), and even careful examination of discussions throughout the history of EBP about how to employ it, stress the equal importance of all three components (Sackett et al., 1997; Dollaghan, 2007).

International Classification of Functioning, Disability, and Health   Because of the detail it adds to information about the individual perspectives described in the ASHA definition of EBP, the ***International Classification of Functioning, Disability, and Health*** (ICF; WHO, 2001) represents another ongoing force moving personal characteristics to the forefront of decision making and research frameworks. Among other things, this classification system seeks to provide standard ways of describing personal characteristics, functions, and key life situations that may lead to the choice of specific outcomes (de Schipper et al., 2016). Consistent with EBP and extending it, ongoing developments to the ICF and its application continue to help shift researchers and clinicians away from a primary focus on biological effects related to the body's structures and functions toward a greater valuing of psychosocial effects related to the individual's specific functional capabilities (e.g., having a conversation, making a meal) and abilities to participate in key life situations (e.g., have friends, work, enjoy public events).

Of particular value for researchers and clinicians interested in people with autism is the recent emphasis on functional outcomes, yielding a greater role for functional outcomes in assessment and intervention goal planning (e.g., Gan et al., 2013; Mahdi et al., 2018; Schiarti et al., 2018). Powerful outcomes such as friendship or satisfying employment can be tackled more directly rather than indirectly, as is done when a linguistic goal (e.g., more well-formed simple sentences) is targeted based on the assumption that progress on that goal will indirectly lead to more satisfying and effective conversations and thus to stronger friendships and other relationships. Recent research using the ICF is also advancing the ideal of focusing not just on weaknesses but on acknowledging and leveraging strengths, such as attention to detail, honesty, creative talents associated with looking at the world differently, visual perception, and others (see de Schipper et al., 2016, Table 6).

Treatment Characteristics

Looking at the complexity and variety of components described for interventions in this book provides a window into the many moving parts—also called *ingredients* or *elements*—that need to work together to support valued outcomes for people with ASD. Intervention chapter authors provided considerable information about the elements included in their interventions in chapter sections Theoretical Basis and Key Components. Before diving into their insights, we review a few fundamental terms that describe the inner workings of interventions. Among these are *dose, active ingredient, mechanism of action*, and *fidelity.* Some of these terms are widely used by chapter authors.

Most people probably are familiar with the idea of dose from their experience in taking the prescribed one or two aspirins for a headache. Taking the correct dose can be expected to produce the desired effect (e.g., headache reduction) with minimal side effects (e.g., gastric upset). Also familiar is the idea that active ingredients in the aspirin are those that have the therapeutic effect, not those that cause the pill to conform to a particular shape, maintain that shape long enough to be swallowed, be palatable enough to be tolerated, and so on. Aspirin dosage, then, is based on the amount of the active ingredient scientifically demonstrated to be needed to achieve the desired effect of reducing headache pain for a person of a given size, age, and so on. In the case of a pharmaceutical agent, such as aspirin, the **mechanism of action** consists of the processes by which the drug produces its therapeutic effects. This friendly analogy breaks down a bit when it comes to terms comparable to the actions the physician and patient need to take so that the aspirin is correctly prescribed and consumed; these are often referred to as safe prescribing and patient adherence or compliance, respectively.

Now, let's consider more directly how these concepts might apply to behavioral interventions. In the context of behavioral interventions, **active ingredients** include any procedures, stimulus sets, activities, materials, and so on, that must be in place for desired outcomes to occur. Because it is assumed that active ingredients promote positive outcomes, there's also a need to identify those ingredients as well as those that are neutral or that might even undermine the intended outcome. Although *active ingredient* is the term often used hypothetically rather than on the basis of evidence, we use the term **elements** to refer to prominent components of an intervention to which positive effects have not yet been empirically attributed.

Application of the concept of dose in behavioral interventions is still in the early stages. In a groundbreaking paper, Warren and colleagues (2007) suggested that **dosage,** or intensity, as it is also called, depends on the sum of variables, including how often the therapy is offered each week (e.g., two times per week for 1 hour), how many separate occasions the identified or presumed active ingredients are available during those therapeutic intervals (e.g., 50 conversational turns in which procedures are used), and how long the intervention is pursued (e.g., 9 months). Given that most behavioral interventions are likely to have many active ingredients (Reichow et al., 2011) and that not all the time spent in therapy will be devoted to them, it has become clear that the concept of dosage should reflect the extent to which the active ingredients are actually delivered when the intervention is offered (Justice, 2018; Warren et al., 2007; Yoder et al., 2012). In fact, the actual dose received by a recipient of the intervention may depend on a number of personal and interventionist factors (e.g., amount of time spent addressing a child's challenging behaviors, setting up the environment so that an activity can be carried out, etc.; Justice, 2018; Justice et al., 2016). As a substitute for the physician's safe prescribing and the patient's adherence to instructions about how to take a medication, **fidelity** encompasses the interventionist's knowledgeable and skilled delivery of active ingredients of an intervention as it has been described, researched, and validated. In this behavioral realm, as in medicine, mechanism of action is the processes by which the identified or presumed active ingredients produce positive outcomes. Active ingredients and mechanisms of action are often suggested in theoretical discussions supporting behavioral interventions, and the purpose of many single case experimental designs and group experimental designs is to rule out the likelihood that something other than the treatment caused observed outcomes. However, subcomponents of interventions have less commonly been subjected to such scrutiny.

Researchers' Perspectives on Personal Characteristics   When examined from the lens of the concepts just described, chapter authors' discussions of next steps for their interventions seem to fall into three categories: 1) adding intervention elements or using combinations of interventions, 2) determining effective dosage, and 3) identifying active ingredients and mechanisms of action.

Adding Intervention Elements or Combining Interventions   Improving outcomes by adding new intervention elements to existing interventions or combining interventions was touched on earlier in this chapter, under Personal Characteristics. However, we confined the discussion to instances in which distinct interventions were added to address co-occurring conditions affecting the person with ASD or their family (e.g., ADHD, parental pessimism). Related strategies are being explored as a means of improving outcomes for communication and social interaction, frequently in recognition that as skills improve, new strategies may be needed. Several explorations of this kind are currently underway for JASPER (Chapter 9) and EMT (Chapter 10). Not only is research underway to investigate JASPER and EMT, but combinations that include JASPER, EMT, and discrete trial training (DTT; Chapter 6) and JASPER, EMT, and the use of speech-generating devices (SGDs) to promote spoken word use are also being investigated. Examining theoretically motivated combinations of interventions such as these represents an important step toward understanding the best way to develop interventions.

Determining Effective Intervention Dosage   Although one might think that more is always better in the case of any intervention for people with ASD, research in language interventions for related populations (e.g., children with developmental language disorders) suggests that more is *not* always better and may even be worse (e.g., Justice, 2018; Meyers-Denman & Plante, 2016; Plante et al., 2019). It seems likely that the same may be true for specific ASD interventions. Empirical determination of appropriate dosages for specific objectives and interventions could pave the way for more effective *and* efficient interventions. In turn, these developments might allow for additional time to be devoted to interventions targeting other goals, reduce intervention costs, or both—steps that could increase access to intervention for many families and children affected by ASD.

Research on the search for effective dosages was mentioned by several chapter authors in their discussions of future directions for research. In Chapter 4, on augmentative and alternative communication (AAC), Wegner mentions the need to examine instructional strategies and intensity as one of AAC's three most important areas for future research. In Chapter 5, on the ESDM, Howard and Dawson describe ongoing efforts to compare two levels of dosage (15 vs. 25 hours per week of one-to-one therapy) along with two teaching methods (DTT vs. routines and play-based teaching). In Chapter 9, on JASPER, Kasari and Sterrett indicate that finding variables that predict necessary dosage represents an important next step. Further, in Chapter 10, Kaiser and Heidlage note efforts to identify optimal dosage for EMT when used alone or combined with other interventions. Finally, in Chapter 16, on Social Stories, Hutchins poses several questions that relate to aspects of dosage as next steps for that intervention. For example, she suggests directions for research that considers how outcomes might be affected by different schedules according to which Social Story is reviewed, how long it might be used, and whether using several different readers across settings might improve initial outcomes and generalization.

Identifying Active Ingredients and Mechanisms of Action to Understand How Interventions Work   Although no chapter authors used the actual terms active ingredients and *mechanisms of action* in their Future Directions sections, one chapter's authors, Prelock and Brien (Chapter 15), use the *key ingredient* in their description of the need for effective social skills interventions to engage parents as a future direction. All of the authors described future research on components of interventions that might inform evolving understandings of which elements of the intervention actually are active ingredients as well as how they work to produce positive outcomes. Specifically, Howard and Dawson (Chapter 5) use *active ingredient* in their discussion of empirical bases when they point to the need to "demonstrate active ingredients" as a step toward wider international application of the ESDM. In their Future Directions section, Kasari and Sterrett mention the need for studies of JASPER (Chapter 9) that would involve "teasing apart various components of the intervention." Then, under Suggested Readings, they summarize a study demonstrating that a particular parent strategy in JASPER acted as "an active ingredient of the JASPER treatment" (Gulsrud et al., 2016, p. 606). Although it remains to be seen to what extent the *active ingredients* and *mechanisms of action* become more commonly used in ASD intervention research (e.g., Levac et al., 2012), that trend seems likely, given larger trends toward a shared vocabulary across scientific fields devoted to improving personal and societal outcomes.

Larger Trends Affecting Attention to Intervention Characteristics   Over the past few decades, researchers and clinicians interested in advancing the development of interventions of all kinds have begun to push for 1) more attention to research quality and detailed descriptions of interventions in research and 2) development of theories and classification systems to better understand the inner workings of and relationships among interventions. Combined, these developments should support existing efforts to understand how intervention elements work and how they work together to produce positive change.

Improving Transparency, Accuracy, and Reliability of Published Research   A widely known expectation of empirical research is that it involves carefully conceived methods designed to reduce the possibility that a chance result is mistakenly viewed as meaningful. A perhaps less widely known but equally important expectation is that a study should be described in sufficient detail so that its method can be replicated by others to provide equivalent data as a means of further reducing the possibility of erroneous conclusions. In a historical account of developments in medicine, Altman and Simera (2016) report that alarm bells about the poor quality of such research began to be rung in the mid-20th century, with reviews of medical journal articles suggesting that many articles came to erroneous conclusions due to errors in design, analysis, and interpretation. For example, one group of medical researchers (Glasziou et al., 2008) observed that medical interventions were so poorly described that study results could not be replicated, generalized to clinical decision making, or thoroughly judged for quality. Since then, not only has the quality of the research being conducted in medicine and many other disciplines come under fire, but the way research is reported has drawn increasing scrutiny across diverse intervention-oriented disciplines. Similar concerns began and continued to be raised about research in speech-language pathology (e.g., Ludemann et al., 2017) as well as other social and behavioral sciences (e.g., Michie et al. 2011; Open Science Collaboration, 2015).

The essence of the concern about poor reporting is that without knowledge of what was done in a particular study, researchers can neither replicate it fully nor generalize from its findings—thus depriving both researchers and consumers of research with solid foundations on which to build despite all the hard work that went into that previous research. Such concerns about the quality of research reports provided the impetus for the development of **reporting guidelines** for different research designs. Initially, reporting guidelines were designed for use in the review of manuscripts for publication, but now they also are viewed as research planning tools that can alert researchers to issues that require attention at the beginning rather than just the end of the research process (Altman & Simera, 2014). The EQUATOR (Enhancing the Quality and Transparency of Health Research) Network provides a compendium of more than 200 guidelines and associated checklists for almost any research design. A more streamlined set of guidelines for quantitative research designs, Journal Article Reporting Standards (JARS), is described by Applebaum and colleagues (2018) and is available in the latest version of the *Publication Manual of the APA* (American Psychological Association, 2020). Interested readers may want to look at JARS before diving into the more complete sets of guidelines offered by the EQUATOR Network.

Despite these dramatic advances designed to improve reporting of many research methods, guidance regarding how to describe interventions in research has been slower to arrive. Initially, interventions were addressed using single items on a couple of reporting guidelines for randomized trial reporting and protocols: respectively, CONSORT (Schultz et al., 2010) and SPIRIT (Chan et al., 2013). More recently, a 12-item guideline called TIDieR (**T**emplate for **I**ntervention **D**escription and **R**eplication; Hoffman et al., 2014) has been developed. Template items call upon study authors to provide information—in the body of an article or an alternative location, such as a related article or accessible manual—that include the name of the intervention, rationales for essential elements of the intervention, procedures, intervention providers, location(s) where the intervention is provided, and fidelity efforts and results.

In 2017, Ludemann and her colleagues used TIDieR items to evaluate 162 treatment descriptions in recent randomized controlled trials of speech-language pathology interventions. They found that none of the interventions they looked at had complete descriptions—even when secondary sources were used to augment information taken from the article. These researchers concluded that research with such descriptive holes has limited value for researchers wishing to replicate it or clinicians wishing to use it to arrive at intervention decisions. When asked to choose between five possible barriers preventing more detailed description of interventions, 40% of authors who responded cited length limitations posed by journals, 19% indicated they saw no barriers, 13% indicated that reviewers favored the elimination of some of the required information or that they did not have a means of sharing additional information (e.g., a dedicated website), and 6% indicated that copyrighted material related to the intervention prevented further disclosure or that it was prevented by a variety of other barriers, including intervention complexity.

Structural Descriptions of Interventions: Taxonomies and Other Classification Methods   In the autism literature, several intervention categorizations have been proposed. For example, Howlin and colleagues (2009) proposed three strands of interventions: 1) those focusing on communication, 2) those using developmental/educational strategies, and 3) those emphasizing the use of behavioral principles. These same strands have also been described as behavioral, social communication focused, and multimodal developmental interventions (Tachibana et al., 2017). Other distinctions among interventions for ASD have included *focused interventions* versus *comprehensive interventions*, where focused interventions address a limited set of deficits or skills (e.g., Bejarano-Martín et al., 2020) and comprehensive treatments address broader learning and developmental issues (e.g., National Research Council [NRC], 2001; Wong et al., 2015). Particularly relevant, given the interventions discussed in this book, is yet another category of interventions—*Naturalistic Developmental Behavioral Interventions*, which include behavioral strategies implemented in line with insights from developmental science (Schreibman et al., 2015). These interventions "are implemented in natural settings, involve shared control between child and therapist, utilize natural contingencies and use a variety of behavioral strategies to teach developmentally appropriate and prerequisite skills" (Schreibman et al., 2015, p. 2411). Each of these proposed categories appears related to intervention goals, types of strategies being deployed to effect change, or both.

To our knowledge, no classifications of autism interventions have been undertaken that consider a wider range of intervention characteristics (including verified versus putative active ingredients). The sheer range and complexity of interventions designed to address the many core difficulties and coexisting problems facing families and people with ASD may well explain this. However, this state of affairs contrasts with the more comprehensive classifications that are currently being developed and used in several areas of speech-language pathology, including speech-sound disorders, rehabilitation, aphasia, and voice (Baker et al., 2020; Baker et al., 2018; Turkstra et al., 2016; Van Stan et al., 2015). Although there are many types of classification systems (Stavri & Michie, 2012), those currently being developed in relation to speech-language pathology interventions are described as taxonomies, which can be defined as systems for organizing and naming things, often on the basis of shared characteristics.

Looking further afield, the development of classification systems has burgeoned over the past decade, in education, in medicine, and particularly in the area of behavior change—an interdisciplinary field that draws upon health psychology, public health, and virtually any discipline designed to help change human behaviors for the good of the individual and the society (e.g., Abraham & Michie, 2008; De Silva et al., 2014; Embry & Biglan, 2008; Michie et al., 2011; Whyte et al., 2014). Many of the techniques in behavior change research are focused on changing the habits of large groups of individuals and can involve a great many interventionists, participants, contexts, and stakeholders deeply invested in the outcomes. Therefore, it is perhaps natural that this field has in many ways created and led interest in the development and use of such classifications (e.g., Abraham & Michie, 2008; Michie et al., 2011; Michie et al., 2015) as a means of clearly communicating their structure, comparing and improving them, and training new interventionists to use them. As a group, behavior change interventions can be seen as complex interventions, a characterization that also seems applicable to many ASD interventions.

Complex interventions have been defined in terms of the "number of interacting components within both experimental and control interventions; the number and difficulty of behaviors required by those delivering or receiving the intervention, the number of groups or organizational levels targeted by the intervention, the number and variability of outcomes, and the degree of flexibility or tailoring of the intervention permitted" (Craig et al., 2008, p. 2). The development of a taxonomy for interventions used for people with ASD could probably yield similar benefits to both research and practice as those being realized in these other fields. Specifically, one might anticipate clearer descriptions and comparisons of intervention structures and how elements within the interventions work to achieve positive outcomes as well as more effective imparting of key components to those who need to learn the intervention in order to deliver it.

Interventionist Characteristics

The scope of individuals providing treatment related to communication and social skills for individuals with ASD covers scores of professional and semiprofessional interventionists (e.g., SLPs, educators, psychologists, behavioral analysts, aides) and nonprofessional interventionists (e.g., parents, siblings, other family members, peers, and other conversation partners)—as well as teams comprising differing constellations of professionals and nonprofessionals. Consequently, as interventions move out of the hands of expert clinicians who may be researchers focused on a single intervention in a laboratory and into the hands of individuals and teams of interventionists in more real-world settings, interventionist characteristics rise in stature as contributors to successful outcomes. In fact, success can depend in part on 1) interventionists' general and intervention-specific knowledge and skills and 2) ongoing supports such as continuing education and coaching.

Researchers' Perspectives on Interventionist Characteristics The need to address intervention selection, training, and other supports to facilitate better treatment outcomes for people with ASD is a recurring theme across the Future Directions sections of the intervention chapters. Although other nonprofessionals or paraprofessionals work with individuals with ASD, given the focus of this book, the two groups of nonprofessionals we discuss are caregivers and peers.

Parents Research needs related to better training of and support for caregivers, especially parents, are frequently mentioned in the intervention chapters in which parents were at least sometimes directly involved in interventions, either as co-interventionists or interventionists who were supported by SLPs or other professionals (i.e., Chapters 4, 5, 7, 9, 10, 11, 15). Parent interventionists face special challenges because not only will they almost always lack relevant previous education and training, but they will be balancing their new role as interventionists with their primary role as parent, bringing with that role many stresses that alone constitute major directions for future research (e.g., Hayes & Watson, 2013).

Particular needs identified in specific chapters include identifying key competencies of interventions and methods to instill them (Chapter 4 on AAC, Chapter 11 on early social interaction), determining how well caregivers actually execute the intervention (Chapter 10 on EMT), determining how to further support their efforts after initial training (Chapter 8 on FCT), and ways to engage them so that they can support behavior change in the home setting (Chapter 15 on social skills interventions). Among the strategies mentioned to address these needs are the use of Internet-accessible training and refresher materials (Chapter 11) and ongoing consultation and coaching (Chapters 11 and 15). In Chapter 8, Durand and Moskowitz suggest incorporating additional treatment elements to bolster parental optimism as a means of promoting better outcomes and greater persistence in the family's use of the intervention.

Research on parents as interventionists is especially important for several reasons. First, principles of family-centered care recognize parents as presenting the greatest expertise about their child, their child's needs, and how that child fits within his or her social world (Beatson, 2006; Prelock & Hutchins, 2008). Second, brain and behavioral development are powerfully affected by experience, especially in the first years of life; thus, the earlier intervention begins, the better, a context that further highlights the importance of parents (e.g., Bradshaw et al., 2015; NRC, 2001). Third, using parents and nonprofessionals as interventionists is seen as a practical necessity in order to achieve broader generalization of skills beyond treatment settings (e.g., Schreibman et al., 2015) as well as levels of intervention intensity (i.e., at least 25 hours per week) that are recommended but would be cost-prohibitive if only professionals served as interventionists (e.g., Maglione et al., 2012; Morgan et al., 2014). Thus, it should be no surprise that parental involvement is strongly recommended by the recent National Standards Report (National Autism Center, 2015; Wong et al., 2015) and, in the United States, is consistent with principles embodied in the Individuals with Disabilities Education Act (IDEA) of 2004, Part C.

According to an international survey, Gillon and colleagues (2017) found that 80% of the SLPs taking the survey reported that they often or always involved families in intervention practices. The use of parents in implementing intervention is especially common in early intervention designed for children from birth to age 3 years (Bradshaw et al., 2015; McConachie & Diggle, 2007), with interventions for children 2 and under growing in frequency (Bradshaw et al., 2015). Research into the effectiveness of parent-implemented interventions is somewhat mixed in terms of the size of effects achieved by parents, but it is promising nonetheless (e.g., Bejarano-Martín et al., 2020; Bradshaw et al., 2015; McConachie & Diggle, 2007; Oono et al., 2013; Sandbank et al., 2020). Over the next few years, as identification of risks and diagnoses are made at ever-earlier ages, research into parent-implemented interventions, and particularly, how to support parents to achieve the best possible outcomes (e.g., Woods et al., 2011) will surely grow in importance.

Peers   Peers represent another group whose place in the social world of individuals with ASD make them a natural ally in efforts to improve social interaction and, perhaps, language and communication skills as well. Peer interaction and support seems particularly valuable during later childhood, adolescence, and adulthood, developmental periods when home may no longer be the chief venue in which social skills naturally develop. Thus, arguments similar to those advocating for more research to assist parents as interventionists can be made to advocate for more research into how to better choose, train, and support peers. Admittedly, peers will not necessarily be involved as intensively as parents or have roles across as wide an array of outcomes, but their promise as interventionists involved in improving social-interaction outcomes and quality of life looms large. Not surprisingly, the chapter that addresses their needs most specifically is Chapter 12, on peer-mediated support interventions. Carter, the chapter's author, outlines not only the need for improving selection, training, and support but also the need to move research contexts beyond studies of primary and secondary students to include the use of peers in higher education and work contexts. Chapter 15 also highlights the crucial role of socially competent peers to support positive engagement of children, adolescents, and young adults with ASD in several social contexts, from having conversations during play to talking with friends at a social gathering to knowing what to say on a date. In addition, as in research involving parents as interventionists, there is the need to maximize benefits experienced not only by the recipients of the intervention but also by the peer interventionists.

Speech-Language Pathologists and Other Professionals   Certainly, as a group, SLPs can be expected to have more knowledge about autism and its treatment than do parents or peers. SLPs treat a wide range of communication and swallowing disorders and consequently receive generalist rather than highly specialized education and clinical training as part of their preparation for certification or licensure. Although formal courses in autism are increasingly available, most SLPs may have little direct experience in intervention for ASD in their clinical practice (Plumb & Plexico, 2013). Consequently, most SLPs must acquire additional and ongoing training beyond their degree to be effective with even a few of the well-researched intervention options that are available. Research further confirms that practicing SLPs in the United States differ greatly in their baseline knowledge of autism and best practices in intervention as well as in their levels of confidence about treating individuals with ASD (Plumb & Plexico, 2013; Schwartz & Drager, 2008).

The intervention chapters sections on Future Directions frequently mention research needs related to nonprofessionals, but they somewhat less often mention research needs related to SLPs or other professionals. When mentioned, the most important identified needs appear to be in research examining the extent to which SLPs can faithfully execute interventions outside of the context of a research study (Chapters 9 and 11). More elaborately, Woods and colleagues (Chapter 11) indicate the need to identify competencies underpinning successful implementation and to develop effective and readily available continuing education and mentoring resources to support continuing success.

Investigations of whether and how a wide range of professionals (e.g., teachers, SLPs, medical personnel) can consistently reproduce interventions as intended and studied (and thus supported) fit under the topic of fidelity (Kadaravek & Justice, 2010), or as it was originally termed, *intervention reliability* (Billingsley et al., 1980). At first, fidelity was primarily discussed in research contexts, referring to the need for researchers to demonstrate that the intervention they wanted to claim had caused an outcome was being consistently delivered by all intervention providers. With increasing attention to how interventions could be implemented beyond the laboratory as part of evidence-based practice, fidelity concerns have been raised specifically with regard to interventionists treating individuals with ASD (e.g., Dunst et al., 2013; Reichow et al., 2011).

Larger Trends Affecting Attention to Interventionist Characteristics Three larger trends shaping research to address and shape interventionist characteristics that can affect outcomes are 1) **adult learning theories and practices,** 2) **behavior change theories and techniques,** and 3) efforts to provide more cohesive and effective interdisciplinary teams through **interprofessional education and interprofessional collaborative practice (IE/IP).** Adult learning theories (Dunst et al., 2010; Mukhalalati & Taylor, 2019) and behavior change theories (Abraham & Michie, 2008; Michie et al., 2015) are two somewhat loosely intertwined but influential sources of ideas about how to help people change their behaviors, including their professional practices. Despite differences in their philosophical origins and the disciplines that these theories and methods influence most, both are relevant here because they share some tenets and techniques that are increasingly influencing researchers and organizations seeking to bring well-studied practices into everyday use.

Adult Learning Theories and Techniques In the last decade or so, theories of adult learning have begun to affect some aspects of professional development, particularly in relation to efforts designed to support evidence-based practice. Trivette and colleagues (2009) summarized a set of four principles that have affected current work on improving learning among adult interventionists, based on ideas drawn from earlier work by Knowles (1984). The assumptions described by Trivette and colleagues (2009) are that adults are highly motivated to learn, are self-directed, and learn best through active participation and when learning is directed toward problem solving. Methods associated with these principles include 1) the use of role playing and practice exercises; 2) one-to-one or small-group coaching that includes cycles of shared planning, modeling by the coach, performance by learners, followed by self-analysis and coach feedback; 3) an emphasis on the development of problem-solving and meta-cognitive skills; and 4) readily available continuing support of problem solving. More recent steps in the methods being used to support professionals have included manuals (Kadaravek & Justice, 2010) and checklists as two strategies for highlighting what is most important to be learned as well as for serving as reminders of what needs to be done once practices are put into place (Dunst, 2017; Dunst et al., 2013).

In their 2009 study, Trivette and her colleagues also synthesized the results of 79 group studies (using randomized controlled trials or comparison group designs) to evaluate a number of training methods associated with adult learning theory. Effect sizes, which measure the magnitude of differences between groups (e.g., results obtained by those who did vs. those who did *not* receive coaching), were used to determine how effective these methods were. The four kinds of outcomes they examined were learners' 1) knowledge, 2) skills, 3) attitudes toward their training experience, and 4) self-efficacy beliefs (e.g., belief that they could effectively carry out the methods they had learned through the training). Put succinctly, what the researchers found was that "adult learning method practices that more actively involved learners in using, processing, and evaluating their knowledge and skills as part of learning and mastering new information practices were most effective" (Trivette et al., 2009, p. 9). Trainings that involved smaller groups (<34) and longer periods of time (i.e., >10 hours) were also found to be the most effective.

Adult learning theories and methods continue to be studied extensively for use with professionals across a variety of fields, including medicine (e.g., Min et al., 2015; Mukhalalati & Taylor, 2019), teaching (e.g., Kraft et al., 2018), and early intervention (e.g., Dunst, 2017; Friedman et al., 2012). Not surprisingly, it seems that the effectiveness of any of the adult-learning methods—for example, coaching—cannot be viewed as a foregone conclusion; rather, it requires considerable effort to truly meet the needs of the interventionist-learner while capturing the actual key ingredients of the intervention or practice being taught (e.g., Piasta et al., 2020). In this context, improving our identification and description of an intervention's active ingredients and implementation strategies will need to develop together.

Behavior Change Theories and Techniques   Already mentioned because of their role in driving the development of taxonomies to describe complex interventions, behavior change theories and techniques represent another widely influential source of ideas regarding how to address the faithful application of evidence-based interventions deployed on a large scale. These theories and techniques may be best known in health psychology and health sciences, in which people, often adults, are targeted as recipients of interventions to promote health, for example, to help people stop smoking, eat better, or exercise more (Lippke & Ziegelmann, 2008; van Achterberg et al., 2010). In this context (as is the case in many interventions discussed in this volume), there are often two levels at which behavior changes are needed—at the level of the end recipient of the intervention and at the level of the interventionist who must implement the intervention with fidelity to manifest the active ingredients intended by the developers. Unsurprisingly, therefore, advocates of behavior change theories and techniques have also liberally applied them to the challenge of promoting evidence-based practice in health care personnel and others (e.g., Chauhan et al., 2017; Huis et al., 2012).

To date, the application of behavioral change theories and techniques to communication disorders interventions has been limited. Thus, a groundbreaking project by early literacy researcher Laura Justice and her colleagues is mentioned here.

The project involved 128 caregiver dyads in a caregiver shared-reading intervention for children with language impairment (Justice et al., 2015; Justice et al., 2018; Justice et al., 2020). The project examined mechanisms by which carefully selected behavior change techniques (viz., rewards, feedback, encouragement, modeling) affected caregivers' fidelity and attrition as well as child outcomes. Of particular importance is the authors' focus on behavior change techniques as an additional reservoir of strategies to support interventionists—strategies that may well be applied to the many kinds of interventionists whose work can contribute to better outcomes for children and older individuals with ASD.

Interprofessional Education and Practice   The growth of IE/IP is yet another trend that may help shape future research to support interventionists' roles in social-interaction and communication interventions for ASD. IE/IP refers to initiatives taken by educational institutions and professional groups to improve the quality of collaborations between teams of professionals who work in educational and health care settings. Therefore, unlike EBP, which is influencing future directions related to understanding interventionist characteristics for both professionals and nonprofessionals alike, efforts related to supporting IE/IP center more narrowly on professional interventionists. The World Health Organization (WHO) has led the way for this work in medicine and health care as a means of addressing worldwide workforce challenges and improving the quality of health outcomes (WHO, 2010). Given similar challenges that can interfere with effective collaboration in schools, IE/IP initiatives have now been extended to address educational settings as well. By receiving education and training experiences with students or colleagues from different professions, advocates of IE/IP working in the area of ASD hope that outcomes can be maximized for individuals receiving care or education (Prelock et al., 2017; Potvin et al., 2017).

Over the past decade, ASHA has strived to deepen its commitment to principles of IE/IP related to both education and health care. Highpoints in this deepening commitment have included the organization's 2017 joining of the Interprofessional Education Collaborative, which recommends core competencies for IE/IP practice (Interprofessional Education Collaborative, 2016), and its 2018 commitment to including elements related to IE/IP in 2020 certification standards for both audiologists and SLPs (https://www.asha.org/Practice/IPE-IPP-Activities-and-Collaborations). In a 2019 survey completed by ASHA members on the topic, key findings were that 84% of SLPs in health care settings and 91% of SLPs in educational settings reported active engagement in interprofessional practice, but only 44% and 43%, respectively, reported feeling "very prepared for this practice." Across the professional groups, the majority (71%) reported no formal training (ASHA, 2019). Internationally, Gillon and colleagues (2017) reported frequent involvement with teachers, occupational therapists, other SLPs, and psychologists. Thus, efforts to support IE/IP, including research into how collaborations can work best to produce improved outcomes for people with ASD, represent important forces affecting future research and practice.

Contextual Characteristics

Contextual characteristics, the fourth main component of the model shown in Figure 18.1, is perhaps best discussed last—not because it is least important but in order to emphasize the crucial, but sometimes underappreciated, role it plays in outcomes. One large set of contextual characteristics concerns the physical and organizational realm in which intervention is carried out—for example, at home through early intervention programs, in educational systems as varied as preschool to higher education, and in medically oriented settings such as hospitals or clinics. A second set of these characteristics consists of how the intervention is delivered—for example, who beyond the recipient is involved, how directly others are involved, and with probably increasing frequency, whether the interactions are in person or conducted synchronously over the Internet. Different countries vary substantially in what settings may be most used or even available as well as in the resources and philosophies that prevail, further intensifying the complexity of contextual characteristics globally.

Intervention developers and researchers often see contextual characteristics as barriers to overcome in order for treatments that have been shown to be efficacious in laboratory settings to be disseminated and adopted broadly, then used effectively in a sustained manner in the real world. All of the concerns related to fidelity that were mentioned in previous sections are relevant here, because contexts other than those used during the intervention's development create some of the biggest threats to fidelity.

Researchers' Perspectives on Contextual Characteristics   In their sections on Future Directions, chapter authors propose research efforts in two areas: expanding the contexts in which the intervention can be used and using technology to increase the effectiveness or efficiency of intervention delivery.

Expanding Intervention Settings   Having an evidence-based intervention used in settings beyond those in which it was developed should increase its impact on a wider range of individuals, including those in younger and older age groups who are currently so badly underserved (Bishop-Fitzpatrick et al., 2013; Steinbrenner et al., 2020). When the research goal of serving a wider range of people with ASD was described earlier in the chapter under Personal Characteristics, it was not by chance that settings and delivery models were often mentioned as well. After all, age is generally a major determinant in societal expectations about where people will spend their time and where educational or therapeutic interventions might be offered. Not surprisingly, therefore, extending interventions to new settings and delivery modes associated with them seems to encompass a single goal. For example, Laurent and colleagues (Chapter 14) mention the need for more study of SCERTS in public schools as a means of better serving school-age children because that is the context in which many children of that age will be served. Similarly, although noting that JASPER (Chapter 9) is currently being *studied* in a variety of settings, Kasari and Sterrett point to the need to determine whether it can be adopted into "community settings with fidelity." When it comes to using peer-mediated interventions to serve older individuals, Carter (Chapter 12) recommends research in environments such as inclusive college programs and integrated workshops. In addition to calls for a better understanding of characteristics of the different environments in which FCT (Chapter 8) may be used, Durand and Moskowitz propose a very specific and quite different research direction for FCT. Because the primary focus of FCT is on the replacement of challenging behaviors by more acceptable communications, those authors recommend assessing environments to determine if one over another might be more accepting and therefore more appropriate for the individual.

Using Technology to Increase Effectiveness or Efficiency   Technology is particularly important for two interventions that often or always depend on relatively complex technological components—AAC (Chapter 4, Wegner) and video modeling (Chapter 17, Buggey). In her discussion of future directions for AAC, Wegner proposes a research focus on AAC system design to better integrate communication and curricular content as a way of enhancing learning as well as finding ways to capitalize on the availability of tablet computers and software, developments that increase the practicality of AAC in many environments. Given that technology lies at the heart of video modeling, it is understandable that Buggey discusses a greater number of future research options related to technology than do other chapter authors. One option he mentions involves increasing the variety of model sources for peer and self-modeling through models based on photographs of oneself or other people (or even one's pet) or digital avatars. In these applications, not only might the nature of the model change, but the ability to demonstrate a wider range of skills could be possible through digital enhancement. Other options include the use of cell phone displays to allow videos to be used as portable reminders of target behaviors and the use of educational television channels to share relevant video across intervention recipients. Finally, although this option appears to be somewhat farther in the future, Buggey mentions the possibility of virtual reality to enrich the training of social and functional skills through point-of-view modeling.

Although not mentioned specifically in future directions, Prelock and Brien, in Chapter 15, highlight two recent social skills interventions, Virtual Reality-Social Cognition Training and Mind Reading, that specifically emphasize the use of technology for adolescent and young adult populations. These social skills interventions focus on enhancing particular elements of theory of mind, such as emotion or affect recognition and complex social judgement, via practice with computer-based vocal and facial expressions and social scenarios. Use of technology, in this context, allows adolescents and adults to learn and practice application of their social skills via computer-illustrated social situations.

The topic of technology in future research on intervention research in ASD is discussed in this section on context rather than as a characteristic of interventions because the creation of new contexts through telehealth represents a particularly powerful and timely capability that depends on technology. In their Future Directions section, two authors mention future directions in research targeting telepractice. Telehealth is defined by ASHA as "the application of telecommunications technology to the delivery of speech-language pathology and audiology professional services at a distance by linking clinician to client or clinician to clinician for assessment, intervention and/or consultation" (ASHA, n.d.-b).

In Chapter 5, Howard and Dawson indicate that future research plans for the ESDM include looking into adaptations to that intervention achieved through telehealth and other technologically assisted modifications. Through a web platform, Woods and colleagues (Chapter 11) describe the development of online courses and video libraries for a wide range of audiences, such as parents, paraprofessionals, professionals, and multidisciplinary teams, to help teach basic strategies of the ESI model and how to embed those strategies in natural routines. Although these resources themselves do not fit within the definition of telepractice used by ASHA, they have the potential to facilitate more efficient coaching, thus helping to increase the fidelity needed to make telepractice more efficient and effective. Although, until recently, discussions of telepractice have emphasized its particular value to rural or poor families who experience reduced access to early intervention services (Meadan et al., 2016), the heightened risks and challenges associated with in-person meetings during the 2020 pandemic may make the development and use of such resources a truly urgent research priority.

The state of research on telepractice, especially as it relates to interventions for people with ASD, is still in its infancy. Two systematic reviews that considered both assessment and intervention research have been completed to date (Boisvert et al., 2010; Sutherland et al., 2018). Because the more recent review also included the eight articles that were identified in the first review, only the second review is sum-marized here. Using the ASHA definition of telehealth, Sutherland and colleagues found only 14 articles up to 2018 that met inclusion criteria, with some 26 additional articles having been rejected because they lacked a comparison condition as a dem-onstration of scientific control. The 284 participants with ASD consisted of 23 adults and 261 children who ranged in age from 19 months to early adolescence. Only the adults and 18 children were directly involved in the telehealth sessions—17 children in a single group study of 11 year olds receiving anxiety intervention. The remain-ing children were considered involved in telehealth because of participation by their teachers ($n = 49$) or parents ($n = 211$) who were working toward outcomes related to the child's functioning.

Three of the 14 studies reviewed by Sutherland and colleagues (2018) focused on assessment, including a single study in which adults with ASD were participants. The remaining 11 intervention studies, therefore, were all directed toward children, although they addressed a variety of purposes. Specifically, 6 of the 11 were early intervention studies (one focused on imitation and the other five on communica-tion). Other topics that were addressed included anxiety intervention (one study), functional behavioral assessment and functional communication training (two stud-ies), and achievement of individualized goals (a school-based study in which teach-ers worked with school-age children; goals were not specified in the study). Finally, there was one language intervention study of an 11-year-old boy with ASD. Nota-bly, Sutherland and colleagues also reported that whereas the 23 adult participants and 18 older children with ASD in these studies were directly engaged during the telepractice, only the 11-year-old receiving language intervention participated in the telehealth session without an adult facilitator (e.g., parent) in the room (Boisvert et al., 2012). Sutherland and colleagues (2018) interpreted their findings as indi-cating that telehealth delivery resulted in outcomes equivalent to those obtained conventionally, including outcomes related to client satisfaction. However, given the small number of studies overall and smaller numbers focused on specific intervention types, Sutherland and her colleagues appropriately called for further research, which might now be seen as a practical imperative.

Larger Trend Affecting Attention to Contextual Characteristics—Implementation Science

Implementation science can be defined as "the scientific study of methods to promote the systematic uptake of research find-ings and other evidence-based practices into routine practice" (Eccles & Mittman, 2006, p. 1). During the past decade or so, many theoretical approaches have been developed that can be seen as fitting under the umbrella of implementation sci-ence (Esmail et al., 2020)—all of them addressing a problem variously called the research-to-practice gap, knowledge transfer, and the scaling up of evidence-based practices, among others (Olswang & Prelock, 2015). Manifestations of this problem include the slow uptake of research into practice (e.g., an estimated 17 years in medical research; Olswang & Prelock, 2015), the outright failure of many interventions with strong evidence bases to enter widespread use, and the continued use of less well-studied interventions. Not surprisingly, implementation science has sometimes been seen as a response to the "disappointing results" (Fixsen et al., 2009) of the evidence-based practice movement in not leading directly to widespread strengthening of clinical and educational practices.

In relation to autism, Dingfelder and Mandell (2011) described the problem of inadequate implementation by pointing grimly to the undeniable reality that "efficacious interventions for autism are rarely adopted, implemented, and maintained in community settings," largely because of concerns about "the perceived fit between the intervention and the needs and capacities of the setting" (p. 497). Using one of the oldest approaches to implementation science, diffusion of innovation theory (Rogers, 1962, 2003), Dingfelder and Mandell described four stages of implementation: dissemination, adoption, implementation, and maintenance. They called particular attention to factors affecting the final stages in which the new intervention or practice must be embraced by end users and reconciled with its ultimate community context. Important factors included the end user's perceptions of the relative advantage of new innovation (i.e., practice or intervention) over the status quo, its compatibility with setting characteristics, and its complexity, that is, how difficult its use seemed to be. Recognizing the many contextual challenges posed by implementation in addition to these, Dingfelder and Mandell called for the pursuit of strategies for "linking intervention development and the settings in which we hope interventions ultimately be used" (p. 607). Some of the strategies they called upon autism intervention researchers to pursue were earlier involvement of end users of an intervention, greater attention to early development of materials that will be used during everyday application of the intervention, improved documentation of what demands and benefits may actually be associated with implementation, and the placement of greater value on studies examining feasibility of an intervention's use in a particular setting.

Despite taking a variety forms (Nilsen, 2015), many implementation theories can serve as the basis for research designed to identify and deploy strategies similar to those called for by Dingfelder and Mandell (2011). For example, Fixsen and colleagues (2009) identify core implementation components to support individual interventionists and their organization, that can then serve as targets for support. Also called *implementation drivers*, these components include "staff selection, preservice and in-service training, ongoing coaching and consultation, staff evaluation, decision support data systems, facilitative administrative support, and systems interventions" (Fixsen et al., p. 533). Related ways to develop strategies include the identification of barriers that can be removed or mitigated or facilitators that can be promoted (Nilsen, 2015; Olswang & Prelock, 2015). Numerous sources have identified potential categories of strategies, often tailored to meet the special demands of educational or health care settings—both of which serve individuals with ASD (e.g., Campbell & Douglas, 2017; Odom et al., 2013; Powell et al., 2012). Numerous strategies designed to address barriers related to end users, such as their need for effective training and ongoing support, were mentioned in earlier sections of this chapter on adult learning and behavior change theories. Additional sources describing the intricacies of implementation research may also prove helpful (e.g., Olswang & Prelock, 2015; Wilson & Landa, 2010).

In this section of the chapter, we have primarily emphasized the ways in which implementation science can address the role that context plays in optimizing outcomes for individuals with autism. However, implementation science and research endeavors can also be expected to cast light on the complex interactions of individual, intervention, interventionists, and contextual characteristics that can affect outcomes. Therefore, it is likely that this trend in intervention research will continue and perhaps gain further momentum.

Conclusions

Although the model pictured in Figure 18.1 is quite simple, readers may recall that it is intended to capture the idea that best outcomes can result when well-equipped interventionists choose and effectively use the most well-developed treatments in places and situations that can best facilitate that treatment, given the particular strengths, facilitators, difficulties, and interests of the person receiving it. This is such an important idea that if, as details of the chapter up to this point fade, the reader remembers just the model, the overriding purpose of this section has been achieved. In the second major section of this chapter, we turn from a focus on readers interested in intervention research to the very particular needs of specific groups of readers.

FUTURE DIRECTIONS FOR READERS

This portion of the chapter considers future directions for each of three main audiences: families, professionals, and students and their professors. In particular, we suggest how they might continue their quest for information about issues affecting treatment decisions for people with ASD. Although the specific kinds of decisions required, the backgrounds, and the information needs of these three audiences can differ substantially, they also converge to a great extent. Consequently, although we have organized our discussions according to the three audiences, all readers can benefit from reading the entire section. Before diving into the specifics for each audience, we briefly consider the complexities associated with seeking information to aid in our future decision making.

The unending avalanche of new information on autism challenges anyone seeking guidance by making it difficult to determine which information is both relevant and useful. Although the challenge exists regardless of the type of information source (i.e., research publication, popular books, magazine articles), it can seem heightened in the case of websites because, despite their apparent dominance, they are still an extraordinarily new source of information. The number of potentially relevant websites is growing exponentially, with many including both downloadable, printable resources as well as structured sets of video demonstrations of the behaviors or techniques being described. Websites providing online printable materials can greatly reduce the burden of sharing information with others or can point to or remind viewers of concepts or strategies they do not want to forget. Websites that include video material can lead to those ah-ha moments we can get when we see something in action rather than simply read about it. Indeed, websites can be friendly, accessible, and potentially irreplaceable sources of information for all of us. In fact, along with personal recommendations from professionals and families with similar problems, families in particular value websites as easily accessible, if sometimes overwhelming, sources of information (Carlon et al., 2013; Grant et al., 2016).

Quotes taken from Grant and colleagues' qualitative study illustrate this complicated situation. In their study of 23 parents of children with ASD examining information preferences, Grant and colleagues (2016) found parents vividly expressed the benefit of Internet accessibility. One parent offered this insight: "I mainly prefer the Internet, because I can do it at night in my own time, without having to wait for business hours to call somebody or—especially chasing two small kids" (p. 130). Another parent highlighted the possible downside: "I found the Internet overwhelming and too much" (p. 130). Thus, although there is much to invite us to use websites as information sources, we must be cautious when doing so.

Besides potentially swamping us with too much information to deal with, evidence pretty clearly suggests that many autism-related websites provide information of questionable value (e.g., Reichow et al., 2012; Grant et al., 2015). In their 2015 study, Grant and her colleagues identified 20 autism-related health websites that appeared frequently across three different search engines, then rated them for the presence of valuable treatment information. The researchers found that almost none of the websites they reviewed included information regarding treatment risks or no treatment as an option, and only 30% provided research references. In a summary of two studies of the availability and quality of information regarding interventions contained in autism websites, Reichow and colleagues (2012) came to similar conclusions and suggested the best websites for high-quality information are those with the domains with .gov or .edu. Those researchers further advised parents that they should use such information as a "supplement, not a replacement to information they obtain from professionals (e.g., pediatrician, psychologist, psychiatrist, special educator)" (p. 1270). We would add SLPs to that list as well.

Of course, not just parents or people with ASD, but professionals as well, including SLPs, students and their professors, should be equally concerned about the quality of website information about treatment they consume. Therefore, Tables 18.2, 18.4, and 18.5 suggest websites that may serve as places to start. Each website listed is connected to a well-known educational (.edu), not-for-profit (.org), or governmental (.gov) organization that is likely to do its best to ensure the quality of the information provided. Through these carefully selected resources, we hope the problem of knowing where to look for credible information is at least a bit reduced.

Whatever the website, we also suggest that anyone using Web sources for information gathering strongly consider evaluating the quality of information on it. At least one formal research-focused tool has been developed to evaluate websites providing consumer health information (e.g., the DISCERN; Charnock, 1998), which has been used to evaluate website quality in a variety of medically related areas (e.g., Cerminara et al., 2014; Khazaal et al., 2009). Recently, researchers interested in autism have begun to use them for that purpose, as we indicated previously (e.g., Grant et al., 2015). Instead of reproducing the DISCERN in its entirety instrument here, we drew on it and several additional sources (e.g., National Institutes of Health, 2011; Rogers et al., 2012) to create Table 18.1, which explains five characteristics readers should look for when evaluating websites (most of which also apply to evaluating any information sources). Pending the development of systems for regular expert evaluation of websites for autism, we recommend keeping the questions contained in that table in the back of your minds throughout your work but asking them explicitly when the information being sought concerns consequential decisions. Such decisions may be related to purchasing materials, choosing an intervention, or changing significant routines in households or practices in schools or clinics.

Table 18.1.   Desirable characteristics for a website

Characteristic	Questions you should ask to assess the presence of the characteristic
Evidence-based	If a website claims to be evidence based, does it provide references to research so you can review any research claims that are made? Does it include more information from systematic research than from personal testimonials?
Current	Can you find dates for specific sources of information contained in the website? If so, are they current?
Unbiased	Does the website present multiple points of view or identify possible options rather than focus on only a single point of view?
Trustworthy	Was the website created and is it maintained by an individual or organization that seems likely to have the best interests of the users at heart? Does it contain content that seems designed primarily to *sell* you a product, assessment, or treatment?
Reasonable	Does the website discuss shorter- and longer-term *risks* as well as benefits? Are the described outcomes sensible or practical rather than grandiose?

Resources for Families of Individuals With ASD

Table 18.2 lists four books and seven websites to share with families. A huge number of books are now available for people with ASD and their families, about which many of the websites in the table offer recommendations. Rather than try to choose just a few to cover all the ages, circumstances, difficulties, and strengths that you might be interested in, we decided to choose books that can provide families with a deeper and perhaps more readable dive into several of the interventions described in this book. Consequently, the four books included are written by authors or coauthors of intervention chapters in this book and are aimed at a popular rather than academic or professional readership. The four interventions for which such books were available are the ESDM (Chapter 5), FCT (Chapter 8), PRT (Chapter 13), and the SCERTS Model (Chapter 14).

The seven websites in Table 18.2 are affiliated with the professional organization associated with SLPs in the United States, four U.S. associations dedicated to serving people with ASD, a triad of related websites affiliated with research into ESI (Chapter 11), and one governmental agency—the Department of Health and Human Services. Both the professional website and the governmental agency represent the tip of the iceberg in that different countries have similar associations, and there are many agencies within the U.S. government that address issues related to ASD. Similarly, the autism organizations and research-related websites we chose are not the only ones of their kind in the United States but were selected because they seemed to offer a promising and safe start for information seekers.

Despite our efforts to winnow down the vast number of available resource repositories, the complexity of even one of them can be daunting. Therefore, we again face this question: How can you make use of these resources without being overwhelmed? As one answer, we propose that you choose either an issue-based or a one-website-at-a-time approach as a means of focusing your efforts. In an issue-based approach, you would first choose a single issue (e.g., helping teens deal with sexuality, approaching employment challenges, dealing with sleep problems). Then you would search for resources related to that issue on two or three promising-looking websites listed in Table 18.2 to see what turns up. In a one-at-a-time approach, you would first choose a single appealing website, then search it for

Table 18.2. Resources primarily for parents and other family members but also for students and in-place professionals

Source	Brief description
Books about interventions mentioned in this text	
Durand, V. M. (2011). *Optimistic parenting: Hope and help for you and your challenging child*. Paul H. Brookes Publishing Co.	In this book, Victor Durand, a specialist in challenging behavior and a parent, addresses parents whose children with autism spectrum disorder (ASD) whose behaviors perplex, distress, and truly challenge them. After exploring the origins of these behaviors and their effects on parents, the author presents strategies designed to result in more satisfying outcomes for both parents and children. In Chapter 8, he discusses research on functional communication training, the source of these strategies.
Koegel, R. L., & Koegel, L. K. (2012). *The PRT pocket guide: Pivotal response treatment for autism spectrum disorders*. Paul H. Brookes Publishing Co.	Aimed at parents and teachers, this book describes strategies and specific activities based on Pivotal Response Treatment (PRT) that they may find particularly useful. It also provides an in-depth description of this intervention. PRT is described in Chapter 13.
Prizant, B. M., with Fields-Meyer, T. (2016). *Uniquely human: A different way of seeing autism*. Simon & Schuster.	The central premise of this book is that because autism is just a different way of being human, not an illness, people with autism need understanding, not "fixing." Drawing on his research, clinical work as a speech-language pathologist, and friend of many articulate adults with autism, Barry Prizant and his coauthor make a powerful argument for that premise. The SCERTS Model, which Prizant has studied for decades, is described in Chapter 14.
Rogers, S. J., Dawson, G., & Vismara, L. A. (2012). *An early start for your child with autism: Using everyday activities to help kids connect, communicate, and learn*. Guilford Press.	Drawing on their knowledge as experienced clinicians and researchers, these authors use composite stories capturing children and families they have known, recommendations, and countless examples to help caregivers learn how to use everyday activities to help their children thrive. The strategies they incorporate come from the Early Start Denver Model described in Chapter 5.
Web-based resources	
American Speech-Language-Hearing Association (https://www.asha.org)	The ASHA Practice Portal, www.asha.org/Practice-Portal/Clinical-Topics/Autism, provides a basic overview of what is known about the nature of ASD and the relationship of speech-language pathologists (SLPs) to its assessment and intervention, including their roles and responsibilities. It also provides links to other areas of the website offering more technical information and research. A list is included that describes state insurance mandates related to ASD: https://www.asha.org/Advocacy/state/States-Specific-Autism-Mandates
Autism Society https://www.autism-society.org/about-the-autism-society An organization dedicated to improving "the lives of all affected by autism" through "advocacy, education, information and referral, support, and community at national, state, and local levels"	**Living With Autism** is a series of brief (4–12 page) publications that can be downloaded for free. They cover topics that are useful to families, such as supporting appropriate behavior, preparing for college, puberty, positive sleep patterns, and transitioning to adult. https://www.autism-society.org/about-the-autism-society/publications/resource-materials **Background information and materials for sharing with other professionals**, including teachers and professionals who may be associated with criminal safety issues, such as child abuse counselors; advocates, attorneys and judges; social workers and counselors; domestic violence and sexual assault counselors; paramedics and emergency room staff, can be found at https://www.autism-society.org/about-the-autism-society/publications/resource-materials

(continued)

Table 18.2. *(continued)*

Source	Brief description
Web-based resources	

Autism Speaks https://www.autismspeaks.org/about-us Perhaps the most well-known of organizations supporting people with autism and their families with major goals of their mission including "advocacy and support," increasing "public understanding and acceptance," and "advancing research into causes and better interventions"	**A parent's guide to autism: An Autism Speaks family support tool kit** is a downloadable 17-page PDF that includes topics such as 10 things parents can do to help their child with autism, building a support network, taking care of yourself, and strategies for supporting your other children. https://www.autismspeaks.org/tool-kit/parents-guide-autism **A guide for accessing website resources,** with tailoring of searches made possible using filters specifying geographic location, types of service (e.g., schools, employment supports, professional group), life stage (age group), and level of support required (some, moderate, intensive): https://www.autismspeaks.org/resource-guide **More than 40 online tool kits** are available for specific family members as well tool kits meant for others, such as employers, educators, health care professionals, and even hairstylists.
First Words Project (described in Chapter 11) Working in collaboration with the First Words Project, a number of organizations have contributed to creating several websites focused on young children with typical or atypical social communication development.	**First Words Project** resources for parents of young children include https://firstwordsproject.com • Two photographic lookbooks identifying social-communication landmarks: 16 gestures by 16 months and 16 actions with objects by 16 months • **Growth charts** showing social-communication milestones developing from 7 to 24 months that allow parents to explore or chart a child's development in the areas of language, play, social interaction, emotional regulation, and self-directed learning • **A series of brief downloadable and printable** documents related to imparting understanding and observation of children's early social-communication development, many in several languages besides English, including Spanish, Portuguese, Canadian French, Creole and Arabic **Baby Navigator** provides access to many of the same resources as those available through the First Words Project website. Support is available to both parents interested in promoting development who have no concerns about their young child and to parents who have concerns, and many video examples are available: https://babynavigator.com • **Smart Early Screening for Early Autism and Communication Disorders (Smart ESAC),** a screening tool for parents based on parent report, can provide recommendations about contacting professionals who can further screen or provide a diagnosis for ASD. It also connects parents whose child shows signs indicating a possible risk to the Autism Navigator website. **Autism Navigator and A Seamless Path for Families** (https://autismnavigator.com/wp-content/uploads/2016/11/Seamless-Path-for-Families.pdf), a one-page handout that orients users to five major resources: three unique resources for families whose children screen positive for ASD or who suspect that the child has ASD and two Web-based courses—About Autism in Toddlers, How-To Guide for Families, and an interactive ASD Video Glossary.

Table 18.2.   *(continued)*

Source	Brief description
Web-based resources	
Organization for Autism Research (OAR) https://researchautism.org An organization with a "singular focus on applied research and the quality and practical value of its resource materials"	**Kit for kids** includes materials to facilitate teaching elementary and middle school students about peers with ASD; the kit comprises an introductory video, 20 booklets "What's Up with Nick?" supportive instructional materials, and a printable poster and workbooks. • **Eight Life Journey into Autism guidebooks** are available as downloadable PDFs, with some associated websites that include topics of interest to individuals with ASD, parents, and professionals. Examples include the following: ○ *Navigating the Special Education System* (2012) (106 pages) ○ *A Guide to Safety* (2014) (146 pages); Think Safety website ○ *Transition Guide to Adulthood* (2006) (86 pages) ○ *A Guide for Military Families* (2019) (98 pages); Operation Autism website
National Autism Association https://nationalautismassociation.org A parent-run advocacy organization whose stated mission involves responding to "the most urgent needs of the autism community," addressing issues related to autism safety, autism abuse, crisis prevention, and autism-related wandering prevention and response	**Autism Training Resources, Information, and Materials (ATRIUM)** offers recorded webinars, training resources, information, and materials, primarily for parents but also for educators and first responders, including police: https://nationalautismassociation.org/family-support/programs/autism-atrium The **Give A Voice program** provides communication devices for nonverbal and minimally verbal people with autism: https://nationalautismassociation.org/family-support/programs/naas-give-a-voice-program **NAA Big Red Safety Box** consists of three sets of resources to help address wandering or elopement issues and are available for three different audiences: caregivers, educators, and first responders. In addition to brochures, fact sheets, and checklists, the kits include other practical materials, emotion identification cards, and child identification kits from the National Center for Missing and Exploited Children. A similar safety toolkit is also available for teachers. https://nationalautismassociation.org/big-red-safety-box
U.S. Department of Health and Human Services (HHS) https://www.hhs.gov/programs/topic-sites/autism/index.html	This website provides • Information about HSS's perspectives on autism • Links to governmental organizations that ○ Track the occurrence of autism (Centers for Disease Control) ○ Fund autism-related research (National Institute of Mental Health, National Institute of Neurological Disorders and Stroke, and National Human Genome Research Institute) ○ Describe national legislation affecting health plans and insurance affecting people with autism

information across several areas relevant to the person inspiring your search. The authors of *An Early Start for Your Child with Autism* (Rogers et al., 2012) suggest that Autisms Speaks may be a good place to start. Still, looking at the description of alternatives listed in Table 18.2 may suggest a different choice that better fits your needs and interests.

Resources for Speech-Language Pathologists and Other Professionals

Acknowledging that professionals can find themselves in the same quandary as that of families and people with ASD, we offer Table 18.3. There is much information of varying quality and much competition for what needs to be learned, yet little guidance and time available for crafting and pursuing a self-designed syllabus for ongoing learning. We hope that the descriptions of interventions in this book advanced your learning in a practical fashion by helping you find out a bit more about how the interventions have been developed thus far and what additional refinements are needed. Furthering this work through additional information gathering can help fuel your ongoing journey to achieve more effective person/family-centered work with people with ASDs as *they* navigate toward improved communication and social interaction outcomes.

Table 18.3.   Resources for speech-language pathologists, students, faculty, and other professionals

Profession	Organization resources	Selected resources
Speech-language pathologists (SLPs)	American Speech-Language-Hearing Association (https://www.asha.org) The professional association for SLPs in the United States	**Evidence Maps—Autism.** This area of the ASHA website identifies and describes published articles falling within three domains that mirror the major types of evidence to be considered in evidence-based practice: external scientific evidence, clinical expertise, and client perspectives. https://www2.asha.org/evidence-maps/
		Practice Portal—Autism. This area of the ASHA website presents information written in a more informal style to address topics that include incidence and prevalence information, signs and symptoms, causes, the special roles and responsibilities of SLPs in autism, assessment, treatment, resources, and references. https://www.asha.org/Practice-Portal/Clinical-Topics/Autism
	Ohio Center on Autism and Low Incidence Disorders (OCALI) (https://ocali.org)	The **Autism Center of OCALI** provides a variety of online print and video resources, primarily for educational settings but also for parents (e.g., a series of social narratives designed to support families during the 2020 COVID-19 pandemic). https:/ocali.org/center/autism
	General goal is to improve access to opportunities for people with disabilities, including autism	**Autism Internet Modules (AIM)** offers 48 modules that include online case studies, instructional videos, pre- and post-assessments, and a glossary. Many of the modules are related to specific intervention strategies (including at least 24 identified as evidence-based practices; Odom et al., 2013). Although the modules are available at no cost, payment is required for certificate and credit options that document module completion. Methods for obtaining continuing education credits are in development. (https://autisminternetmodules.org/)

Table 18.3. *(continued)*

Profession	Organization resources	Selected resources
	National Autism Association (https://nationalautismassociation .org) Mission is to address the "most urgent needs of the autism community"	**Autism Training Resources Information and Materials** (ATRIUM) is a digital library that provides access to regularly scheduled online webinars, downloadable toolkits, and brochures primarily for parents but also for educators, clinicians, and first responders (e.g., police and emergency room staff). Topics that seem particular to this organization include wandering and elopement and autism abuse. https://nationalautismassociation .org/family-support/programs/autism -atrium
	The National Autism Center (https://www.nationalautism center.org/resources) Dedicated to identification and dissemination of information about evidence-based practices	The following are book-length reports based on the Center's efforts to promote evidence-based practice. They are available for downloading after signing up for access. National Autism Center. (2015). *Findings and conclusions: National Standards Project, Phase 2. Addressing the need for evidence-based practice guidelines for autism spectrum disorder.* https://www .nationalautismcenter.org/resources. This report updates the review from Phase 1 to studies conducted up to 2012 and includes studies for adults, which was not in the earlier phase. National Autism Center. (2015). *Evidence-based practice and autism in the schools: An educator's guide to providing appropriate interventions to students with autism spectrum disorder.* https://www.nationalautismcenter.org /resources
	National Professional Development Center on Autism Spectrum Disorder (https://autismpdc.fpg.unc.edu /national-professional -development-center-autism -spectrum-disorder) Seeks to promote comprehensive professional development at state and local levels	**Autism Focused Intervention Resources and Modules** (AFFIRM) provides modules requiring 1.5–2 hours to complete about 27 practices identified as evidence-based (Steinbrenner et al., 2020), including specific practices and manualized interventions, such as Functional Communication Training, Picture Exchange Communication System, Pivotal Response Training, social skills training, and video modeling. Requires creating an account and logging in. An overview of these materials can be found at AFIRM (Sam et al., 2020). https://afirm.fpg.unc.edu **Evidence-based practices for children, youth, and young adults with autism** (Steinbrenner et al., 2020) is a 140-page PDF reporting on an updated systematic review of intervention studies to identify evidence-based practices. https://ncaep.fpg.unc.edu/sites/ncaep .fpg.unc.edu/files/imce/documents /EBP%20Report%202020.pdf

(continued)

Table 18.3.   *(continued)*

Profession	Organization resources	Selected resources
Educators	National Education Association (https://www.nea.org)	National Education Association. (n.d.). *Teaching students with autism: A guide for educators.* A 96-page pdf available at https://www.nea.org/sites/default /files/2020-06/Autism_Guide_final.pdf **Autism Resources for Teachers** provides informational links; links to instructional methods, activities, and materials; and links to specialty publishers.
	National Center for Pyramid Model Innovations (https://challengingbehavior .cbcs.usf.edu) Center funded to support implementation of multitiered supports promoting social-emotional competence for children from birth to age 5 at risk for or with identified developmental disabilities	**National Center for Pyramid Model Innovations** provides a searchable resource library containing a wide range of materials (e.g., training modules, videos, visual supports, scripted stories, forms, guides, handouts), including ones related to the 2020 COVID-19 pandemic (e.g., helping children understand the need for social distancing, hand washing). Intended for educators, related professionals, and families of children from birth to age 5 at risk for or with identified developmental disabilities. https://challengingbehavior.cbcs.usf.edu /resources/index.html
Occupational therapists	American Occupational Therapy Association (https://www.aota.org)	***Occupational therapy practice guidelines for individuals with autism spectrum disorder*** (Tomchek & Patten Koenig, 2016); available for purchase on the AOTA website and from a variety of other online stores. Autism resources webpage provides PDFs and links to topics related to ASD and occupational therapy, such as fact sheets on the role of occupational therapy, tips for educators, and addressing issues related to sensory integration. https:// www.aota.org/Practice/Children-Youth /Autism.aspx
Pediatricians	American Academy of Pediatrics (https://www.aap.org).	Harrington, J. W., & Allen, K. (2014). The clinician's guide to autism. *Pediatrics in Review, 35*(2), 62–77. Hyman, S. L., Levy, S. E., Myers, S. M., & Council on Children with Disabilities, Section on Developmental and Behavioral Pediatrics. (2020). Identification, evaluation, and management of children with autism spectrum disorder. *Pediatrics, 14*(1), e20193447. American Academy of Pediatrics web site addresses pediatrician's role with autism (e.g., how pediatricians screen for ASD and ASD diagnosis). https://www .healthychildren.org/English/health-issues /conditions/Autism/Pages/default.aspx
Family Physicians	American Academy of Family Physicians (https://www.aafp.org)	Sanchack, K. E., & Thomas, C. A. (2016). Autism spectrum disorders: Primary care principles. *American Family Physician, 94*(12), 972–979A.

Table 18.3. *(continued)*

Profession	Organization resources	Selected resources
Physical therapists	American Physical Therapy Association (https://www.apta.org)	Downey, R., & Rapport, M. J. K. (2012). Motor activity in children with autism: A review of current literature. *Pediatric Physical Therapy, 24*(1), 2–20.
		Hedgecock, J., Dannemiller, L., Shuie, A., Rapport, M., & Katz, T. (2018). Associations of gross motor delay, behavior, and quality of life in young children with autism spectrum disorder. *Physical Therapy, 98*, 251–259.
		Srinivasan, S. M., Pescatello, L. S., & Bhat, A. N. (2014). Current perspectives on physical activity and exercise recommendations for children and adolescents with autism spectrum disorders, *Physical Therapy, 94*(6), 875–889.
		Physical therapy guide to autism spectrum disorder https://www.choosept .com/symptomsconditionsdetail/physical -therapy-guide-to-autism-spectrum -disorder
Psychologists	American Psychological Association (apa.org)	McGrew, J. H., Rubel, L. A., & Smith, I. M. (2016). Autism spectrum disorder and evidence-based psychology. *Clinical Psychology: Science and Practice, 23*(3), 239–255.
		Soorya, L., Arnstein Carpenter, L., & El Ghoroury, H. (2017). Diagnosing and managing autism spectrum disorder (ASD): How psychologists help with autism spectrum disorder. https://www .apa.org/helpcenter/autism
		Wilkinson, L. E. (2017). *A best practice guide to assessment and intervention for autism spectrum disorder in schools* (2nd ed.). Jessica Kingsley Publishers.
		Autism topics: https://www.apa.org /topics/autism
Social workers	National Association of Social Workers (https://www.socialworkers.org)	Baylot Casey, L., & Elswick, S. E. (2011). The social worker's role in the assessment of autism spectrum disorder. *Children and Schools, 33*(3), 176–183.
		Haney, J. L. (2018). Reconceptualizing autism: An alternative paradigm for social work practice. *Journal of Progressive Human Services, 29*(1), 61–80.
		Haney, J. L., & Cullen, J. A. (2017). An exploratory investigation of social workers' knowledge and attitudes about autism. *Social Work in Mental Health, 16*(2), 201–222.
		Webb, N. B. (2019). *Clinical practice with children, adolescents and families* (4th ed.) [formerly *Social work practice with children and families*]. Guilford Press.

Table 18.3 provides several additional general sources of information that may prove helpful to SLPs and other professional team members supporting people and families affected by ASD. We suggest that you investigate not only those resources related to your own profession but also those offered to members of the professions with whom you may frequently work on ASD-related issues. Doing so may result in your discovery of thought-provoking ideas, practical strategies, and content to share with families and other professionals. In addition, exploring those resources will constitute a foray into interprofessional education, thereby energizing your personal efforts in collaboration, which is a key to maximizing outcomes for individuals with complex needs (Interprofessional Education Collaborative, 2016; WHO, 2010).

Resources in Table 18.3 include articles, books, and websites, usually associated with specific professional groups but sometimes associated with other organizations. In deciding which content to include, we first looked for articles, including position statements or policy documents, books, and other sources that describe how each profession views its work with people with autism and their families. The professions that most clearly indicated more professionally sanctioned documents were pediatrics, occupational therapy, and physical therapy. Table 18.3 also indicates an area of the practice portal website of ASHA, where the roles and responsibilities of SLPs are reported. With the similar goal of defining expected orientations and practices of the professional groups, other relevant articles or books that came up in the search were also included.

Additional resources identified in Table 18.3 include websites associated with a variety of organizations that systematically identify evidence-based practices, often across professional boundaries (the National Autism Center, the National Center for Pyramid Model Innovations, and the National Professional Development Center on Autism Spectrum Disorder). The National Autism Center regularly conducts systematic reviews designed to identify evidence-based practices across disciplines, which contributed to our selection criteria for chapter topics in this book. Audiences who may find valuable content there include not just SLPs but also educators and families. The National Center for Pyramid Model Innovations represents the outgrowth of efforts to support successful programmatic implementation of evidence-based practices supporting children's social and emotional development (Odom et al., 2013; Odom et al., 2014). Consequently, materials shared by this website include not just material for professionals and parents, but community stakeholders as well (Dingfelder & Mandell, 2011; Dunst et al., 2019; Olswang & Prelock, 2015). The National Professional Development Center on Autism Spectrum Disorder grew out of a federally funded grant involving three universities to help develop and disseminate materials for professional development, primarily for professionals in educational settings.

In the last, but far-from-least category of websites mentioned in Table 18.3, there are those offering training materials to support additional learning through modules, online webinars, and toolkits. Many of these include video content that can be especially appreciated through the observation of specific practices featuring real professionals and people with autism. These websites include those associated with the Ohio Center on Autism and Low Incidence Disorders (OCALI), the National Autism Association, the National Professional Development Center on Autism Disorder, and the National Center for Pyramid Model Innovations. They also offer forms, guides, and handouts that may be of immediate use. For any readers unaware of them, these websites may represent the single-most valuable take-away information contained in this chapter.

All professionals who work with children, adults, and families affected by ASD may also benefit from exploring the parent-friendly resources described in Table 18.2. Information there may help them enact client/patient-centered and family-centered care. For example, as part of being family centered, professionals may become involved in helping promote effective communication strategies to achieve individual and family goals (e.g., helping a young child develop a bedtime routine to promote better sleep or helping support an adolescent experiencing bullying or an adult preparing to seek employment). In addition, professionals share resources with parents or other team members who may be unaware of them, thus promoting greater team effectiveness and brighter treatment outcomes.

Resources for Students and Faculty

The resources presented here are primarily to help students deepen their learning and engagement about autism; faculty may be interested in assigning these resources to students. Whereas the other groups of readers may have come to this book with actual individuals firmly in mind (their child, client, student, etc.), speech-language pathology students, and even their professors, may grapple with the issue of treatments for communication and social interaction at a far more abstract level. Consequently, we hope that you will have explored resources described in earlier sections of this chapter, which offer information about the personal and professional landscapes in which treatments are used. Further, after having read earlier chapters in the book, we hope and expect that student readers will have gained a basic sense of how such interventions are developed and studied and how they may fit the needs of individuals and their families. Nonetheless, we recognize that your continuing growth in decision making will depend on the *application* of what you have been learning. Therefore, in this section, we offer a few more resources to deepen your understanding of the lived experience of autism, then suggest a series of exercises designed to stretch your integration and application skills.

Table 18.4 lists two types of resources that can extend your involvement with the experiences of people who live with autism: 14 memoirs and two student organizations.

Many people love memoirs because they tell us not only about what people do but also about their "essence"—to quote a 16th-century writer, De Montaigne (1580/2017, Book 2, chapter 6, para. 14). Thus, memoirs can allow people who are neurotypical to take a deep dive into what it might feel like to be a person with autism and can allow people with autism a deep dive into the struggles and triumphs of *another* person on the spectrum. Authors of such memoirs in the autism community have generally been diagnosed with Asperger syndrome. In fact, 7 of the 14 authors whose books are listed in Table 18.4 describe themselves as having Asperger syndrome, two no longer believe they have autism, and one has had his authorship questioned because of concerns that other demonstrations of his verbal skills do not seem to match those on display in the memoir (Fein & Kamio, 2014). In the book *Uniquely Human* (2016), the autism researcher and SLP Barry Prizant includes a chapter called The Real Experts, by which he means speakers and authors who themselves have been diagnosed with Asperger syndrome. Prizant counters objections that insights from this group may not fairly represent the experiences of others with autism and more severe impairments by observing that their shared difficulties may nonetheless allow them a far better chance of approximating

Table 18.4. Resources for students and their professors

Books containing personal accounts of living with autism	**Barron, J., & Barron, S. (2002).** *There's a boy in here: Emerging from the bonds of autism.* **Future Horizons.**
	In this book, you hear the voice of both a young man with autism and his mother, and they reflect on their experiences and life living with autism from both a personal and family perspective. Diagnosed as a preschooler, it was not until he was 17 that he understood he had autism and engaged in efforts to create a life that would allow him to thrive in the neurotypical world he had struggled to manage as a child.
	Finch, D. (2012). *The journal of best practices: A memoir of marriage, Asperger syndrome, and one man's quest to be a better husband.* **Scribner.**
	A very upbeat memoir by a man with Asperger syndrome who decides to take on the difficult work of finding ways around his difficulties with understanding what other people need and want so that he can become the perfect husband for his wife and the perfect father for his children.
	Fleisher, M. (2003). *Making sense of the unfeasible: My life with Asperger syndrome.* **Jessica Kingsley Publishers.**
	This author shares how he made the most of his life in spite of having autism. He highlights the value of support from family and the services provided to him that led him to pursuing college degrees in mathematics.
	Grandin, T. (1996, 2006). *Thinking in pictures: And other reports from my life with autism.* **Vintage Books.**
	As one of the earliest of its kind, this book is a classic memoir by one of the most famous (and articulate) people with autism living today, Temple Grandin. In her first and a series of more recent books, including a second edition of this book in 2006, Dr. Grandin, a professor of animal behavior, delves into not only her life but issues of research and experience affecting the broader autism community. She speaks to how she managed the challenges of autism to function in the "outside world."
	Higashi, N. (2007). *The reason I jump: The inner voice of a thirteen-year-old boy with autism* **(K. Yoshida & D. Mitchell, Trans. [2013]). Random House.**
	This best-selling book was purportedly written by a boy with severe autism describing his life experiences. Although widely viewed as offering a very compelling window into the world of individuals not usually represented in first-person accounts, serious concerns about the veracity of its authorship and the implications of that have been raised (Fein & Kamio, 2014).
	Nazeer, K. (2006). *Send in the idiots: Stories from the other side of autism.* **Bloomsbury Publishing.**
	In this memoir, Nazeer reports on the lives of four adults he met as children in the early 1980s when they all attended an at-the-time innovative private school for children with autism and were dubbed the "idiots" by one of their members. Although he no longer considers himself to have autism, Nazeer's personal observations and his accounts of his classmates' outcomes make for compelling reading.
	O'Toole, J. (2018). *Autism in heels: The untold story of a female life on the spectrum.* **Skyhorse Publishing.**
	In this memoir, O'Toole vividly chronicles her life on the spectrum, a life that included many successes but also bullying, an eating disorder, feelings of isolation, and a diagnosis that did not occur until she was 34 years old.
	Prince-Hughes, D. (2004). *Songs of the gorilla nation: My journey through autism.* **Harmony Books.**
	In a thought-provoking memoir, this author chronicles her personal journey through no diagnosis to self-discovery. She describes her inability to connect with others in meaningful ways and her tendency to self-isolate. When she responds to her fascination with gorillas by studying them, she learns how to connect in new ways.

Table 18.4. *(continued)*

	Purkis, J. (2006). *Finding a different kind of normal: Misadventures with Asperger syndrome.* **Jessica Kingsley Publishers.** In her personal journey with autism, this author shares the difficulty she had with accepting her diagnosis, which did not occur until she was 20. This is a powerful read for both people with ASD and the families who live with them.
	Robison, J. E. (2008). *Look me in the eye: My life with Asperger's.* **Three Rivers Press.** In this personal account, Robison describes the social challenges he experienced as a young boy and teenager, as he avoided eye contact, offered irrelevant statements in the classroom, and fixated on his desire to dismantle radios. He speaks to the challenges of a late diagnosis, when he was in his 40s, and shares his journey of self-exploration.
	Schneider, E. (1999). *Discovering my autism: Apologia pro vita sua (with apologies to Cardinal Newman).* **Jessica Kingsley Publishers.** This author, initially misdiagnosed as having schizophrenia, reflects on his difficulties with relationships and inattention in his childhood and adolescent years and speaks to his revelation of having autism and attention deficit disorder. This is a powerful read for individuals with ASD, professionals, and parents.
	Schneider, E. (2002). *Living the good life with autism.* **Jessica Kingsley Publishers.** As a follow-up to his 1999 memoir, this author continues his story, comparing what he knows to be true and not true, right and wrong. He describes his attitudes toward relationships, religion, politics, and health and offers ways for those affected by ASD to enrich their lives.
	Shore, S. (2003). *Beyond the wall: Personal experiences with autism and Asperger syndrome* **(2nd ed.). Autism Asperger Publishing.** This is an honest autobiography in which the author adds to his previous edition of his personal experiences with insights on getting ready for college and his more public engagement in autism-related issues.
	Willey, L. H. (1999). *Pretending to be normal.* **Jessica Kingsley Publishers.** This book offers the personal reflection of a young woman with Asperger syndrome who experiences much self-doubt throughout her life. When she finally accepted her diagnosis, she found joy and hope in her future. She offers encouragement to young people with autism, their families, and the professionals who support them.
Student organizations	**Autism Science Foundation (ASF) Student Clubs** (https://autismsciencefoundation.org/get-involved/student-clubs) Student clubs disseminate information about autism in their communities and conduct fund-raising to support ASF, an organization aimed at supporting both current and future researchers as well as individuals and families affected by autism.
	Autism Speaks U (https://www.autismspeaks.org/autism-speaks-u) This program of Autism Speaks came into existence in 2008. With more than 30 local chapters, college students host awareness, advocacy, and fund-raising events while supporting their local autism communities.

their reality than insights offered by people with neurotypical development. Reading even one of these 14 books will undoubtedly increase your understanding of the complicated diversity of what autism means to a person's life and may further whet your appetite for learning more and contributing through research, clinical practice, or advocacy.

At the end of Table 18.4, we list two student organizations in expectation that they can offer you an alternative, more direct avenue for learning about autism than you might get from reading articles and books or visiting websites. These student groups, and the larger organizations to which they are connected, have strong connections to people with autism and their families as well as to researchers and clinicians who serve them. Awareness, fund-raising, and advocacy activities may constitute contexts in which you can forge relationships and develop skills that can further guide your future learning goals.

Returning to the idea that learning is only solidified when one can integrate various pieces of information and use them to solve problems, derive novel insights, to make practical decisions, we close this section with some exercises that we hope will allow you to test your learning.

1. Reread the section Application to a Child or Application to an Adolescent or Adult for one of the treatments that you found particularly interesting or that you had already known something about. Then consider whether one of the *other* approaches discussed in the book might have been selected as an alternative or an additional one to use for that individual. What advantages and disadvantages might have been anticipated had the other approach been used or added to the individual's program? What other family members or professional groups, if any, might have been consulted to arrive at even better outcomes?

2. In a classic article by Reichow and colleagues (2008), the authors proposed quality indicators for individual research articles and for what constitutes a reasonable evidence for an intervention to claim status as an evidence-based intervention. After reading that article, choose a *research* article on an intervention that interests you and see how it stacks up. Alternatively, choose and evaluate *two* intervention studies: one that used a group research design and another that used a single case experimental design. The paper by Reichow and colleagues is considered especially valuable because it proposes criteria for both types of designs—something uncommon in other evaluation systems but vital to autism research, which more often uses single case experimental designs (Wong et al., 2015).

3. Identify one of the interventions that seemed especially intriguing to you, looking carefully at what research had already been conducted to support its potential efficacy and what the author(s) described as needed areas of additional study. Considering what you have learned about how interventions are developed, design a study that would constitute a reasonable next step for that approach.

4. Read one of the books listed in Table 18.4, making note of the continuing challenges reported by these very successful adults. What challenges, if any, were addressed, and what interventions or services were used? Which of these challenges might have been, or still could be, addressed by the treatments described in this book? Which could not be? What professions would be most helpful in addressing them? What do these authors write that helps you appreciate why they would or would not take part in such interventions if they had access to them?

5. Look at a case study provided describing intervention with a child or adult with ASD—choose from either the shorter accounts included in the applications sections of chapters in this book or the longer ones contained in the companion book (Prelock & McCauley, 2021). Then visit one of the websites identified in this chapter to locate several resources (e.g., worksheets, handouts, toolkits,

videos) that might have been useful for that person, the person's family, or his or her team.

CONCLUDING THOUGHTS

Autism is frequently characterized as a puzzle, especially to those of us who are outsiders to the lived experience of people with ASD—even when we are their parents, family members, clinicians, friends, or daily acquaintances. Difficulties in communication and social interaction are among the core features of this puzzle and thus are a focus of ever-increasing efforts to develop, disseminate, and support effective interventions intended to alleviate the core impairments in autism while acknowledging the strengths unique to each person. Knowledgeable collaborations of all of the groups addressed in this book and participating in its preparation—family members, professionals, students and their instructors, and researchers—will be needed to solve this puzzle in the many forms faced by individuals with ASD. Their individual and group efforts will surely culminate in better outcomes for individuals, families, and communities affected by ASD.

REFERENCES

Abraham, C., & Michie, S. (2008). A taxonomy of behavior change techniques used in interventions. *Health Psychology, 27*(3), 379–387.

Altman, D. G., & Simera, I. (2014). Using reporting guidelines effective to ensure good reporting of health research. In D. Moher, D. G. Altman, K. F. Schulz, I. Simera, & E. Wager (Eds.), *Guidelines for reporting health research: A user's manual* (pp. 32–40). Wiley.

Altman, D. G., & Simera, I. (2016). A history of the evolution of guidelines for reporting medical research: The long road to the EQUATOR Network. *Journal of the Royal Society of Medicine, 109*(2), 67–77.

American Psychiatric Association. (2013). *Diagnostic and statistical manual of mental disorders, fifth edition* (DSM-5). Author.

American Psychological Association. (2020). *Publication manual of the American Psychological Association* (7th ed.) Author.

American Speech-Language-Hearing Association (2020). Demographic profile of ASHA members providing bilingual services, year-end 2019. Available from www.asha.org

American Speech-Language-Hearing Association. (2019). *Interprofessional practice survey results.* https://www.asha.org/uploadedfiles/2019-interprofessional-practice-survey-results.pdf

American Speech-Language-Hearing Association. (n.d.-a). *Evidence-based practice.* https://www.asha.org/research/ebp/evidence-based-practice

American Speech-Language-Hearing Association. (n.d.-b). *Telepractice.* https://www.asha.org/practice-portal/professional-issues/telepractice

Applebaum, M., Cooper, H., Klein, R. B., Mayo-Wilson, E., Nezu, A. M., & Rao, S. M. (2018). Journal article reporting standards for quantitative research in psychology: The APA Publications and Communications Board Task Force Report. *American Psychologist, 73*(1), 3–25.

Baker, E., McCauley, R. J., Williams, A. L., & McLeod, S. (2020). Elements in phonological intervention: A comparison of three approaches using the Phonological Intervention Taxonomy. In E. Babatsouli & M. J. Ball (Eds.), *On under-reported monolingual child phonology* (pp. 375–399). Multilingual Matters.

Baker, E., Williams, A. L., McLeod, S., & McCauley, R. (2018). Elements of phonological interventions for children with speech sound disorders: The development of a taxonomy. *American Journal of Speech-Language Pathology, 27*(3), 1–30.

Beatson, J. (2006). Preparing speech-language pathologists as family-centered practitioners in assessment and program planning for children with autism spectrum disorder. *Seminars in Speech and Language, 27*(1), 2–9.

Benevides, T. W., Lee, J., Nwosu, N. A. O., & Franks, J. (2019). Understanding the family impact of autism spectrum disorder in racially and ethnically diverse sample: Findings from the National Survey of Children with Special Health Care Needs. *Maternal and Child Health Journal, 23*, 951–960.

Bejarano-Martín, A., Canal-Bedia, R., Magán-Maganto, M., Fernández-Àlvarez, C., Lóa-Jonsdóttir, S., Saemundsen, E., Vincente, A., Café, C., Rasga, C., García-Primo, P., & Posada, M. (2020). Efficacy of focused social and communication intervention practices for young children with autism spectrum disorder: A meta-analysis. *Early Childhood Research Quarterly, 51*, 430–445.

Billingsley, F., White, O., & Munson, R. (1980). Procedural reliability: A rationale and an example. *Behavioral Assessment, 2*, 229–241.

Bishop-Fitzpatrick, L., Minshew, N. J., & Eack, S. M. (2013). A systematic review of psychosocial interventions for adults with autism spectrum disorders. *Journal of Autism and Developmental Disorders, 43*, 687–694.

Boisvert, M., Hall, N., Andrianopoulos, M., & Chaclas, J. (2012). The multi-faceted implementation of telepractice to service individuals with autism. *International Journal of Telerehabilitation, 4(2)*, 11–24.

Boisvert, M., Lang, R., Andrianopoulos, M., & Boscardin, M. L. (2010). Telepractice in the assessment and treatment of individuals with autism spectrum disorders: A systematic review. *Developmental Neurorehabilitation, 13*(6), 423–432.

Bradshaw, J., Steiner, A. M., Gengoux, G., & Koegel, L. K. (2015). Feasibility and effectiveness of very early intervention for infants at-risk for autism spectrum disorder: A systematic review. *Journal of Autism and Developmental Disorders, 45*(3), 778–794.

Campbell, W. N., & Douglas, N. F. (2017). Supporting evidence-based practice in speech-language pathology: A review of implementation strategies for promoting health professional behavior change. *Evidence-Based Communication Assessment and Intervention, 11*(3–4), 72–81.

Carlon, S., Carter, M., & Stephenson, J. (2013). A review of declared factors identified by parents of children with autism spectrum disorders (ASD) in making intervention decisions. *Research in Autism Spectrum Disorders, 7*, 369–381.

Cerminara, C., Santarone, M. E., Casarelli, L., Curatolo, P., & El Mahany, N. (2014). Use of the DISCERN tool for evaluating web searches in childhood epilepsy. *Epilepsy & Behavior, 41*, 119–121.

Chan, A.-W., Tezlaff, J. M., Altman, D. G., Laupacis, A., Gøtzsche, P. C., Krleža-Jeric, K., Hrøbjartsson, A., Mann, H., Dickerson, K., Berlin, J. A., Dore, C. J., Parulekar, W. R., Summerskill, W. S. M., Groves, T., Schulz, K. F., Sox, H. C., Rockhold, F. W., Rennie, D., & Moher, D. (2013). SPIRIT 2013 Statement: Defining standard protocol items for clinical trials. *Annals of Internal Medicine, 158*(3), 200–207.

Charnock, D. (Ed., 1998). *The DISCERN handbook: Quality criteria for consumer health information on treatment choices*. University of Oxford and The British Library. Retrieved from https://a-f-r.org/wp-content/uploads/sites/3/2016/01/1998-Radcliffe-Medical-Press-Quality-criteria-for-consumer-health-information-on-treatment-choices.pdf

Chauhan, B. F., Jeyaraman, M., Mann, A. S., Lys, J., Skidmore, B., Sibley, K. M., Abou-Setta, A., & Zarychanski, R. (2017). Behavior change interventions and policies influencing primary healthcare professionals' practice: An overview of reviews. *Implementation Science, 12*, 1–16.

Committee on Hospital Care and Institute for Patient- and Family-Centered Care. (2012). Patient-and Family-centered care and the pediatrician's role. *Pediatrics, 129*(2), 394–404.

Craig, P., Dieppe, P., Macintyre, S., Michie, S., Nazareth, I., & Petticrew, M. (2008). Developing and evaluating complex interventions: The new Medical Research Council guidance. *British Medical Journal, 337*, a1655.

De Montaigne, M. (1580/2017). *The complete essays* (C. Cotton, Trans.; W. C. Hazlit, Ed.) [Ebook]. Digireads.com Publishing.

de Schipper, E., Mahdi, S., de Vries, P., Granlund, M., Holtmann, M., Karande, S., Almodayfer, O., Shulman, C., Tonge, B., Wong, V. V. C. N., Zwaigenbaum, L., & Bölte, S. (2016). Functioning and disability in autism spectrum disorder: A worldwide survey of experts. *Autism Research, 9*, 959–969.

De Silva, M. J., Breuer, E., Lee, L., Asher, L., Chowdhary, N., Lund, C., & Patel, V. (2014). Theory of change: A theory driven approach to enhance the Medical Research Council's framework for complex interventions. *Trials, 15*, 267–279.

de Vries, A. L. C., Noens, I. L. J., Cohen-Kettenis, P. T., van Berckelaer-Onnes, I. A., & Doreleijers, T. A. (2010). Autism spectrum disorders in gender dysphoric children and adolescents. *Journal of Autism and Developmental Disorders, 40*(8), 930–936.

Dingfelder, H. E., & Mandell, D. S. (2011). Bridging the research-to-practice gap in autism intervention: An application of diffusion of innovation theory. *Journal of Autism and Developmental Disorders, 41*, 597–609.

Dollaghan, C. A. (2007). *The handbook for evidence-based practice in communication disorders.* Paul H. Brookes Publishing Co.

Dunst, C. J. (2017). Research foundations for evidence-informed early childhood intervention performance checklists. *Education Sciences, 7*(4), 78.

Dunst, C. J., Trivette, C. M., & Hamby, D. W. (2010). Meta-analysis of the effectiveness of four adult learning methods and strategies. *International Journal of Continuing Education and Lifelong Learning, 3*(1), 91–112.

Dunst, C. J., Trivette, C. M., & Raab, M. (2013). An implementation science framework for conceptualizing and operationalizing fidelity in early childhood intervention studies. *Journal of Early Intervention, 35*(2), 85–101.

Dyches, T., Wilder, L. K., Sudweeks, R. R., Obiakor, F. E., & Algozzine, B. (2004). Multicultural issues in autism. *Journal of Autism and Developmental Disorders, 34*(2), 211–222.

Eccles, M. P., & Mittman, B. S. (2006). Welcome to *Implementation Science. Implementation Science, 1*(1), 1–3.

Embry, D. D., & Biglan, A. (2008). Evidence-based kernels: Fundamental units of behavioral influence. *Clinical Child and Family Psychology Review, 11*, 75–113.

Esmail, R., Hanson, H. M., Holroyd-Leduc, J., Brown, S., Strifler, L., Straus, S. E., Niven, D. J., & Clement, F. M. (2020). A scoping review of full-spectrum knowledge translation theories, models, and frameworks. *Implementation Science, 15*(11), 1.

Fein, D., & Kamio, Y. (2014). Commentary on *The reason I jump* by Naoki Higashida. *Journal of Developmental and Behavioral Pediatrics, 35*, 539–542.

Fixsen, D. L., Blasé, K. A., Naoom, S. F., & Wallace, F. (2009). Core implementation components. *Research on Social Work, 19*(5), 531–540.

Friedman, M., Woods, J., & Salisbury, C. (2012). Caregiver coaching strategies for early intervention providers: Moving toward operational definitions. *Infants & Young Children, 25*(1), 62–82.

Fulcher-Rood, K., Castilla-Earls, A., & Higginbotham, J. (2020). What does evidence-based practice mean to you? A follow-up study examining school-based speech-language pathologists' perspectives on evidence-based practice. *American Journal of Speech-Language Pathology, 29*, 688–704.

Gan, S., Tung, L., Yeh, C., & Wang, C. (2013). ICF-CY based assessment tool for children with autism. *Disability and Rehabilitation, 35*(8), 678–685.

Gillam, S. L., & Gillam, R. B. (2006). Making evidence-based decisions about child language intervention for schools. *Language, Speech, and Hearing Services in Schools, 37*, 304–315.

Gillon, G., Hyter, Y., Fernandes, F. D., Ferman, S., Hus, Y., Petinou, K., Segal, O., Tumanova, T., Vogindroukas, I., Westby, C., & Westervelt, M. (2017). International survey of speech-language pathologists' practices in working with children with autism spectrum disorder. *Folia Phoniatrica et Logopaedica, 69*, 8–19.

Glasziou, P., Meats, E., Heneghan, C., & Shepperd, S. (2008). What is missing from descriptions of treatment in trials and reviews? *BMJ, 336*, 1472–1474.

Grant, N., Rodger, S., & Hoffman, T. (2015). Evaluation of autism-related health information on the web. *Journal of Applied Research in Intellectual Disabilities, 28*, 276–282.

Grant, N., Rodger, S., & Hoffmann, T. (2016). Intervention decision-making processes and information preferences of parents of children with autism spectrum disorders. *Child: Care, Health, and Development, 42*, 125–134.

Gulsrud, A. C., Hellemann, G., Shire, S., & Kasari, C. (2016). Isolating active ingredients in a parent-mediated social-communication intervention for toddlers with autism spectrum disorder. *Journal of Child Psychology & Psychiatry, 57*(5), 606–613.

Guthrie, W., Wineford, L. B., Nottke, C., & Wetherby, A. M. (2013). Early diagnosis of autism spectrum disorder: Stability and change in clinical diagnosis and symptom presentation. *Journal of Child Psychology and Psychiatry, 54*(5), 582–590.

Hambly, C., & Fombonne, E. (2012). The impact of bilingual environments on language development in children with autism spectrum disorders. *Journal of Autism and Developmental Disorders, 42*, 134–1352.

Hayes, S. A., & Watson, S. L. (2013). The impact of parenting stress: A meta-analysis of studies comparing the experience of parenting stress in parents of children with and without autism spectrum disorder. *Journal of Autism and Developmental Disorders, 43*, 629–642.

Hoffman, L. M., Ireland, M., Hall-Mills, S., & Flynn, P. (2013). Evidence-based speech-language pathology practices in schools: Findings from a national survey. *Language, Speech, and Hearing Services in Schools, 44*(3), 266–280.

Hoffman, T. C., Glasziou, P. P., Boutron, I., Milne, R., Perera, R., Moher, D., Altman, D. G., Barbour, V., Macdonald, H., Johnson, M., Lamb, S. E., Dixon-Woods, M., McCulloch, P., Wyatt, J. C., Chan, A., & Michie, S. (2014). Better reporting of interventions: template for intervention description and replication (TIDieR) checklist and guide. *BMJ, 348*, g1687. https://doi.org/10.1136/bmj.g1687

Howlin, P., Magiati, I., & Charman, T. (2009). Systematic review of early intensive behavioral interventions for children with autism. *American Journal of Intellectual and Developmental Disabilities, 114*(1), 23–41.

Huis, A., van Acterberg, T., de Bruin, M., Grol, R., Schoonhoven, L., & Hulscher, M. (2012). A systematic review of hand hygiene improvement strategies: A behavioural approach. *Implementation Science, 7*, 92. https://www.implementationscience.com/content/7/1/92

Individuals with Disabilities Education Improvement Act (IDEA) of 2004, PL 108-446, 20 U.S.C. §§ 1400 *et seq.*

Interprofessional Education Collaborative. (2016). *Core competencies for interprofessional collaborative practice: Report of an expert panel.* Interprofessional Education Collaborative. Retrieved on February 15, 2021 from https://nebula.wsimg.com/2f68a395 20b03336b41038c370497473?AccessKeyId=DC06780E69ED19E2B3A5&disposition=0&alloworigin=1

Johnson, C. (2006). Getting started in evidence-based practice for childhood speech-language disorders. *American Journal of Speech-Language Pathology, 15*, 20–35.

Justice, L. M. (2018). Conceptualising "dose" in paediatric language interventions: Current findings and future directions. *International Journal of Speech-Language Pathology, 20*, 318–323.

Justice, L. M., Logan, J., Jang, H., & Schmitt, (2016). Algorithm-drive dosage decisions (AD[3]): Optimizing treatment for children with language impairment. *American Journal of Speech-Language Pathology, 26*, 57–68.

Justice, L. M., Chen, J., Jiang, H., Tambyraja, S., & Logan, J. (2020). Early-literacy intervention conducted by caregivers of children with language impairment: Implementation patterns using survival analysis. *Journal of Autism and Developmental Disorders, 50*, 1668–1682.

Justice, L. M., Chen, J., Tambyraja, S., & Logan, J. (2018). Increasing caregivers' adherence to an early-literacy intervention improve the print knowledge of children with language impairment. *Journal of Autism and Developmental Disorders, 48*(12), 4179–4192.

Justice, L. M., Logan, J. R., & Damschroder, L. (2015). Designing caregiver-implemented shared-reading interventions to overcome implementation barriers. *Journal of Speech, Language and Hearing Research, 58*, S1851–S1863.

Kadaravek, J. N., & Justice, L. M. (2010). Fidelity: An essential component of evidence-based practice in speech-language pathology. *American Journal of Speech-Language Pathology, 19*, 369–379.

Khazaal, Y., Chatton, A., Cochand, S., Coquard, O., Fernanez, S., Khan, R., Billieux, J., & Zullino, D. (2009). Brief DISCERN, six questions for the evaluation of evidence-based content of health-related websites *Patient Education and Counseling, 77*, 33–37.

Knowles, M. S. (1984). *Andragogy in action: Applying modern principles of adult education.* Jossey-Bass.

Kraft, M. A., Blazar, D., & Hogan, D. (2018). The effect of teacher coaching on instruction and achievement: A meta-analysis of the causal evidence. *Review of Educational Research, 88*(4), 547–588.

Lai, M., Lombardo, M. V., Auyeung, B., Chakrabarti, B., & Baron-Cohen (2015). Sex/gender differences and autism: Setting the scene for future research. *Journal of the American Academy of Child and Adolescent Psychiatry, 54*(1), 11–24.

Levac, D., Rivard, L., & Missiuna, C. (2012). Defining the active ingredients of interactive computer play interventions for children with neuromotor impairments: A scoping study. *Research in Developmental Disabilities, 33*, 214–223.

Lever, A. G., & Geurts, H. M. (2016). Psychiatric co-occurring symptoms and disorders in young, middle-aged, and older adults with autism spectrum disorder. *Journal of Autism and Developmental Disorders, 46*, 1916–1930.

Lim, N., O'Reilly, M. F., Sigafoos, J., & Lancioni, G. E. (2018). Understanding the linguistic needs of diverse individuals with autism spectrum disorder: Some comments on the research literature and suggestions for clinicians. *Journal of Autism and Developmental Disorders,48*, 2890–2895.

Lippke, S., & Ziegelmann, J. P. (2008). Theory-based health behavior change: Developing, testing and applying theories for evidence-based interventions. *Applied Psychology, 57*(4), 698–716.

Ludemann, A., Power, E., & Hoffmann, T. C. (2017). Investigating the adequacy of intervention descriptions in recent speech language pathology literature: Is evidence from randomized trials useable? *American Journal of Speech-Language Pathology, 26*(2), 443–455.

Maenner, M. J., Shaw, K. A., Baio, J., Washington, A., Patrick, M., DiRienzo, M., Christensen, D. L., Wiggins, L. D., Pettygrove, S., Andrews, J. G., Lopez, M., Hudson, A., Baroud, T., Schwenk, Y., White, T., Robinson Rosenberg, C., Lee, L.-C., Harrington, R. A., Huston, M., Hewitt, A., . . . Dietz, P. M. (2020). Prevalence of autism spectrum disorder among children aged 8 years—Autism Developmental Disabilities Monitoring Network, 11 Sites, United States, 2016. *Morbidity and Mortality Weekly Report Surveillance Summary, 69*(No. 22-4), 1–12.

Maglione, M. A., Gans, D., Das, L., Timbie, J., & Kasari, C. (2012). Nonmedical interventions for children with ASD: Recommended guidelines and further research needs. *Pediatrics, 130*(Suppl. 2), S169–S178.

Mahdi, S., Albertowski, K., Alomodayfer, O., Arsenopoulou, V., Carucci, S., Dias, J. C., Khalil, M., Knüppel, A., Langmann, A., Briciet Lauritsen, M., Rodrigues da Cunha, G., Uchiyama, T., Wolff, N., Selb, M., Granlund, M., de Vries, P. J., Zwaigenbaum, L., & Bölte, S. (2018). An international clinical study of ability and disability in autism spectrum disorder using the WHO-ICF framework. *Journal of Autism and Developmental Disorders, 48*, 2148–2163.

McConachie, H., & Diggle, T. (2007). Parent implemented early intervention for young children with autism spectrum disorder: A systematic review. *Journal of Evaluation in Clinical Practice,13*, 120–129.

Meadan, H., Snodgrass, M. R., Meyer, L. E., Fisher, K. W., Chung, M. Y., & Halle, J. W. (2016). Internet-based parent-implemented intervention for young children with autism: A pilot study. *Journal of Early Intervention, 38*(1), 3–23.

Meyers-Denman, C. N., & Plante, E. (2016). Dose schedule and enhanced conversational recast treatment for children with specific language impairment? *Language, Speech, and Hearing Services in Schools, 47*, 334–346.

Michie, S., Abraham, C., Eccles, M. P., Francis, J. J., Hardeman, W., & Johnson, M. (2011). Strengthening evaluation and implementation by specifying components of behavior change interventions: A study protocol. *Implementation Science, 6*, 10.

Michie, S., Wood, C. E., Johnson, M., Braham, C., Francis, J. J., & Hardeman, W. (2015). Behaviour change techniques: The development and evaluation of a taxonomic method for reporting and describing behavior interventions (A suite of five studies involving consensus methods, randomized controlled trials and analysis of qualitative data). *Health Technology Assessment, 19*(99).

Min, H., Morales, D. R., Orgill, D., Smink, D. S., & Yule, S. (2015). Systematic review of coaching to enhance surgeons' operative performance. *Surgery, 158*(5), 1168–1191.

Morgan, L. J., Rubin, E., Coleman, J. J., Frymark, T., Wang, B. P., & Cannon, L. J. (2014). Impact of social-communication interventions on infants and toddlers with or at-risk for autism: A systematic review. *Focus on Autism and Other Developmental Disabilities, 29*(4), 246–256.

Mukhalalati, B. A., & Taylor, A. (2019). Adult learning theories in context: A quick guide for healthcare professional educators. *Journal of Medical Education and Curricular Development, 6.* https://doi.org/10.1177/2382120519840332

National Autism Center. (2015). *Evidence-based practice and autism in the schools* (2nd ed.). Author.

National Institutes of Health. (2011). *How to evaluate health information on the Internet: Questions and answers.* https://ods.od.nih.gov/Health_Information/How_To_Evaluate _Health_Information_on_the_Internet_Questions_and_Answers.aspx

National Research Council. (2001). *Educating children with autism.* National Academy Press.

Nilsen, P. (2015). Making sense of implementation theories, models, and frameworks. *Implementation Science, 10,* 53.

Nordahl-Hansen, A., Cicchetti, D. V., & Øien, R. A. (2019). A review update on gender dysphoria and ASD and response to corrections. *Journal of Autism and Developmental Disorders, 49,* 1745–1748.

Odom, S. L., Cox, A. W., & Brock, M. E. (2013). Implementation science, professional development, and autism spectrum disorders. *Exceptional Children, 79*(2), 233–251.

Odom, S. L., Duda, M. A., Kucharczyk, S., Cox, A. W., & Stabel, A. (2014). Applying an implementation science framework for adoption of a comprehensive program for high school students with autism spectrum disorder. *Remedial and Special Education, 35*(2), 123–132.

Øien, R. A., Cicchetti, D. V., & Nordahl-Hansen, A. (2018). Gender dysphoria, sexuality, and autism spectrum disorders: A systematic map review. *Journal of Autism and Developmental Disorders, 48,* 4028–4037.

Olswang, L. B., & Prelock, P. A. (2015). Bridging the gap between research and practice: Implementation science. *Journal of Speech, Language, and Hearing Research, 58*(6), 1–9.

Open Science Collaboration. (2015). Estimating the reproducibility of psychological science. *Science, 349*(6251). https:// doi.org/10.1126/science.aac4716

Oono, I. P., Honey, E. J., & McConachie, H. (2013). Parent-mediated early intervention for young children with autism spectrum disorders (ASD). *Cochrane Database of Systematic Reviews, 4.* https://doi.org/10.1002/ebch.1952

Pallathra, A. A., Cordero, L., Wong, K., & Brodkin, E. S. (2019). Psychosocial interventions targeting social functioning in adults on the autism spectrum: A literature review. *Current Psychiatry Reports, 21*(5).

Piasta, S. B., Farley, K. S., Mauck, S. A., Ramirez, P. S., Schachter, R. E., O'Connell, A. A., Justice, L. M., Spear, C. F., & Weber-Mayrer, M. (2020). At-scale, state-sponsored language and literacy professional development: Impacts on early childhood classroom practices and children's outcomes. *Journal of Educational Psychology, 112*(2), 329–343.

Plante, E., Mettler, H. M., Tucci, A., & Vance, R. (2019). Maximizing treatment efficiency in developmental language disorder: Positive effects in half the time. *American Journal of Speech-Language Pathology, 28*(3), 1233–1247.

Plumb, A. M., & Plexico, L. W. (2013). Autism spectrum disorders: Experience, training, and confidence levels of school-based speech-language pathologists. *Language, Speech and Hearing Services in Schools, 44,* 89–104.

Powell, B. J., McMillen, J. C., Proctor, E. K., Carpenter, C. R., Griffey, R. T., Bunger, A. C., Glass, J. E., & York, J. L. (2012). *Medical Care Research and Review, 69,* 123.

Potvin, M. C., Prelock, P. A., & Savard, L. (2017). Supporting children with autism and their families: A culturally-responsive family-driven interprofessional process. *Pediatric Clinics of North America, 65,* 47–57.

Prelock, P. A., & Hutchins, T. (2008). The role of family-centered care in research: Supporting the social-communication of children with autism spectrum disorder. *Topics in Language Disorders, 28*(4), 323–339.

Prelock, P. A., & McCauley, R. J. (Eds.). (2021). *Case studies for the treatment of autism spectrum disorder.* Paul H. Brookes Publishing Co.

Prelock, P. A., Melvin, C., Lemieux, N., Melekis, K., Velleman, S., & Favro, M. A. (2017). One team: Patient, family, & healthcare providers—An IPE activity providing collaborative and palliative care. *Seminars in Speech and Language, 38*(5), 350–359.

Prizant, B. M., with Fields-Meyer, T. (2016). *Uniquely human: A different way of seeing autism.* Simon & Schuster.

Reichow, B., Doehring, P., Cicchetti, D. V., & Volkmar, F. R. (2011). *Evidence-based practices and treatments for children with autism.* Springer.

Reichow, B., Halpern, J., Steinhoff, T., Letsinger, N., Naples, A., & Volkmar, F. R. (2012). Characteristics and quality of autism websites. *Journal of Autism and Developmental Disorders, 42,* 1263–1274.

Reichow, B., Volkmar, F. R., & Cicchetti, D. V. (2008). Development of the evaluative methods for evaluating and determining evidence-based practices in autism. *Journal of Autism and Developmental Disorders, 38,* 1311–1319.

Richmond, A. S. (2011). Autism spectrum disorder: A global perspective. *Perspectives on Global Issues in Communication Sciences and Related Disorders, 1,* 39–46.

Rogers, E. M. (1962). *Diffusion of innovations.* Free Press.

Rogers, E. M. (2003). *Diffusion of innovations* (5th ed.). Free Press.

Rogers, S. J., Dawson, G., & Vismara, L. A. (2012). *An early start for your child with autism: Using everyday activities to help kids connect, communicate, and learn.* Guilford Press.

Sackett, D. L., Richardson, W. S., Rosenberg, W., & Haynes, R. B. (1997). *Evidence-based medicine: How to practice and teach EBM.* Churchill Livingstone.

Sam, A. M., Cox, A. W., Savage, M. N., Waters, V., & Odom, S. L. (2020). Disseminating information on evidence-based practices for children and youth with autism spectrum disorder: AFIRM. *Journal of Autism and Developmental Disorders, 50*(6), 1931–1940.

Sandbank, M., Bottema-Beutel, K., Crowley, S., Cassidy, M., Feldman, J. I., Canihuante, M., & Woynaroski, T. (2020). Intervention effects on language in children with autism: A Project Aim meta-analysis. *Journal of Speech-Language-Hearing Research, 63,* 1537–1560.

Schiarti, V., Mahdi, S., & Bolte, S. (2018). International classification of functioning, disability, and health core sets for cerebral palsy, autism spectrum disorder and attention-deficit-hyperactivity disorder. *Developmental Medicine and Child Neurology, 60,* 933–941.

Schreibman, L., Dawson, G., Stahmer, A. C., Landa, R., Rogers, S. J., McGee, G. G., Kasari, C., Ingersoll, B., Kaiser, A., Bruinsma, Y., McNerney, E., Wetherby, A., & Halladay, A. (2015). Naturalistic developmental behavioral interventions: Empirically validated treatments for autism spectrum disorder. *Journal of Autism and Developmental Disorders, 45*(8), 2411–2428.

Schultz, K. F., Altman, D. G., Moher, D., & the CONSORT Group (2010). CONSORT 2010 Statement: Updated guidelines for reporting parallel group randomized trials. *BMC Medicine, 8,* 18.

Schwartz, H., & Drager, K. D. R. (2008). Training and knowledge in autism among speech-language pathologists: A survey. *Language, Speech, and Hearing Services in Schools, 39,* 66–77.

Soke, G. N., Maenner, M. J., Christinensen, D., Kurzius-Spenser, M., & Schieve, L. A. (2018). Prevalence of co-occurring medical and behavioral conditions/symptoms among 4- and 8-year-old children with autism spectrum disorder in selected areas of the United States in 2010. *Journal of Autism and Developmental Disorders, 48*(8), 2663–2676.

Stavri, Z., & Michie, S. (2012). Classification systems in behavioural science: Current systems and lessons from the natural, medical, and social sciences. *Health Psychology Review, 6*(1), 113–140.

Steinbrenner, J. R., Hume, K., Odom, S. L., Morin, K. L., Nowell, S. W., Tomaszewski, B., Szendrey, S., McIntyre, N. S., Yücesoy-Özkan, S., & Savage, M. N. (2020). *Evidence-based practices for children, youth, and young adults with autism.* National Clearinghouse on Autism Evidence and Practice. https://ncaep.fpg.unc.edu/sites/ncaep.fpg.unc.edu/files/imce/documents/EBP%20Report%202020.pdf

Sutherland, R., Trembath, D., & Roberts, J. (2018). Telehealth and autism: A systematic search and review of the literature. *International Journal of Speech-Language Pathology, 20,* 324–336.

Tachibana, Y., Miyazaki, C., Ota, E., Mori, R., Hwang, Y., Kobayashi, E., Terasaka, A., Tang, J., & Kamio, Y. (2017). A systematic review and meta-analysis of comprehensive interventions for preschool children with autism spectrum disorder (ASD). *PLoS ONE 12*(12), e0186502. https://doi.org/10.1371/journal.pone.0186502

Thompson, T., Caruso, M., & Ellerbeck, K. (2003). Sex matters in autism and other developmental disabilities. *Journal of Learning Disabilities, 7*(4), 345–361.

Trivette, C. M., Dunst, C. J., Hamby, D. W., & O'Herin, C. E. (2009). Characteristics and consequences of adult learning methods and strategies. *Research Brief, 3*(1), 1–33.

Turkstra, L. S., Norman, R., Whyte, J., Dijkers, M. P., & Hart, T. (2016). Knowing what we're doing: Why specification of treatment methods is critical for evidence-based practice in speech-language pathology. *American Journal of Speech-Language Pathology, 25*(2), 164–171.

U.S. Department of Education. (2016). *Thirty-eighth annual report to Congress on the implementation of the Individuals with Disabilities Education Act.* Office of Special Education and Rehabilitative Services. https://www2.ed.gov/about/reports/annual/osep/2016/parts-b-c/index.html

van Achterberg, T. V., Huisman-De Waal, G. G. J., Ketelaar, N. A. B. M., Oostendorp, R. A., Jacobs, J. E., & Wollersheim, H. C. H. (2010). How to promote healthy behaviors in patients? An overview of evidence for behaviour change techniques. *Health Promotion International, 26*(2), 148–162.

Van Stan, J. H., Roy, N., Awan, S., Stemple, J., & Hillman, R. E. (2015). A taxonomy of voice therapy. *American Journal of Speech-Language Pathology, 24*(2), 101–125.

Van Wingaarden-Cremers, P. J. M., van Eeten, E., Groen, W. B., Van Deurzen, P. A., Oosterling, I. J., & Van der Gaag, R. J. (2014). Gender and age differences in the core triad of impairments in autism spectrum disorders: A systematic review and meta-analysis. *Journal of Autism and Developmental Disorders, 44,* 627–635.

Wang, M., Jegathesan, T., Young, E., Huber, J., & Minhas, R. (2018). Raising children with autism spectrum disorders in monolingual versus bilingual homes: A scoping review. *Journal of Developmental and Behavioral Pediatrics, 39,* 434–446.

Warren, S. F., Fey, M. E., & Yoder, P. J. (2007). Differential treatment intensity research: A missing link to creating optimally effective communication interventions. *Mental Retardation and Developmental Disabilities Research Reviews, 13,* 70–77.

Webb, N. B. (2019). *Clinical practice with children, adolescents and families* (4th ed.) [formerly *Social work practice with children and families*]. Guilford Press.

Whyte, J., Dijkers, M. P., Hart, T., Zanca, J. M., Packel, A., Ferraro, M., & Tsaousides, T. (2014). Development of a theory-driven rehabilitation treatment taxonomy: Conceptual issues. *Archives of Physical Medicine and Rehabilitation, 95*(Suppl. 1), 524–532.

Wilson, K. P., & Landa, R. J. (2019). Barriers to educator implementation of a classroom-based intervention for preschoolers with autism spectrum disorder. *Frontiers in Education, 4.* https://doi.org/10.3389/feduc.2019.00027

Wong, C., Odom, S. L., Hume, K. A., Cox, C. W., Fettig, A., Kurcharczyk, S., Brock, M. E., Plavnick, J. B., Fleury, V. P., & Schultz, T. R. (2015). Evidence-based practices for children, youth, and young adults with autism spectrum disorder: A comprehensive review. *Journal of Autism and Developmental Disorders, 45,* 1951–1966.

Woods, J. J., Wilcox, M. J., Friedman, M., & Murch, T. (2011). Collaborative consultation in natural environments: Strategies to enhance family-centered supports and services. *Language, Speech, and Hearing Services in Schools, 42*(3), 379–392.

World Health Organization. (2001). *International classification of functioning, disability and health.* Author.

World Health Organization. (2010). *Framework for action on interprofessional education and collaborative practice.* Author. https://apps.who.int/iris/bitstream/handle/10665/70185/WHO_HRH_HPN_10.3_eng.pdf

Yoder, P., Fey, M. E., & Warren, S. F. (2012). Studying the impact of intensity is important but complicated. *International Journal of Speech-Language Pathology, 14*(5), 410–413.

Zhou, V., Munson, J. A., Greenson, J., Hou, Y., Rogers, S., & Estes, A. M. (2019). An exploratory longitudinal study of social and language outcomes in children with autism in bilingual home environments. *Autism, 32*(2), 394–404.

Glossary

active ingredients The elements of an intervention that contribute to the positive effect of the intervention on outcomes; ideally, they are empirically verified rather than simply asserted.

aggression Behavior that is directed at others and frequently results in pain and/or injury to other individuals.

aided augmentative and alternative communication (AAC) systems The use of a tool or equipment external to the person to replace or supplement oral communication. Such systems include a way to represent meaning, a way to access the meaning represented, and a way to share that meaning with others (Beukelman & Mirenda, 2013). Aided AAC systems can be low tech, such as communication books with symbols, or high tech, such as speech generating devices.

alternate assessment Formal educational assessments designed for students with significant cognitive impairments who cannot participate in general state assessments even with accommodations.

alternative solution thinking The ability to find solutions to interpersonal challenges.

applied behavior analysis A science that relies on the application of the principles of behavior to make socially significant and meaningful changes in a learner's life (Steege et al., 2007).

augmentative and alternative communication (AAC) Any means that supplements or replaces oral communication. It includes gestures, signs, symbols, and speech-generating devices.

augmentative and alternative communication (AAC) systems A collection of tools and strategies used to support the communication of individuals who do not speak verbally or in ways that are easily understood.

augmented language input The use of speech paired with an aided communication system by the communication partner. This technique enhances the user's comprehension and provides a model for aided augmentative and alternative communication use.

autism spectrum disorder (ASD) Disorder that emerges in early childhood, characterized by deficits in social relatedness, nonverbal and verbal communication, and various interests and behaviors. These deficits can cause pervasive impairment in thinking, language, feeling, and the ability to relate to others.

behavior change theories and techniques Theories, best known in health psychology and health sciences, targeted to promote health and potentially change behavior at two levels—the recipient of the intervention and the interventionist implementing the intervention.

behavioral cusp Skills that lead to improved access with new reinforcers, contingencies, and environments (Bosch & Fuqua, 2001).

challenging behaviors Behaviors that may be inappropriate (e.g., shouting in a public place) or even dangerous to others or to the individual with autism (e.g., hitting others or oneself) but that may serve a communicative function (e.g., requesting attention).

challenging/problem behavior Behaviors that in some form interfere with a student's educational and/or social progress.

child choice Allowing the child to choose the activities or materials involved in teaching.

consequence Change in the environment that occurs following a behavior that either increases or decreases the likelihood of the behavior occurring in the future under similar conditions.

consequential thinking The ability to recognize and understand the impact of one person's behavior on another's behavior.

contemporary behavioral interventions Behavioral approaches that give children choices, provide shared teaching opportunities between the interventionist and the child, and incorporate the child's preferred activities and materials.

contingent reinforcement Providing an immediate and contingent reward after the correct response.

core vocabulary Vocabulary that is used frequently and by a variety of people. Core vocabulary can be obtained from word lists based on individual characteristics such as age, aided augmentative and alternative communication use, and contexts.

cultural competence Having awareness of your own cultural beliefs and biases and how they may be different from those of people who have a different cultural background.

Curriculum Checklist   The criterion-referenced tool that is used to develop teaching objectives for intervention, administered every 12 weeks in a play-based, interactive fashion and incorporating information gained from parents and others working with the child; provides developmental sequences of skills in multiple developmental domains.

Daily Data Sheet   A tool used by the therapist in the intervention session to track periodic recordings of child performance; guides the therapist on which teaching step is currently being targeted (updated from session to session) and includes a short version of each objective as well as a short version of each teaching step.

Developmental, Individual-Difference, Relationship-Based (DIR) model   The model representing a paradigm to be used for the assessment of and intervention for children with developmental challenges. Three components are addressed in the DIR paradigm: the child's functional emotional developmental level, the child's individual processing profile, and the relationship between the child and his or her caregivers.

discrete trial instruction   Instructional approach to teach subcomponents of a skill using manageable components. Four components are 1) discriminative stimulus, 2) response, 3) consequence, and 4) intertrial interval (Steege et al., 2007).

discriminative stimulus (S^D)   Cue or brief instruction provided by the practitioner to initiate a discrete trial.

dosage   A complex concept in the behavior intervention literature related to the level of an individual's exposure to the number of procedurally effective teaching/learning experiences provided within a given intervention session as well as across all sessions over a period of time.

ecomap   A graphic tool used to situate families in terms of the organizations and situations affecting access to and use of resources as well as potential sources of stress.

elements   Components of an intervention, such as goals, procedures used by the intervention, and materials, that distinguish it from other interventions and nontherapeutic interactions.

emotional regulation (ER)   The developmental domain of The SCERTS Model that supports an individual's ability to regulate arousal and emotional state to attain and maintain a state of active engagement in the social and physical environment.

engagement   The duration of the child's attentional focus involving people and objects, ranging from unengaged to coordinated joint engagement (shifting focus with communicative intent between a person and event/objects).

Enhanced Milieu Teaching (EMT)   A third generation of naturalistic teaching strategies, building on the principles of milieu teaching and systematically adding principles for responsive conversational skills and language modeling in everyday communication contexts.

environmental arrangement   One of six core components of Enhanced Milieu Teaching that includes procedures for organizing and managing the child's environment to increase requesting behavior and provide adults with language prompting and scaffolding opportunities.

episodic memory   A special kind of autobiographical memory for personally experienced events.

error correction   Teaching technique that increases the likelihood of correct future performance when a mistake is made on a given trial (see Table 6.2 for listing of error-correction procedures and description of steps for each error correction method).

everyday routines and activities   Activities that typically occur in the context of a child and family's daily routine. They typically occur in the same manner each day, have a specific sequence of steps, and have specific outcomes.

evidence-based practice (EBP)   Clinical practice in which clinicians integrate the best available external research evidence; information they obtain about client needs, values, and preferences; and their clinical expertise and practice-internal evidence.

executive functions   a set of cognitive processes and resources including working memory, inhibition, focused attention, attention shifting and planning—all of which operate to control and guide behavior.

family centered care   Assessment and intervention in which clinicians are working with families to meet their needs and those of their child or adult with autism while understanding their unique set of values, beliefs, and practices.

feed-forward   A term coined by Peter Dowrick (1983) to describe the process in video self-modeling whereby people see themselves performing beyond their present ability, providing them a view of their futures. The term was meant to be the opposite of *feedback*. Feed-forward applies to novel or newly emerging skills.

fidelity of implementation   The degree to which an intervention is delivered as intended.

fidelity   The extent to which an intervention is being implemented as intended.

Floortime   A therapeutic strategy that is specific to the Developmental, Individual-Differences, Relationship-Based (DIR) approach. Floortime describes the spontaneous, developmentally appropriate, one-to-one interactions during which the six functional emotional developmental levels (FEDLs) are mobilized.

form–content relation   The intersection between ideas about objects, events, and relations (content or semantics) and the phonological, morphological, and syntactic coding (form) of those ideas in language (Lahey, 1988).

fringe vocabulary Vocabulary to be used in an augmentative and alternative communication system that is specific to the individual. This vocabulary might include names of people, pets, or activities.

functional analysis A form of functional behavior assessment that involves manipulating antecedents and/or consequences to determine if and how they are influencing behavior.

functional behavioral analysis (FBA) A problem-solving process designed to identify the purpose of a behavior and interventions to address it.

functional behavioral assessment A class of techniques used to assess the variables that appear to be influencing a behavior or behaviors. Usually involves assessing immediate antecedents and consequences as well as more distant events (setting events).

functional communication training (FCT) An intervention strategy for addressing challenging behavior that relies on replacing problem behavior with functionally equivalent alternative communication.

Functional Emotional Assessment Scale (FEAS) An assessment tool used to determine the child's functional emotional developmental levels (FEDLs) as well as the nature of the interactions between the child and his or her caregivers. This determination leads, in turn, to creating a treatment plan based on the child's individual profile and provides a baseline for measuring his or her progress.

functional emotional developmental levels (FEDLs) A construct for conceptualizing increasingly more complex emotional development while considering all of the components of development, including cognition, language, and motor skills. The FEDLs "serve as the orchestra leader that enables all the developmental components to work together in a *functional* manner" (Greenspan et al., 2001, p. xiii).

functional equivalence The concept that describes how two behaviors can serve the same function for a student and therefore can replace each other in a student's behavioral repertoire.

genogram A graphic tool indicating the family composition, presence of illness or disabilities, and other aspects of family history.

graphic symbols A way to represent meaning in an aided augmentative and alternative communication system. This representation can include pictures, photographs, line drawings, Blissymbols, printed words, and traditional orthography.

I Can Problem Solve (ICPS) dialoguing Two-way adult–child conversation fostering active participation in problem solving; teachers capitalize on concepts taught formally in the training to everyday social problems that might occur during the school day to help children make connections between what they do and how they are thinking.

implementation fidelity Extent to which the independent variable (i.e., intervention) is implemented consistently and accurately (Jenkins et al., 2015).

implementation science "The scientific study of methods to promote the systematic uptake of research findings and other evidence-based practices into routine practice" (Eccles & Mittman, 2006, p. 1).

inclusive education An educational approach in which students with and without disabilities participating fully, meaningfully, and collaboratively in the breadth of social and learning opportunities that take place in and through a school.

individualized education program (IEP) A written statement describing the educational program that is personalized to meet a child's individual needs in school and is updated at least annually.

individually assigned paraprofessionals An educational assistant who is not a certified teacher and who provides one-to-one support to a student with a disability.

Interdisciplinary Council on Developmental and Learning Disorders—Diagnostic Manual for Infants and Young Children (ICDL-DMIC) A developmentally based classification system for infants and young children with developmental disorders. The comprehensive classification system can be used to describe challenges in emotional, speech-language, cognitive, regulatory-sensory, and motor capacities.

International Classification of Functioning, Disability and Health A framework developed by the World Health Organization to describe and organize information on the impact of diseases and other health conditions on individuals' functioning in society.

interpersonal support (IS) Category of transactional support that refers to communication partners' therapeutic use of self and interactive style modifications to scaffold learning and engagement.

interprofessional education and interprofessional practice (IE/IP) Educational offerings in which students from different professions share learning opportunities with the intent of fostering effective interprofessional collaboration as a means of improving health outcomes.

intertrial interval Period of time between the conclusion of one discrete trial and the presentation of the next trial.

joint attention (JA) Critical capacity in the domain of Social Communication. Refers to the reasons that an individual communicates (e.g., the *why* of communication). Gestures and words used for sharing a topic or event between two social partners. Initiations of joint attention involve the use of gesture and spoken words to coordinate the attention of a social partner to an event or topic of conversation, whereas responding to joint attention refers to responding to the sharing gestures of another person.

joint engagement   Maintaining a state (duration) of actively attending and coordinating one's attention between an object and another person with communicative intent.

language expansions   One of the six Enhanced Milieu Teaching core strategies aimed to scaffold language for more complex vocabulary, grammar, and syntax by responding to child communication with a slightly more advanced language model, either by adding one to three words or by changing the grammar to be more complex or correct.

language modalities   Aspects of early development that are considered central to the process of acquiring language and being a successful communicator. Although overlapping at the very early stages with the functional emotional developmental levels, the language modalities are considered specifically as they relate to the ability to learn to comprehend and produce a language system (i.e., a system of phonology, morphology, syntax, semantics, and pragmatics).

language modeling   One of the six core components of Enhanced Milieu Teaching that includes specific procedures for providing the child models of language that are salient for the child and match the language level of the child so that the child is primed for imitation.

learned helplessness   A condition in which a person behaves as if he or she is helpless by not responding or by infrequently responding.

learning support   Category of transactional supports that refers to communication partners' modification of activities and environments to scaffold learning and development.

manual signs   An unaided form of augmentative and alternative communication in which the user has no external equipment or tool. There are several sign language systems commonly used in the United States, including American Sign Language (ASL) and Signing Exact English (SEE).

means–end thinking   The ability to plan a goal and understand the challenges that may serve as barriers to achieving that goal.

mechanism of action   The processes by which active ingredients of an intervention effect desired outcomes.

milieu teaching   A naturalistic approach to teaching communication skills in everyday communication contexts, which uses environmental arrangement, specific natural prompts for language, and functional consequences to increase the frequency and complexity of children's communication.

minimally verbal   Based on a National Institutes of Health workshop consensus meeting (Tager-Flusberg & Kasari, 2013), minimally verbal applies to individuals who are past age 5 years with fewer than 20 functional words in their spoken language repertoire and have been exposed to early interventions.

modular   A type of targeted intervention that can be implemented independently of the other services that a child is receiving. These interventions should complement children's other interventions, including school, and often address specific challenges not met by more general interventions.

Motivation Assessment Scale (MAS)   A form of functional behavior assessment. Includes 16 questions about the antecedents and consequences of the target behavior.

mutual regulation (MR)   Critical component in developmental domain of Emotional Regulation within The SCERTS Model. Refers to skills and abilities for regulation of arousal and emotional state that occur within the context of interactions with others.

natural communities of reinforcement   The concept that behaviors can be taught to gain access to reinforcers that are naturally occurring in the environment (e.g., teacher's praise).

natural environments   The settings where infants and toddlers with and without delays and disabilities, and their families, live and learn in the context of everyday routines and activities that are important to them.

natural language paradigm   The original form of Pivotal Response Treatment, which incorporated motivational components into the language intervention for children with ASD.

natural rewards   Providing a reward that is directly and functionally related to the child's response.

natural support   The reliance on ordinary supports that already exist in a particular setting and are unpaid.

Naturalistic Developmental Behavioral Interventions (NDBI)   According to Schreibman and colleagues, these interventions are "implemented in natural settings, involve shared control between child and therapist, utilize natural contingencies, and use a variety of behavioral strategies to teach developmentally appropriate and prerequisite skills" (2015).

naturalistic intervention   Creating opportunities for learning during naturally occurring everyday situations.

object-focused joint activities   Materials provide the play theme, and both the child and adult attend to actions on objects; primary foci include parallel actions with objects, communication about objects, and taking turns with objects.

parent coaching   Collaborating with parents to help them facilitate their child's learning, a method central to several intervention approaches, including the Developmental, Individual-Differences, Relationship-Based (DIR) approach and the Early Start Denver Model.

parent implemented   Interventions with the child that are implemented primarily by the parent or caregiver with support and coaching from professionals.

peer network interventions   A cohesive social group of three to six students that meets formally and informally across an entire semester or school year and emphasizes social connections for students with ASD beyond the classroom.

peer partners   Students without significant disabilities who provide academic, social, and/or behavioral support over time and with guidance from an educator.

peer support arrangements   Individually tailored interventions that involve equipping two or more peers without disabilities to provide academic and social support to a classmate with ASD throughout the semester in a general education classroom.

peer-mediated interventions   Equipping and engaging similar-age students without disabilities to provide ongoing social, academic, and or other support to their schoolmates with disabilities.

percentage of non-overlapping data (PND)   A controversial method of evaluating single-participant research designs in which the highest performance from baseline stages is compared to lower levels of performance during treatment and maintenance stages. It was encouraged in the early 21st century to add a statistical element to single-participant data analysis. It has been widely criticized for diminishing apparent improvement because several data points during treatment equaling the high baseline score can greatly skew data irrespective of overall gains.

perspective taking   The ability to recognize and understand the feelings of others.

pivotal area   An area of a child's development that, when targeted, produces broad and collateral gains in nontargeted areas.

Pivotal Response Treatment® (PRT)   An empirically validated, play-based intervention approach, which utilizes applied behavior analysis techniques and a developmental approach to target the core deficits of autism (PRT also refers to Pivotal Response Training, Pivotal Response Teaching, Pivotal Response Therapy, and Pivotal Response Intervention).

play level   The highest type of play at which a child can independently complete at least three types of play according to a developmental play scale (e.g., Lifter et al., 1993).

play routine   Natural and social play interactions between two individuals that involve a sequence of play steps and contains communication within the various steps.

point-of-view (PoV) modeling   A form of video modeling shot from the viewer's perspective.

prompt   External support that increases the likelihood of correct performance (See Table 6.3 for a list of prompts).

recognizing mixed emotions   The ability to recognize that people can have different feelings about the same thing.

regulation   The child's ability to regulate his or her attention and behavior while being interested in the full range of sensations (sights, sounds, smells, his or her own movement patterns, etc.). Children who are regulated can attend to and process their environment, filter out distractions, engage with others, and focus on play or tasks (e.g., pay attention in the classroom).

reporting guideline   "A checklist, flow diagram, or structured text to guide authors in reporting a specific type of research, developed using explicit methodology." (Equator Network, n.d.).

response   Behavior exhibited that can be strengthened or reinforced on the basis of the outcome delivered immediately following it.

responsive interaction   One of the six core components of Enhanced Milieu Teaching that includes a set of strategic behaviors, including following the child's lead, mirroring and mapping, responding to initiations, and providing meaningful semantic feedback that maintains child interest in conversations.

rewarding attempts   Rewarding the child's clear attempts rather than rewarding only responses that were as good as or better than the previous response.

SCERTS®   A child- and family-centered, activity- and curricular based, developmentally grounded assessment and intervention approach (Prizant et al., 2006a, b). It targets the most significant challenges faced by children with ASD in the domains Social Communication (SC) and Emotional Regulation (ER). Goals and objectives in the Transactional Supports (TS) domain are targeted for the communication partners (i.e., parents, siblings, peers) to support learning in the natural environment.

schema   A conceptual framework for understanding events, thoughts, and behaviors.

scoping review   A structured review of the literature that analyzes a research literature but, unlike a systematic review, may not assess the quality of individual studies; instead, it describes the current state in a research area, identifies gaps, provides a summary of major findings, or helps researchers prepare for a systematic review (Levac et al., 2012).

scripted language (scripts)   The use of phrases, sentences, and longer strings of language that are repeated, often verbatim, from movies, books, television shows, and so forth. For some children, scripted language reflects challenges in the comprehension and/or production of language.

self-efficacy   A term coined by Albert Bandura to describe a person's belief that he or she can succeed at a task.

self-injurious behavior   Behaviors that are directed at oneself and often result in injury to the person.

self-observation   The use of raw video to evaluate performance, as in football films. This has also been used by teachers and parents to demonstrate how children with ASD behave in their respective environments, often depicting negative behaviors. In this respect, it is the antithesis of video modeling, which depicts only positive behavior, and is *not* recommended for therapeutic use.

self-regulation (SR)   Critical component in developmental Emotional Regulation domain of The SCERTS Model. Refers to skills and abilities that an individual is able to employ on his or her own to regulate arousal and emotional state.

sensory social routines   Dyadic, joint activity routines whereby each partner's attention is focused primarily on the other person, rather than on objects, and where the play is characterized by mutual pleasure and engagement; the primary theme of the activity is social exchange (e.g., lap games, song routines with motions, movement routines, adult-operated objects such as bubbles/balloons/pinwheels), and these activities teach children to communicate in order to initiate, maintain, and end social interactions.

short-term learning objectives   Measurable objectives designed to be mastered over the 12 weeks following the curriculum assessment, spanning all developmental domains.

SMART design   A multistage randomized research design that can be used to evaluate and build adaptive treatments (individualized sequences of treatment progression).

social cognition   The process by which people make sense of the self and others and acquire, use, and understand social knowledge.

Social Communication (SC)   The developmental domain in The SCERTS Model that includes an individual's abilities to initiate, respond to, and maintain interactions. It is the foundation of social engagement and participation.

social competence   Skills necessary to engage in social interactions as well as the insights required in managing various social encounters.

social motivation   The ability to experience pleasure in seeking out social interactions.

Social Stories™   Short stories that adhere to a specific format and guidelines to objectively describe a person, skill, event, concept, or social situation.

social-pragmatic developmental interventions   Interventions that follow the child's lead, foster initiation and spontaneity, and reinforce contingent responses.

SPACE Assessment   An approximately 15- to 20-minute naturalistic, semi-structured, and play-based evaluation of children's communication, play, engagement, and regulation. It is used within JASPER to identify and monitor treatment progress.

speech-generating device (SGD)   An aided form of augmentative and alternative communication that provides voice output when activated. These systems provide synthesized or digitized voice and are computer based.

storyboard   A drawing that divides a movie or activity step-by-step scenes (cells).

suprasegmental aspects of speech production   Characteristics of speech that may extend over several segments, such as intonation, lexical stress, or overall pitch.

symbol use   Critical component of the Social Communication domain of The SCERTS Model. Refers to the means that an individual uses to communicate (e.g., the *how* of communication).

symbolic play (SP)   Play that involves pretense; pretending that an object or another person is something else. Examples include actions such as pretending a block is piece of food, pretending to be a chef, making dolls or other inanimate objects come to life.

tantrums   Typically describe a combination of behaviors such as screaming, running around, and a variety of other behavioral disruptions.

task variation   Interspersing previously mastered (maintenance) tasks with the target, more difficult (acquisition) task.

Teaching Fidelity Rating System   Assesses therapist's and/or caregiver's mastery of the teaching practices of the Early Start Denver Model (e.g., management of child attention, quality of behavioral teaching, quality of dyadic engagement, adult sensitivity and responsivity to child communicative cues).

theory of mind   The ability to reason about the inner mental worlds of self and others and to understand that others may have perspectives that differ from our own.

time delay   A language elicitation strategy used to get children to communicate more frequently while reducing potential of prompt dependence. This nonverbal strategy includes holding up choices, pausing in a familiar routine, and setting up a situation in which the child needs assistance.

traditional behavioral interventions   Teach skills one-to-one with a predetermined correct response and a highly prescribed teaching structure.

Transactional Support   A domain of The SCERTS Model, which consists of evidence-based supports and strategies implemented by communicative partners to help scaffold development in social communication and emotional regulation for individuals with ASD across environments.

unaided augmentative and alternative communication (AAC)   A form of AAC that requires no external tool or equipment. Unaided forms of AAC include sign language, gestures, vocalizations, and facial expressions.

understanding motives   The ability to recognize the reasons for the behaviors people demonstrate.

verbal behavior   Behavior reinforced through the mediation of others (Skinner, 1957).

video peer modeling (VPM)   A video depicting others performing a task that would be helpful for a viewer. Adult video modeling is often included in this category.

video self-modeling (VSM)   A type of video modeling in which the individual acts as both model and viewer. Requires video editing to make it appear a person is performing at higher level or more appropriately.

visual scene display   A picture or scene that represents an activity, experience, or situation. Specific objects or people in the scene are programmed to speak a word or message when they are activated.

weak central coherence   A cognitive style, believed to be present in ASD, in which the processing of parts takes precedence over the processing of wholes.

REFERENCES

Beukelman, D. R., & Mirenda, P. (2013). *Augmentative and alternative communication: Supporting children and adults with complex communication needs* (4th ed.). Paul H. Brookes Publishing Co.

Bosch, S., & Fuqua, R. W. (2001). Behavioral cusps: A model for selecting target behaviors. *Journal of Applied Behavior Analysis, 34*, 123–125.

Dowrick, P. W. (1983). Self-modeling. In P. W. Dowrick & J. Biggs (Eds.), *Using video: Psychological and social applications* (pp. 105–124). Wiley.

Eccles, M. P., & Mittman, B. S. (2006). Welcome to *Implementation Science. Implementation Science, 1*(1), 1–3.

EQUATOR Network. (n.d.) What is a reporting guideline? http://equator-network.org/about-us/what-is-a-reporting-guideline/

Greenspan, S. I., De Gangi, G. A., & Wieder, S. (2001). *The Functional Emotional Assessment Scale (FEAS) for Infancy and Early Childhood: Clinical and research applications.* ICDL Press.

Jenkins, S. R., Hirst, J. M., & DiGennaro-Reed, F. D. D. (2015). The effects of discrete-trial training commission errors on learner outcomes: An extension. *Journal of Behavioral Education, 24*(2), 196–209.

Lahey, M. (1988). *Language disorders and language development.* Wiley.

Levac, D., Rivard, L., & Missiuna, C. (2012). Defining the active ingredients of interactive computer play interventions for children with neuromotor impairments: A scoping study. *Research in Developmental Disabilities, 33*, 214–223.

Lifter, K., Sulzer-Azaroff, B., Anderson, S. R., & Cowdery, G. E. (1993). Teaching play activities to preschool children with disabilities: The importance of developmental considerations. *Journal of Early Intervention, 17*(2), 139–159.

Prizant, B., Wetherby, A., Rubin, E., Laurent, A., & Rydell, P. (2006a). *The SCERTS® model: A comprehensive educational approach for children with autism spectrum disorders. Vol. I: Assessment.* Paul H. Brookes Publishing Co.

Prizant, B., Wetherby, A., Rubin, E., Laurent, A., & Rydell, P. (2006b). *The SCERTS® model: A comprehensive educational approach for children with autism spectrum disorders. Vol. II: Program planning and intervention.* Paul H. Brookes Publishing Co.

Schreibman, L., Dawson, G., Stahmer, A. C., Landa, R., Rogers, S. J., McGee, G. G., Kasari, C., Ingersoll, B., Kaiser, A. P., Bruinsma, Y., McNerney, E., Wetherby, A., & Halladay, A. (2015). Naturalistic Developmental Behavioral Interventions: Empirically validated treatments for autism spectrum disorder. *Journal of Autism and Developmental Disorders, 45*(8), 2411–2428. https://doi.org/10.1007/s10803-015-2407-8

Skinner, B. F. (1957). *Verbal behavior.* Prentice Hall.

Steege, M. W., Mace, F. C., Perry, L., & Longenecker, H. (2007). Applied behavior analysis: Beyond discrete trial teaching. *Psychology in the Schools, 44*(1), 91–99.

Index

Tables and figures are indicated by *t* and *f* respectively.

Notes

Notes

Notes

Notes

Notes

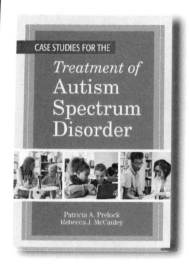
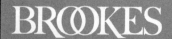